The Electroencephalogram

The Electroencephalogram
Its Patterns and Origins

John S. Barlow

A Bradford Book
The MIT Press
Cambridge, Massachusetts
London, England

© 1993 Massachusetts Institute of Technology

All rights reserved. No part of this book may be reproduced in any form by any electronic or mechanical means (including photocopying, recording, or information storage and retrieval) without permission in writing from the publisher.

Set in Palatino by Asco Trade Typesetting Ltd., Hong Kong.
Printed and bound in the United States of America.

Library of Congress Cataloging-in-Publication Data

Barlow, John S., 1925–
  The electroencephalogram: its patterns and origins / John S. Barlow.
    p.   cm.
  "A Bradford book."
  Includes bibliographical references and index.
  ISBN 0-262--02354-7
  1. Electroencephalography.   I. Title.
  [DNLM: 1. Electroencephalography.   WL 150 B528e 1993]
  QP376.5B37   1993
  612.8'22—dc20
  DNLM/DLC
  for Library of Congress   92-48443
                                                                 CIP

For Sibylle Jahrreiss Barlow, patient wife, without whose support in more ways than one this work could not have been completed.

Contents

Preface   xi

1 Introduction   1

I The Hypothesis and Methods of Testing It; Simulation Results

2 The Hypothesis and the Oscillator Model   13

3 Approaches, Methods, and EEG Database for Testing the Hypothesis   23

4 Simulation of EEG Patterns   33

II Tests of Predictions from the Hypothesis for Normal and Abnormal EEGs

5 The Waking EEG   53

6 The Normal EEG during Sleep   71

7 Normal and Abnormal Random Slowing in the Waking State   85

8 Epileptiform Patterns   103

9 Reconstitution of EEGs from Extrema and Slopes   115

10 Appraisal and Revision of the Extrema-Slopes Hypothesis on the Basis of Tests   127

III Appraisal of the Hypothesis in Relation to Anatomy, Physiology, and Pathophysiology of the EEG; Other Models; Overall Appraisal

11	Some Aspects of Neocortical Anatomy	137
12	The Physiological Basis of the EEG	147
13	Pathophysiology of the EEG	175
14	Other Models of the EEG, and Related Models	189
15	Comparisons with Some Other Models of the EEG	213
16	The Significance of the Extrema-Slopes Hypothesis: A Formulation	221
17	Implications for, and Applications to, Computerized EEG Analysis	237
18	Limitations of the Scope of the Present Work	273
19	A Methodological Note on the Wiener Clock Hypothesis for the Alpha Rhythm	277
20	Résumé	281

IV Technological Chapters

21	Introduction to Technological Chapters	291
22	The Oscillator Model	293
23	Precision Full-Wave Rectifier; Transversal Filter; Tapped Delay Line	307
24	Basic Measures	317
25	Derived Measures	319
26	Photo-Optical Scanner for Data Retrieval from EEG Ink Recordings	335

27 Time-Scale Converter ("Time Machine") 341

28 Random-Noise Generators 345

29 Instantaneous Envelopes of the EEG and of Its First Derivative; Interfacing with the Oscillator Model 355

Appendixes

A Some Traditional Methods of EEG Analysis: On-Line Real-Time Analog Implementation 383

B Eliminating or Minimizing Artifact by Paired Sampling and by Coherent Rejection; Analog Adaptive Signal Processing 393

C Placement of Scalp Electrodes 409

Glossary 411
Bibliography 417
Index 449

Preface

A new, comprehensive hypothesis for the patterns in the human electroencephalogram is advanced in this book. In essence, according to the hypothesis, the entire range of EEG patterns in humans of every age (including very early premature infants), in every normal state (including alert wakefulness and the various stages of sleep), and in every type of brain pathology (whether localized or generalized) can be modeled by an oscillator of a new type that can be modulated in two independent ways.

The four principal types of wave patterns obtainable from the oscillator model can be compared with four major types of EEG activity: rhythmic activity, irregular "slow waves" (both normal and abnormal), the EEG activity of epilepsy, and the EEG patterns of irregular waves. The simulation of such a wide range of EEG patterns is made possible by the modulation of intrinsic oscillations both as to their extrema and as to their slopes; the corresponding hypothesis is thus termed the *extrema-slopes hypothesis*.

For testing the hypothesis, three different approaches are developed: simulation of EEG patterns, testing of hypothesis-based predictions of features of specific EEG patterns by means of a battery of methods especially designed for this purpose, and reconstitution of EEGs on the basis of their primary features as specified by the hypothesis.

As background for an evaluation of the significance of the extrema-slopes hypothesis, and for a formulation based on that hypothesis and related to fundamental EEG-generating mechanisms in terms of cortical excitatory and inhibitory processes, the relevant fields of brain anatomy, physiology, and pathophysiology of the EEG are reviewed, as are other models of these and related phenomena.

A large number of new techniques have been developed specifically for testing the hypothesis. Brief descriptions of these are included in the primarily scientific portion of the book (parts I–III); the details are given in the primarily technological chapters (part IV).

The book, which represents a new departure in the field of electroencephalography, is written from the perspective of extensive experience in the computer analysis of EEGs and in the design of equipment for that purpose, and, at the same time, from the perspective of long experience in clinical electroencephalography.

The material is arranged in such a way that chapters or sections can be omitted or read out of sequence according to the reader's interests. A quick survey can be obtained from chapters 1, 2, 3, 10, 16, and 20, or, even more expeditiously, from chapter 20 alone. Chapter 1 is, however, essential to an understanding of the plan of the book.

Except for a brief abstract (Barlow 1989) and a chapter in a symposium volume (Barlow 1993), this material (which dates from early 1986) has not been previously published. It seemed sensible to gather all aspects of it in one place: the basic hypothesis, the testing of it (and the extensive associated methodology), and its ramifications and implications, considered from a broad perspective. (Seminars concerning an early phase of the work were presented at several West and East European centers in the spring of 1988.)

Early experience with some of the methods (in particular, the development of the Spectral Purity Index as a measure of EEG rhythmicity) was gained during a collaborative study in the summer of 1988 in Moscow with Irina I. Goncharova (now at the Brain Institute of the Russian Academy of Sciences), who also pointed out to me the significant advantages of the Coefficient of Variation as an indicator of EEG variability.

For many helpful comments and suggestions, I am indebted to a number of colleagues who read parts or all of an interim draft of the manuscript: Reginald Bickford of the University of California at San Diego, Mary Brazier of East Falmouth, Massachusetts (who originally introduced me to the EEG); Theodore Bullock of the University of California at San Diego; Pierre Gloor and Jean Gotman of the Montreal Neurological Institute and Hospital; Eli Goldensohn of the Montefiore Medical Center in New York; Charles Henry of the Medical College of Virginia in Richmond; Donald Klass of the Mayo Clinic; John Knott of Iowa City; Harold Shipton of Washington University in St. Louis; Mircea Steriade of Laval University in Québec; Donald Walter of the University of California at Los Angeles; and especially James Frost, Jr., of Baylor University/Methodist Hospital in Houston. I am indebted to the late Bernard Saltzberg of Houston for encouragement at a very early stage of this work.

A wide variety of electroencephalograms, which were essential for testing the hypothesis, were generously made available from several laboratories, as detailed in chapter 3.

Grateful acknowledgment is made to the large number of publishers and authors who have given permission for reproducing illustrations originally published elsewhere, as noted in the individual legends.

A few words about the manner in which this work has been carried out: Circumstances have necessitated that expenses be minimal. The necessary pieces of standard laboratory equipment for the work were already on hand from prior research supported by the National Institutes of Health. The relatively inexpensive analog techniques that were developed especially for the work, and with which the analyses were carried out, were in an area in which I had had appreciable prior experience. Indeed, the technological aspects of this work can ultimately be traced back to the early 1950s, to a collaboration (in which I had the good fortune to be a participant) on the study of EEGs by some of the methods of statistical communications theory (in the specific form of an analog correlator system for brain potentials) between the then-new Laboratory of Communications Biophysics of Walter Rosenblith, in the Research Laboratory of Electronics at MIT, and the then-new Neurophysiological Laboratory of Mary Brazier, at the Massachusetts General Hospital. (The collaborative project was spurred on by the interest of Norbert Wiener, who had originated much of the body of statistical communications theory, on which the project was based. It reflected a broad perspective on the part of the director of the Research Laboratory of Electronics, Jerome Wiesner, and the Chief of the Neurology Service at the Massachusetts General Hospital, Raymond Adams.) More recently, the Massachusetts General Hospital and its Department of Neurology generously continued to make laboratory space available in the absence of outside funding.

Essential early guidance concerning the preparation of the manuscript on a personal computer was provided by my daughter Lisa and my son Robert. The facilities and the expertise at the Computer Resource Center for Harvard Arts and Sciences Faculty, under the direction of Andrew McKinney, are gratefully acknowledged.

It has been a pleasure to work with the staff of The MIT Press, in particular Fiona Stevens and Paul Bethge, on this book.

A Note Concerning the Figures

For the sake of authenticity, the figures were reproduced from the best available masters, without redrafting or enhancement.

The Electroencephalogram

1 Introduction

THE PRESENT STATUS OF ELECTROENCEPHALOGRAPHY

Although the electroencephalogram was discovered in rabbits more than a century ago (Caton 1875), and the first report concerning the human EEG appeared more than 60 years ago (Berger 1929; see also Gloor 1969), much remains to be clarified about the nature and the origin of the EEG. Nonetheless, very soon after its discovery in humans the EEG became an important diagnostic tool, and it has remained so.

In a sense, however, clinical electroencephalography has become frozen in time. The specialty has been taught by the apprentice method and has been practiced as visual inspection of the ink-written trace by trained experts. Experimental advances in electrophysiology have had relatively little impact on the clinical practice of electroencephalography, which has advanced mainly through technical developments such as a progressive increase in the number of simultaneously recorded channels. With the exception of the analysis of brain potentials evoked by sensory stimuli (by means of averaging or summation techniques) and the automatic detection of epileptiform EEG patterns, computer techniques have not come into routine use in clinical electroencephalography despite quite a large amount of exploratory work. Perhaps the reason for this state of affairs is that the computer techniques come with their own built-in assumptions, usually based on mathematical approaches rather than on the EEG itself.

In electroencephalography the "revolution of computerization" has not turned out to be as far-reaching and enduring as the revolution in neuroimaging brought about by computerized axial tomography (CAT), magnetic-resonance imaging (MRI), and positron-emission tomography (PET). And yet, as a non-invasive clinical tool for evaluating brain function, the EEG continues to be very useful, especially in the evaluation of epilepsy and of sleep disorders. It is truly remarkable that the most complex organ so far known to exist in the universe is so arranged as to make listening in on its most closely guarded whisperings so easy. The essentials for such eavesdropping include a few electrodes placed on the scalp with a conducting medium (electrode paste), several channels of a relatively simple amplifier, and some type of write-out.

There is an enormous diversity of EEG patterns. In a normal waking EEG (i.e., one within the empirically established normal range), there is the whole sequence of maturational changes, from the particular and even unique evolution of patterns in the premature infant through infancy, childhood, adolescence, and adulthood. The different types of sleep (e.g., rapid-eye-movement patterns, non-REM patterns, and transitional patterns) in the various age groups add another dimension. There are the normal-variant patterns, some of which must be distinguished from abnormal ones. And finally there is the vast range of abnormal patterns for every age group; these can be quite different in the premature infant from those in the child, and different again from those in the adult.

Historically, one method of approaching a mass of disparate data has been to develop models in an attempt to lend some organization to the data; the more consistent the predictions of a model relative to the actual data, the more satisfactory the model for characterizing a phenomenon succinctly. Thus, the Ptolemaic geocentric model of epicycles upon epicycles for describing the motions of the sun and the planets about the earth was ultimately unsatisfactory, despite its longevity, because there were too many discrepancies between predictions and actuality. Thus, the Ptolemaic model gave way to Copernicus' heliocentric view and to Kepler's three laws of planetary motion, based on Newton's three laws of motion, which left only very small discrepancies. But even small discrepancies can ultimately become intolerable, and so Newton's laws, which seemed immutable, gave way to Einstein's more exact general relativity theory of 1915, which accounted correctly for the long-known precession of the perihelion of the planet Mercury and for the gravitational bending of light rays. (The latter prediction was confirmed, with great fanfare, by astronomical observations during the solar eclipse of 1919.)

On the other hand, none of the mathematical models (theories), including Einstein's general relativity, has explained the gravitational attraction that keeps the planets in their orderly progressions. Indeed, gravity (along with its putative messenger, the graviton) remains an enigma, perhaps to be elucidated by a still-elusive grand unified theory of physics.

What is the comparable stage of our understanding of the EEG? Will there ultimately be a grand unified theory of it? In some respects, perhaps the Ptolemaic comparison is the closest one. Are the multiple frequencies that emerge from our sophisticated methods of spectral analyses of EEG the counterpart of the structure of cycles, epicycles, and epi-epicycles of the Ptolemaic approach, based as those methods are on the intrinsic assumption of spectral analysis that gives its results in terms of superpositions of continuous fixed-amplitude sine waves (the individual spectral components being comparable to the Ptolemaic cycles originating from a geocentric model)? Perhaps we need a new perspective on electroencephalography—one that is EEG-oriented rather than analysis-oriented, and one that accounts for the vast diversity of EEG patterns in terms of a few simple principles.

In any event, in the face of the enormous diversity of EEG patterns, all of them dynamic rather than static with time, it is perhaps not very surprising that no single model has been advanced which is specifically intended to encompass the entire range of this diversity by generating or simulating the full panoply of EEG patterns. The model for the EEG that is proposed in this book is intended as such a comprehensive model.

Is so comprehensive a model bound to be meaningless and even trivial? More specifically, can it contribute anything toward a further understanding of the EEG? The latter question is approached in two steps, which are consonant with the subtitle of the book (*Its Patterns and Origins*). First, accepting the premise that the EEG originates from the brain (more specifically, from the cerebral cortex), the EEG is considered as a signal from a "black box"—that is, without regard to its generating mechanisms—and an attempt is made to characterize it in terms of a specific model. Such a first step is appropriate and even necessary, since if the fit of the model to actual EEG patterns should be found to be largely unsatisfactory there would be little or no point in pursuing possible implications of the model in relation to basic EEG-generating mechanisms. It is for this reason that the reader will find little mention of brain mechanisms until after the validity of the model has been rather extensively tested and the results of the tests have been reviewed—i.e., until after chapter 10.

In fact, the model (which can be considered basically to have only two parameters), and its associated hypothesis, were found to be surprisingly satisfactory in accounting for a large variety of EEG patterns, including alpha activity, the low-voltage irregular pattern of the "desynchronized" EEG of the alert eyes-open state, the EEG in certain stages of sleep, epileptiform EEG patterns, the emergence of certain unexpected features of alpha activity and of its relationship to the "desynchronized" EEG, and an unanticipated relationship between spike and slow-wave components of epileptiform patterns. Therefore, the second step of the two-step plan is to explore the implications of the model for EEG-generating mechanisms. Existing information concerning anatomical, physiological, and pathophysiological aspects of the EEG is summarized as a preliminary to exploring the implications (necessarily speculative) of the model.

Relating the basic hypothesis to existing information concerning EEG-generating mechanisms of the brain is difficult and the reader may be disappointed by the few speculations on this question (in particular, on the exact physiological counterparts of the electronic components of the model) in the later chapters. On the other hand, the suggestion is advanced (on the basis of a detailed consideration of the features of the model, the characteristics of the EEG, and the known aspects of the physiology of the cerebral cortex) that the envelope of the EEG may be an indication of summary inhibitory effects, and the envelope of the first derivative of the EEG an indication of summary excitatory effects, within some not-very-precisely-defined area of the cortex the activity of which is reflected at given scalp electrodes. Further, although the question explored in this book is that of the single-channel EEG, and the multi-channel EEG is not explored, the possibility of simulating the interactions of the electrical activity from different cortical areas (e.g., mutual entrainment and lesser degrees of coherence) is inherent in the nonlinear nature of the basic model.

SOME ASPECTS OF THE MODULATION OF WAVES

Since the present hypothesis evidently entails a previously undescribed oscillator capable of two distinct but simultaneous forms of modulation, some familiar types of modulation will be considered first.

Amplitude Modulation and Frequency Modulation

In an EEG, the alpha rhythm of about 10 Hz characteristically increases and decreases in amplitude with relatively little change in the frequency of the individual alpha waves—that is, the waves appear to be amplitude modulated. Figure 1.1A illustrates a 10-Hz triangular wave modulated in amplitude by a 1-Hz triangular wave.

Alpha waves also may exhibit a slight decrease in their frequency in the second or so following their reappearance after eye closure. Figure 1.1B illustrates a 10-Hz wave modulated in frequency by a 1-Hz triangular wave.

Extrema Modulation

The modulation of extremes, which was introduced into this work in order to simulate certain EEG patterns, is illustrated in figure 1.1C. The characteristic feature of this evidently new type of modulation is that the slopes of the individual waves (in the case of the triangular waves shown in figure 1.1C) or the running mean slope (in the case of sinusoidal waves—see chapter 2) remain(s) constant; hence the term *constant-slope waves*, meaning waves of relatively constant slope, will be used. In contrast to the constancy of slope, both the amplitude and the frequency (or its inverse, the period) of the modulated waves vary.

Dual Modulation

In principle, combined (simultaneous) amplitude modulation and frequency modulation could be carried out on the same wave train. But such combined or dual modulation is evidently not ordinarily used in practice, and it is not apparent in the EEG save perhaps in the slight variations in alpha frequency (e.g., a slight decrease immediately after eye closure, or the small decrease that may become evident in some subjects with minimal drowsiness) that occur at the same time as the characteristic waxing and waning of the alpha amplitude.

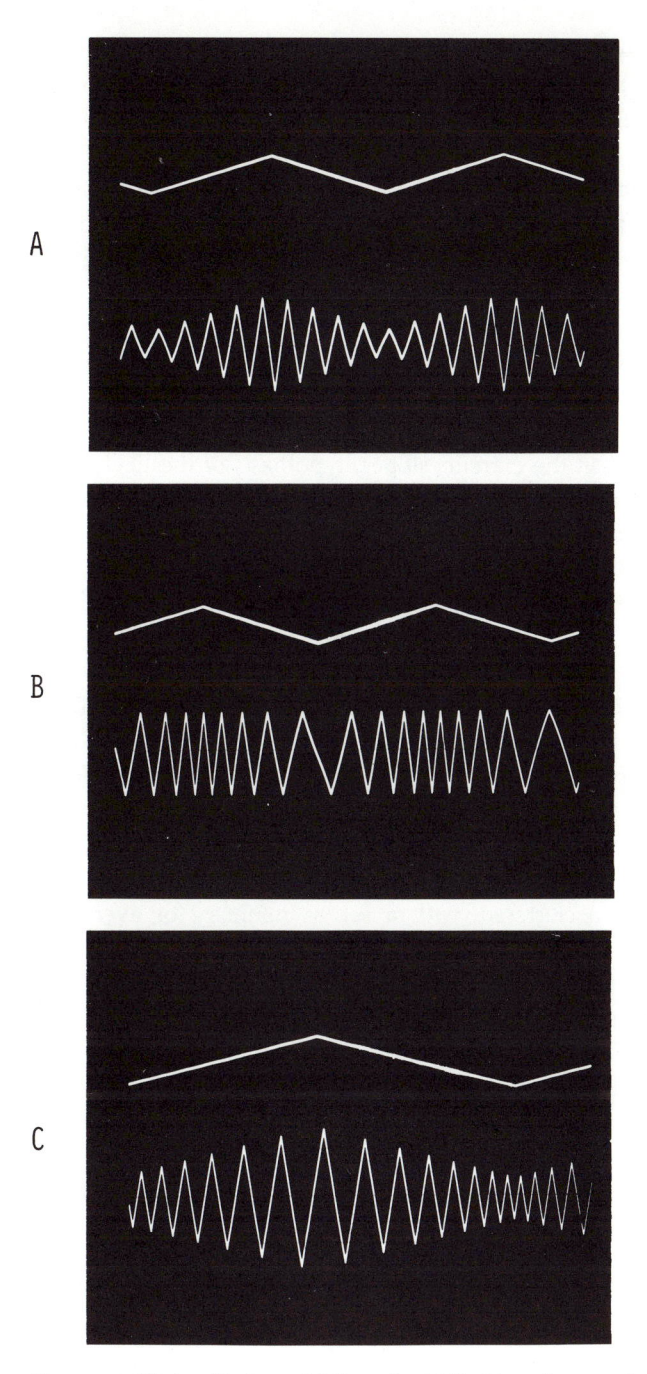

Figure 1.1 (A) Amplitude modulation of a 10-Hz triangular wave by a 1-Hz triangular wave. The duration of the individual waves remains constant whereas their amplitude varies. (B) Frequency modulation of a 10-Hz triangular wave by a 1-Hz triangular wave. The duration (and the slopes) of the individual waves varies whereas their amplitude remains constant. (C) Extrema modulation (modulation of extremes) of a 10-Hz triangular wave by a 1-Hz triangular wave (the time base is expanded by a factor of 2 in comparison with A and B). The slopes of the waves remain the same (hence the term *waves of constant slope*, or *constant-slope waves*), but both the amplitudes (peak excursions) and the durations of the waves vary.

Introduction

The oscillator model developed in chapter 2 as a generalized model for EEG activity may be new in two respects: it entails the modulation of extrema, and it employs two completely different forms of modulation simultaneously (namely, the aforementioned modulation of extremes in combination with modulation of slopes). The modulation of slopes is similar to although not identical with frequency modulation, since the slopes-modulating signal can take on negative as well as positive values. The interesting question arises of whether dual modulation in the particular form just described (employed in the present oscillator model) is a unique feature (at least until now) of the oscillatory systems of the brain, in particular the cerebral cortex, or at least of living systems. A substantiated affirmative answer might be of no small interest.

Inherent in the extrema-slopes hypothesis of the EEG is that the two significant parameters of any single EEG signal are its amplitudes (more exactly, its positive and negative extremes) and its slopes (i.e., the steepnesses of the individual waves). Expressed more precisely: According to the extrema-slopes hypothesis of the EEG, the two important parameters are the envelope of the EEG and the envelope of its first (time) derivative.

THE ORIGINS OF THE EXTREMA-SLOPES HYPOTHESIS

The hypothesis arose from chance observation made in early 1986 in the course of some work on adaptive segmentation of the EEG. This was a technique whereby different patterns of activity within the same recording (e.g., background activity and paroxysmal activity) could be separated or segmented and clustered, with a set of summary or average amplitude and frequency characteristics given for like segments (Praetorius et al. 1977; Bodenstein and Praetorius 1977; Michael and Houchin 1979; Barlow et al. 1981; Creutzfeld et al. 1985). The segmentation and clustering processes were based on running measures of amplitude and frequency and of the mean amplitude and mean frequency of the segments, respectively—the amplitude and frequency measures having been obtained by use of the autocorrelation function. The computer calculation of the autocorrelation function was, however, relatively time-consuming, and therefore more expeditious methods of obtaining running measures of amplitude and of frequency were sought.

A running measure of amplitude was obtained, with relative ease, as the running mean absolute amplitude of the EEG (i.e., with all half-waves made positive, followed by some smoothing). The method devised to measure the running frequency of a fixed-amplitude sine wave was based on the fact that the absolute amplitude (after smoothing) of the output of a differentiator for such a constant-amplitude sine-wave input is directly proportional to the frequency of the sine wave. A measure of the running mean frequency of a signal with variable amplitude could thus be obtained as the quotient of the running mean slope (i.e., the running mean amplitude of the first derivative of the signal) to the running mean amplitude of the signal itself:

$$\underline{\dot{f}} = k(\underline{\bar{s}}/\underline{\bar{a}}),$$

where $\bar{f}$, $\bar{s}$, and $\bar{a}$ are the running means of frequency, slope, and amplitude, respectively, and k is a constant that requires evaluation at only one frequency, so that the expression yields the correct frequency. (Small amplitudes need not imply high frequencies, since frequency, according to the hypothesis, is determined by the quotient of amplitude and slope, so that lower amplitudes in combination with lower slopes in the EEGs of lower vertebrates can result in frequencies in the same range as in the human EEG.)

Experimental tests of the electronic implementation of this system yielded satisfactory results for a clinical EEG having a prominent alpha rhythm. However, by chance, a section of drowsiness (Stage 1 slow-wave sleep) followed the alpha-activity portion, and it became evident that, in contrast to the parallel fluctuations of amplitude and slope of the alpha portion of the EEG, the fluctuations of slope appeared, at least intermittently, to be less than the fluctuations of amplitude (figure 1.2). In other words, there seemed to be a tendency for waves of relatively constant slope to appear during drowsiness. (In addition to "good" alpha waves and a pattern of drowsiness, the same EEG, as it happened, also showed a 3-Hz spike-wave pattern, so this particular clinical EEG turned out to include a trove of interesting features in relation to this work at a very early stage.)

It then seemed of interest to develop an electronic model capable of generating waves of constant slope, which was promptly accomplished by modulating the extrema of the intrinsic oscillations of the model, as illustrated in figure 1.1C. But since the test EEG also included alpha activity—waves of relatively constant frequency but variable amplitude (i.e., the characteristic waxing and waning of alpha activity), the question immediately arose of whether the alpha could be simulated by some modification of the constant-slope oscillator, instead of by the more conventional amplitude modulation (figure 1.1A), therefore enabling a single oscillator to simulate both EEG patterns (i.e., waves of constant slope and waves of constant frequency, corresponding to the drowsiness and the alpha patterns, respectively). After brief exploration, it was found that such waves of constant frequency but variable amplitude could be generated by simultaneous and identical modulation of both the extrema and the slopes of the intrinsic waves of the oscillator.

After these initial steps, the full-fledged dual-modulation (i.e., extrema and slopes) oscillator model emerged. In time this model was found to be capable of simulating a wide range of normal and abnormal EEG patterns. Indeed, it was found to be capable of on-line real-time instantaneous reconstitution of EEGs (within certain limitations), given the appropriate input modulation signals, the latter being derived from actual EEGs.

THE ORGANIZATION OF THE CHAPTERS

The overall organization of the book is as follows: Parts I and II describe and establish the validity of the extrema-slopes hypothesis. In part III the hypothesis is evaluated from a wider perspective. The technical details of the methodologies developed to test the hypothesis are discussed in part IV. In

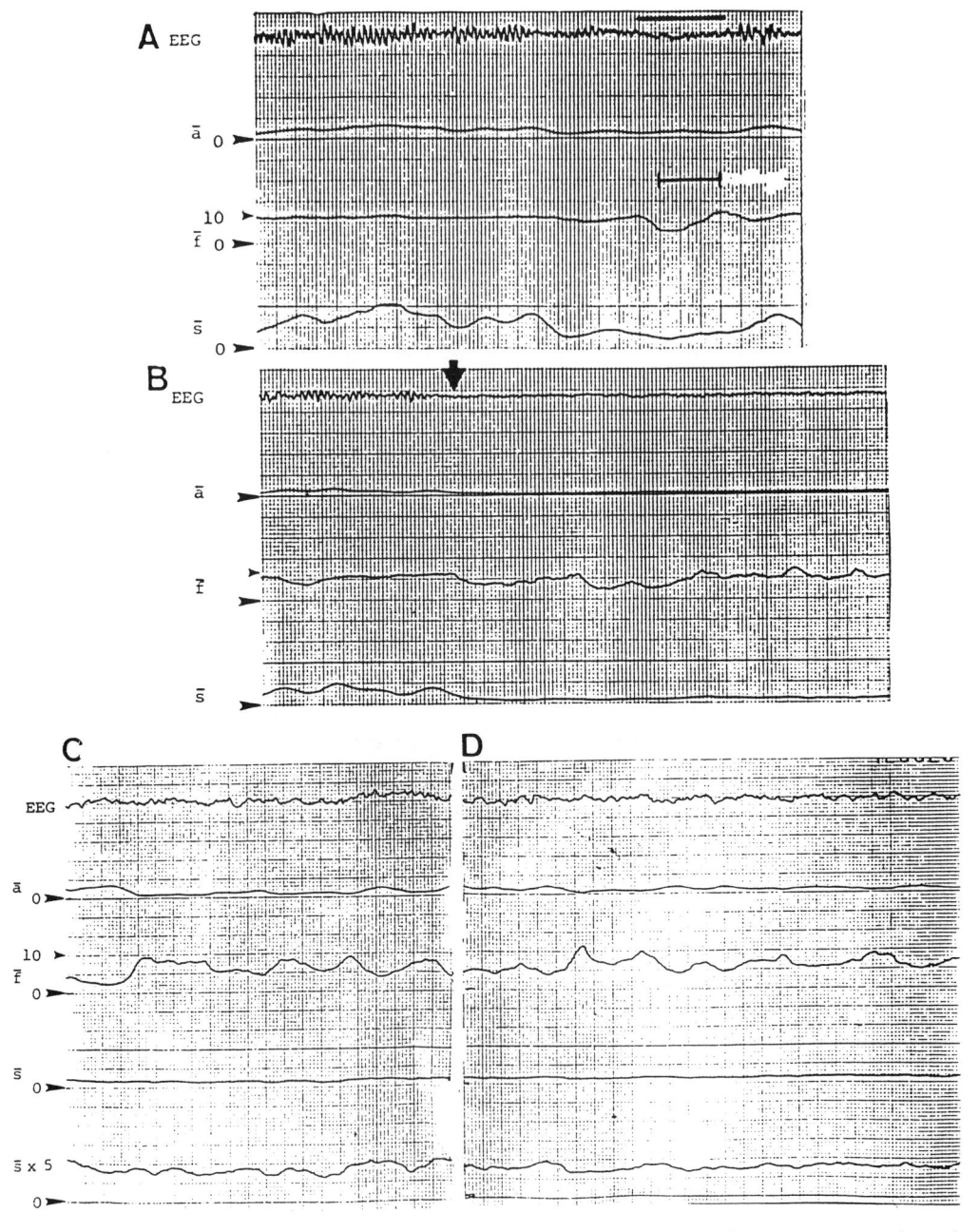

Figure 1.2 Sample early results with the circuit for mean-running-frequency (trace 3), derived from the quotient of the mean running slope (trace 4) and the mean running amplitude (trace 2), suggesting less variability of the mean running slope than of the mean running amplitude or frequency during periods of drowsiness in the EEG (trace 1). A and B show transitions from wakefulness (with variable amplitude and slope, but relatively constant frequency) to drowsiness (variable frequency and amplitude but, suggestively, less variable slope). Drowsiness is indicated in A by the bar at the top, the onset of drowsiness in B is indicated by the arrow. C and D show drowsiness, with the mean running slope displayed on a magnified scale (trace 5), suggesting a smaller variability of slope than of frequency (and, by inference, of amplitude). Parieto-occipital EEG recording. Baselines indicated by large arrows; 10-Hz calibration by small arrow. Time marker: 1 sec.

the first two parts the EEG is treated phenomenologically, as a signal from a "black box" (the brain); accordingly, there is little mention of brain mechanisms until part III.

Part I

The hypothesis and its associated model are developed in chapter 2. The three-pronged approach to testing the hypothesis—(1) simulating EEG patterns, (2) testing predictions based on the hypothesis, and (3) reconstituting EEGs from their essential elements, the latter being the instantaneous envelope of the EEG and of its first derivative (as prescribed by the hypothesis)—is presented in chapter 3. In chapter 4, simulations of several types of EEG patterns are compared with actual EEGs of the same type.

Part II

The results of tests of the hypothesis with various types of normal and abnormal EEG patterns are presented in chapters 5–9. In chapter 10 the hypothesis is appraised in relation to the experimental tests of it.

Part III

Selective reviews of the anatomy, physiology, and pathophysiology of the EEG and of EEG models are presented in chapters 11–14. The hypothesis is appraised from these perspectives in chapters 15 and 16, and in relation to other computer techniques of EEG analysis in chapter 17. Some limitations of the work are detailed in chapter 18. In view of the relevance of the extrema-slopes hypothesis to it, Norbert Wiener's concept of the alpha rhythm as a brain clock is revisited methodologically in chapter 19. A comprehensive overview of the nontechnological chapters is presented in chapter 20.

Part IV

The technical details of the methodologies and of the oscillator model itself are discussed in chapters 21–29. The development of the techniques and the electronic circuitry for this work has engendered some powerful new on-line real-time analog approaches to some conventional methods of EEG data processing (e.g., averaging, correlation, spectral analysis in the form of compressed spectral arrays, artifact minimization). These, placed in the perspective of some relevant earlier developments, are the subjects of appendixes A and B. A diagram of the scalp electrode placements specified by the International Federation of Societies for Electroencephalography and Clinical Neurophysiology is given in appendix C as a reference for the clinical EEG patterns reproduced throughout the book. A glossary follows the appendixes.

More general reference works that are relevant include Kandel et al. 1991 (a standard comprehensive neuroscience text in which there appears a chapter on electroencephalography by Martin); standard reference works on clinical electroencephalography by Tyner et al. (1983, 1989), Niedermeyer and Lopes da Silva (1987, 1993), and Daly and Pedley (1990); specialized treatments of drowsiness (Santamaria and Chiappa 1987) and of sleep (Carskadon and Rechtschaffen 1989); and books on EEG technology (Cooper et al. 1981) and on computer analysis of the EEG (Lopes da Silva et al. 1986; Gevins and Rémond 1987).

I The Hypothesis and Methods of Testing It; Simulation Results

2 The Hypothesis and the Oscillator Model

MODULATION OF EXTREMA

The suggestive finding that the EEG during drowsiness could exhibit relatively constant slope compelled, for its modeling, the introduction of an apparently previously undescribed type of modulation: the modulation of the extrema (the peaks and valleys) of waves. It is apparent that this modulation changes both the amplitude and the duration of the waves (figure 1.1C). The slope of the individual waves, however, remains constant. That extrema modulation changes *both* the amplitude *and* the duration (and thus the frequency) of waves contrasts sharply with the effect of amplitude modulation, which changes *only* the amplitude of the modulated waves, and with the effect of frequency modulation, which changes *only* the frequency (and thus the duration) of the modulated waves.

DUAL MODULATION OF EXTREMA AND SLOPES

In the oscillator model about to be described, which was mandated by the characteristics of EEG patterns themselves, the above-described principle of modulation of extrema is combined with modulation of slopes to form a simultaneous dual-modulation arrangement. (It will become apparent that the principle employed in the modulation of slopes is the same as that employed in frequency modulation—at least, if only triangular waves are considered.) However, the term *frequency modulation* is not used, since this term implies that only the frequency of the waves is varied; instead, the term *slopes modulation* is retained.)

THE BASIC HYPOTHESIS

The basic hypothesis of this book is that any EEG pattern can be considered as though it were made up of oscillations the waves of which have been modulated independently with respect to their extrema (i.e., positive and negative maxima, hereafter sometimes referred to less accurately as their amplitudes) and with respect to their slopes. The hypothesis can thus be termed the *extrema-slopes hypothesis*. The aforementioned two independent variations,

1. CONSTANT SLOPE,
   INCREASING HEIGHT
   (FREQUENCY DECREASES)

2. CONSTANT HEIGHT,
   INCREASING SLOPE
   (FREQUENCY INCREASES)

3. INCREASING SLOPE AND
   INCREASING HEIGHT
   (FREQUENCY CONSTANT)

4. SLOPE AND HEIGHT
   INDEPENDENTLY VARIABLE
   (FREQUENCY VARIABLE)

   (NOT ILLUSTRATED)

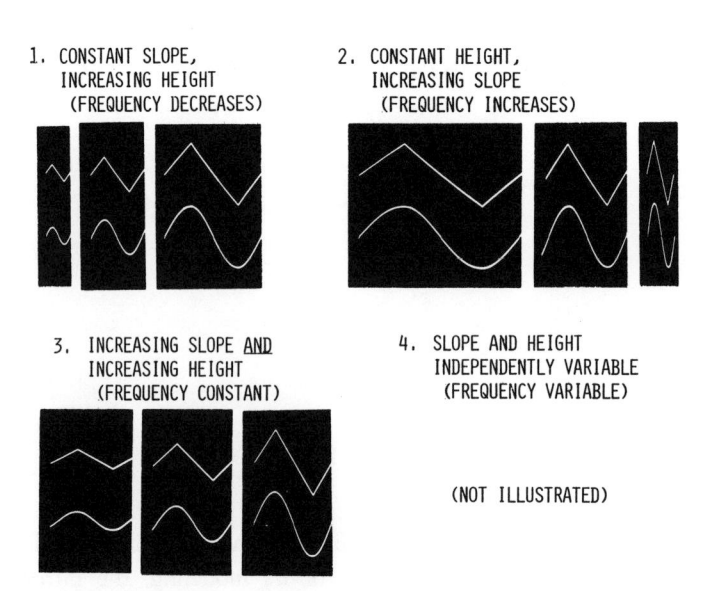

Figure 2.1 Sequences of Type 1, Type 2, and Type 3 waves according to the extrema-slopes hypothesis of the EEG. Type 4 waves are not illustrated, since they cannot be depicted as a single progressive sequence as can the others. (See figure 2.2.)

alone and in different combinations, can give rise to four basic types of waves, three of which are illustrated in figure 2.1.

In part 1 of figure 2.1, three triangular waves having the same slope or steepness but of progressively increasing height are shown together with their sine-wave counterparts; these are Type 1 waves. It is apparent that, as the distance between the extrema and the baseline increases, the frequency of the waves decreases, and correspondingly the duration of the waves increases. In the present hypothesis, these are termed *constant-slope* waves. (Occasional reference to the glossary may be useful for the following discussion.) An essential part of the hypothesis is that, for Type 1 waves, extrema (or amplitude) and duration vary together, or covary. Correspondingly, amplitude and frequency vary inversely.

Part 2 of figure 2.1 shows a series of three triangular waves whose extrema or amplitude are the same but whose slopes increase progressively. These are Type 2 waves, which are termed *constant-extrema* or *constant-amplitude* waves. It is apparent that for Type 2 waves the frequency increases as the slope increases.

Part 3 of figure 2.1 shows a set of waves for which both the extrema and the slopes increase progressively and conjointly, in such a way that the frequency remains constant. These are Type 3 waves, and they are termed *constant-frequency* waves.

Waves varying independently in their extrema and in their slopes are termed Type 4 waves. These are not illustrated in figure 2.1, because there is no single sequence of the kind shown for the other types of waves. (A three-dimensional display would be required for the dual sequence resulting from the dual independent modulation in Type 4 waves.)

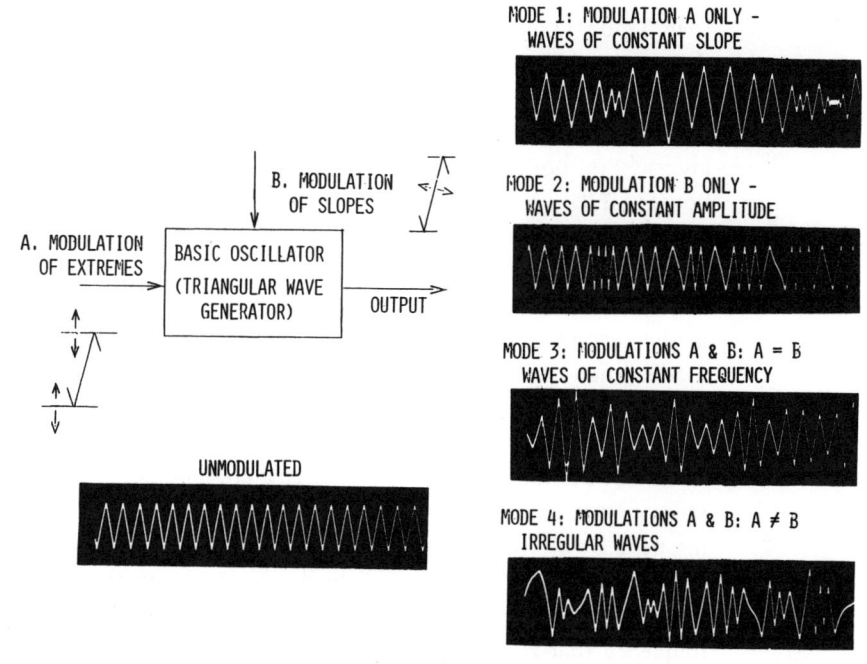

Figure 2.2 Schema and illustrations of the four modes of operation of the dual-modulation oscillator model or EEG-pattern simulator (further details are given in chapter 22). The unmodulated triangular-wave output is shown at the lower left, and the effect of modulation of extremes (modulation A) and modulation of slopes (modulation B) are indicated at the left center. The sequence of four traces on the right shows the output of the oscillator for these two modulations separately (modes 1 and 2), and in combination, congruently (mode 3) (i.e., identical signals to both modulating inputs) and incongruently (mode 4) (i.e., non-identical signals to the two modulating inputs). The resultant waves are (1) of constant slope, (2) of constant amplitude, (3) of constant frequency, and (4) completely irregular.

THE OSCILLATOR MODEL

The model that corresponds to the hypothesis, termed the *oscillator model*, has been implemented in analog electronic form. Its output waves can be modulated independently with respect to their extrema and their slopes. The oscillator model can be used to simulate various types of EEG patterns, from which simulations inferences can be made about the nature of the constituent waves in the corresponding actual EEG patterns. As will become apparent, the oscillator model can also be used to reconstitute EEGs on the basis of their extrema and slopes. Details of the oscillator model are given in chapter 22.

As is indicated on the left in figure 2.2, the basic oscillator in the oscillator model is a triangular-wave generator, the triangular-wave output of which in unmodulated form is shown. The use of two independent input modulations, A and B, makes possible the aforementioned four separate modes of oscillation, which correspond to the four types of waves shown on the right side of the figure. (In addition to the four principal modes, there are any number of mixed modes of operation, as will be discussed further below.)

In Mode 1, the slope (Modulation B) is kept constant while the extrema (Modulation A) are varied. The resultant waves are the constant-slope waves shown at the top right in figure 2.2. In this mode of the oscillator model, the amplitude of the output waves is directly proportional to their duration (i.e., inversely proportional to their frequency). The amplitude is therefore proportional to $1/f$.

In Mode 2, only the slope of the triangular waves is modulated (i.e., Modulation B varies), their extrema (positive and negative peaks) being kept constant (Modulation A constant). A sample train of the resulting waves is shown in the second trace on the right in figure 2.2. In this mode, the oscillator model functions essentially as a conventional FM (frequency-modulation) device, or Voltage-Controlled Oscillator (VCO), a common laboratory device. The resulting waves are constant-amplitude waves.

In Mode 3, the slopes and the extrema are modulated congruently, i.e., the same modulating signal is fed to Modulation A and to Modulation B inputs (figure 2.2, left), and a sample of the output waves is shown in the third trace on the right in figure 2.2. In this mode, an increase in frequency that would result from an increase in slope is just counterbalanced by a decrease in frequency that would result from an increase in the extrema, with the result that such congruent modulation results in waves of variable amplitude but constant frequency. The generation of waves of constant frequency by such dual congruent modulation of extrema and slopes is an essential feature of the oscillator model. The result is equivalent to that obtained by conventional amplitude modulation (compare figure 1.1A). The frequency of Mode 3 oscillations indicates the intrinsic frequency of the oscillator model (compare the third right trace with the bottom left trace in figure 2.2).

In Mode 4 of the oscillator model, the slopes and the extremes are modulated independently, i.e., different signals are fed to Modulation Input A and to Modulation Input B (figure 2.2, left). The resulting waves (figure 2.2, bottom right) are completely irregular; neither extrema (amplitudes), nor slope, nor frequency is constant.

In addition to the four basic types of waves corresponding to the four modes of operation depicted in figure 2.2, mixed modes are possible. These include the following:

(a) primarily modulation of slopes (Mode 2), but with a small amount of modulation of extrema (Mode 1).

(b) primarily modulation of extrema, but with a small amount of modulation of slopes—i.e., the converse of (a).

(c) unequal degrees of modulation of slopes and extrema, using the same modulating signal (i.e., modified Mode 3).

(d) partially congruent, partially independent modulation of slopes and of extrema (i.e., a mix of Modes 3 and 4).

(A special case is that of identical waveforms but opposite polarities of the two input modulations, in which case the amplitude of the output waves of the oscillator model is inversely proportional to the square of their frequency, instead of inversely proportional to the first power of their frequency as in Mode 1 operation.)

The basic triangular-wave oscillator model can be considered as a form of relaxation oscillator (van der Pol 1926) having two independent possibilities of modulation. (The term *relaxation oscillator* originally stemmed from the term *time of relaxation*; see chapter 14.)

CONVERSION OF TRIANGULAR WAVES TO QUASI-SINUSOIDAL FORM

In the lower traces in figure 2.1, the sine-wave counterpart of each of the types of waves (except for Type 4) is included below the respective triangular wave, since ordinarily (although not invariably) EEG waves are more rounded or sinusoidal than triangular. It might seem that conventional low-pass filtering could serve to convert the triangular waves to sinusoidal form. Only for Type 3 waves, of constant frequency, would this procedure be feasible, since for all of the other types of waves the frequency is variable from one wave to the next, and hence no single setting of a low-pass filter would suffice.

The procedure illustrated on the left in figure 2.3 was therefore employed for conversion of the triangular-wave output of the basic oscillator to a quasi-sinusoidal form. In essence, the latter waveform is obtained by joining together at the baseline a series of parabolic curves fitted to the successive upper and lower halves of the triangular waves. (The details of this procedure are given in chapter 22.) The right side of figure 2.3 shows the four types of waves for the four basic modes of operation of the oscillator model in their triangular and smoothed forms. (In actual practice, it is possible to select any arbitrary equal-amplitude mixture of triangular waves and quasi-sinusoidal ones simply by adjusting the relative contributions of the two to the final output of the system.)

It would be possible in principle to build an oscillator model whose output would itself be essentially sinusoidal, thus eliminating the need for the special process just described for converting triangular to sinusoidal waves. The end result would, however, be the same. The two-stage process just described—generating first the triangular wave, and then from it the sine wave—was used because of its relative simplicity.

From inspection of the waves for Mode 1 (figure 2.3), it is evident that, in contrast to the constant slope (except for sign) of the triangular waves in the course of a single cycle, the slope of the quasi-sinusoidal version varies in the course of a single cycle. Hence, reference will be made subsequently to the *running mean slope*, a shortened form of the more accurate and more complete term *running mean absolute* (i.e., irrespective of sign) *slope*, the mean being taken over some short interval (nominally, 0.5 sec) or window that moves progressively along the signal (e.g., an EEG) in question.

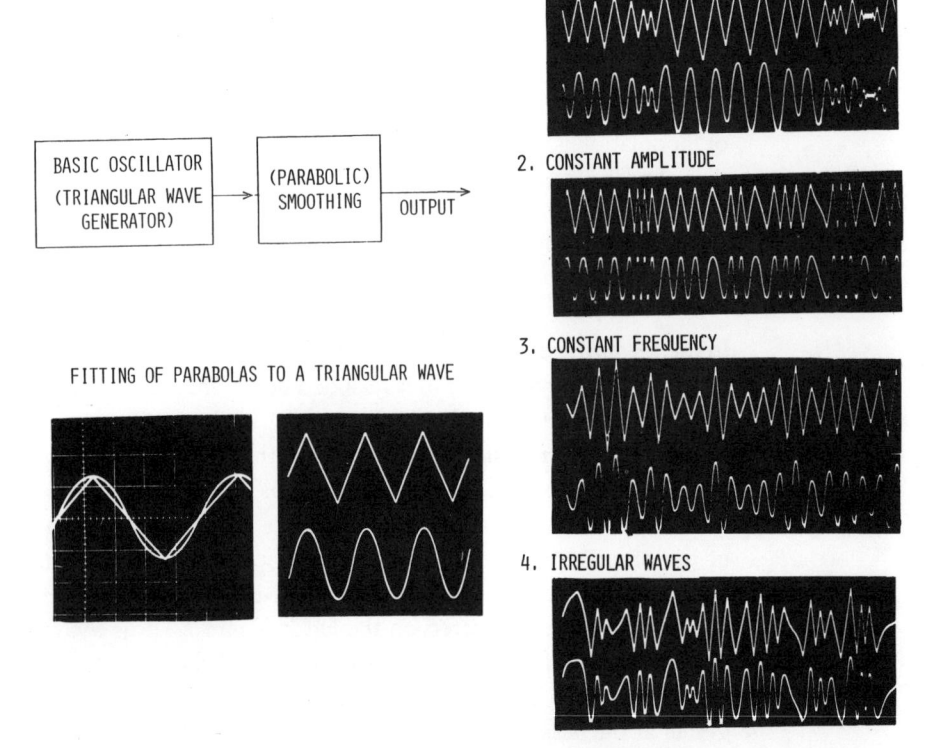

Figure 2.3 Left: Schema of conversion of triangular waves to quasi-sinusoidal form by fitting a parabola to each half-wave (positive and negative) of the triangular wave, so that the successions of parabolas join at the baseline. Right: Same sequence of triangular waves for modes 1–4 of the oscillator model as shown in figure 2.2 together with their quasi-sinusoidal versions.

SPECIAL FEATURES OF THE FOUR TYPES OF OUTPUT WAVES OF THE OSCILLATOR MODEL

Type 1 waves, in which only the extrema are modulated and which have a constant running mean slope, have the particular characteristic that the modulation results in a simultaneous and reciprocal variation in amplitude and in frequency; i.e., the amplitude of the waves is inversely proportional to their frequency. Sine waves having this characteristic can be obtained by passing frequency-modulated waves through an integrator; the effect of the integrator is to impose a $1/f$ amplitude characteristic on the conventional frequency-modulated waves. Modulated waves with this specific characteristic, and the corresponding oscillator-modulator, however, may not have been previously described.

Type 2 waves, in which only the slopes are modulated, are the same as the waves resulting from conventional frequency modulation (for example, in a voltage-controlled oscillator), with the exception that in the latter the modulation is not normally negative.

Type 3 waves, in which extrema and slopes are congruently or conjointly modulated by a single input modulating signal, and which are of constant frequency but variable amplitude, are the equivalent of conventional amplitude-modulated waves (obtained, for example, by means of a fixed-frequency oscillator in combination with a multiplier).

Type 4 waves, in which extrema and slopes are independently modulated, are random or irregular in amplitude, frequency, and slope, appear not to have been previously described, and may be unique to the present oscillator model.

COMPARISON OF COMBINED EXTREMA-SLOPES MODULATION WITH COMBINED AMPLITUDE-FREQUENCY MODULATION

It might be supposed that it would be possible to generate waves of constant slope (an essential aspect of the present hypothesis) by means of combined amplitude-frequency modulation. That this is not the case is evident from figure 2.4, in which a single modulating signal (top trace) has been used to frequency modulate a triangular wave (second trace) and then to amplitude modulate the latter (third trace). The waves of the third trace may appear superficially to be of constant slope, but that this is not the case is evident from the fourth trace, which shows the slope (first time derivative) of the doubly modulated wave train. For this trace, the relative magnitudes of the frequency and amplitude modulations were chosen such that the slopes would be the same (i.e., the width of trace 4 would be the same) at the two extremes of modulation. The very noticeable bowing of the fourth trace indicates that it is not possible to generate waves of constant slope by means of combined amplitude and frequency modulation.

CONSTANT-SLOPE WAVES CAN NOT BE OBTAINED
BY A COMBINATION OF CONVENTIONAL
FREQUENCY AND AMPLITUDE MODULATION

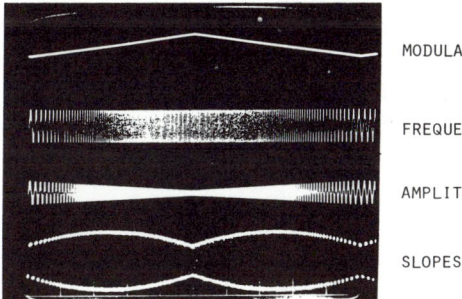

MODULATING SIGNAL

FREQUENCY MODULATION
+
AMPLITUDE MODULATION

SLOPES (D/DT)

Figure 2.4 Frequency modulation (trace 2) of triangular waves followed by amplitude modulation (trace 3) of the already frequency-modulated waves, using the same low-frequency triangular modulating wave (trace l) for both. Trace 4 shows the first time derivative of trace 3, the doubly modulated waves. The relative levels of the frequency and amplitude modulations were adjusted so that trace 4 had the same amplitude for the positive and negative extrema of the modulating low-frequency triangular wave. The variation in the width of trace 4 indicates the impossibility of obtaining true constant-slope waves by combined amplitude and frequency modulation.

THE 1/f AMPLITUDE CHARACTERISTIC OF TYPE 1 WAVES

It was noted above that for Type 1 waves of the oscillator model there is an inverse relationship between the amplitude of the output waves and their frequency, which can be termed a *1/f amplitude characteristic*. It should be pointed out, however, that this 1/f amplitude characteristic is not the same as the so-called 1/f characteristic of noise signals from certain electronic components, such as germanium filaments (McWhorter 1957; Walma 1980); the 1/f characteristic in such instances refers not to amplitude (as for the present Type 1) but to power, the latter being proportional to the square of amplitude. Further, in a spectrum of amplitude (or log power) versus frequency, the "noise" component (i.e., excluding peaks corresponding to rhythmic activity such as alpha) of an EEG may have the appearance of decreasing linearly with increasing frequency. Actually, for waves having a 1/f amplitude characteristic, a linear relationship is present only on a plot of log amplitude vs. log frequency (a log-log plot), not on a plot of log amplitude vs. frequency (a semi-log plot). This question is considered further in chapters 7 and 15.

POSSIBLE EEG CORRELATES OF THE FOUR BASIC TYPES OF WAVES OF THE OSCILLATOR MODEL

In preliminary reports concerning the extrema-slopes hypothesis of the EEG (Barlow 1989, 1993), it was suggested that the output waveforms for the different modes of operation of the oscillator model might constitute model

TYPE:
1. CONSTANT SLOPE

2. CONSTANT AMPLITUDE

3. CONSTANT FREQUENCY

4. IRREGULAR WAVES

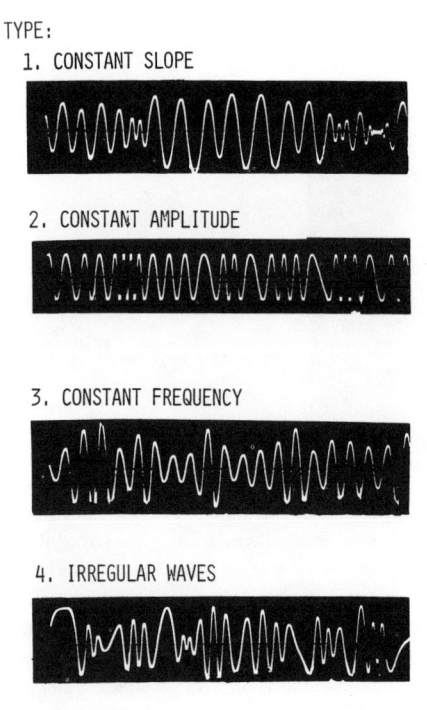

Figure 2.5 The four types of waves in their quasi-sinusoidal forms.

waveforms for particular types of EEG patterns. For this purpose, the quasi-sinusoidal forms of the four types of waves are brought together in figure 2.5. The suggestions or predictions (which do not include mixed-mode possibilities from the oscillator model) were as follows:

Type 1 (constant slope, variable amplitude) waves: non-REM sleep (excepting sleep spindles and vertex sharp waves); abnormal irregular slowing (polymorphic delta slowing); hyperventilation-induced slowing; the EEG in the deeper stages of general anesthesia (prediction not tested)

Type 2 (constant amplitude, variable slope) waves: some epileptiform patterns, e.g., the 3-Hz spike-wave pattern

Type 3 (constant frequency) waves: rhythmic activity, e.g., alpha activity; slow posterior rhythm; sleep spindles; only alpha activity has been tested

Type 4 (irregular) waves: the "desynchronized" EEG (i.e., low-voltage irregular activity) of the alert eyes-open waking state (in some individuals, also with eyes closed); the EEG during REM sleep.

These four principal types of patterns, and the prediction that each pattern can be a model for certain specific types of EEG activity, constitute one method of testing the basic extrema-slopes hypothesis. This method, and two others, will be considered in the next chapter.

3 Approaches, Methods, and EEG Database for Testing the Hypothesis

Three approaches to testing the extrema-slopes dual-modulation hypothesis of the EEG have been employed; these are listed in the order in which they were developed and used:

• simulation of EEG patterns, using the basic oscillator model in conjunction with standard and specially constructed signal-generating equipment

• testing of specific predictions, made on the basis of the hypothesis, concerning particular features of specific EEG patterns

• evaluation of the degree of similarity between original EEGs and their reconstituted versions, the latter generated by means of the oscillator model, using as the modulating inputs for the latter, for a given EEG, the instantaneous envelope of the latter together with the instantaneous envelope of the first derivative of the EEG.

These approaches, of which the third is the most powerful and the most comprehensive, are illustrated schematically in figure 3.1.

SIMULATION OF EEG PATTERNS (METHOD 1)

For simulation of EEG patterns by means of the oscillator model (figure 3.1, upper section), considerable use was made of low-frequency random signals of various frequency characteristics (bandwidths), for which a standard low-frequency noise source (Elgenco) was used, in conjunction with a two-channel variable electronic filter (Spencer Kennedy Laboratories), to generate modulating signals for the oscillator model. In some instances in which two independent noise signals having the same characteristics were required, a special multi-channel random low-frequency noise generator was constructed (chapter 28).

Some examples of simulated patterns were presented in chapter 2, and additional ones will be presented in subsequent chapters. These simulated patterns are presented for visual comparison, to give an indication of the capabilities of the oscillator model for simulating a variety of actual EEG patterns; no quantitative comparisons between simulated and real patterns are attempted.

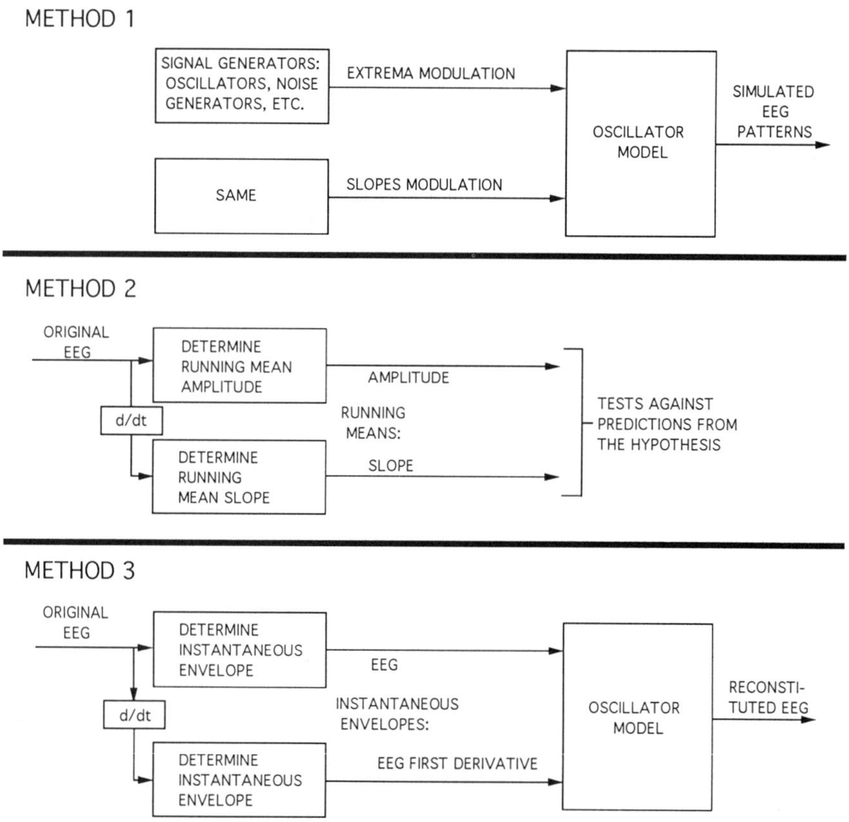

Figure 3.1 Block diagrams of the three approaches to testing the extrema-slopes hypothesis.

TESTING FOR PREDICTED CHARACTERISTICS OF EEG PATTERNS (METHOD 2)

For the evaluation of the predictions made on the basis of the extrema-slopes hypothesis in relation to actual EEG patterns (figure 3.1, middle section), as enumerated in chapter 2, a large battery of EEG data-processing techniques were employed, most of them implemented especially for this purpose. All these procedures were carried out on line in real time, the processed results being displayed on an oscilloscope or written out on a multi-channel inkwriter (polygraph) adjacent to the write-out of the EEG signal under analysis. The results appear in chapters 5–8, in which the EEG patterns are arranged in a conventional sequence (normal EEG awake and asleep, normal and abnormal slowing, epileptiform patterns) rather than according to the principal types of wave patterns of the oscillator model.

The determinations include the following:

• running mean (moving average) of (absolute) amplitude, evaluated over a "window" of (e.g.) 0.5 sec that moves progressively along the EEG with time

- running mean (absolute) slope
- running mean frequency
- running Spectral Purity Index, a measure of the degree of regularity (sinusoidality) of an EEG
- Coefficient of Variation of running mean amplitude
- slope
- frequency
- the Pearson Product-Moment Correlation Coefficient, and its square
- the Coefficient of Determination.

Of the preceding determinations, the running mean amplitude and the running mean slope provide smoothed envelopes of the EEG and of its first (time) derivative, and also provide the basic measures with which the predictions made from the extrema-slopes hypothesis can be tested. The running mean frequency and the running Spectra Purity Index provide information concerning the mean frequency and the frequency spread of an EEG. (The Spectral Purity Index gives information that can be compared with the spectral width of an EEG spectrum; for a pure sine wave, its value is 1.0.) The Coefficient of Variation, defined as the quotient of the standard deviation to the mean, provides a quantitative index of the relative variability of a given measure; the relative variability of two measures is conveniently given by the logarithm of the ratios of their respective Coefficients of Variation. The Pearson Product-Moment Correlation Coefficient and its square, the Coefficient of Determination, provide a measure of the degree of similarity between, e.g., the running mean amplitude and the running mean slope.

The principles employed in the above-listed computations are summarized below; the details of the methods are given in chapters 24 and 25.

The *running mean amplitude* entails use of a three-step procedure. For the first step, the absolute value of the EEG is obtained; i.e., negative values are changed to positive ones (a process that is accomplished electronically by full-wave rectification). Short-time R-C (resistance-capacitance) filtering (nominally 0.1 sec) follows, to provide preliminary smoothing. The resulting signal is then averaged over a moving time window of nominally 0.5 sec by means of a transversal or rectangular filter (the details of the latter are given in chapter 23). The transversal or rectangular filter (sometimes also termed a *boxcar filter*) differs from RC filtering in that the data points within the moving window (nominally 16 sample points) are equally weighted, whereas in an RC filter the progressively more recent points are given progressively greater weights (i.e., the curve of the weighting factor is an exponentially decaying curve toward the past).

The *running mean slope* is determined in the same way as just described for the running mean amplitude, except that the determination is carried out on the first derivative of the EEG rather than on the EEG itself.

The *running mean frequency* is obtained simply as the quotient of the running mean slope to the running mean amplitude, with a constant of proportionality calibrated to yield the correct frequency for a sine wave of precisely known frequency. (The logic behind this determination is detailed in chapter 25.)

The *running Spectral Purity* Index (Goncharova and Barlow 1990) is a new measure of the degree of sinusoidality or regularity (rhythmicity) of a signal. It has the value of 1.0 for a sine wave, even if it varies in amplitude, irrespective of the amplitude and the frequency. The more irregular a signal, the closer the Spectral Purity Index to its maximum value of 1.0. Its evaluation entails a combination of the running mean amplitude, the running mean slope, and also the running mean curvature or sharpness; the latter is evaluated in the same way as the running mean slope, except that the determination is carried out on the second (time) derivative of the EEG instead of on its first derivative. The value of the running Spectral Purity Index is given as the quotient of the square of the running mean absolute slope to the product of the running mean absolute curvature and the running mean absolute amplitude, normalized to a value of 1.0 for a sine wave. For a signal that waxes and wanes, such as successive alpha spindles, the information given by the Spectral Purity Index differs in an important way from that given by the width of the spectrum in spectral analysis, as follows. Assume that a 10-Hz sine wave is modulated by a 1-Hz sine wave, resulting in such a waxing and waning pattern. The spectrum of such a signal will indicate the presence of two sine waves, at 9 and 11 Hz, the two sine waves the sum of which will produce such a pattern. However there will be no component in the spectrum at 10 Hz, although the mean frequency for the spectrum will be correct at 10.0 Hz. (Spectral analysis intrinsically assumes that the signal being analyzed is represented as the sum of a combination of sine waves, each of a particular fixed amplitude.) The corresponding spectral width is 2 Hz, the difference between the two components. The Spectral Purity Index for such a modulated signal, on the other hand, is 1.0, since only a single (albeit modulated) frequency (10 Hz) is present. In the case of EEG alpha spindles, spectral analysis would thus indicate the combination of fixed-amplitude sine waves that would summate to result in the spindle pattern, whereas the Spectral Purity Index would indicate, by a value close to 1.0, that a single sine wave was being modulated to result in the spindle pattern.

The *Coefficient of Variation* (which is computed for the three running means itemized above) is defined as the ratio of the standard deviation to the mean, multiplied by 100; it is thus a normalized measure of variability, rendered as a percentage (Goncharova and Barlow 1990). Its minimum value is 0, its maximum 100%. For quantitative comparison of the relative variability of two variables (e.g., the relative variability of the mean running values for amplitude and for slope), the quotient of the logarithms of their respective Coefficients of Variation can be taken. A linear scale of their relative variability results; thus, a value of 1.0 for the quotient indicates that the two are equally variable, and a quotient of 2.0 or 0.5 indicates that the amplitude is twice or half as variable as the slope, respectively. For evaluating the Coefficient of Variation, a moving window width of generally 4 times the width of the averaging window for the running means was used—e.g., 2 sec, as compared with 0.5 sec.

The computation of the *Pearson Product-Moment Correlation Coefficient* is similar to that for the ordinary correlation coefficient, r, for a zero-mean (i.e., no DC component) signal, except that the mean, or DC component, is first removed. This is an essential step in comparing the running means of amplitude and of slope, since these are, by definition, positive quantities, and hence a DC component will be present in them. The Pearson Product-Moment Correlation Coefficient can range in value between $+1.0$ (indicating that the two signals being compared—e.g., running means—are identical) and -1.0 (indicating that the two signals are identical except for an inversion in polarity for one of them).

The *Coefficient of Determination*, which is the square of the Pearson Product-Moment Correlation Coefficient, ranges in value between zero and 1.0. It gives a measure of the similarity between the two signals being compared, regardless of their relative polarity. As will become evident in chapter 9, the Coefficient of Determination can be useful for comparing the envelopes (i.e., the extrema and the slopes) of a reconstituted EEG with the respective envelopes of the original EEG.

All these determinations are carried out essentially by analog means, on line, in real time, and the results can be written out alongside the original EEG on a multi-channel polygraph.

EVALUATION OF PREDICTIONS FROM THE HYPOTHESIS WITH THE AID OF THESE MEASURES (METHOD 2)

The use of the above-described measures in the testing of the predictions made on the basis of the extrema-slopes hypothesis in relation to actual EEG patterns (figure 3.1, middle section) will now be considered. As a preliminary, some abbreviations will be introduced: the running mean amplitude, slope, and frequency will be denoted respectively by $\bar{a}$, $\bar{s}$, and $\bar{f}$. (The latter is given by the quotient of $\bar{s}/\bar{a}$, as previously mentioned.) Since $\bar{a}$ and $\bar{s}$ are means of absolute (all-positive) numbers, $\bar{a}$ and $\bar{s}$ are themselves always positive (as is $\bar{f}$, of course).

Figure 3.2 schematizes, in "phase-plane" plots, the types of $\bar{a}$ vs. $\bar{s}$ scatter diagrams corresponding to the waves generated by the four modes of the oscillator model. Thus, for Type 1 waves (corresponding to Mode 1 of the oscillator model) the variability of slope (s) is rather less than that of amplitude (a), and hence the term *constant slope* is used. (The latter term refers both to the absence of a trend and to a minimal moment-to-moment variability, as measured with the Coefficient of Variation.) This type of relationship was predicted to characterize the EEG during non-REM sleep (i.e., Stages 1–4). For such EEG patterns, a smaller variability of the running mean slope (hereafter referred to simply as *slope*) than of the running mean amplitude (hereafter termed simply *amplitude*) is thus expected. Further, a low value of the Coeffi-

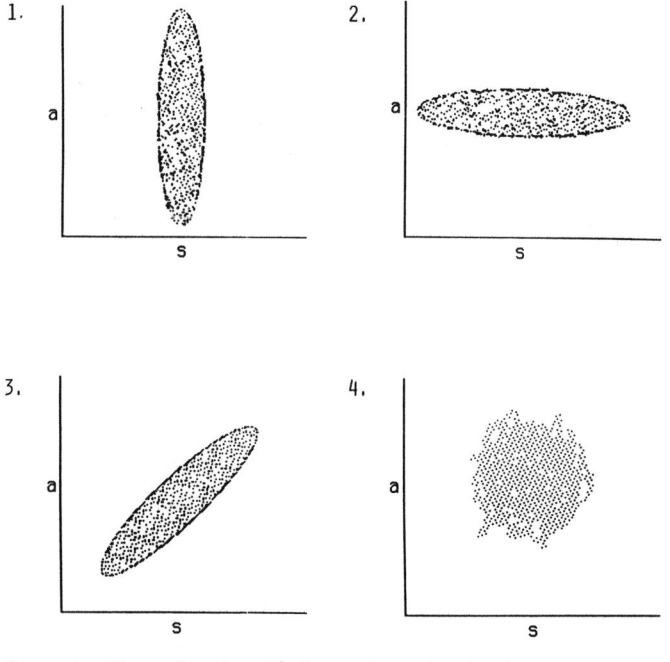

Figure 3.2 Phase plots (amplitude vs. slope) for the four types (1–4) of waves from the oscillator model.

cient of Determination for the running means of amplitude and slope should occur, indicating their relative independence.

For Type 2 waves (corresponding to Mode 2 of the oscillator model), amplitude is rather less variable than slope—a relationship that was predicted to characterize the 3-Hz spike-wave EEG pattern. Further, the value of the Coefficient of Determination should be close to 0 for this EEG pattern.

For Type 3 waves (Mode 3), amplitude and slope are correlated (and are about equally variable)—a relationship that was predicted to characterize rhythmic activity in the EEG, alpha activity and sleep spindles in particular. In addition, the Pearson Product-Moment Correlation Coefficient (and the Coefficient of Determination) is expected to be close to 1.0.

For Type 4 waves (Mode 4), amplitude and slope are uncorrelated and about equally variable—a relationship that was predicted to characterize irregular EEG activity, such as the waking "desynchronized" EEG and the EEG of REM sleep. Further, the Pearson Product-Moment Correlation Coefficient (and the Coefficient of Determination) is expected to be near 0.

RECONSTITUTION OF EEG PATTERNS FROM THEIR ENVELOPES AND THOSE OF THEIR FIRST DERIVATIVES (METHOD 3)

In the first of the three methods for testing the extrema-slopes hypothesis of the EEG, the oscillator model is used to simulate various types of patterns that resemble specific types of EEG patterns. In the second of the three methods, actual EEGs are analyzed for characteristics predicted on the basis of the extrema-slopes hypothesis, using techniques of analysis from among those just described. But if the features of amplitude and of slope are really of primary importance for the EEG, then it should in principle be possible to dissociate an EEG into the putative modulating signals for extremes and for slopes, feed this pair of signals into the oscillator model, and reconstitute the original EEG. As a first approximation, the running mean amplitude and the running mean slope could be used for this purpose, but these signals are obtained by time-averaging over a running 0.5-sec window (interval). Such a pair of signals might suffice for attempting to reconstitute an EEG consisting of long alpha spindles, but not for more irregular EEGs and certainly not for epileptiform patterns of very brief duration (e.g., of the order of 100 msec or less).

Consequently, reconstituting a variety of EEG patterns required an entirely different procedure—namely, deriving the instantaneous envelope of the EEG and that of its first derivative as the pair of modulating signals for extremes and slopes, respectively, of the oscillator model, as indicated in the bottom section of figure 3.1. The accuracy of the reconstitution could be evaluated by visual inspection and by applying the same tests to the reconstituted version to determine whether the same results are obtained as for the original EEG. Further, the Coefficient of Determination could be used to determine how closely, for example, the instantaneous envelope of the reconstituted EEG matches that of the original. The instantaneous envelope of a signal (or, as it is known technically, the magnitude of the *analytic signal*), and methods for obtaining it (including one especially developed for the present investigation) are considered in detail in chapter 29, where some applications by others of the "instantaneous envelope" are also discussed.

It is very important to note that the process of deriving the pair of instantaneous envelopes of an EEG and of its first derivative, and the reconstitution process carried out by the oscillator model using this pair of signals as modulating inputs, are carried out without reference to the four types of output waves that were the focus of the first type of test of the hypothesis or to the corresponding four particular types of EEG patterns that were the focus of the second type of test of the hypothesis. The adequacy of the model *for any arbitrary EEG* (pattern) can therefore be tested with this third method.

The results of this third type of test of the extrema-slopes hypothesis appear primarily in chapter 9.

EEG DATABASE

In the second and third methods of testing the hypothesis, actual EEGs are employed. For this purpose, normal and abnormal EEGs from a number of sources were employed; all these EEGs had been interpreted clinically.

A digitized library of 65 normal and abnormal clinical EEGs (four channels each, on floppy disks) was donated to this project by Otto Creutzfeldt of the Department of Neurobiology of the Max Planck Institute for Biophysical Chemistry in Göttingen. The computer program for reconverting these digitized EEGs to analog form was written by Klaus Bauer, preliminary analysis of data from those recordings for the present study was carried out by Jutta Tolksdorf, and extensive consultations concerning the computer programs for adaptive segmentation were provided by Dieter Michael, all of the Max-Planck-Institut in Göttingen.) Selected examples of these digitized EEGs were reconverted to analog electrical form for processing by means of a Plessey Corporation equivalent of the Digital Equipment Corporation PDP 11/23 computer.

Ink-written clinical EEG recordings were generously provided for this project by the following individuals in Boston: Keith Chiappa, John Stakes, and Margaret Merlina of the Massachusetts General Hospital; Thomas M. Browne and Carol Herbert of the Veterans' Administration Medical Center; Bruce Ehrenberg and Kathleen Corbett at the New England Medical Center; and Gregory Holmes, at Children's Hospital. These clinical EEG ink recordings were supplemented by research recordings of normal subjects recorded during drowsiness and during reading, kindly made available by Keith Chiappa, Director of the EEG Laboratory at the Massachusetts General Hospital. For the analyses, selected channels of the EEG ink recordings (after microfilming) were reconverted to electrical form by photo-optical scanning (chapter 26) as the recordings were rerun through a Grass Model 8 electroencephalograph, which has generously been on long-term loan from the Grass Instrument Company. The photo-optical scanning technique permits direct visual selection of the portions of an EEG recording to be analyzed, thus avoiding the problem of artifact, which otherwise could entail separate processing for minimization or elimination (Barlow 1986).

POSSIBLE SIGNIFICANCE AND IMPLICATIONS OF CONFIRMATORY RESULTS FOR THE HYPOTHESIS

From the foregoing discussion, it is evident that three types of evidence in favor of the extrema-slopes hypothesis could emerge, commensurate with the three types of tests: Specific EEG patterns could indeed be simulated on the oscillator model, using appropriate input modulating signals for it. Second, predictions made on the basis of the hypothesis for particular EEG patterns could indeed be confirmed. Third, reconstituted EEGs of a variety of types could indeed resemble closely or even be identical to the respective originals. It can be held that such positive results would be consistent with the hypothesis, as opposed to providing confirmation for it.

Such confirmatory evidence would indeed concern only the scalp EEG as a signal, without regard to its origin, although the question of waves of relatively constant mean slope, as well as the particular form of the oscillator model that has the capability of generating (among others) waves of constant slope, has apparently not previously arisen in electronics, physics, or biology. As previously mentioned, this latter circumstance raises the question of whether waves of relatively constant mean slope are peculiar to the brain.

On the other hand, confirmatory evidence for the extrema-slopes hypothesis may be useful of itself if it provides a unifying perspective for a large variety of EEG patterns, if it gives rise to new and useful methods of analyzing EEGs, and if it engenders "design specifications" that are relevant to the anatomy and physiology of EEG-generating mechanisms. After the experimental results are examined and considered (chapters 4–10), and some anatomical, physiological, and pathophysiological aspects of the EEG are considered (chapters 11–13) together with some previous models of the EEG (chapters 14 and 15), the extrema-slopes hypothesis will be appraised (chapters 16–18) in relation to these several perspectives.

4 Simulation of EEG Patterns

In chapter 2, possible EEG counterparts of the four types of waves were suggested. These were principally as follows.

• for Type 1 waves (constant-slope waves, for which amplitude is proportional to duration or inversely proportional to frequency): non-REM sleep (i.e., stages 1–4) and abnormal random or polymorphic (delta) slowing

• for Type 2 waves (of constant amplitude but variable slope and frequency): certain epileptiform patterns, in particular the 3-Hz spike-wave pattern

• for Type 3 waves (of constant frequency but variable amplitude): rhythmic patterns, such as alpha activity

• for Type 4 waves (of independently variable amplitude, frequency, and slope): the waking "desynchronized" EEG and the EEG of REM sleep.

From inspection of the top trace of figure 2.5, a resemblance between Type 1 (constant slope) waves, on the one hand, and at least stages 3 and 4 of non-REM sleep and random pathological slowing, on the other hand (see, for example, traces E and F of figure 6.1, for which the slower waves are generally of higher amplitude) seems evident. Similarly, a resemblance between constant-frequency Type 3 waves, on the one hand, and alpha activity (e.g., figures 5.2 and 5.3) and sleep spindles (e.g., figure B.4), on the other, would appear to be apparent. Further, there appears to be at least some superficial resemblance between the irregular pattern of Type 4 waves and the irregular pattern of the waking "desynchronized" EEG (e.g., figure 9.5). A parallel between Type 2 waves and epileptiform patterns is, however, perhaps not immediately evident. This chapter will therefore focus particularly on epileptiform patterns, but also on certain normal-variant patterns that have some features not entirely unlike those of epileptiform patterns. In addition, certain other features of particular types of waves will be included, as well as special modifications of the waves to simulate (e.g.) EEG waves that are asymmetrical about the baseline (such as the mu rhythm, a normal arcuate-shaped rhythm seen in the EEG overlying the motor areas of the cerebral cortex). Other normal variant patterns will also be simulated.

For simplicity and clarity, only the basic waveforms in each case will be illustrated; such refinements as spindling and wave-to-wave variability will

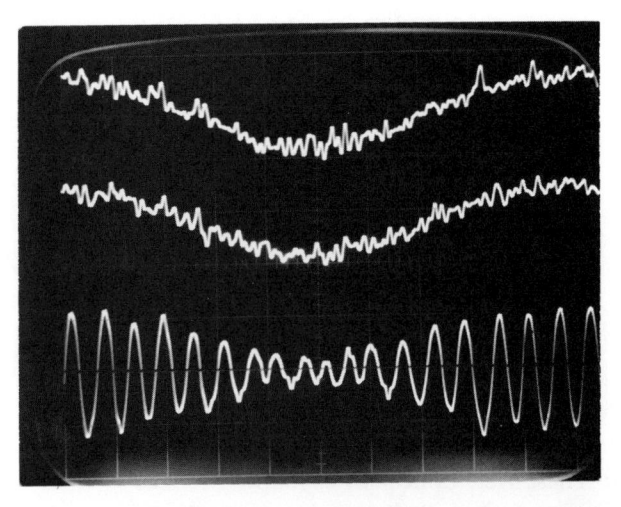

Figure 4.1 The addition of some independent noise to the modulations for extrema (trace l) and for slopes (trace 2) results in the simulation of slightly irregular rhythmic activity (trace 3), which is most evident at the lowest amplitude of the rhythmic activity.

not be included. In most cases, the resemblance between the simulation patterns and the real ones is not very close; rather, the examples illustrate the principles by which the operating parameters of the oscillator model can be altered to produce the general features that characterize actual EEG patterns.

SIMULATED RHYTHMIC ACTIVITY—SPECIAL FEATURES

As was discussed in chapter 2, Type 3 waves from the oscillator modulator, which are of constant frequency, result when the modulations of extrema and of slopes are identical. Figures 4.1–4.4 illustrate some effects of small differences in the two modulations of different types.

The rhythmic waves (Type 3) that are illustrated in the third trace of figure 2.5 are very smooth in their contour—a feature that is rarely seen in actual EEGs, in which at least some small irregularities are evident. In figure 4.1, the addition of some non-identical noise of relatively high frequency (which perhaps can be compared with "synaptic noise") to each of the identical sine waves used to modulate the extremes (trace 1) and the slopes (trace 2) results in a somewhat irregular rhythm (trace 3), particularly at low amplitudes.

Small amplitude differences between the modulation for extrema and the modulation for slopes, illustrated in figure 4.2, give rise to differences in the frequency of waves during the minimum of a spindle as compared with those at the maximum of a spindle; figure 4.3 shows predicted scatter diagrams for this effect for actual EEGs. (Evidence for just such an effect for the alpha rhythm in a series of EEGs is presented in chapter 5.)

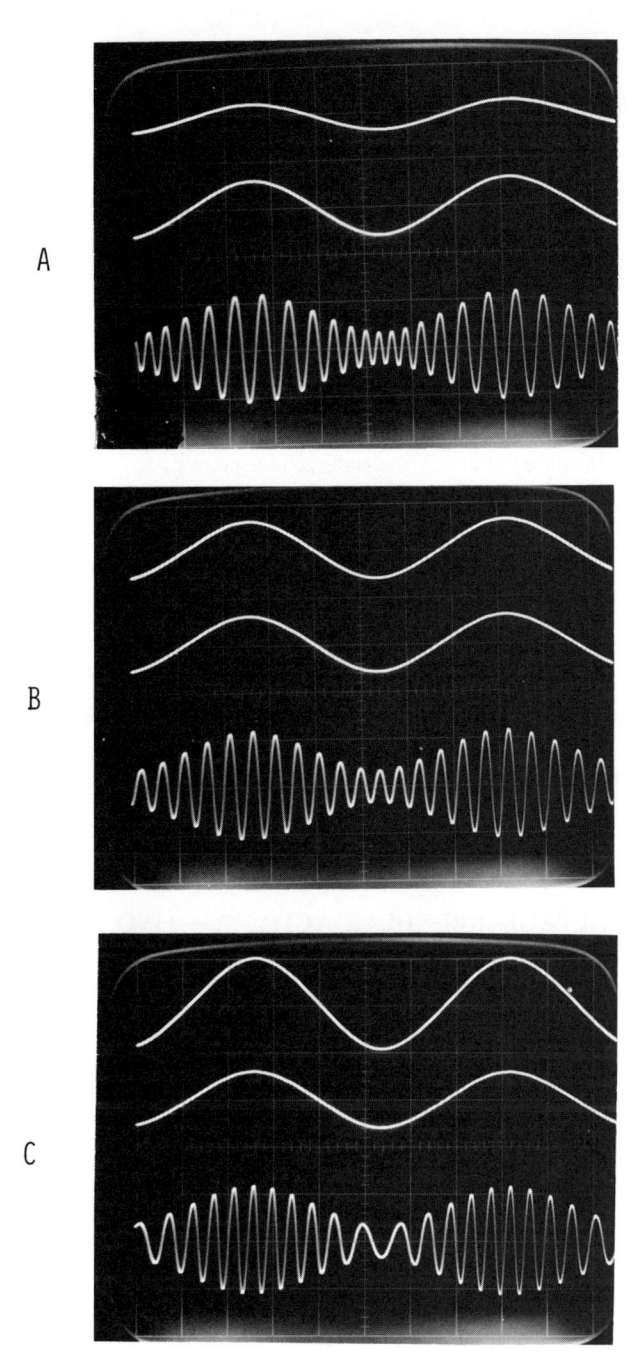

Figure 4.2 Effect of small differences in amplitude between the modulations for extrema (second trace in each instance) and for slopes (first trace in each instance). The control is shown in B, for which the two modulations are identical; waxing and waning spindles of constant-frequency waves result. In A, a small decrease in the amplitude of the slopes modulation (first trace) (the extrema modulation—second trace—remaining unchanged) results in waves of slightly lower frequency during the maximum of a spindle, and in waves of slightly higher frequency during the minimum of a spindle. In C, the reverse effect is apparent: a small increase in the amplitude of the slopes modulation (top trace) results in waves of slightly higher frequency during the maximum of a spindle, and in waves of slightly lower frequency during the minimum of a spindle.

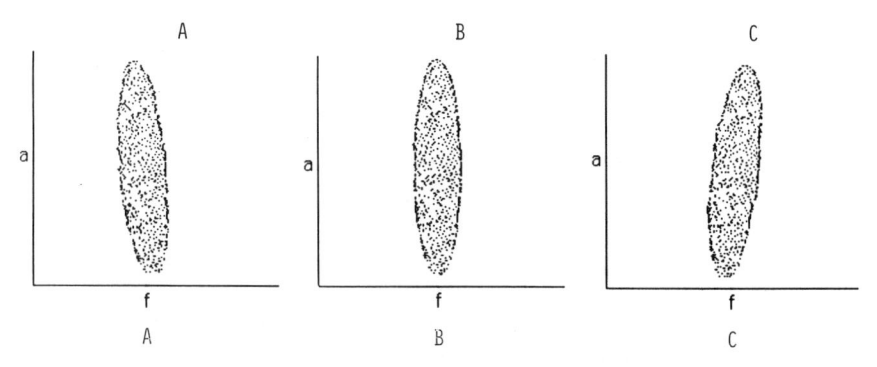

Figure 4.3 Schema for scatter diagrams for the amplitude-frequency relationship of individual waves of spindles of EEG alpha activity predicted on the basis of the simulated results shown in figure 4.2. The three scatter diagrams correspond respectively to parts A, B, and C of figure 4.2.

The effect of a small phase difference between the modulations for extrema and for slopes is illustrated in figure 4.4. Advancing the phase of the extrema modulation and delaying the phase of the slopes modulation (figure 4.4A) results in a pattern in which there is a slight slowing of the rhythm during the rising or waxing phase of individual spindles and a slight acceleration of the rhythm during the falling or waning phase of individual spindles. On the other hand, if the two phase-shifted input modulations are reversed (figure 4.4B), there is an acceleration of the rhythm during the waxing phase of the spindles and a slowing during the waning phase. Such variations of frequency are occasionally encountered in spindles of normal alpha activity.

LOW-VOLTAGE IRREGULAR ACTIVITY—TWO MODELS

It is evident from figure 2.5 that Type 1 (constant-slope) and Type 4 (irregular) waves are variable both in amplitude and in frequency. In contrast, Type 2 (constant-amplitude) waves are variable only in frequency, and Type 3 (constant-frequency) waves are variable only in amplitude. There are two possibilities, then, for models of low-voltage irregular EEG patterns, i.e., Type 1 and Type 4 waves. These are illustrated in figure 4.5, where the low-voltage pattern made up of Type 4 waves appears to be more irregular than that made up of Type 1 waves.

In actual EEGs, low-voltage irregular patterns can occur in at least two conditions: during alertness in the "desynchronized" EEG, and during Stage 1 sleep (i.e., drowsiness) (compare traces A and C in figure 6.1). In chapter 2 it was suggested that Type 4 waves could be a model for the "desynchronized" EEG (simulated in figure 4.5B), and that Type 1 waves could be a model for the EEG in drowsiness (simulated in figure 4.5A). These predictions are tested in chapters 5 and 6, respectively.

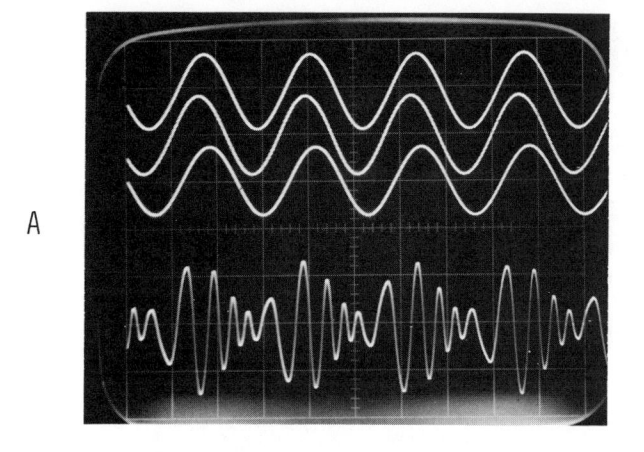

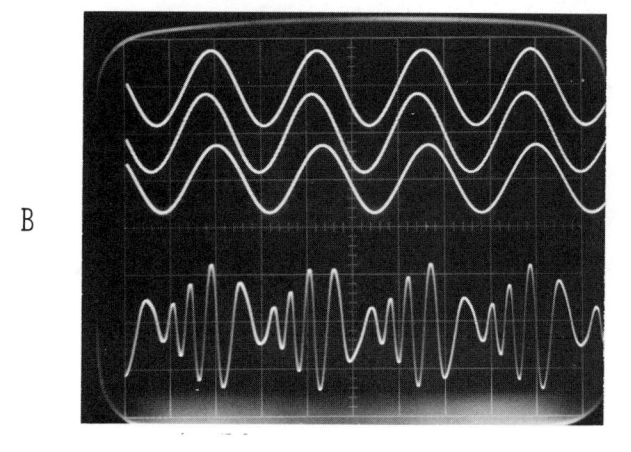

Figure 4.4 Effect on simulated rhythmic activity of relative phase shifts between the extrema-modulation signal and the slopes-modulation signal. Of the three traces at the top in part A, the first is to indicate a reference phase with respect to which the extrema modulation (second trace) is advanced, and the slopes modulation (third trace) is delayed in phase. As a result, the frequency of the waves during the rising phase of the spindles is somewhat decreased, whereas during the falling phase the frequency is somewhat increased. For the results shown in part B, the two input modulating signals to the oscillator model were interchanged (i.e., the second of the three traces as slopes modulation and the third as extrema modulation), with the result that the frequency is somewhat lower during the falling phase (instead of during the rising phase) and is somewhat higher during the rising phase (instead of during the falling phase).

Simulation of EEG Patterns

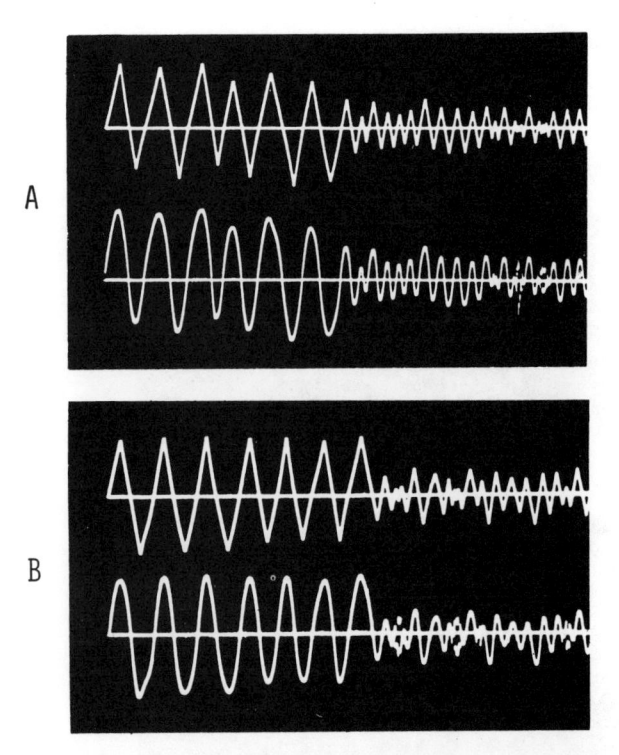

Figure 4.5 Simulated low-voltage activity (following an interval of quasi-rhythmic activity) for Type 1 (constant-slope) waves (A) and for Type 4 (irregular) waves (B). The triangular form is included as the top trace of each, to distinguish the two (note that all triangular waves in part A have the same slope, whereas the slopes of the triangular waves in part B are variable). Although the two types of waves are rather similar at higher amplitudes, the Type 4 waves appear to be more irregular at lower amplitudes. (There are some minor imperfections in the smoothed versions.)

INTERMITTENT PATTERNS

In certain types of EEG patterns, the voltage of the EEG falls to relatively low levels for varying periods of time. In preliminary work, it was found that such discontinuous EEG patterns could be simulated if the extrema modulation fluctuated not around some positive value but around zero, the negative swings being clipped or eliminated (figure 4.6). The EEG counterparts include the severely abnormal "suppression-burst" (or "burst-suppression") pattern of children and adults (figure 4.7) and the normal *tracé discontinu* or discontinuous pattern of the early premature infant (Lombroso 1987; Hrachovy et al. 1990). (It was from such a simulation, as illustrated in figure 4.6, that the idea originated for the development of the system whereby an EEG could be reconstituted by using its instantaneous envelope and the instantaneous envelope of its first derivative as the extremes-modulation input and the slopes-modulation input of the oscillator model, providing the basis of the third method of testing the extrema-slopes hypothesis, as described in chapter 3.)

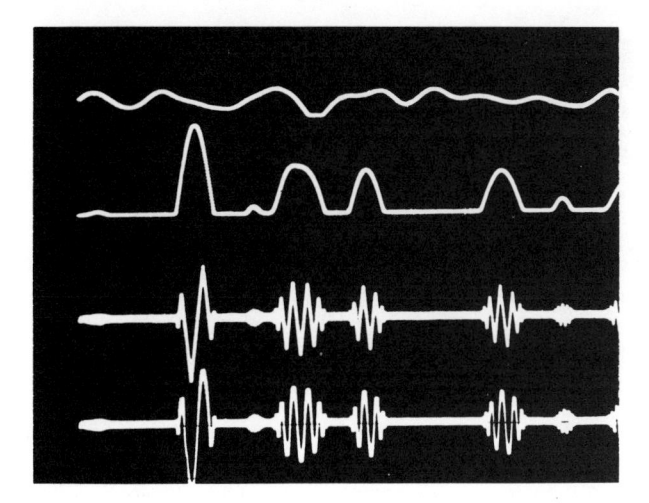

Figure 4.6 Approach to simulating intermittent or suppression-burst EEG patterns (illustrated in figure 4.7) by using an extrema-modulation waveform (trace 2) whose maximal negative swing corresponds to zero extrema modulation. Note that the extrema modulation signal is just the envelope of the output of the oscillator model (trace 3 for the triangular version and trace 4 for the smoothed version). The low-amplitude slopes modulation (trace 1) has relatively little effect in this instance.

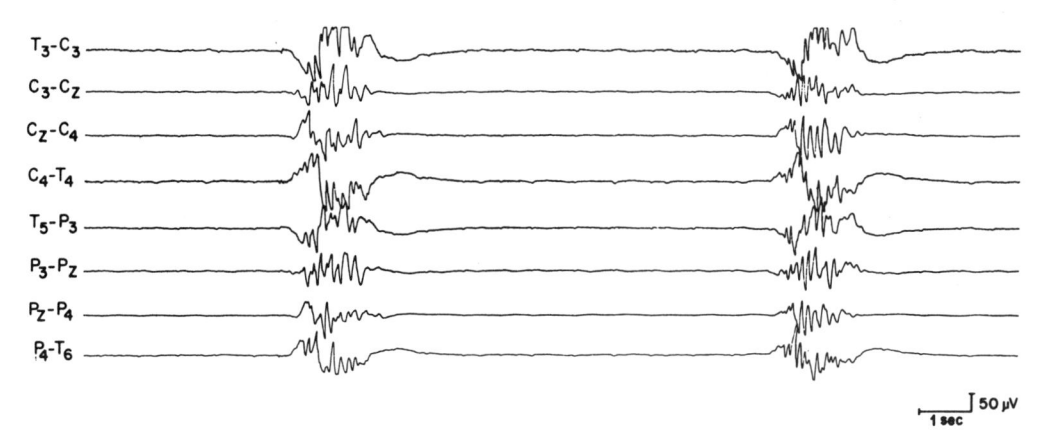

Figure 4.7 Suppression-burst EEG pattern. (Electrode placements for this and subsequent EEGs are shown in figure C.1.) (From Vas and Cracco 1990.)

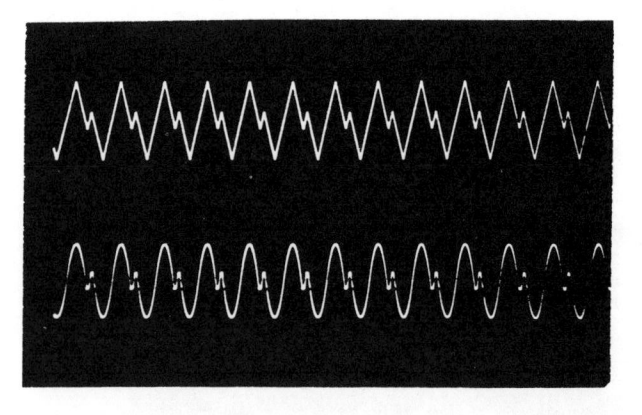

Figure 4.8 The effect of brief reversal of the slopes modulation is to introduce a notch; the resulting waveform has some resemblance to the normal-variant pattern of rhythmic temporal theta bursts of drowsiness (psychomotor variant pattern) (figure 4.9). Note that the brief reversals will result in a small increase in the duration of the waves and, correspondingly, a slight decrease in their frequency.

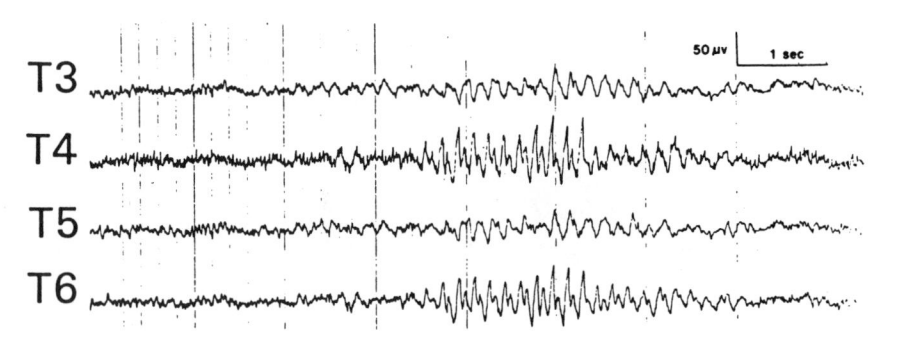

Figure 4.9 EEG pattern of rhythmic temporal theta bursts of drowsiness. (From Santamaria and Chiappa 1987.)

BRIEF SLOPE REVERSAL

If the slopes modulation in Type 3 (constant-frequency) waves is briefly reversed in the vicinity of the baseline, as illustrated in figure 4.8, a notched waveform appears. This waveform has some resemblance to the normal-variant pattern termed "rhythmic temporal theta bursts (of 5–7-Hz waves) of drowsiness" (figure 4.9) (Westmoreland 1990), sometimes known by its earlier name: the "psychomotor variant" pattern.

EEG PATTERN SIMULATION WITH BASELINE OFFSETS AND PERIOD ALTERNATIONS

In the description of the oscillator model in chapter 2, it was pointed out that the basic triangular waves were smoothed by means of fitting a parabola to three points on the positive half-wave of each triangular wave (the apex and

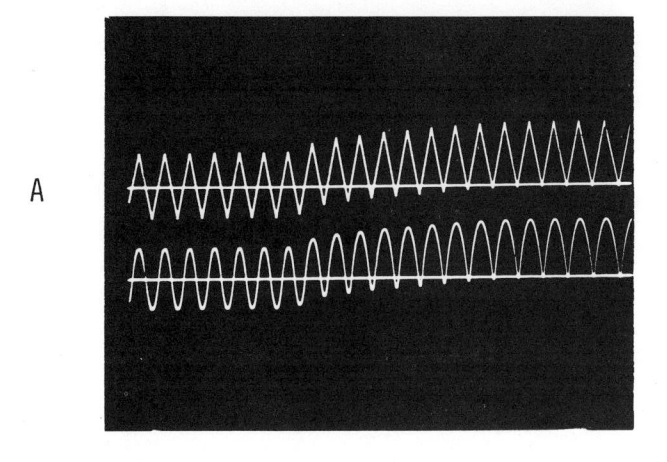

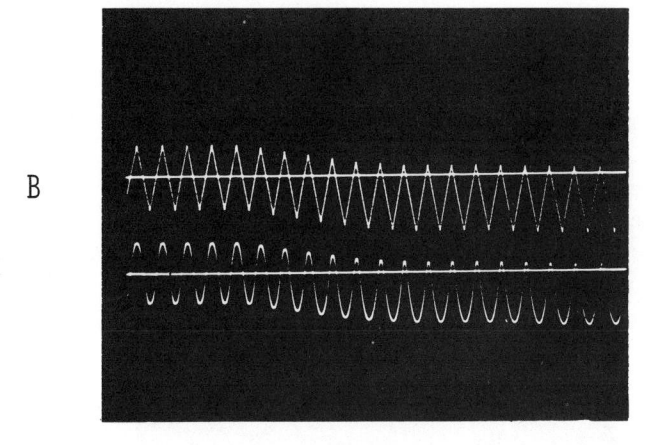

Figure 4.10 Effect of a DC offset (baseline shift) on the smoothing process. As the DC (baseline) level of the triangular wave is shifted upward (A) or downward (B), the parabola-fitting process continues until only positive or negative parabolas, respectively, are evident. The resulting waveforms have a resemblance to that of the EEG mu rhythm (figure 4.11).

the two baseline intercepts), and similarly for the negative half-wave of the triangular wave. The two parabolas (to which a further fourth-order or quartic correction was subsequently added) were continuous across the baseline. It had not originally been anticipated, but it soon became apparent, that such smoothing was equally effective if the triangular wave had a DC offset. This effect is apparent in parts A and B of figure 4.10. The resulting asymmetrical waveform (lower traces) is rather similar to the EEG mu rhythm (figure 4.11) (so called because of its resemblance to the Greek letter μ), a normal pattern that appears in recordings from electrodes overlying the motor cortex and is suppressed by movement of an opposite extremity (Niedermeyer 1987a; Kellaway 1990). It is a rhythm that is independent of the (posterior) alpha rhythm although of much the same frequency range. Such an asymmetrical waveform serves as the basis of simulation of additional EEG patterns, as is evident from figures 4.12–4.20.

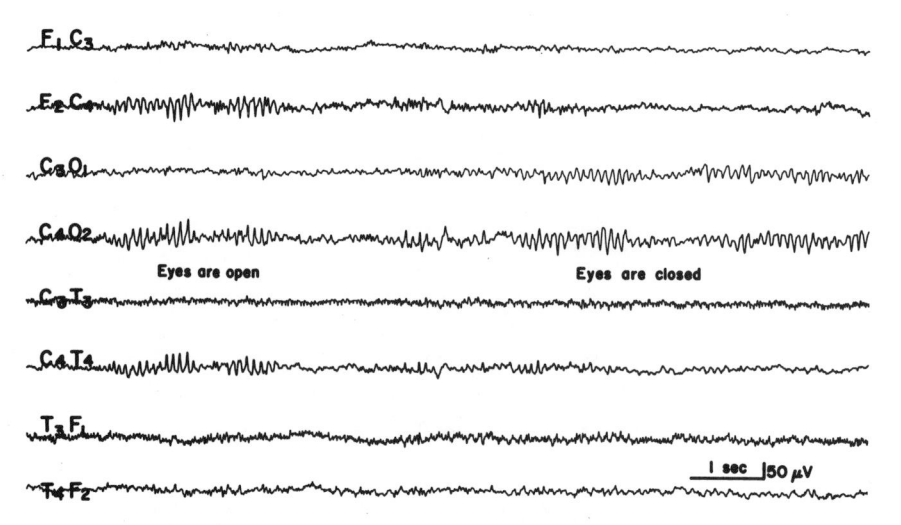

Figure 4.11 Mu rhythm appearing at C4 with eyes open. (From Kellaway 1990.)

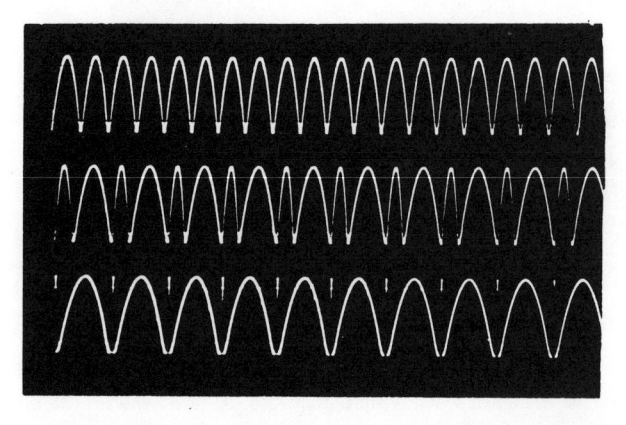

Figure 4.12 Effect of DC or baseline offset alone (trace 1, same as figure 4.10A) and in combination with an alternation of the duration of the successive cycles (trace 2 and trace 3). Trace 2 and trace 3 have some resemblance to the 14- and 6-Hz positive spikes pattern (figure 14.3) and the 6-Hz spike-wave EEG patterns, respectively.

In trace 1 of figure 4.12 the basic effect of an upward shift is shown again, and traces 2 and 3 indicates the effect of alternation of the durations of successive cycles of the asymmetrical waves in such a way that the mean duration in each case remains the same. The second trace, when inverted, has some resemblance to the "14- and 6-Hz positive bursts" (figure 4.13) (note that the mean frequency remains at 10 Hz), sometimes known by the earlier term "14- and 6-Hz positive spikes." In the third trace of figure 4.12 the difference between the durations of successive waves is even greater, and the resultant pattern has some resemblance to the "6-Hz spike-and-wave" pattern or "phantom spike-wave" pattern (figure 4.14). Both this and the 14- and 6-Hz positive burst pattern have been considered as normal

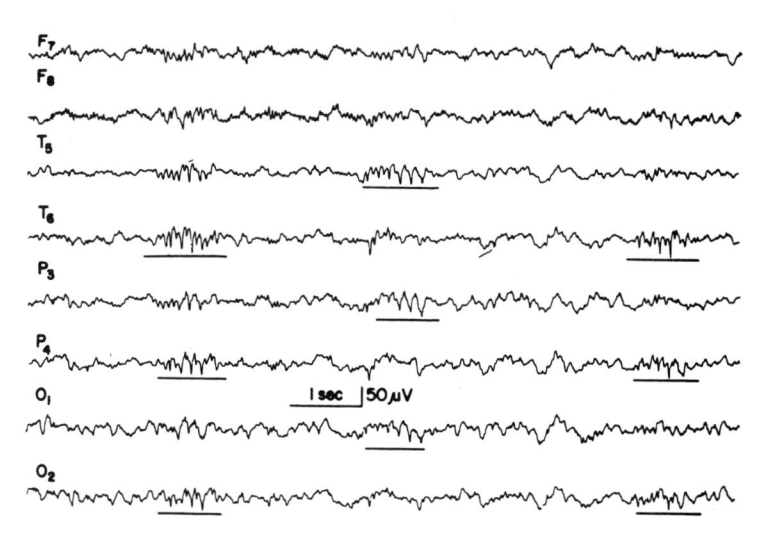

Figure 4.13 Examples of 14- and 6-Hz positive spikes (underlined). (From Niedermeyer 1987c.)

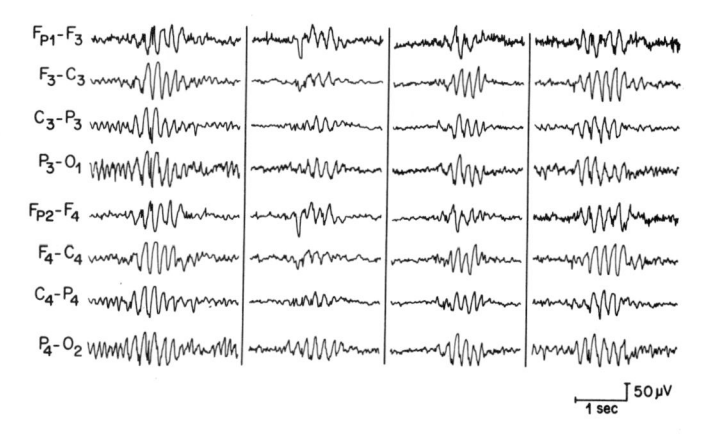

Figure 4.14 Six-Hz spike-and-wave pattern. (From Westmoreland 1990.)

variant or benign patterns with an "epileptiform morphology" (Westmoreland 1990).

A further modification arises if the slopes are kept constant and the positive extrema and negative extrema are shifted by different amounts, as is illustrated in figure 4.15A. For the upper trace in that figure, the modulation of the extrema was simultaneously increased and shifted upward, resulting in an increase in the duration of these constant-slope waves. With the alternation of the duration of successive waves (figure 4.15B) and of the duration of successive half-waves (figure 4.15C), alternating the modulation of slopes produces spike-wave patterns that have some resemblance to the classical 3-Hz spike-wave pattern of primary generalized epilepsy of the absence type (figure 4.16) and to the slow spike-wave pattern of the Lennox-Gastaut syndrome (figure 4.17). In relation to the DC shift apparent in figures 4.15A and 4.15B, it is of particular interest to note that, when the 3-Hz spike-wave pattern is recorded

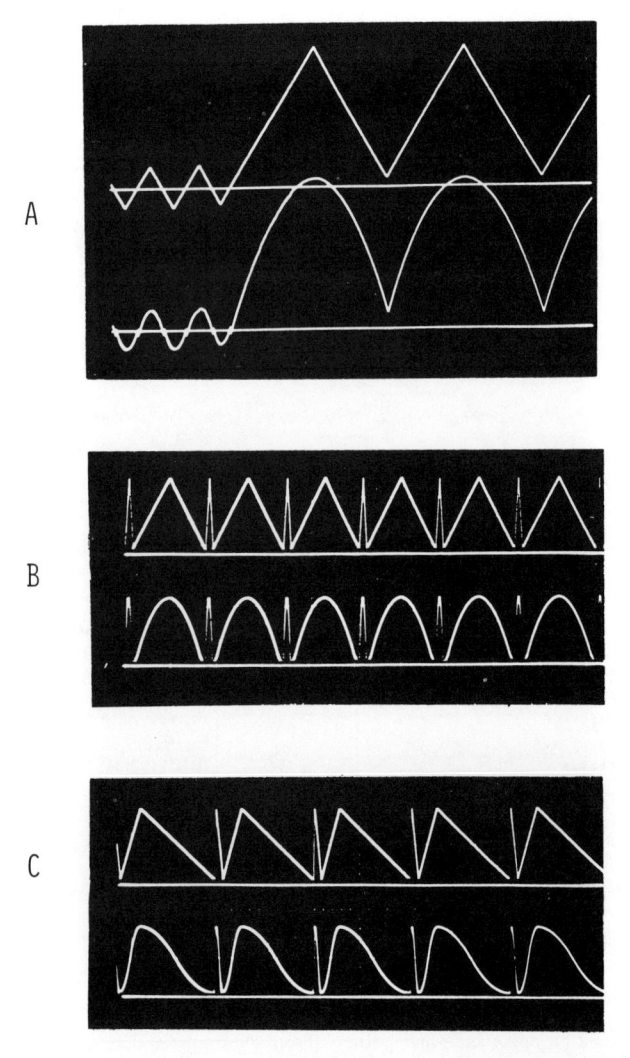

Figure 4.15 Simulating spike-wave patterns with symmetrical (B) and asymmetrical (C) wave components by diverging upward shifts of the positive and negative extrema (A) and alternating the duration of successive cycles (B, C). (Note that part A is on different time and amplitude scales than parts B and C.) The lower trace in part C has some resemblance to the classical 3-Hz spike-wave pattern (figure 4.16), including its characteristic DC shift when recorded with DC amplifiers. The lower trace in part C has some resemblance to the slow spike-wave pattern of the Lennox-Gastaut syndrome (figure 4.17).

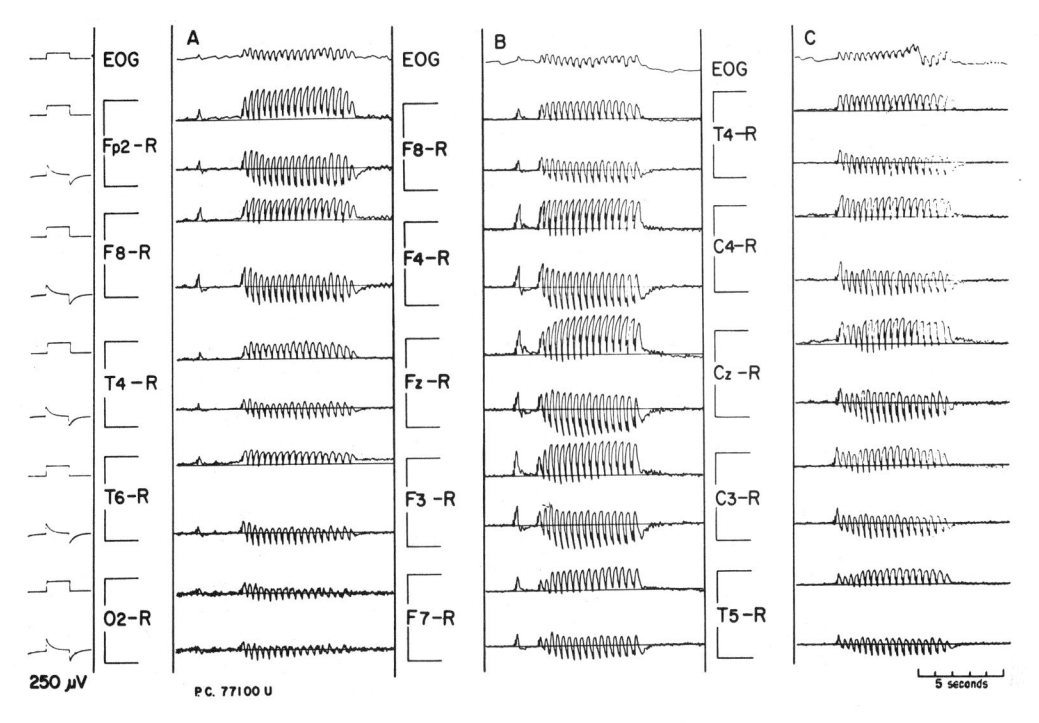

Figure 4.16 Three examples of 3-Hz spike-and-wave patterns in one patient. Alternate EEG channels were recorded with DC and AC amplifiers. (From Chatrian et al. 1968.)

with DC amplifiers instead of the usual AC-coupled amplifiers (alternate traces in figure 4.16) used in clinical electroencephalography, a baseline or DC shift is observed during the spike-wave events. (DC shifts in epilepsy are considered in chapter 13.)

A different kind of modification results if the slopes are kept constant and the positive and negative extrema are shifted by different amounts so as to narrow the distance between the two, as is illustrated in figure 4.18. For the upper trace, the modulation of the extrema was simultaneously decreased and shifted downward, resulting in a decrease in the duration of these constant-slope waves. The resultant waveform (upper trace) has some resemblance to the electrodecremental EEG pattern (figure 4.19) that may be seen in tonic seizures or infantile spasms (Bickford and Klass 1963; Kellaway et al. 1979; Chatrian et al. 1982) and also in some partial seizures (Blume et al. 1984), although the asymmetrical waveshape that results after smoothing (figure 4.18A, lower trace) is not a part of the electrodecremental pattern. (The asymmetry is, of course, not present if there is no downward DC shift of the triangular waves concurrent with their decreasing amplitude.)

THE SPIKE-AND-SLOW-WAVE COMPLEX

In the simulation of the repetitive 3-Hz spike-wave pattern (figure 4.15B, second trace), the amplitude (or, more exactly, the envelope of the amplitude)

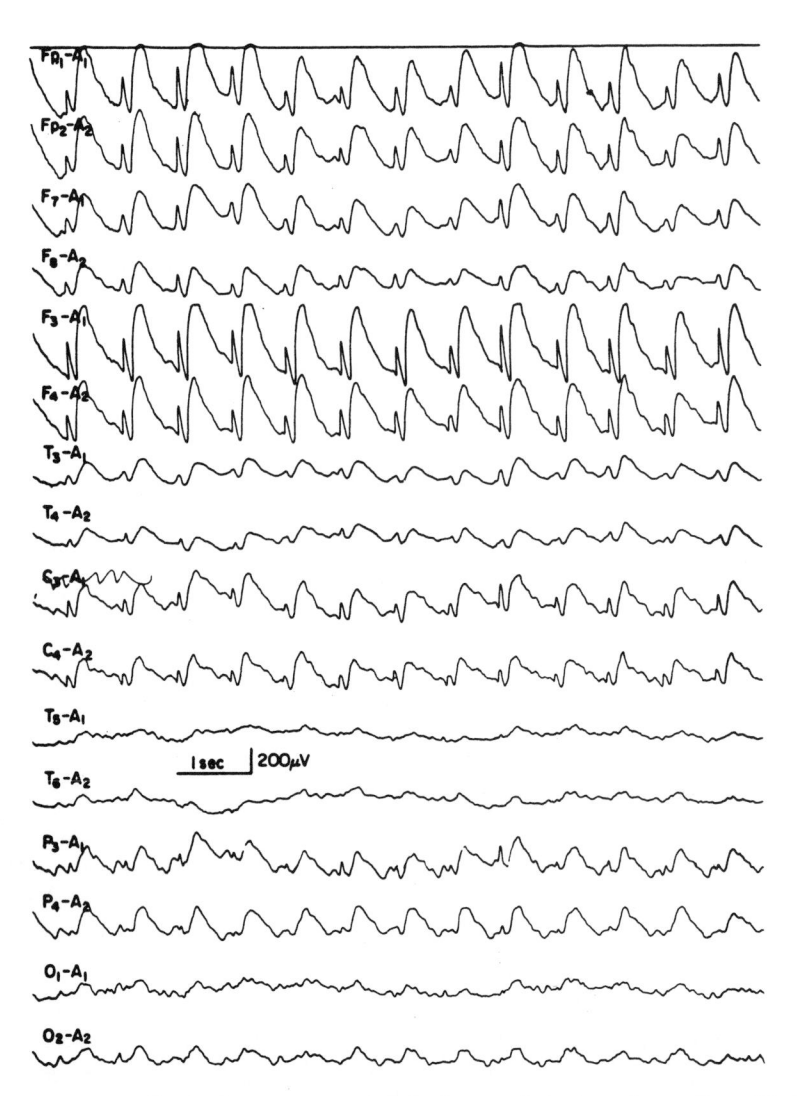

Figure 4.17 Slow spike-wave pattern of the Lennox-Gastaut syndrome. (From Niedermeyer 1987e.)

was assumed to be the same for the spike and for the wave components. However, in the non-repetitive spike-and-slow-wave complex (which is an interictal rather than an ictal or electrical seizure pattern) the slow-wave component is often of smaller amplitude than the spike component, and hence Type 2 (constant-amplitude) waves cannot serve as a model for this type of epileptiform activity. It then became a question of possible simulation of this pattern with Type 4 waves (i.e., waves of independently variable amplitude and slope). With a trial-and-error approach, an appropriate pair of modulating waveforms was found for the oscillator model, consisting of an exponentially decrementing curve (figure 4.20A, trace 1) for the slopes modulation and a rising and falling curve (figure 4.20A, trace 2) for the extrema modulation. (The former curve was obtained as the discharge of a condenser through a

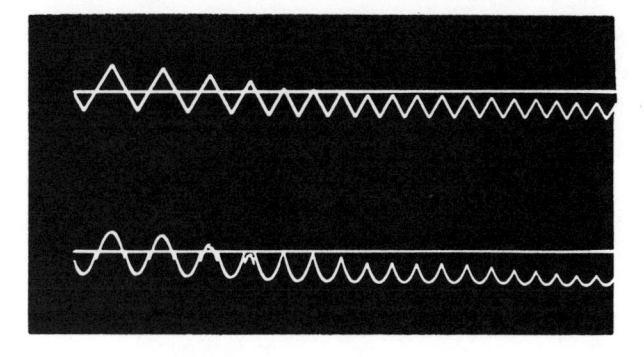

Figure 4.18 (A) Waves generated by converging downward shifts of the positive and negative extrema in waves having constant slope. (Contrast with figure 4.15A.) The resultant decrease in amplitude and increase in frequency bears some resemblance to the low-voltage fast discharge or electrodecremental pattern of onset of some seizures (figure 4.19), although the asymmetrical waveform of the bottom trace is not a characteristic of this EEG pattern.

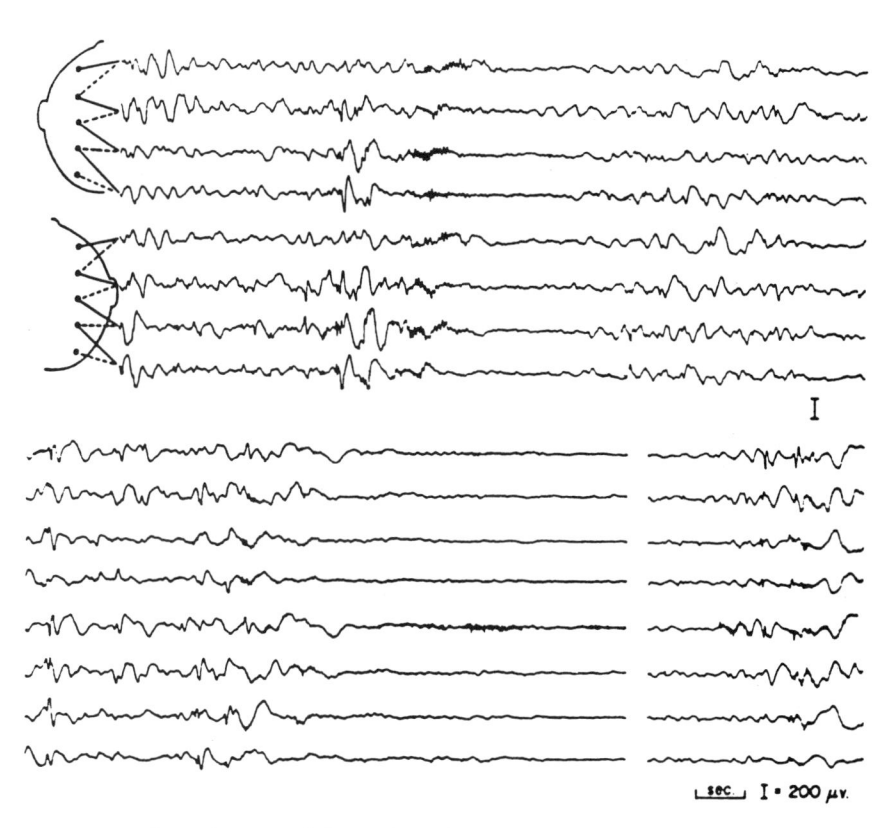

Figure 4.19 Electrodecremental (low-voltage fast) episodes in an EEG. (From Bickford and Klass 1963.)

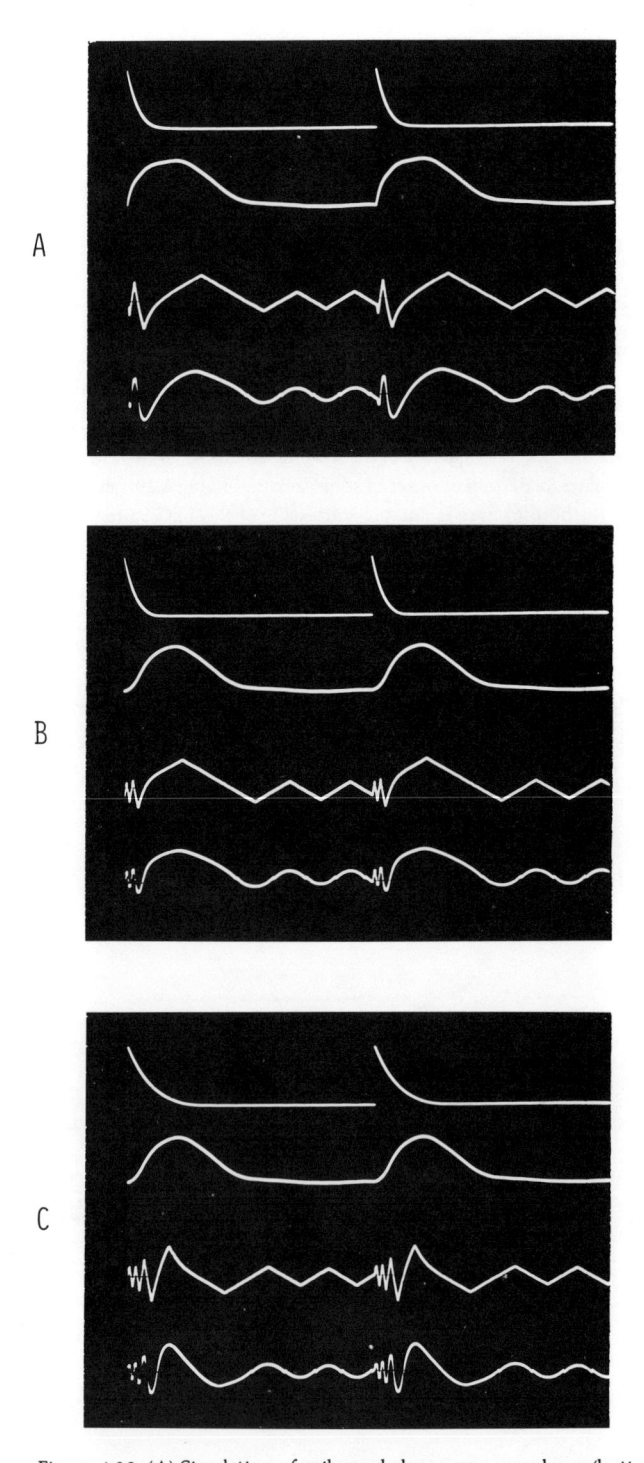

Figure 4.20 (A) Simulation of spike-and-slow-wave complexes (bottom traces) by paired modulation of the slopes of the waves of the oscillator model with a decaying exponential (top traces), and modulation of the extrema with a rising-and-falling curve (second traces). The transient portions of the two modulating waveforms are each superimposed on quiescent levels of modulation that result in a rhythmic background; note the two cycles of a triangular wave (third traces) and the corresponding sine wave (fourth traces) after smoothing. In parts B and C,

48 Chapter 4

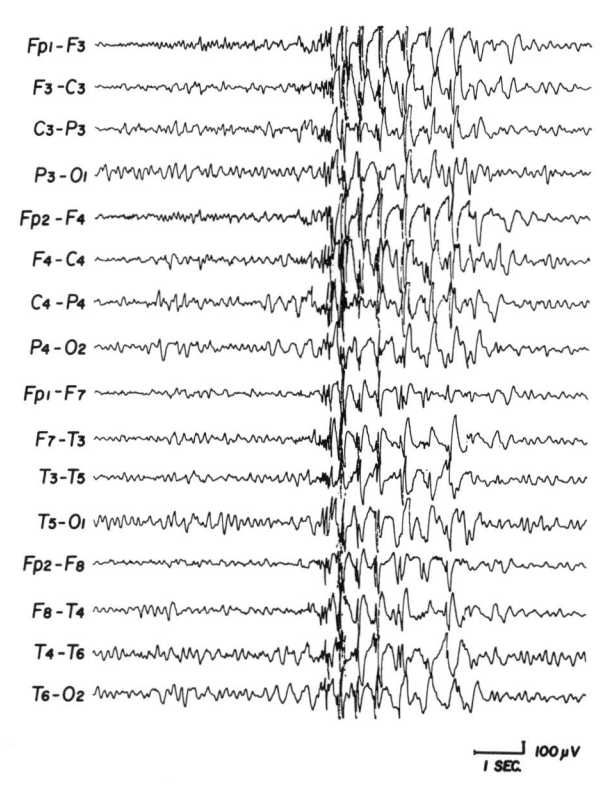

Figure 4.21 Multiple spike-and-slow-wave complexes. (From Daly 1990.)

resistor; the latter curve was formed by means of a specially designed, manually adjusted arbitrary function generator based on a transversal filter, described in chapter 23. The resultant simulated spike-and-slow-wave complexes are shown in figure 4.20A, trace 4.) By increasing the time constant of the decaying exponential (figures 4.20A–C, trace 1) a single spike, two spikes, or three spikes (trace 4 of figures 4.20A, B, and C, respectively) could be obtained. Further, by altering the rise time of the extrema modulation (compare trace 2 in figures 4.20A and 4.20B), the height of the spikes could be varied. Such multiple or polyspike slow-wave complexes are a familiar pattern in the EEGs of epileptics (figure 4.21).

COMMENT

From the preceding figures it is apparent that several rather different normal and abnormal EEG patterns can be simulated approximately by means of

---

the duration of the decaying exponential is progressively increased as compared with part A, resulting in two and in three spikes, respectively. Also, in parts B and C, the rise time of the extrema modulation (second traces) is increased, resulting in lower-amplitude spikes than in part A. The resulting traces have some resemblance to the EEG pattern of multiple-spike-and-slow-wave complexes (figure 14.21).

Simulation of EEG Patterns

appropriate modulation of the extrema and the slopes of the waves of the oscillator model, in one or another of its four modes (i.e., with one or another of its four basic types of waves). To be sure, the selection of EEG patterns that has been simulated is a rather limited one, and the simulations themselves are rather simplified, Nonetheless, in relation to the first of the three major approaches to testing the extrema-slope hypothesis of the EEG as described in chapter 2, it seems evident from the examples given that the oscillator model has a relatively broad capability of simulating EEG patterns beyond the particular ones illustrated, given appropriately chosen input modulation signals (derived from standard laboratory signal-generating equipment, i.e., oscillators or function generators, and electronic noise sources). In brief, the simulation approach appears to offer some corroboration for the extrema-slopes hypothesis of the EEG.

Despite this corroborative evidence, a serious limitation to the simulation approach to testing the extrema-slopes hypothesis is that of evaluating the degree of similarity between actual EEG patterns and the versions simulated with the oscillator model. In the first instance, the evaluation is a visual one. In principle, simulated and actual EEGs could be tested for similar or even identical statistical properties—for example, by comparison of spectra or autocorrelation functions, or by autoregressive modeling. (See chapter 17.)

A solution to this problem is found in the third approach to testing the extrema-slope hypothesis—namely, the approach of reconstituting EEGs with the aid of the oscillator model, using information on extrema and slopes derived from the EEGs themselves (chapter 9). This approach can test the extrema-slopes hypothesis more thoroughly and critically than the simulation approach. Before the latter approach is considered, however, the second approach to testing the hypothesis (the testing of specific predictions about EEG patterns, based on the extrema-slopes hypothesis) will be taken up in the following chapters.

II Tests of Predictions from the Hypothesis for Normal and Abnormal EEGs

5 The Waking EEG

ALPHA ACTIVITY

In chapter 2 it was suggested that Type 3 waves of the oscillator model—i.e., waves of congruently modulated extrema and slopes, with resultant relatively constant frequency—could be a model for rhythmic (quasi-sinusoidal) EEG activity. Instances of such activity would include alpha activity, slow posterior rhythm (i.e., below the alpha frequency range in adults), rhythmic theta activity of drowsiness (in the vicinity of 4–6 Hz), sleep spindles (at about 14 Hz), and rhythmic fast activity in the range of 18–22 Hz induced pharmacologically (e.g, by barbiturates or benzodiazepines). As a representative example of rhythmic types of activity, alpha activity will be considered in some detail.

The analysis of an EEG having a prominent alpha rhythm is shown in figure 5.1, where one can see the close similarity between the running mean amplitude (trace 2) and the running mean slope (trace 3)—both of which are rather variable but virtually identical, as is to be expected for rhythmic activity. The running Coefficients of Variation for the running means of amplitude (trace 5) and slope (trace 6) are also quite similar, and reach appreciable values. The running mean frequency (trace 4) is, however, relatively constant; correspondingly, it exhibits a low running Coefficient of Variation (trace 7).

The results of the analysis of a somewhat irregular alpha-rhythm pattern are shown in figure 5.2, where, in the first eight traces, the features are much the same as in figure 5.1. In trace 9 of figure 5.2, the Spectral Purity Index is shown; note the decreases from a value near 1.0 when the EEG becomes less rhythmic. The analysis of an alpha rhythm having slightly asymmetrical waves is shown in figure 5.3, for which two additional determinations are included: a measure of the relative variabilities of the running means of the EEG's amplitude and slope (trace 1; values greater than zero indicate a relatively greater variability of the running mean amplitude) and a measure of the similarity of the running means of the EEG and of its first derivative in the form of their Coefficient of Determination (trace 11).

Figures 5.1–5.3 are illustrative of the analyses by these methods of a large number of EEG alpha patterns. The results from all these analyses have been quite similar, with very similar running means of amplitude and slope and with a relatively constant (alpha) frequency having a low Coefficient of Variation.

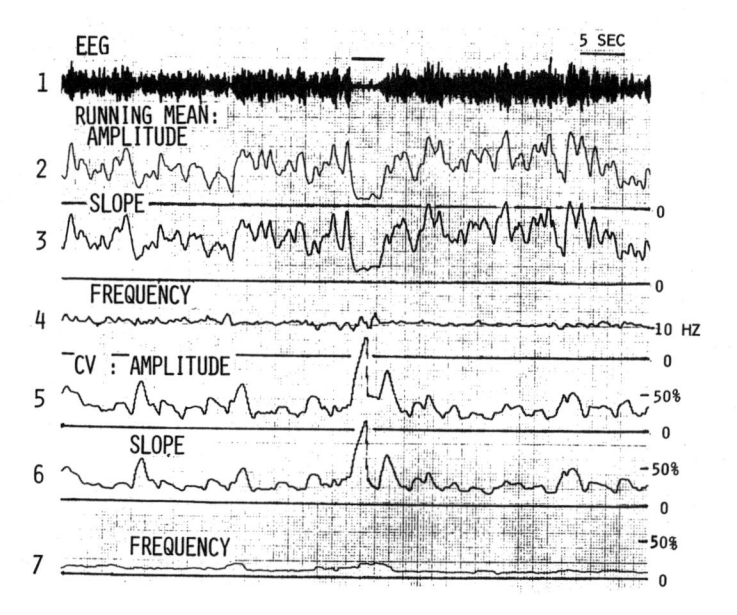

Figure 5.1 Original EEG (trace l) having a prominent alpha rhythm (with brief eye opening indicated by bar at top), running means of its amplitude, slope, and frequency, and Coefficients of Variation (CV) of the latter three parameters, respectively. Note the close resemblance of the running means of amplitude and slope for such quasi-sinusoidal activity having a rather stable frequency at about 10 Hz (note the much lower CV for the running mean frequency than for the running means of amplitude and slope, which parallel one another closely). Note also the marked transients in the CVs of amplitude and slope upon eye opening and again with eye closing. (From Barlow 1993)

These findings are consistent with the dual-modulation hypothesis with congruent modulation of amplitude and slope (i.e., Type 3 waves of the oscillator model).

Of particular interest is the result, according to the extrema-slopes hypothesis, of slight differences in the amplitudes of the two modulating signals. This effect was simulated by means of the oscillator model itself in figure 4.2, and the corresponding three predictions in the form of scatter diagrams of amplitude vs. frequency were shown in figure 4.3 (which, to facilitate comparison in the present discussion, is shown again as figure 5.4).

The prediction from the extrema-slopes hypothesis of a variation of frequency of alpha waves with amplitude was confirmed in a re-review of alpha-type EEGs in a study of EEG patterns by the methods of adaptive segmentation and probability-density-function classification (Creutzfeldt et al. 1985), as shown in figure 5.5. (The methods of adaptive segmentation and probability-density-function classification that were used in the earlier study are described more fully in chapter 17; in brief, the methods automatically sort and classify EEG patterns within a single recording according to the mean frequency and mean amplitude of the individual segments, one of the final results being in the form of a scatter diagram of amplitude (log power) vs. frequency.)

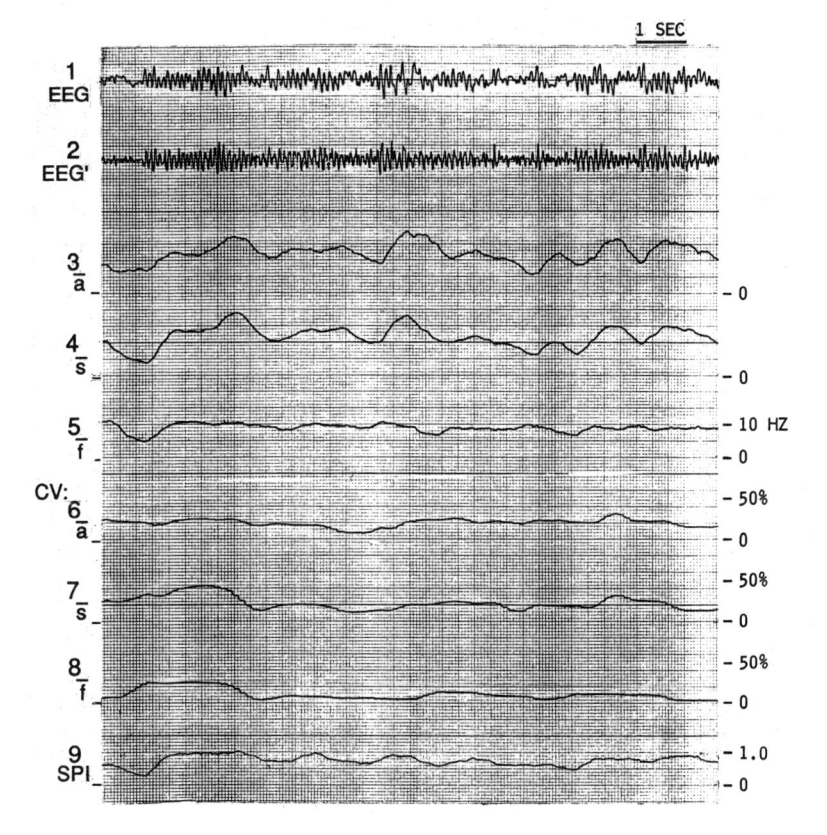

Figure 5.2 Analysis of an EEG having a slightly irregular alpha rhythm. Trace identification: (1) EEG; (2) first derivative of the EEG (EEG'); (3) and (4) running means of amplitude ($\bar{a}$) and slope ($\bar{s}$); (5) running mean frequency ($\bar{f}$); (6–8) Coefficients of Variation (CV) of running means of amplitude, slope, and frequency, respectively; (9) Spectral Purity Index (SPI). (Baselines (zero point) are indicated on both sides of this and subsequent figures.) Note the close parallel between traces 3 and 4, which is reflected in the relatively constant frequency at about 10 Hz (trace 5), except during periods of more irregular EEG activity (extreme left, and middle of trace 1). The CV for frequency is generally appreciably lower than those for amplitude and slope. The Spectral Purity Index is near 1.0 for the most rhythmic portion of the EEG (at the left), and has somewhat smaller, fluctuating values subsequently.

The characterization of EEG activity as rhythmic implies a value of the Spectral Purity Index close to 1.0. However, such a finding would not necessarily constitute specific evidence for the present hypothesis of generation of rhythmic activity as implied by Mode 3 waves of the oscillator model, since the same waveforms could be obtained by conventional amplitude modulation. Somewhat closer to the extrema-slopes model is the demonstration that the running mean amplitude of the EEG and that of its first derivative (i.e., the running mean slope) are quite similar, as is exemplified in the preceding figures; again, such a finding would not necessarily confirm the extrema-slopes hypothesis specifically, since the same similarity would result for conventional amplitude-modulated waves. Indeed, for any narrow-band process (e.g., narrow-band filtered noise), the first derivative of the signal will be quite

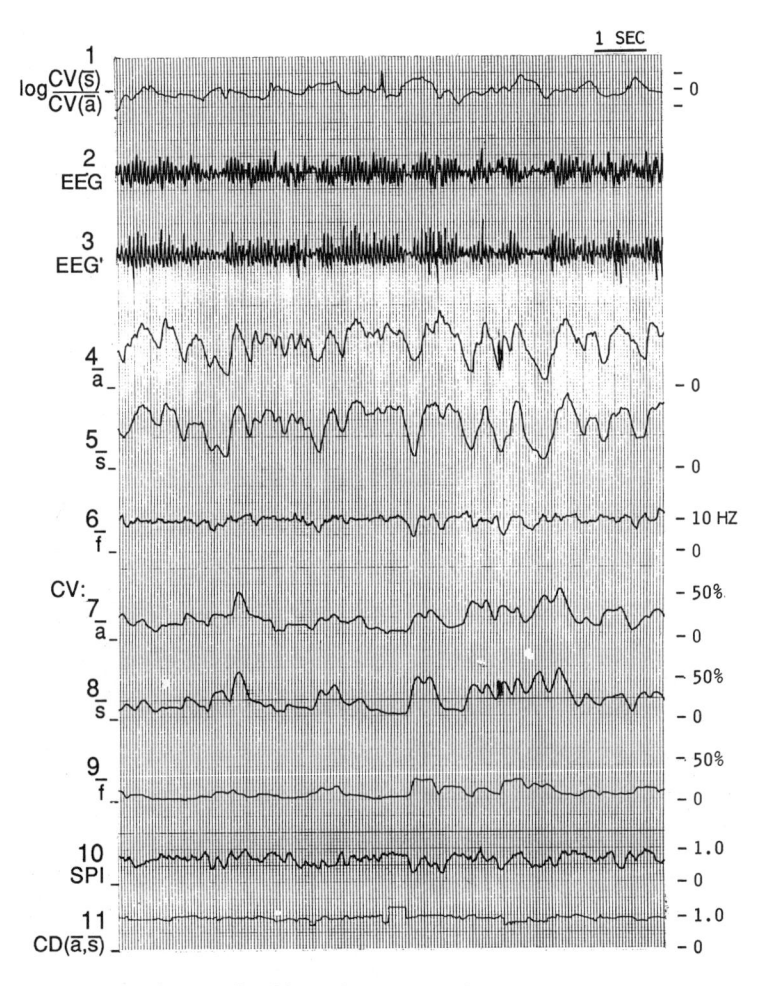

Figure 5.3 Analysis, with additional measures, of an EEG having a somewhat asymmetrical (peaked tops and rounded bottoms) alpha-rhythm pattern. Trace identification: (l) logarithm of the quotient of the Coefficients of Variation of slope and amplitude (a measure of their relative variability); (2) and (3) original EEG and its first derivative; (4–6) running means of amplitude, slope, and frequency; (7–9) Coefficients of Variation of running means of amplitude, slope, and frequency; (10) Spectral Purity Index. (The running means were computed with a shorter averaging window than in figure 5.2.) The Spectral Purity Index (trace 10) fluctuates around a value of about 0.75, reflecting the asymmetrical waves of the alpha activity. The Coefficient of Determination (trace 11) for the running means of amplitude and slope has a value of nearly 1.0, reflecting quantitatively the similarity between the running means of amplitude and slope (traces 4 and 5). The latter two are about equally variable, as reflected in an average value of about zero for the logarithm of the quotient of their Coefficients of Variation (trace 1).

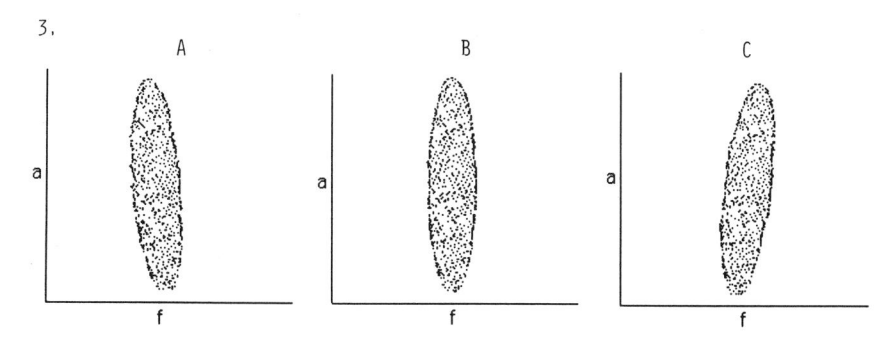

Figure 5.4 Variation of frequency with amplitude for slightly non-congruent modulation of extrema and slopes of the oscillator model (same as figure 4.3): (A) slight decrease in frequency with increasing amplitude, resulting from slopes modulation being slightly less than extremes modulation; (C) slight increase in frequency with increasing amplitude, resulting from slopes modulation being slightly greater than extremes modulation. For comparison, part B shows the case of no change of frequency with increasing amplitude (i.e., for congruent or identical modulation of extremes and slopes).

similar to the original, save for a 90° phase advance, and, correspondingly, their respective running means will be quite similar.

The low value of the running Coefficient of Variation of the running mean frequency can be viewed as confirming the hypothesis that congruent (identical waveshapes) modulation of the amplitude (extrema) and the slope of the basic oscillations of the oscillator model could indeed generate such a rhythm (i.e., strongly rhythmic EEG activity), since the method of derivation of the running mean frequency is based on the quotient of the running means of the slope and the amplitude (i.e., the method itself implies that the signal arose from a congruent modulation system). Nonetheless, such a low Coefficient of Variation for the running mean frequency (the spectral counterpart of which is a narrow spectral peak) does not of itself necessarily indicate that the rhythmic waves are due to extrema-slopes-modulation.

The confirmation of the prediction of the possibility of a slight dependence of the frequency of alpha activity on its amplitude (figures 5.4 and 5.5) offers stronger evidence for the extrema-slopes hypothesis, since such a variation could not be produced by amplitude modulation alone. (A combination of interrelated amplitude and frequency modulation would be required.)

THE "DESYNCHRONIZED" EEG

In chapter 2 it was suggested that Type 4 waves of the oscillator model (i.e., waves modulated both in extrema and in slopes, but by independent or noncongruent signals) could be a model for the irregular (or arhythmic) low-voltage or "desynchronized" EEG pattern.

Two types of EEGs were examined for this purpose: eyes-closed low-voltage irregular posterior activity from normal EEGs in which there was no posterior alpha rhythm, and posterior EEGs recorded from normal subjects during a sustained visual task such as reading. (The latter were kindly made

A

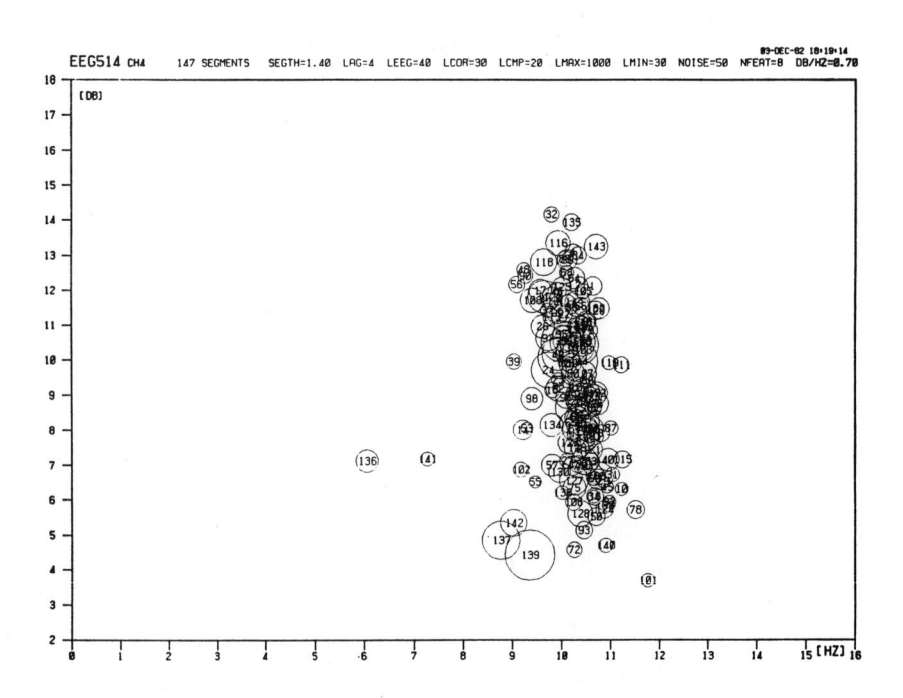

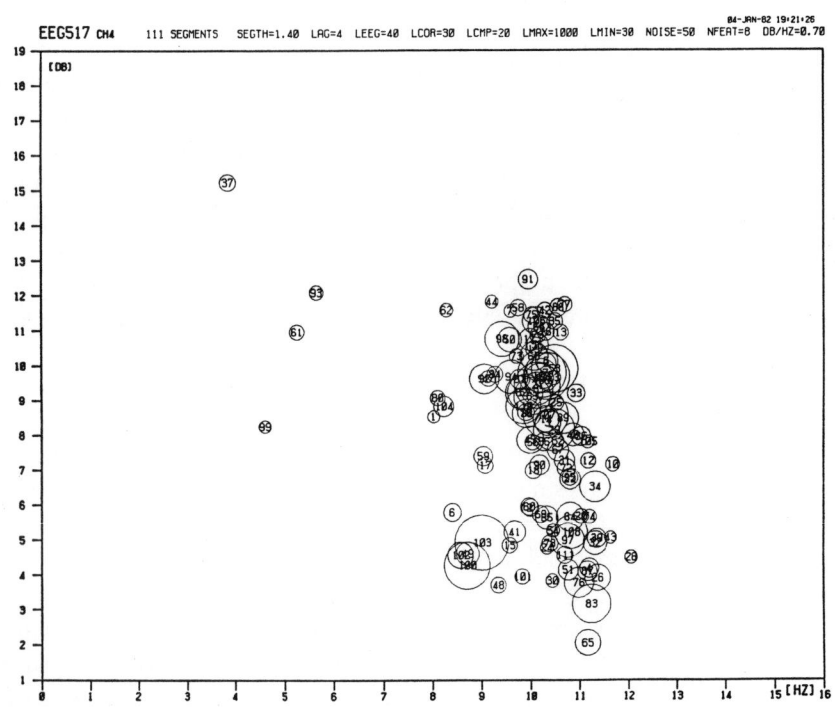

B

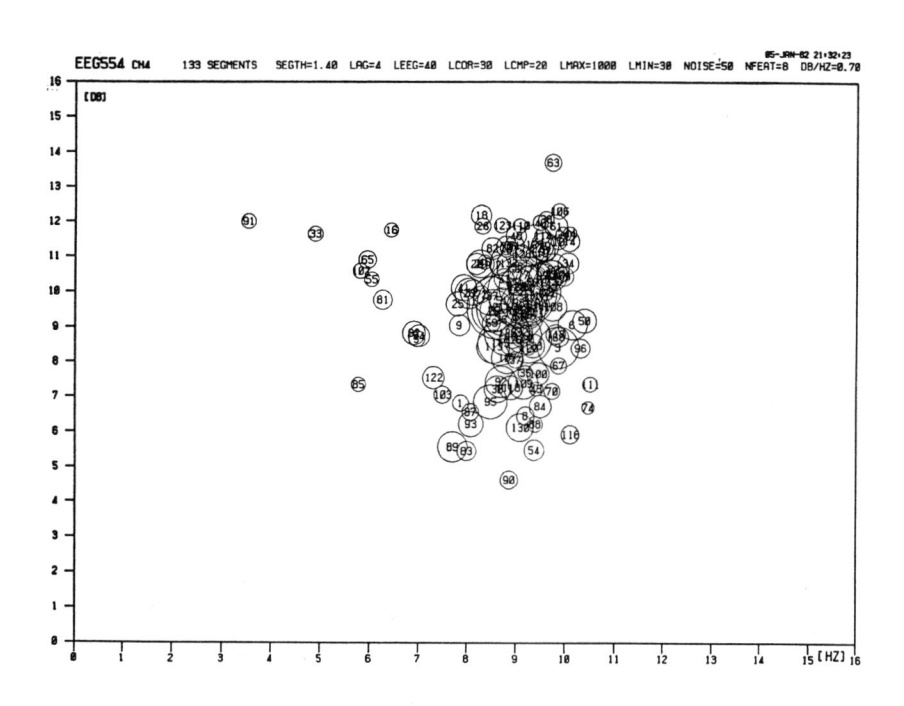

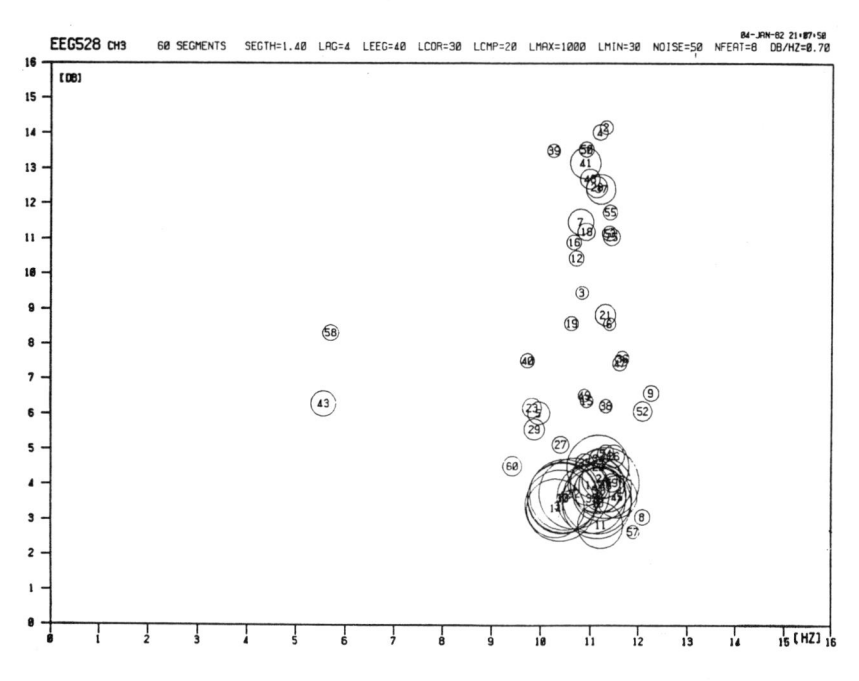

The Waking EEG

C

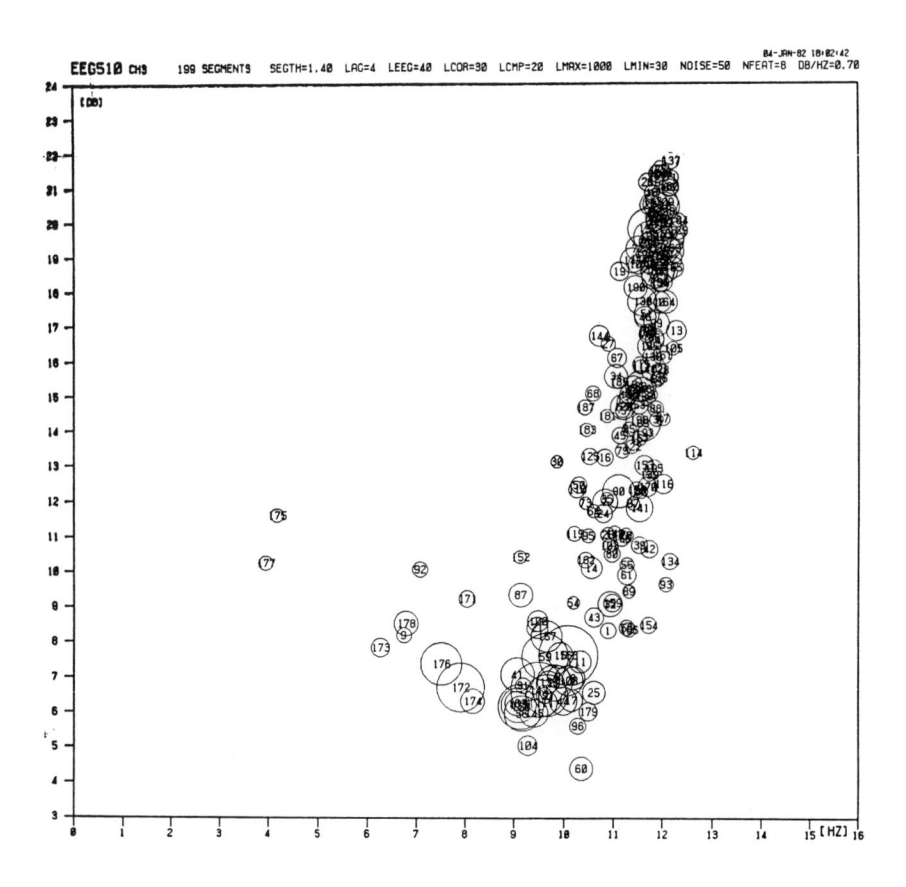

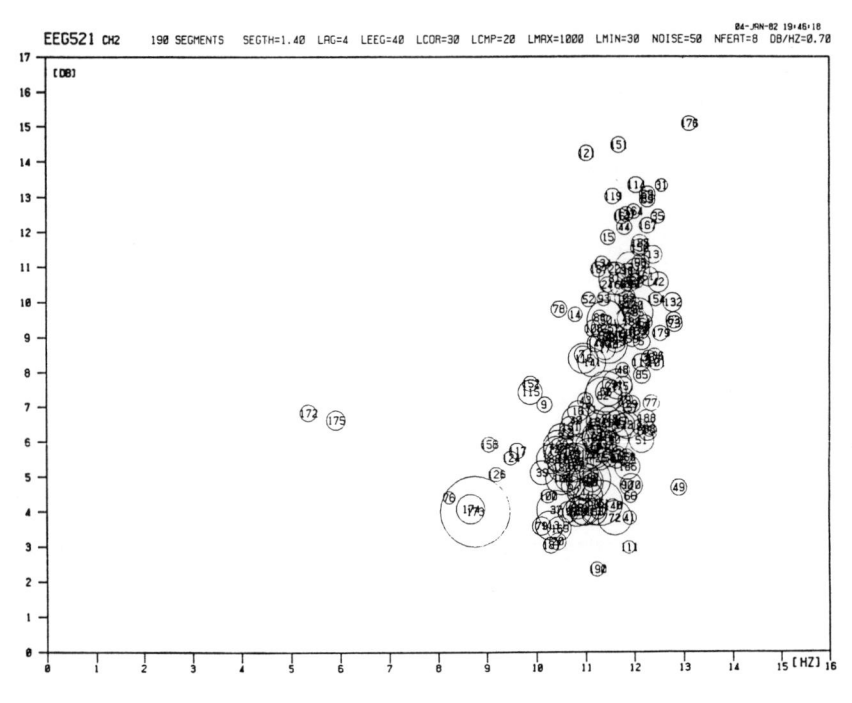

available by Keith Chiappa.) Baseline recordings with eyes closed were also available for these subjects, as were spectra for the EEG during reading and during resting with the eyes closed.

TESTS FOR TYPE 4 WAVES USING THE COEFFICIENT OF DETERMINATION

The primary test used for Type 4 waves of the oscillator model was the Coefficient of Determination for the running mean amplitude and the running mean slope (or, alternatively, of the instantaneous envelopes of the EEG and of its first derivative). As described in chapter 3, the Coefficient of Determination is the square of the Pearson Product-Moment Correlation Coefficient; it provides a quantitative index of the degree of relatedness of two variables, irrespective of their sign or polarity, and ranges in value from 0 to 1.0. (In contrast, the Pearson Product-Moment Correlation Coefficient ranges in value from 1.0 to -1.0; thus, it is sensitive to the polarities of two signals, and for two completely independent signals it would fluctuate around 0.) For completely independent modulations of the amplitude and slope of a signal, as reflected in the envelope of the EEG and of its first derivative, the Coefficient of Determination would in principle be 0; however, because of the squaring of random or statistical positive and negative correlations, it would fluctuate about some value greater than but near to 0.

For comparison with the analyses of the actual EEGs, Type 3 and Type 4 waves were simulated by means of the oscillator model, as was also done for waves of intermediate types (see chapter 28). For these test signals, the corresponding values of the Coefficient of Determination ranged from 1.0 (for Type 3 waves) to near 0 (for Type 4 waves).

Since spectra were available for the group of subjects during reading, the spectra were compared with those for Type 3 and Type 4 waves from the oscillator model.

SPONTANEOUS LOW-VOLTAGE IRREGULAR EEG PATTERNS

In the first group (posterior irregular low-voltage EEGs), where the posterior EEG (bipolar parietal-occipital) was analyzed in six normal EEG recordings, a Coefficient of Determination in the range of about 0.4–0.5 was found, rather

---

Figure 5.5 Log power vs. frequency plots for six EEGs showing three frequency-vs.-amplitude trends (two EEGs are shown—above and below—for each trend) comparable to the three trends simulated in figure 5.4: (A) slight decrease in frequency with increasing amplitude; (B) no change of frequency with amplitude; (C) slight increase of frequency with amplitude. The circles correspond to individual EEG segments, the area of each circle corresponding to the duration. (Outlying segments often indicate artifacts, except for the lower left in the upper plot in part C, which correspond to drowsiness or light sleep.) Parts A, B, and C of this figure correspond to the respective parts of figure 5.4. (Unpublished data from a study reported in Creutzfeldt et al. 1985.)

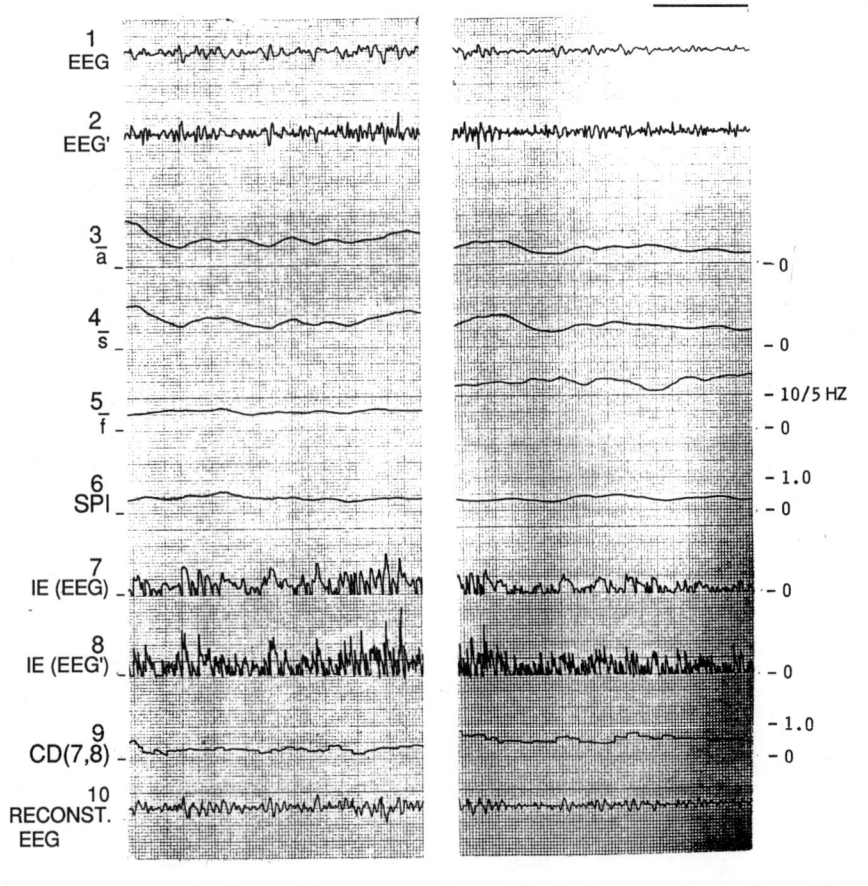

Figure 5.6 Running Coefficient of Determination (trace 9) for the instantaneous envelope of the EEG and of its first derivative (traces 7 and 8) for two EEGs showing irregular low-voltage activity posteriorly with eyes closed. The Coefficient of Determination (trace 9) in each instance is about 0.5. Remaining traces: (2) EEG first derivative; (3–5) running means of amplitude, slope, and frequency (note the difference in the frequency scale for the left and right sides.); (6) Spectral Purity Index; (10) reconstituted EEG (see chapter 9). (Bipolar parieto-occipital recordings.)

than the expected value of about 0 (see below), as is illustrated for the two EEGs in figure 5.6.

PROBABILITY-DENSITY-FUNCTION CLASSIFICATION

A different type of approach to testing the posterior low-voltage irregular EEG pattern in relation to Type 4 waves of the oscillator model is that of examining the probability-density function (Bodenstein et al. 1985; Creutzfeldt 1985) for such EEGs. An example is shown in figure 5.7, where an excerpt of the automatically segmented two-channel EEG is shown at the top and the respective contour lines indicating the distribution of the segments by amplitude (log power) and frequency are shown below. The contour

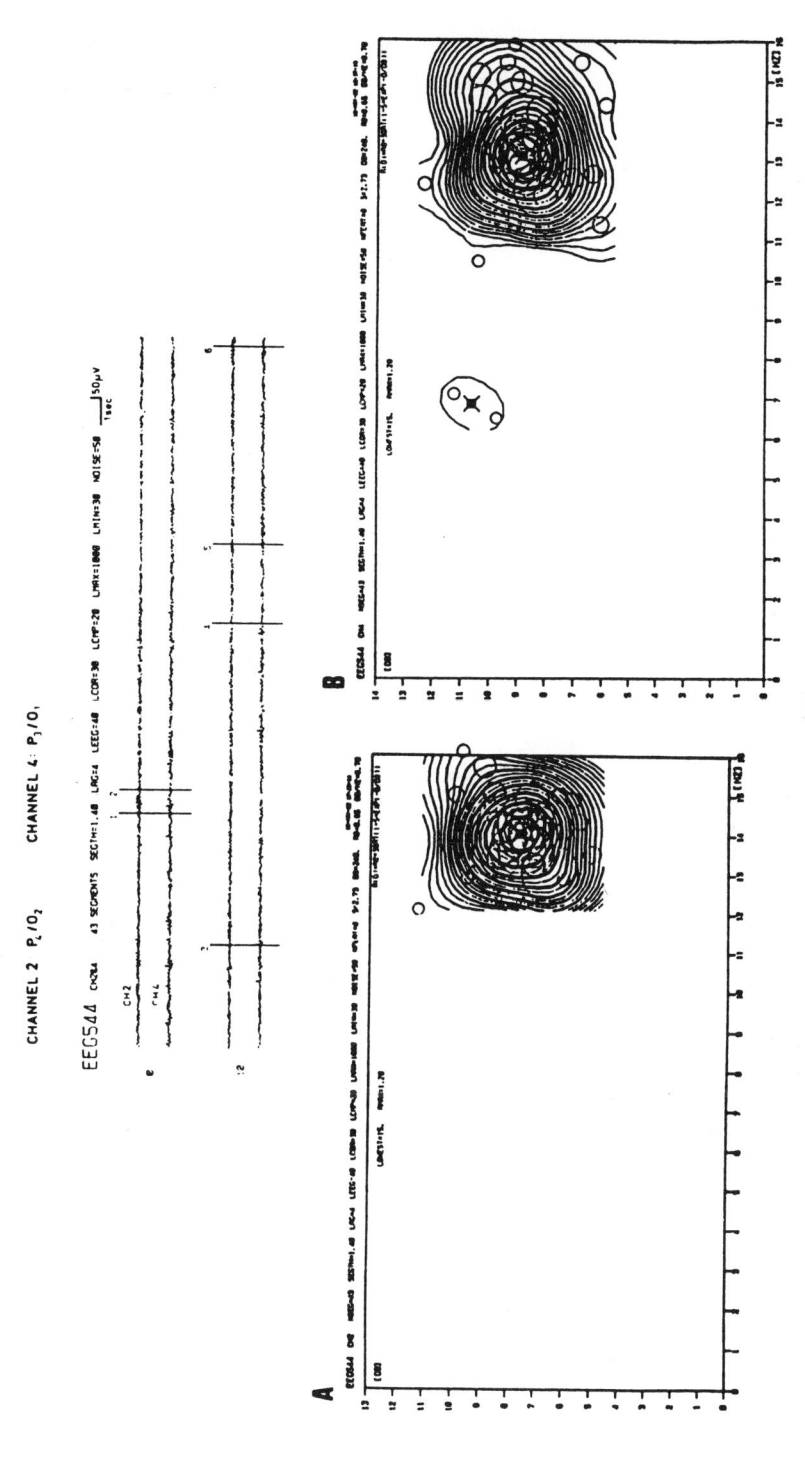

Figure 5.7 Adaptive segmentation (top) and contour plots (bottom) for left and right parieto-occipital EEG (no. 544) showing low-voltage irregular activity. The contour plots indicate a Gaussian, rather than a rectangular, joint probability distribution for amplitude and frequency. (Unpublished results from a study reported in Creutzfeldt et al. 1985.)

The Waking EEG

lines (superimposed on the data points, or rather circles, the diameter of each of which is proportional to the duration of the respective segment) suggest a rounded dome-shaped structure instead of the predicted essentially flat surface. This finding suggests a Gaussian (normal) rather than a rectangular distribution function (see chapter 28) for both the amplitudes and the frequencies of the individual segments in this EEG, which would be expected if the EEG actually consisted of Type 4 waves.

IRREGULAR LOW-VOLTAGE POSTERIOR EEG ACTIVITY DURING READING

Alpha activity is well known to block (i.e., be replaced by low-voltage irregular activity) during a visual task such as reading. (Indeed, alpha blocking, which characteristically occurs upon opening of the eyes, often returns within a few seconds unless there is an ongoing visual task, such as reading.) Some portion of the EEG during reading arises as potentials time-locked to saccadic eye movements—i.e., as "lambda waves" (Barlow 1971). However, such potentials are likely to be small in comparison with the ongoing EEG potentials.

From the EEGs of a larger group of 14 normal subjects, nine EEGs were selected for analysis on the basis of a prominent alpha rhythm in the relaxed eyes-closed state, but without posterior slow (delta and theta) "youth waves" (a normal variant pattern that can be seen up to age 30 or even 35; see Kellaway 1990 and Niedermeyer 1987a). For all nine EEGs, the running Coefficient of Determination for the envelope of the EEG and of its first derivative for the resting alpha rhythm was within the range 0.8–1.0. During reading, the value of the Coefficients of Determination were in the range of about 0.5, as illustrated in figure 5.8.

From the results summarized above, it is evident that values for the Coefficient of Determination around 0.5 are also obtained for the two types of irregular low-voltage EEG patterns. The somewhat surprising point is not that the Coefficient of Determination is smaller for low-voltage irregular EEG activity than for alpha activity (which would be expected), but that it has a value of about 0.5, whereas the expected value for two independent modulating signals for slope and amplitude would be much closer to 0. The possible significance of this finding is discussed below.

SPECTRAL CHARACTERISTICS OF THE POSTERIOR EEG DURING READING

A comparison of the power spectrum (log power) of the EEGs recorded during reading with the spectrum for the same subject resting with the eyes closed disclosed an interesting feature: For seven of the nine subjects, the spectrum during reading was relatively flat up to the resting alpha frequency, beyond which there was a rapid decrease in the power with increasing frequency. Three examples of such spectra are shown in figure 5.9.

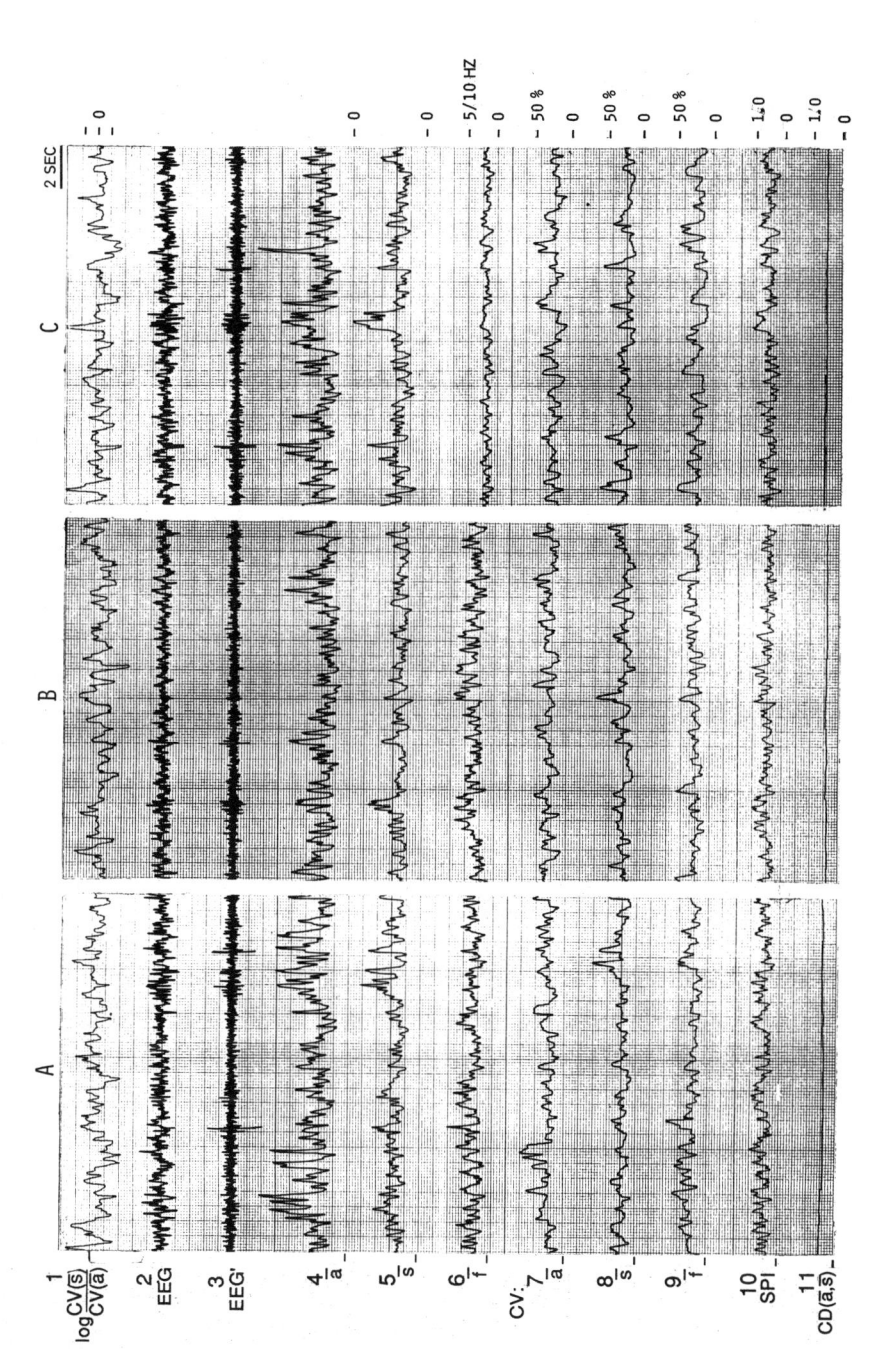

Figure 5.8 Running Coefficient of Determination (trace 11) for running mean of the EEG and of its first derivative for three subjects (A, B, C) during reading. The Coefficient of Determination (64-sec window) in each case is about 0.5. Other traces: (1) log of quotient of Coefficient of Variations for slope and for amplitude; (2) EEG; (3) first derivative of EEG; (4–6) running means of amplitude, slope, and frequency (calibration is 5 Hz for A and B, 10 Hz for C); (7–9) Coefficients of Variation of running means of amplitude, slope, and frequency, respectively; (10) Spectral Purity Index. (Bipolar parieto-occipital recordings.) (Original EEG recordings courtesy of Keith Chiappa.)

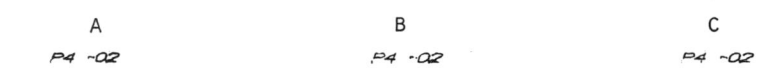

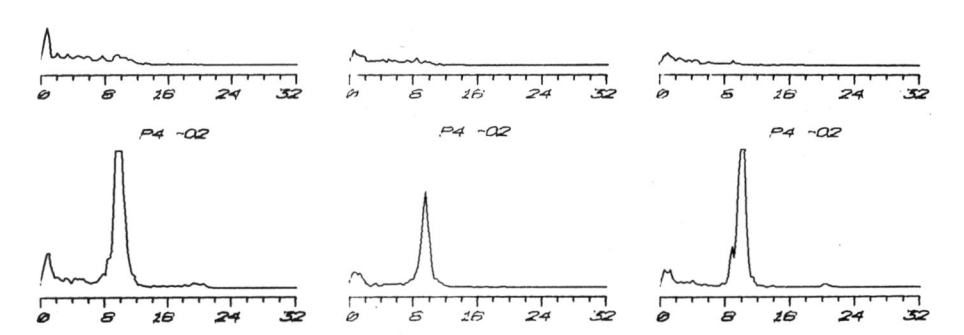

Figure 5.9 Log power vs. frequency for the EEGs of three subjects (A, B, C) while reading (upper spectra) and while resting with eyes closed (lower spectra). Bipolar parieto-occipital recordings. Note that the spectrum during reading is approximately flat up to the frequency that corresponds to the well-demarcated peak for the resting alpha frequency for the respective subject; above this frequency, the power decreases. (Spectra courtesy of Keith Chiappa.)

The relatively flat spectrum of the EEGs during reading led to the exploration of the spectral characteristics of Type 4 waves of the oscillator model, with the goal of determining whether the latter would have the same spectral behavior. As figure 5.10 shows, a similar spectral behavior was in fact found. The spectrum for Type 4 waves from the oscillator model, using incongruent modulation of amplitude (extrema) and slope, was also flat up to the "alpha" frequency (i.e., the frequency of Type 3 waves of the oscillator model); a progressive decline was evident for still higher frequencies.

The unusual and even unanticipated behavior of the spectrum for Type 4 waves illustrated in figure 5.10, in which the spectrum for Type 4 waves of the oscillator model is relatively flat up to the frequency corresponding to that for Type 3 waves but diminishes for still higher frequencies, can be understood from the following consideration in relation to figure 5.11: In the extrema-slopes dual modulation process, modulation of the extremes of waves alters not only their amplitude, but also their duration, and thus their frequency. The resulting change (say, an increase in frequency) can be compensated for by a change in slope, without a change in amplitude, but only up to a certain frequency; that frequency is just the frequency of the Type 3 waves for the same system. This characteristic of extrema-slopes modulation is depicted in figure 5.11.

It is to be emphasized that this spectral characteristic, which is inherent in the extrema-slopes hypothesis and correspondingly in Mode 4 waves of the oscillator model, results from the fact that modulation of extrema results in simultaneous variation of both amplitude and duration (i.e., frequency) of the modulated waves.

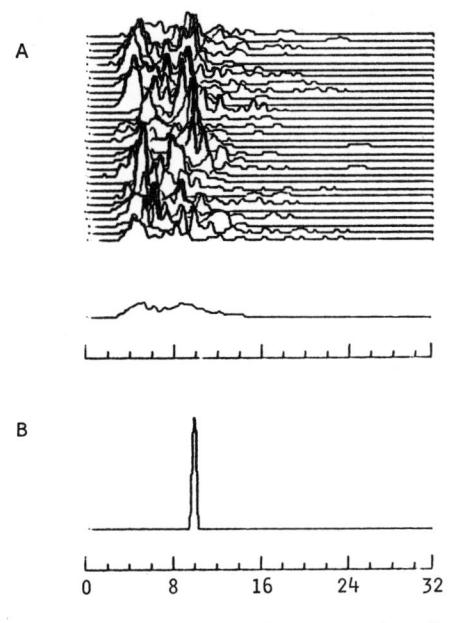

Figure 5.10 Power spectra for output of oscillator model with independent (non-congruent) modulation of extremes and slopes (A), and for no modulation (B). Note that the spectrum in part A is approximately flat up to the unmodulated output frequency of part B and decreases thereafter.

SIGNIFICANCE OF THE RESULTS FOR THE COEFFICIENT OF DETERMINATION

As previously mentioned, the analyses of low-voltage irregular EEGs of different types indicated values of the Coefficient of Determination between the envelope of amplitude and the envelope of slope (i.e., the envelope of the EEG and of its first derivative, respectively) in the range of 0.5, rather than the originally anticipated values nearer 0. This finding indicates a less-than-complete independence of the envelopes of amplitude and of slope, and thus suggests that the low-voltage irregular EEG patterns examined could better be viewed as due to a generator mechanism intermediate between Mode 4 and Mode 3—i.e., partial rather than complete independence of the two modulating signals. It should be mentioned that for Gaussian noise in the frequency range 1.0–10 Hz the Coefficient of Determination was found experimentally to be 0.5 (in contrast to a value close to 1.0 for narrow-band noise centered at 10 Hz). On the other hand, the Coefficient of Determination for Gaussian noise having a $1/f$ dependence of amplitude on frequency (i.e., the equivalent of Type 1 waves of the oscillator model) was found to be about 0.1. (Such a noise characteristic can be obtained by passing Gaussian noise through an integrator, as described in chapter 28.)

The fact that the Coefficient of Determination for low-voltage irregular ("desynchronized") EEGs falls in the range of 0.5 rather than lower may be related to the Central Limit Theorem of statistics (Middleton 1960; Sokal

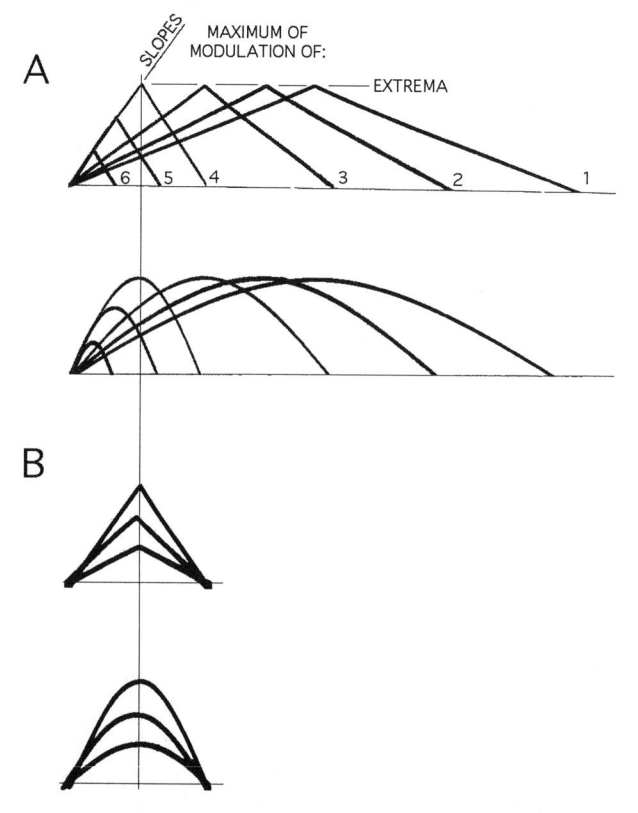

Figure 5.11 Schema to indicate the reason that the spectrum of Type 4 waves (A) of the oscillator model is flat up to the frequency corresponding to Type 3 waves (B), with a progressive decrease in the spectral curve for still higher frequencies. For clarity, only the first upper half cycles of the triangular and sine waves are shown. For the Type 3 waves (B) (congruent modulation of extrema and slope, resulting in constant frequency), a series of three waves, including a wave having the maximum extreme and maximum slope, are shown. For the Type 4 waves, the same maxima are indicated, and a series of waves (1–4) are shown having the same extrema but progressively increasing slope and increasing frequency (decreasing period), the last in this series being identical with wave 4 of the Type 3 series. Of the Type 4 group, waves 5 and 6 have the same slope (i.e., the maximum slope) as that for wave 4, and hence these waves necessarily have lower extrema and are of higher frequency (shorter period) than wave 4. Assuming independent rectangular (as contrasted with a Gaussian) distributions for the extrema and slopes modulations, the spectrum for Type 4 waves should be flat up to the frequency of the Type 3 waves for the same system but should decrease progressively for still higher frequencies, as actually shown in figure 5.10.

and Rohlf 1973), according to which a progressively larger ensemble of any probability distribution function approaches a Gaussian distribution function. (More exactly, "as sample size increases, the means of samples drawn from a population of any distribution will approach the normal (gaussian) distribution" [Sokal and Rohlf 1973, p. 98].) Since the EEG clearly represents the summation of a very large number of individual oscillators or generators (chapter 15), it seems possible or even likely that in such a summation the Central Limit Theorem is operative, and hence a higher Coefficient of Determination than originally expected (i.e., near 0) would result.

6 The Normal EEG during Sleep

It is customary to divide the EEG during various states of consciousness into those of the alert and the relaxed waking state (sometimes termed Stage W), non-REM sleep, and REM sleep (figure 6.1). In the alert waking state with eyes open, an irregular low-voltage pattern is present; in the relaxed waking state with eyes closed, rhythmic alpha activity is usually present posteriorly. Non-REM sleep is subdivided into four stages: Stage 1 (drowsiness), with irregular low-voltage activity, some rhythmic theta waves, and some vertex sharp waves; Stage 2, with vertex sharp waves and sleep spindles (at about 14 Hz) and K complexes (prolonged vertex sharp waves with a slower afterswing, often with superimposed sleep spindles); Stage 3, with delta waves maximal anteriorly of at least 75 microvolts and 2 Hz or less for at least 20 percent but not more than 50 percent of the time, and some sleep spindles; and Stage 4, similar to Stage 3 but with high-voltage slow waves more than 50 percent of the time. Stage 3 and Stage 4 together are sometimes referred to as *slow-wave* sleep. In REM sleep, the EEG pattern is a low-voltage irregular one, with slow "sawtooth waves" occasionally present. Further details, including electro-oculographic (EOG) and electromyographic (EMG) findings in the various states, can be found in Rechtschaffen and Kales 1968, Broughton 1987, Carskadon and Rechtschaffen 1989, and Radke 1990.

As was mentioned in chapter 1, it was the chance observation suggesting that the EEG during drowsiness or Stage 1 sleep might exhibit the constant-slope phenomenon as evidenced by an apparently relatively small variability of the running mean slope that eventually gave rise to the extrema-slopes hypothesis. The original prediction, as indicated in chapter 2, was that the EEG in all stages of non-REM sleep would exhibit the constant-slope phenomenon. If this were the case, then with increasing depth of sleep the running mean amplitude could be expected to show the familiar progressive increase with increasing depth of non-REM sleep, whereas the running mean slope would be expected to remain relatively constant. (Of course, the running mean frequency would be expected to decrease with increasing depth of sleep.)

A simulated EEG exhibiting such a relatively constant slope with a progressively increasing amplitude is shown in trace 2 of figure 6.2. The excursions

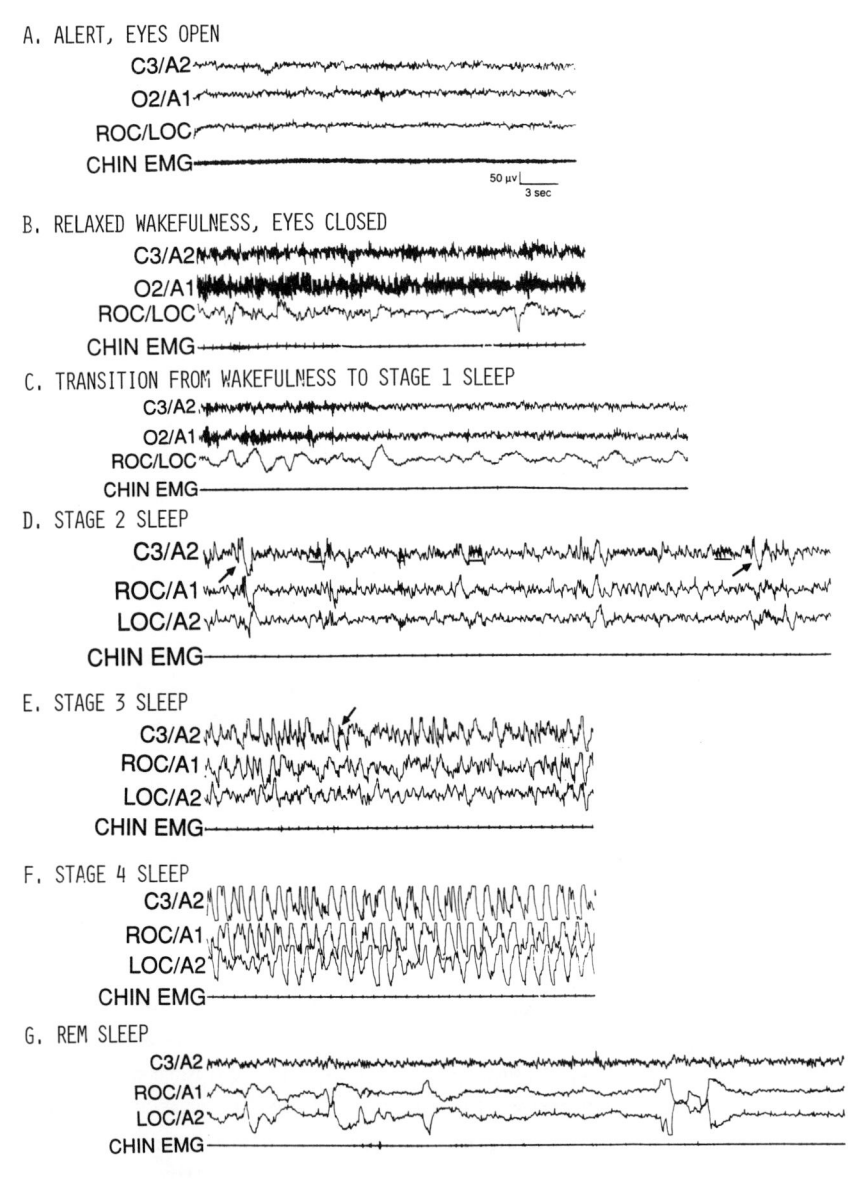

Figure 6.1 Examples of the EEG, electro-oculogram (EOG), and chin electromyogram (EMG) for the several stages of wakefulness and sleep. In part D (Stage 2 sleep), arrows indicate K complexes and underlining indicates sleep spindles. Note that for parts D–G the occipital EEG channel is omitted and the eyes are monitored individually. In part E (Stage 3 sleep), the arrow indicates a sleep spindle. In part G (REM sleep), note the rapid eye movements (second and third traces). EEG and EOG leads: C3/A2, left central (see appendix C) to right ear; O2/A1, right occipital to left ear; ROC/LOC, outer canthus (corner) of right eye to outer canthus of left eye. The calibration applies to all of the EEG traces. Further description of EEG patterns in text. (From Carskadon and Rechtschaffen 1989.)

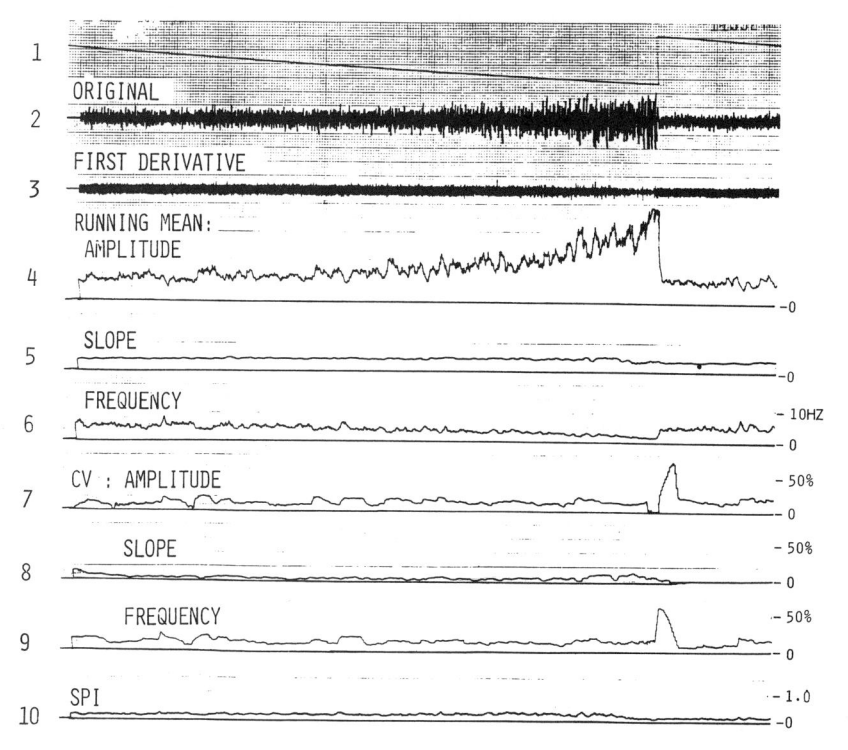

Figure 6.2 Analysis of a signal showing the constant-slope feature. The original signal (the generation of which is described in detail in chapter 28 and schematized in figure 28.11) has the feature that the amplitude of individual waves is inversely related to their frequency—that is, the signal has a $1/f$ frequency characteristic: the lower the frequency, the larger the waves. (Trace 1, which indicates the low-frequency content, can be considered a kind of "depth of (non-REM) sleep" indicator.) Note that the amplitude of the waves (trace 2) increases progressively from left to right, but the first derivative (trace 3) of the signal remains approximately constant, as evidenced by its relatively constant width. Correspondingly, the running mean amplitude (trace 4) increases whereas the running mean slope (trace 5) remains essentially constant. The running mean frequency (trace 6) progressively diminishes, but the Spectral Purity Index (trace 10) remains approximately constant. The Coefficient of Variation for the running mean slope (trace 8) remains consistently below that for the running mean amplitude (trace 7), and the Coefficient of Variation for frequency (trace 9) remains approximately constant.

of the first derivative of the simulated EEG (trace 3) remain relatively constant. These characteristics of the two traces are reflected in the running mean amplitude (trace 3) and the running mean slope (trace 4), respectively, the former progressively rising and the latter remaining essentially level or constant.

STAGE 1 OF NON-REM SLEEP (DROWSINESS)

It was not usually found possible to study Stage 1 sleep in recordings of all-night sleep (see below), because of the relatively short duration of episodes of Stage 1 sleep. Fortunately, records from an independent study of daytime

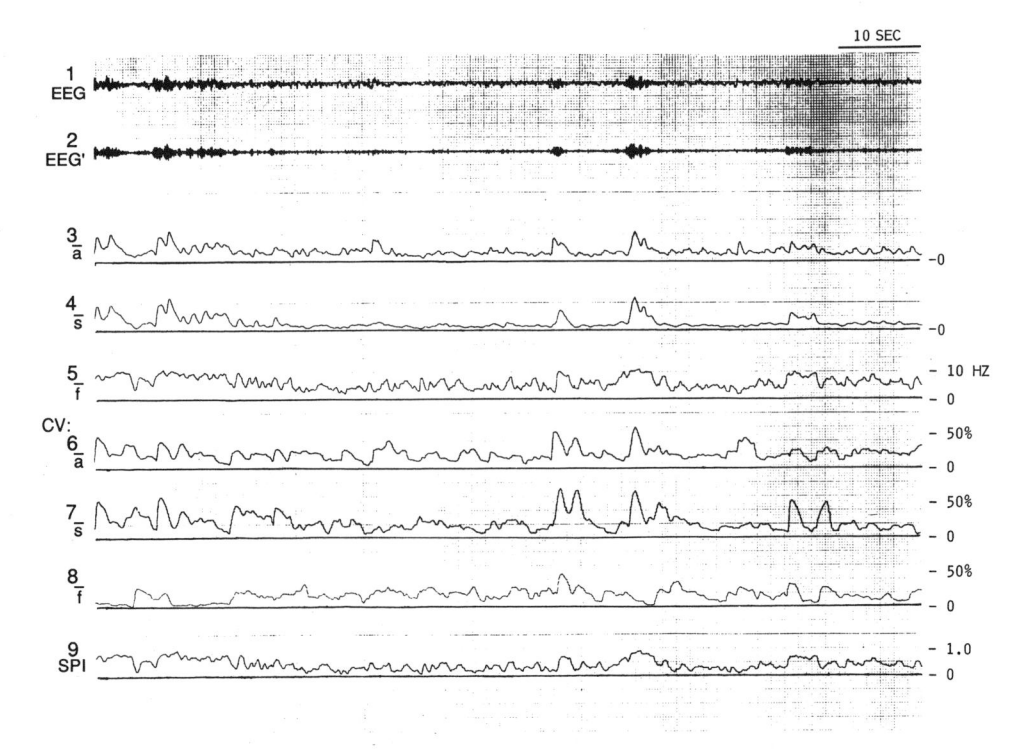

Figure 6.3 EEG (right occipital to right ear) recorded from a subject during the alternations between the waking alpha state and the irregular low-voltage pattern of drowsiness (Stage 1 sleep). Trace identification: (1) EEG (right occipital to right ear); (2) EEG first derivative; (3) running mean amplitude; (4) running mean slope; (5) running mean frequency; (6–8) Coefficients of Variation of these, respectively; (9) Spectral Purity Index. As is indicated by the respective Coefficients of Variation (traces 7 and 8), there is only minimally less variability in the running mean slope than in the running mean amplitude during the periods of drowsiness (the decreases in the width of traces 1 and 2).

drowsiness (Santamaria and Chiappa 1987) were made available for analysis by Keith Chiappa. From this group of EEGs, six that showed a prominent waking alpha rhythm were selected for analysis.

The analysis of these additional EEGs did not confirm the expectation that Stage 1 sleep could be characterized as having constant slope, or at least that the variability of the running mean slope would be less than that of the running mean amplitude. An EEG recorded during the alternations between the alpha activity of the waking state and the irregular low-voltage activity of drowsiness that showed the constant slope phenomenon only to a minimal extent is shown in figure 6.3.

An exception for which a decrease in the relative variability of the running mean slope as compared with that of the running mean amplitude did occur is shown in figure 6.4. The change is evident from comparison of the respective Coefficients of Variation (traces 7 and 8), and also from the write-out of the logarithm of their ratio (trace 1) and the sign of the logarithm (trace 2).

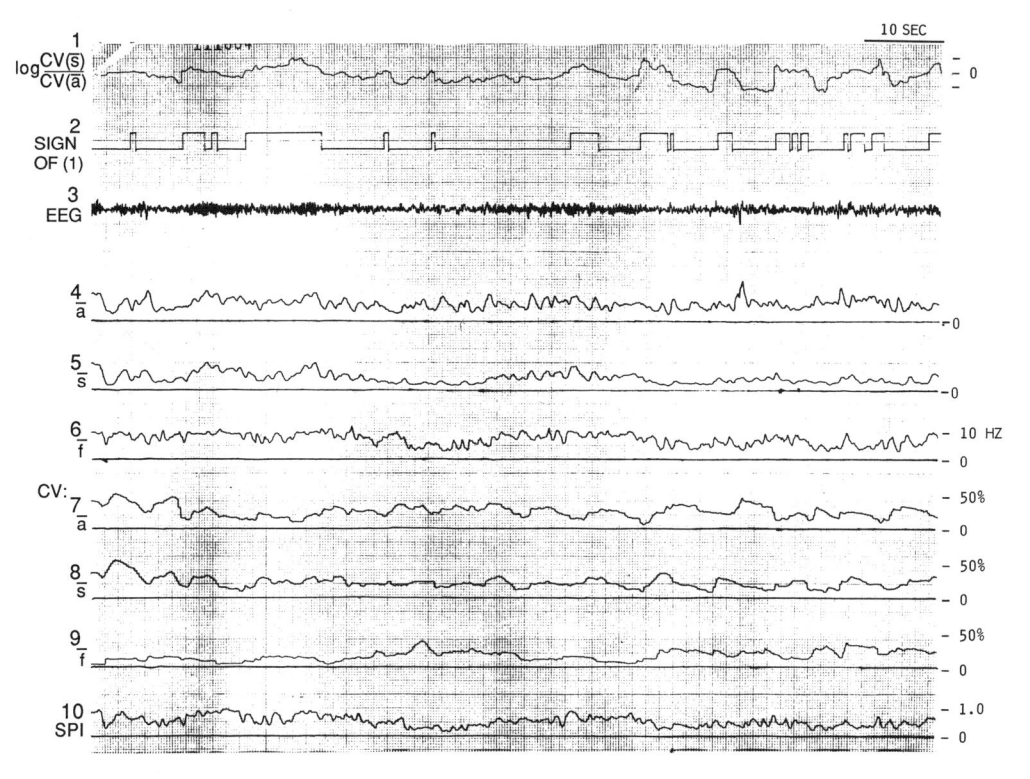

Figure 6.4 EEG (vertex to right ear) during alternations between wakefulness (with alpha) and drowsiness for another subject. Trace identification: (1) logarithm of the quotient of the Coefficients of Variation for slope and amplitude; (2) sign (+ or −) of trace 1; (3) EEG; (4–6) running means of amplitude, slope, frequency; (7–9) Coefficients of Variation of the preceding; (10) Spectral Purity Index. In trace 2, the transitions occur when the logarithm passes through the value of 0, which corresponds to equal Coefficients of Variation for slope and amplitude (since the logarithm of 1.0 is 0). During the periods of drowsiness—indicated by decreased running mean frequency (trace 6) and SPI (trace 10)—a greater decrease is evident in the variability of the Coefficient of Variation for the running mean slope (trace 8) than in that for the running mean amplitude (trace 7). This change is more clearly evident in traces 1 and 2, which swing negatively during drowsiness (one division in the calibrations for trace 1 corresponds to a factor-of-2 difference in the Coefficients of Variation).

STAGES 2–4 OF NON-REM SLEEP

As noted above, a prediction of a characteristic of constant slope was made for all stages of non-REM sleep. To test this prediction for the deeper stages of non-REM sleep, the first non-REM portion of five normal all-night sleep recordings (made available by John Stakes, Director of the Sleep Disorders Laboratory at the Massachusetts General Hospital) were analyzed; all showed the features to be described. Three of the EEGs are shown in figures 6.5–6.7. From inspection of the figures, it is evident that the running mean amplitude (trace 3) tends to increase as the depth of sleep increases (as expected), but the running mean slope tends to reach an upper limit early, and to remain relatively constant thereafter. This behavior provides evidence for the predicted

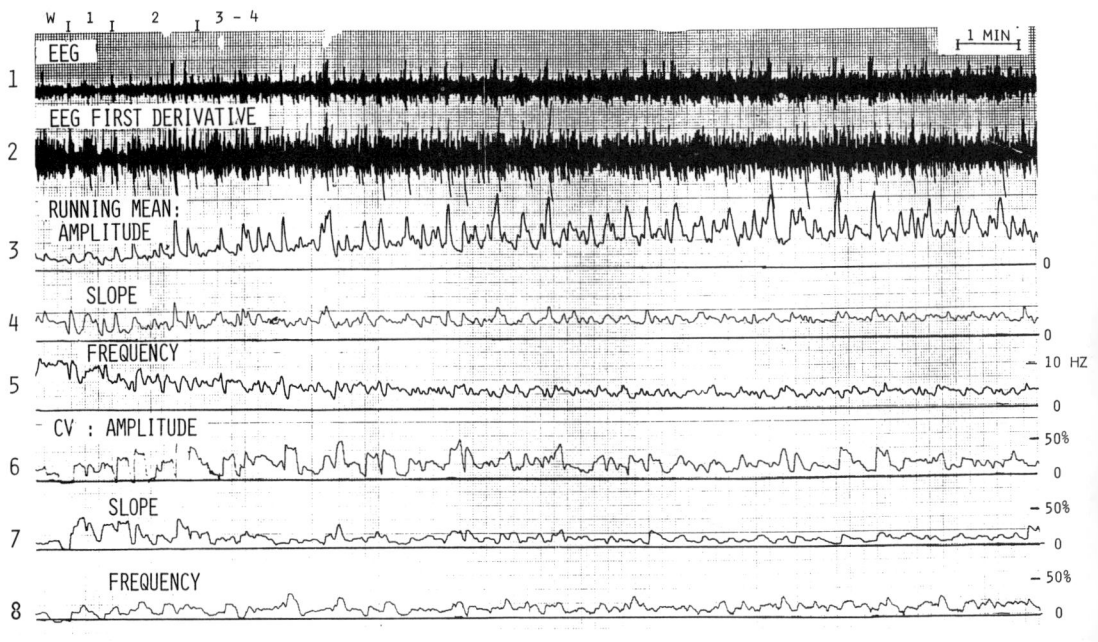

Figure 6.5 Analysis of the first non-REM cycle of a normal all-night sleep EEG recording (vertex to right ear). A brief portion of the waking recording (W) appears at the extreme left, with an alpha frequency of about 10 Hz, and short episodes of Stage 1 and Stage 2 follow. (Stages of sleep indicated by these analyses are shown at the top in this and the following two figures.) The onset of Stages 3 and 4 of sleep (considered together) is marked by a cessation of some resemblance between the curves for the running mean amplitude and running mean slope (traces 3 and 4). After the onset of Stages 3 and 4, the trend of the running mean slope is still upward, whereas the running mean amplitude tends to remain relatively constant, as sleep deepens. After this point, the Coefficient of Variation of the running mean slope is appreciably less than that for the running mean amplitude. After the waking portion of the recording (at the extreme left), the running mean frequency decreases slowly as sleep deepens but its Coefficient of Variation remains at approximately the same level, including during Stage 2. Here and in figures 6.6 and 6.7, the scale for frequency (trace 5) is at the right, and the scale for the Coefficient of Variation (for traces 6–8) is also at the right.

constant-slope characteristic. Further, for all five recordings during Stages 3 and 4 of sleep, the Coefficient of Variation for the running mean slope was rather less than that for the running mean amplitude. (Compare trace 7 with trace 6 in figures 6.5–6.7.) This finding provides corroborative evidence, for Stages 3 and 4 of sleep (i.e., slow-wave sleep), for the constant-slope prediction.

For Stage 2 sleep, the evidence for a constant-slope phenomenon was minimal at best. The reason for the difference between Stage 2 and Stages 3 and 4 appeared to be related not to a possibly greater prominence of sleep spindles during Stage 2 sleep (in fact, sleep spindles appeared to have relatively little effect on these analyses), but rather to the vertex sharp waves during the latter stage; these appeared to behave as single cycles of approximately 5-Hz waves. These brief waves, especially if of some appreciable voltage, tended to be reflected in the traces for both the running mean

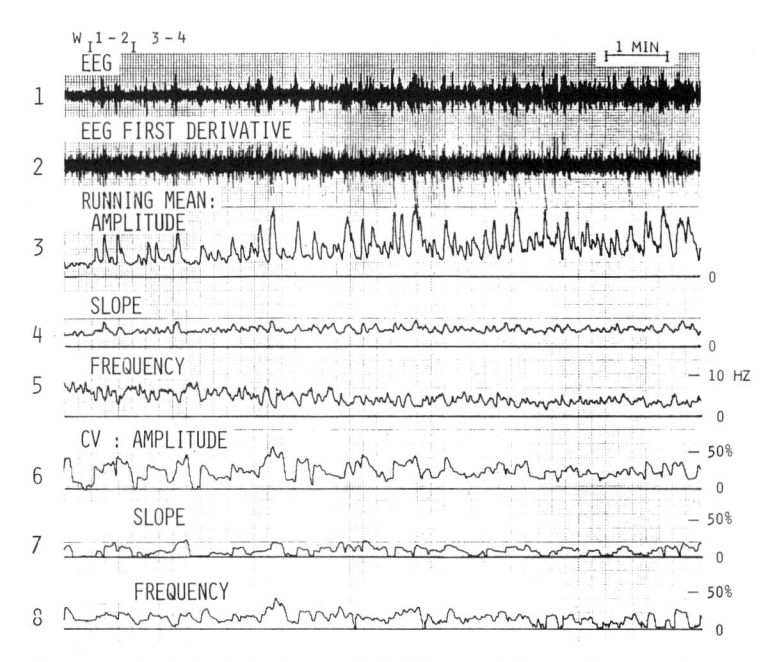

Figure 6.6 Analysis of the first non-REM sleep cycle for another normal EEG (with the same labeling as in figure 6.5.), showing the same findings as the EEG of figure 6.5.

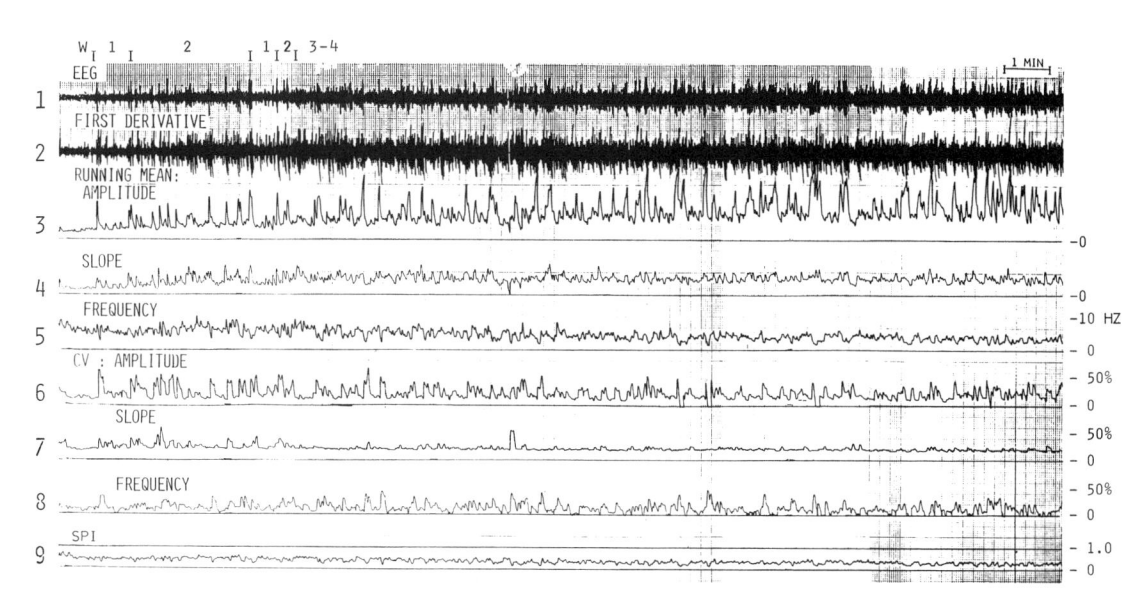

Figure 6.7 Analysis of the first non-REM sleep cycle for a third normal EEG, showing the same findings as for the EEGs of figures 6.5 and 6.6. The labeling is as in figures 6.5 and 6.6, except for the addition of the Spectral Purity Index in trace 9. The latter decreases from about 0.6 at the beginning of the recording to about 0.3 at the end, reflecting the wider span of frequencies in deeper sleep.

The Normal EEG during Sleep

amplitude and the running mean slope (see traces 3 and 4 in figure 6.5). (It is especially noteworthy that the running mean frequency, as well as the instantaneous frequency, which often appears to be about 5 Hz during Stage 1, remained essentially unchanged when vertex sharp waves occurred.) Indeed, the disappearance of transients from the write-out of the running mean slope while transients continued to be evident in the running mean amplitude appeared to be a relatively reliable indication of the onset of Stage 3–4 sleep. This phenomenon may be explainable in terms of the presence of vertex sharp waves in Stage 2 sleep (and also to some extent in Stage 1 sleep) giving way to K complexes of Stage 3 sleep, the duration of K-complexes characteristically being greater than that of vertex sharp transients.

Findings for Stage 1, Stage 2, and Stage 3–4 sleep are shown for the first non-REM cycle of another normal all-night sleep recording in figure 6.8, with the additional inclusion of the logarithm of the ratio of the Coefficients of Variation of running mean slope and running mean amplitude (trace 1), and also the Coefficient of Determination for these two variables (trace 11). During Stage 1 or drowsiness, the logarithm of the ratio of the Coefficients of Variation has a value of about -0.25; during Stage 2 (when there are numerous vertex sharp waves) it is about -0.15, and during Stage 3 it is about -0.4 to -0.5. The respective values for the Coefficient of Determination for Stages 1, 2, and 3 are 0.5, 0.7, and 0.5, approximately. (For comparison, the values for EEGs exhibiting alpha activity were as follows: the logarithm of the ratios of the Coefficients of Variation for slope and amplitude had a value of approximately 0, which indicates that the running mean slope and the running mean amplitude in the case of alpha activity are equally variable; the Coefficient of Determination for alpha activity was close to 1.0, which indicates that the curves for the running mean amplitude and the running mean slope are essentially identical.)

For the EEG of figure 6.8, these results thus indicate the following: For Stage 2 sleep the variability of the running mean slope and that of the running mean amplitude are only slightly different. For Stage 1 the two variabilities differ by a larger amount. For Stage 3 the two variabilities differ by an even larger amount. In all the stages, the variability of the running mean slope is the smaller of the two.

The findings from the EEG shown in figure 6.8 indicate, in agreement with the results of the analyses of other non-REM EEGs discussed above, that the constant-slope characteristic is only minimally evident during Stage 2 sleep (the characteristics of which appear to be those of an "irregularly rhythmic activity," the quasi-rhythmic component being the vertex sharp waves). The constant-slope characteristic is somewhat more evident, though hardly prominent, during Stage 1 sleep, and is more clearly evident during Stage 3 (and Stage 4) sleep.

In summary, in relation to the prediction of constant slope (i.e., Type 1 waves of the oscillator model) for all stages of non-REM sleep, these findings from analyses of the first non-REM cycle of normal all-night-sleep EEG recordings provide corroborative evidence for the constant slope hypothesis

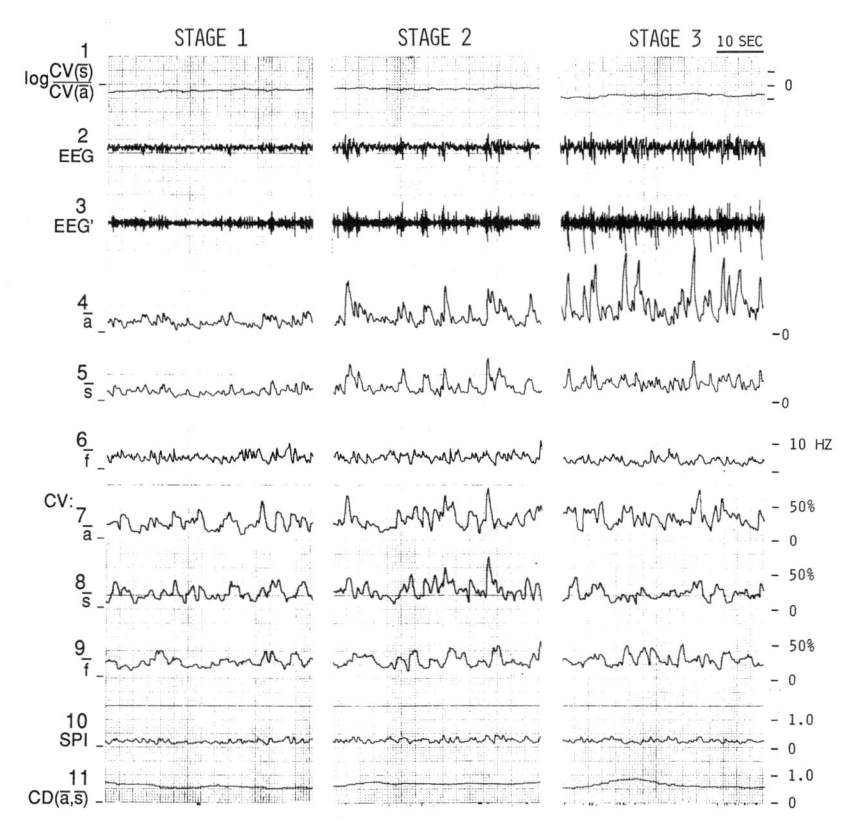

Figure 6.8 Analysis of excerpts from Stages 1, 2, and 3 of sleep from another normal all-night sleep recording (right central to right ear), with inclusion (as trace l) of the logarithm of the quotient of the Coefficients of Variation of the running mean slope and the running mean amplitude (top trace), and also (as trace 11) the Coefficient of Determination (bottom trace) for the running mean amplitude (trace 4) and running mean slope (trace 5). (Traces 2–10 are the same as in figure 6.2.)

for Stages 3 and 4 of sleep, but only minimally or intermittently for Stage 1, and even less for Stage 2. The onset of relatively constant slope invariably marked the transition between Stage 2 and Stage 3.

On the other hand, there were several consistent indications of the presence of Stage 1 or Stage 2 sleep, in comparison with the waking EEG showing an alpha rhythm. These included decreases in the running mean amplitude and frequency and in the Spectral Purity Index. (The latter largely paralleled the decrease in running mean frequency.) Further, the Coefficient of Determination for the running mean amplitude and the running mean slope also decreased. The running mean frequency during Stage 2 sleep was usually about half that of the waking alpha frequency, and it changed little when vertex sharp transients were present. (The question of the nature of the transition from wakefulness to Stage 1 sleep for normal subjects having an irregular low-voltage posterior EEG rather than an alpha rhythm in the waking relaxed state was not explored.)

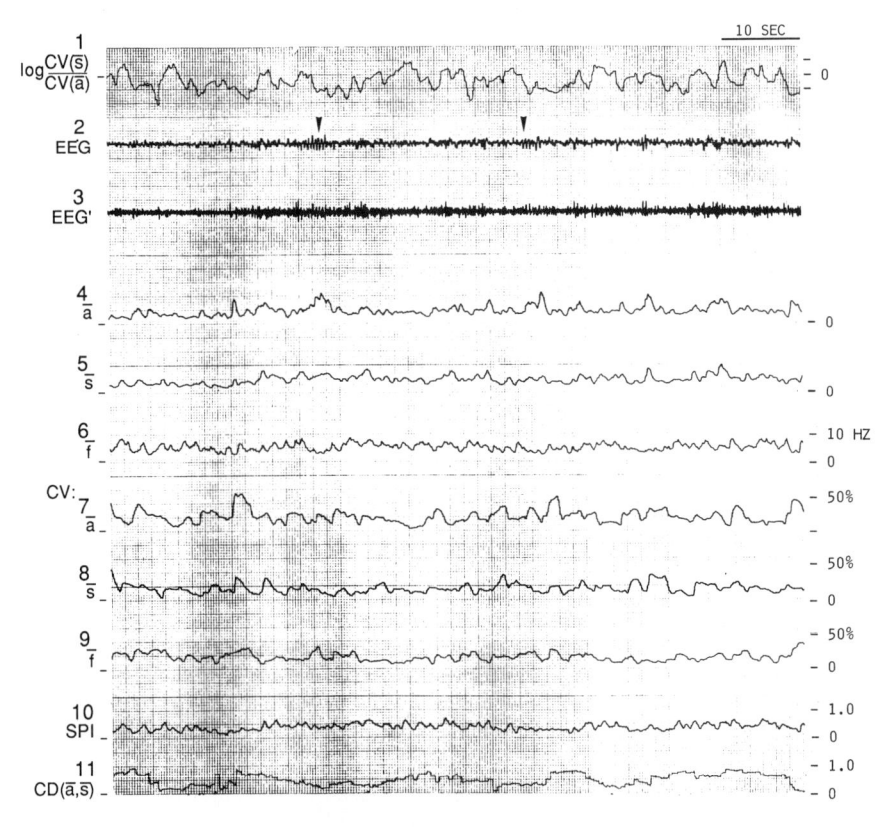

Figure 6.9 Analysis of a section of the first REM period of a normal all-night sleep recording. The top trace, the logarithm of the ratio of the Coefficient of Variation for the running mean amplitude and the running mean slope, fluctuates appreciably, but is generally negative, indicating less variability of running mean slope than of running mean amplitude. Note that the running mean frequency tends to decrease when "sawtooth waves" occur (arrows). The bottom trace shows that the Coefficient of Determination for the running mean amplitude and the running mean slope fluctuates around 0.5.

REM SLEEP

As indicated in chapter 2, it was originally predicted that Type 4 waves of the oscillator model could be a model for the irregular waves of the EEG during REM sleep—i.e., that the modulations of extrema and of slopes would be independent of one another. If this were indeed the case, then the Coefficient of Determination for the running mean amplitude and the running mean slope should be near zero. This prediction was tested with the REM portions of the five all-night-sleep recordings and also with REM EEG portions of positive Multiple Sleep Latency Tests (MSLT), kindly made available by John Stakes and Margaret Merlina of the Sleep Disorders Laboratory at the Massachusetts General Hospital.

Analysis of the REM-sleep recordings did not confirm the predicted complete independence of the running mean amplitude and running mean slope. As an example, for the EEG shown in figure 6.9 the Coefficient of Determina-

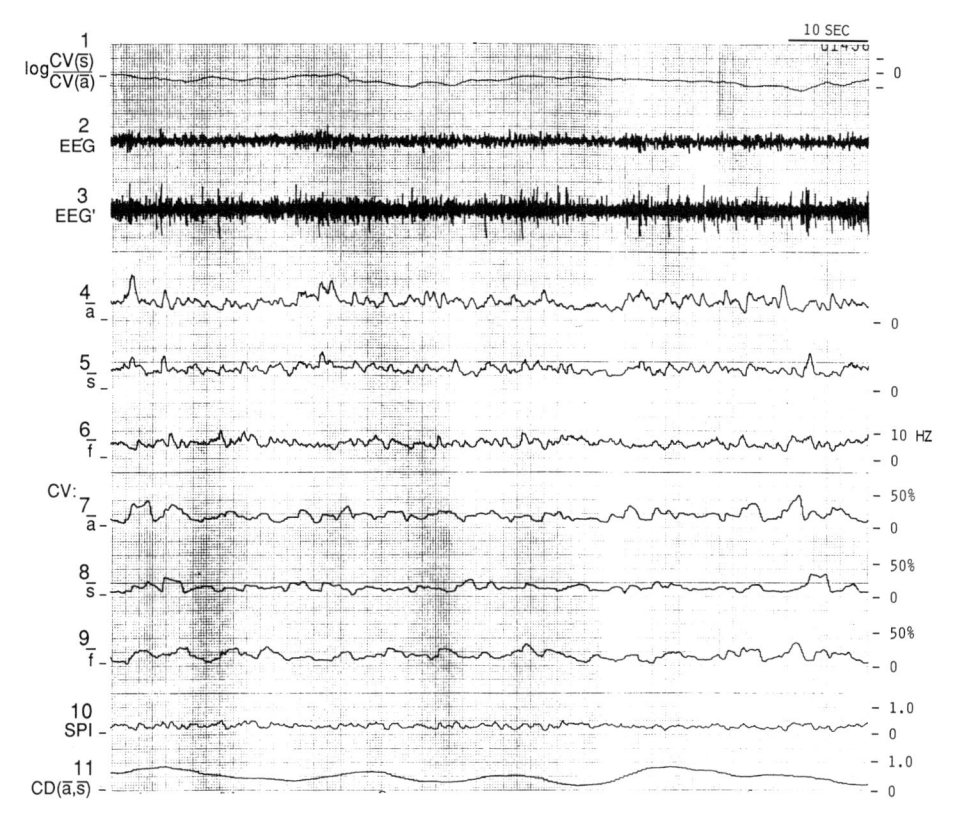

Figure 6.10 Analysis of another normal REM EEG recording, but with longer averaging times for the logarithm of the ratio of the Coefficient of Variation for the running mean amplitude and the running mean slope (trace 1), and for the Coefficient of Determination for the running mean amplitude (trace 4) and running mean slope (trace 5). The results are similar to those of figure 6.9.

tion (trace 11) for these two variables (traces 4 and 5) had values fluctuating around 0.5 instead of near 0. Indeed, comparison of the running mean amplitude and the running mean slope (traces 4 and 5) and of their respective Coefficients of Variation (traces 7 and 8) suggests that the running mean slope is less variable than the running mean amplitude. The write-out of the logarithm of the ratio of the two Coefficients of Variation (trace 1) fluctuates considerably on either side of 0, but the values are predominantly negative, indicating an overall smaller variability of slope than of amplitude—i.e., a tendency toward a constant-slope characteristic. The EEG in figure 6.10, for which a longer averaging time was used for the Coefficient of Determination and the logarithm of the two Coefficients of Variation, indicates the same results.

The clearest indication of a constant-slope effect for the EEG during REM sleep occurred when there were sawtooth waves (Carskadon and Rechtshaffen 1989). This is consistent with the observation that the sawtooth waves in these recordings were generally of somewhat higher voltage and lower frequency than the background REM pattern. (In these respects, sawtooth waves

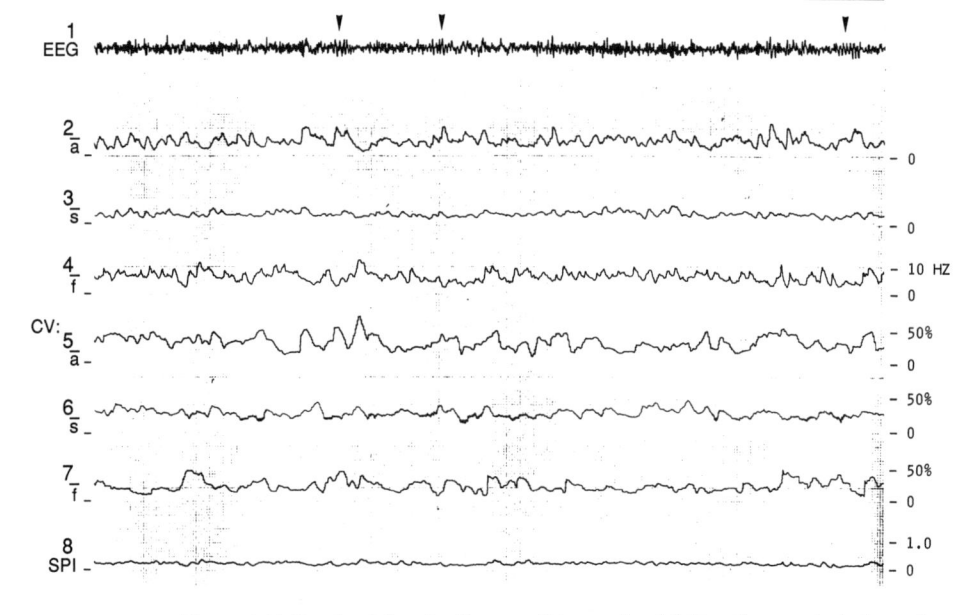

Figure 6.11 Bursts of "sawtooth waves" (arrows) exhibiting the constant-slope phenomenon during REM sleep in a positive Multiple Sleep Latency Test. Note the relative constancy of the running mean slope (trace 3) as compared with the abrupt increases in the running mean amplitude (trace 2) when the "sawtooth waves" appear (arrows). The respective Coefficients of Variation (traces 5 and 6) reflect these effects: generally little change in the Coefficient of Variation for the running mean slope, in contrast to a greater change for the running mean amplitude. The running mean frequency (trace 4) tends to decrease when there are sawtooth waves. The Spectral Purity Index (trace 8) remains relatively constant in the range 0.2–0.4.

can be contrasted with the vertex sharp waves of Stage 2 non-REM sleep, which are of higher voltage but of approximately the same frequency as the background EEG activity during Stage 2 sleep.) The occurrence of sawtooth waves is indicated at the top of figure 6.9, and the associated decrease in running mean frequency is evident in trace 6.

However, when there were sawtooth waves (in some instances, the appearance is more that of triangular waves), the constant-slope effect could be apparent. This is shown in figure 6.11, which is made up of the analysis of REM-sleep episodes from a positive Multiple Sleep Latency (EEG) Test. The constant-slope effect is evident from comparison of the running mean amplitude and the running mean slope during each of the episodes of sawtooth waves (marked by the arrows at the top). The effect is also evident from the relative absence of change of the Coefficient of Variation for the running mean slope, as contrasted with the abrupt increases in the Coefficient of Variation for the running mean amplitude. These instances of relatively constant slope during REM sleep could raise the question of whether sawtooth waves represent "islands" of non-REM sleep in a "sea" of REM sleep.

In summary: These analyses of the EEG waves during REM sleep did not confirm the prediction that they could be modeled by Type 4 waves of the oscillator model (i.e., complete independence of the modulations for extrema and for slope, respectively) . On the contrary, the findings indicate evidence for a constant-slope effect to some degree for the EEG during REM sleep, especially when sawtooth waves were present. Except for the latter, no clear distinction emerged between the characteristics of the EEG during REM sleep and those for the EEG during Stage 1 sleep. The latter finding should perhaps not be surprising in view of reports that the EEG of REM sleep and the EEG of Stage 1 sleep cannot be distinguished by spectra alone (Johnson 1972)— i.e., without added polygraphic measures, such as monitors of eye movements.

7 Normal and Abnormal Random Slowing in the Waking State

In this chapter, the prediction is tested that Type 1 waves of the oscillator model (i.e., waves exhibiting constant slope) could constitute a model for random or irregular slowing—in particular, for abnormal random or polymorphic delta slowing. Also included in this chapter are the results of analyses of normal hyperventilation-induced slowing, for which Type 1 waves were also predicted to be a model.

ABNORMAL RANDOM SLOWING

The primary database for testing this prediction consisted of 14 digitized clinical EEGs showing intermittent or continuous slow-wave activity, selected from a library of 65 normal and abnormal EEGs which had constituted the material for a previous study of EEG characteristics, kindly made available by Otto Creutzfeldt (see Creutzfeldt et al. 1985). Ten of these 14 EEGs were analyzed and are discussed below.

DIRECT TESTS FOR "CONSTANT SLOPE"

An example of an EEG showing intermittent pathological slowing is reproduced in figure 7.1. In addition to the more frequent instances of lower-voltage slowing, there are two occurrences of higher-voltage slowing, during which the amplitude of the EEG increases appreciably (trace 2) whereas the amplitude of its first derivative remains essentially unchanged (trace 3). Correspondingly, the running mean amplitude of the EEG increases appreciably (trace 4), but the running mean slope remains essentially unchanged (trace 5). Further, the Coefficient of Variation for the running mean slope (trace 8) is clearly less than that for the running mean amplitude (trace 7), as is confirmed by a persistently negative value for the logarithm of their quotient (trace 1). The running mean frequency (trace 6) decreases during the slow-wave episodes, and its Coefficient of Variation (trace 9) reflect these events. There is also some decrease in the Spectral Purity Index (trace 10) during the episodes of slowing, which indicates a wider distribution of frequencies during these events. (Were the slow waves truly periodic or monorhythmic, an increase in the Spectral Purity Index would have been expected, since it has a

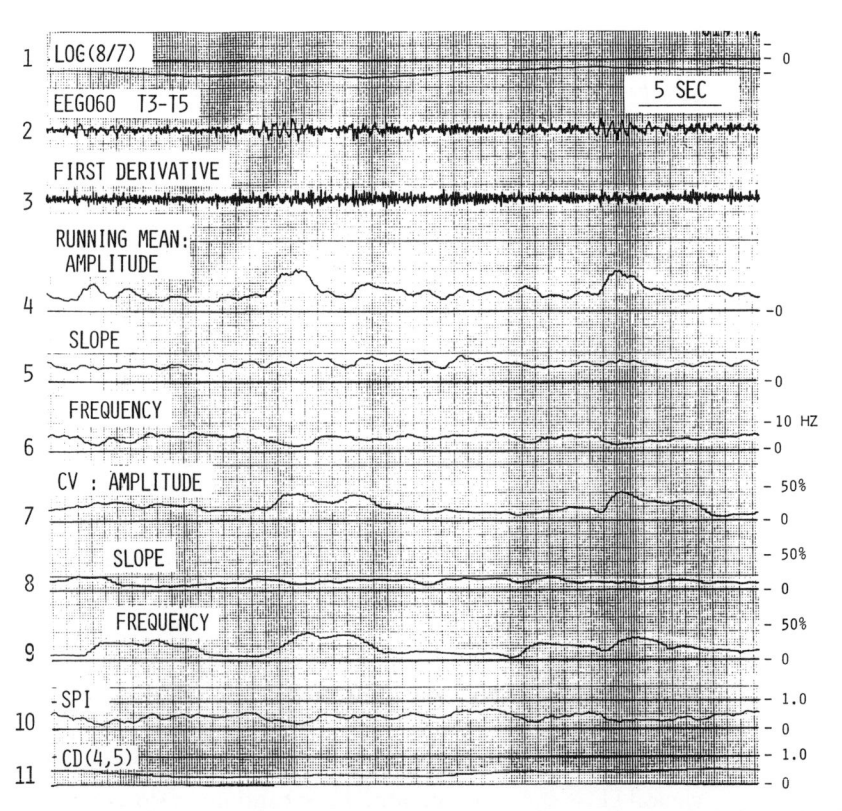

Figure 7.1 Analysis of an EEG (060) showing intermittent slowing, during which the amplitude of the EEG increases (trace 2) but the amplitude of its first derivative (trace 3) remains essentially constant. These findings are paralleled in the respective running means (traces 4 and 5), in the respective Coefficients of Variation for the latter (traces 7 and 8), and also by the negative values of the logarithm of the quotient of the latter two (trace 1). The running mean frequency (trace 6) and the Spectral Purity Index (trace 10) both decrease during the episodes of slowing.

value of 1.0 for a sine wave.) The differences between the running means for amplitude and for slope are also reflected in a value of approximately 0.5 for the Coefficient of Determination for the two (trace 11).

A second example of intermittent slowing is shown in figure 7.2. Again, when there are episodes of slowing with an increase in amplitude of the EEG itself (trace 2) there is relatively little change in the amplitude of its first derivative (trace 3). These findings are also reflected in the respective running means (traces 4 and 5), in the respective Coefficients of Variation (traces 7 and 8), and in the persistently negative value of the log of their ratio (trace 1). The running mean frequency (trace 6) decreases during the intervals of slowing, and these changes are reflected in its Coefficient of Variation (trace 8). The Spectral Purity Index (trace 9) shows a tendency to decrease during the slowing.

Another example of abnormal irregular slowing is shown in figure 7.3. During the periods of prominent slowing, the amplitude of the EEG (trace 2) increases appreciably, as does its running mean (trace 4), but the amplitude of the first derivative of the EEG (trace 3) remains relatively unchanged, as does

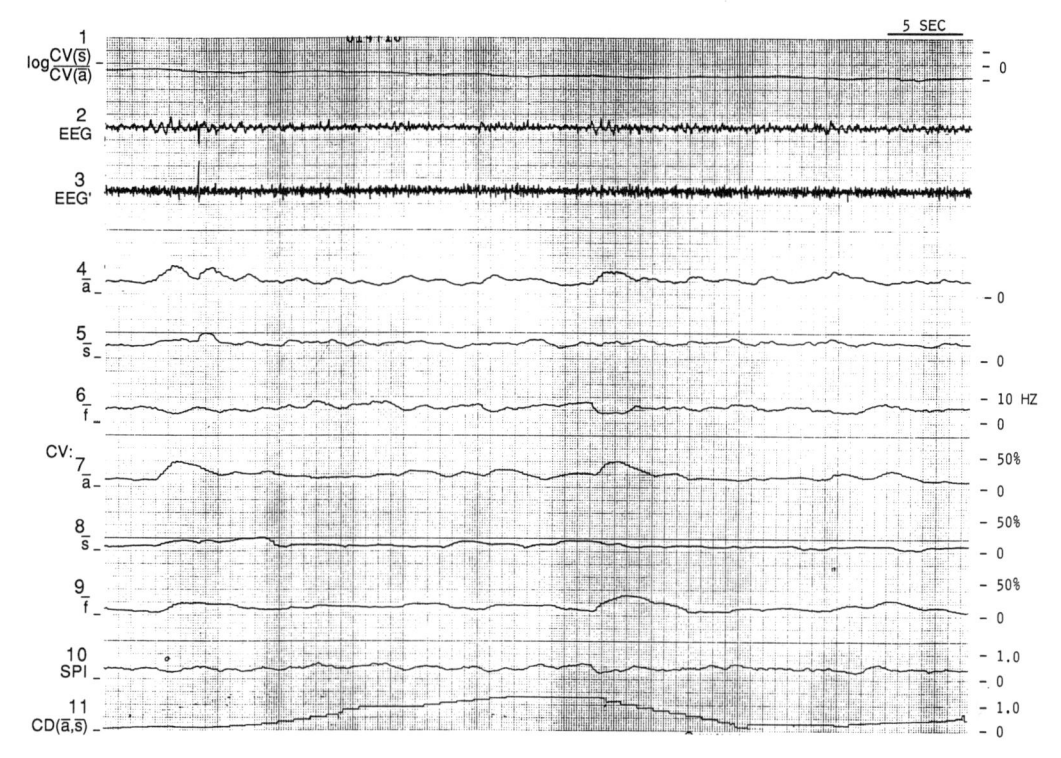

Figure 7.2 EEG (039) showing changes similar to those of figure 7.1 during the slow-wave episodes. The amplitude of the EEG (trace 2), its running mean (trace 4), and the Coefficient of Variation (trace 7) of the latter increase during the slow-wave bursts, whereas the amplitude of its first derivative (trace 3) and its running mean (trace 5), and the Coefficient of Variation of the latter (trace 8) remain essentially constant. Overall, the variability of slope is less than that of amplitude (trace 1). The running mean frequency (trace 6), and its Coefficient of Variation (trace 9), reflect the slowing in the EEG. (The spike at the left in traces 1 and 2 is an artifact in the original EEG.) A value of the Coefficient of Determination for the running means of amplitude and slope exceeding 1.0 (middle of trace 11) indicates that one or the other of this pair of signals was too low during that period to yield an accurate evaluation.

its running mean (trace 5). Correspondingly, the Coefficient of Variation for the running mean amplitude (trace 7) is usually appreciably greater than that for the running mean slope (trace 8); this is confirmed in the logarithm for the quotient of the two (trace 1). The running mean frequency (trace 6) is rather variable, but tends to decrease during the episodes of higher-voltage slowing. The Spectral Purity Index (trace 10) tends to parallel the running mean frequency.

INDIRECT TESTS FOR CONSTANT SLOPE

In the direct test for constant slope, the characteristics of the first derivative of the EEG are examined, as described above. An alternative approach, as outlined in chapter 3, is to test whether amplitude and frequency of the EEG appear to be inversely related, i.e., whether the amplitude of individual waves

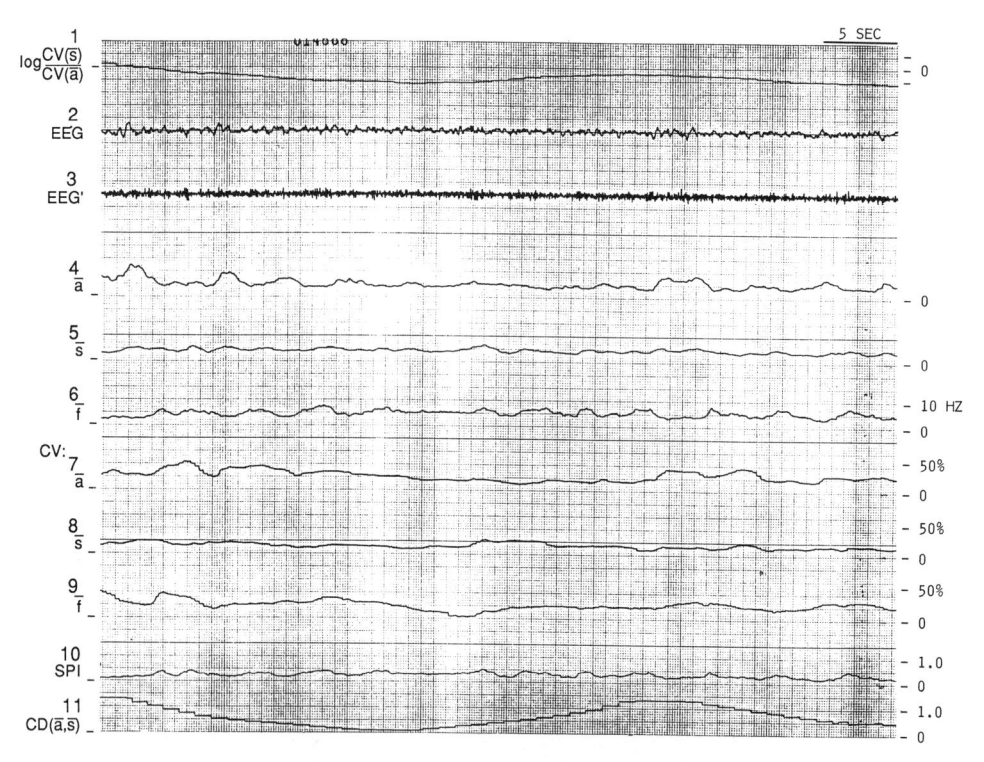

Figure 7.3 EEG (008) showing changes similar to those in figures 7.1 and 7.2 during slowing. As in figure 7.2, error signals (values greater than 1.0) appear in trace 11 (the Coefficient of Determination for the running means of amplitude and slope).

has a $1/f$ characteristic. For this approach, explicit information concerning the first derivative of the EEG is not necessary. The appropriate test for such a relationship between amplitude and frequency is to determine whether a log-log plot of amplitude vs. frequency approximates a straight line. This approach was therefore used with the Göttingen Library of clinical EEGs, for which information about amplitude and frequency was available but not information about slope. For clarity and completeness, the several steps of the original analyses (Bodenstein et al. 1985; Creutzfeldt et al. 1985) and the supplementary tests carried out for the present study will be described in sequence.

An example of the segmentation of an EEGs is shown in figure 7.4. As was mentioned in chapter 5, the boundaries between different patterns of activity appearing within a given channel were identified and demarcated by computer according to predetermined criteria relating essentially to amplitude and frequency. (In actual practice, segmentation was carried out on the basis of five-point autocorrelation functions computed with lag steps of 20 msec.) The location of the center of each of the numbered circles in figure 7.5 corresponds to the amplitude and frequency of a segment (173 in all), the area of the circle being proportional to the duration of the segment.

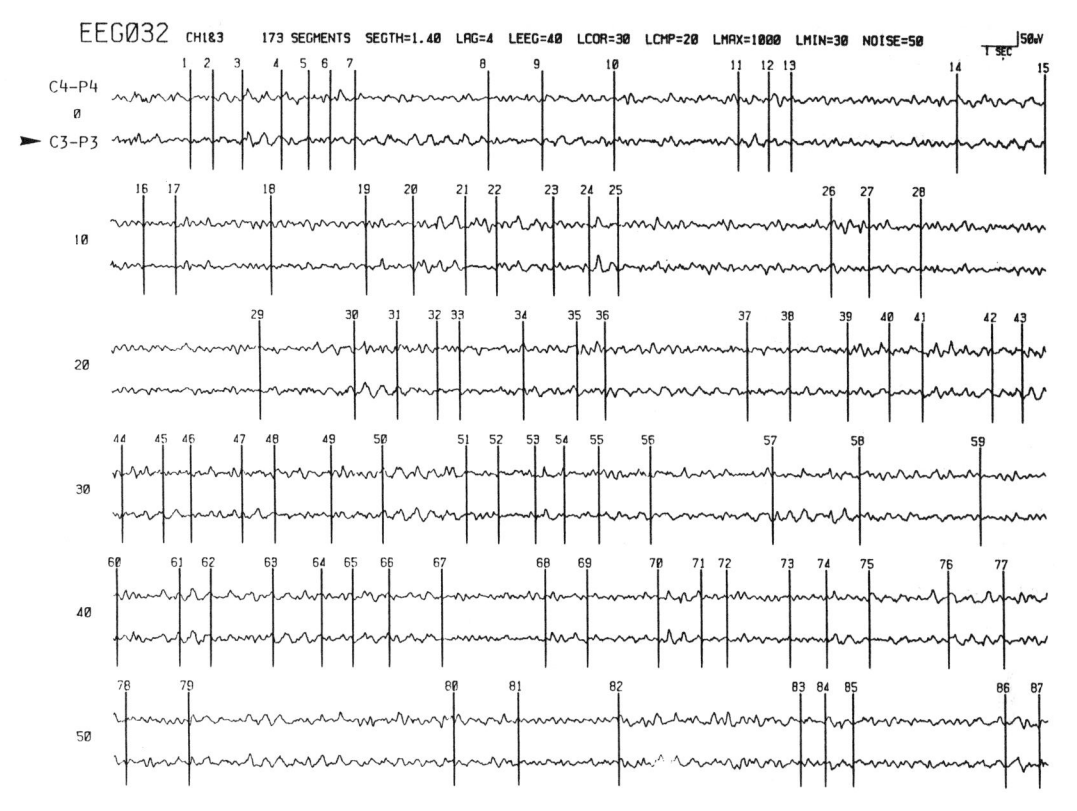

Figure 7.4 Adaptive segmentation of an EEG (032) showing frequent bursts of slow waves. The two channels (C3–P3 and C4–P4) were segmented jointly, i.e., if either channel exceeded the predetermined limits of percentage change of amplitude and/or frequency.

A scatter plot of mean amplitude vs. mean frequency for each segment (such as that shown in figure 7.5, in which the areas of the circles correspond to the durations of the respective segment) should be distinguished from the continuous curve of a power (density) spectral plot, which uses the same coordinate system of log power vs. frequency as the aforementioned scatter plot. An increased preponderance in a recording of EEG activity in the vicinity of a given frequency results, in the scatter plot, in an increased density of points (circles) and/or larger circles, corresponding to segments the mean frequency of which falls at that frequency in the plot, thus reflecting an increased probability of occurrence of activity at that frequency. In the power (density) spectrum, however, an increase in activity at a given frequency results in an increased height of the portion of the curve corresponding to that frequency. Thus, on the scatter plot of mean amplitude vs. mean frequency it is possible to establish a trend of amplitude vs. frequency (as for figure 7.5), whereas it is not possible to establish such a trend from power spectral curves. Further, by constructing contour plots of the densities of points (weighted for duration) from the scatter plots (i.e., two-dimensional representations of probability density functions), different types of EEG activity within a single recording can be classified (clustered) according to the resultant peaks in the

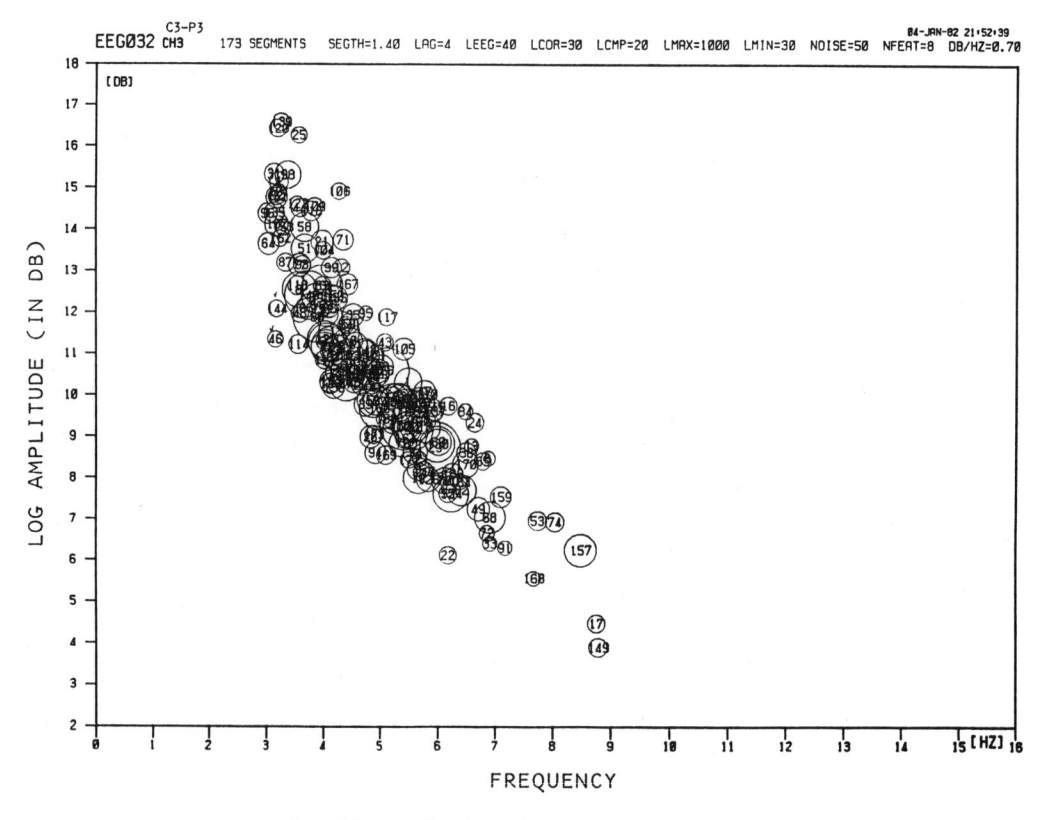

Figure 7.5 Plot of log amplitude vs. frequency (i.e., a semilog plot) for the segments of the second channel (C3–P3, marked by the arrow) of figure 7.4. Note that the trend of the points (circles) is not linear, tending to curve upward at the left.

probability density function (Bodenstein et al. 1985; Creutzfeldt et al. 1985). In short, the scatter plot permits activity of a given frequency to be sorted according to amplitude (which is essential for the present purpose of determining the relationship between amplitude and frequency), whereas such a sorting is not possible in the spectral plot, since all activity at a given frequency is lumped together, irrespective of amplitude. The spectral plot can thus be considered to represent, approximately, a plot of the integral or summation, over all amplitudes, for a given frequency in the scatter plot. The qualification "approximately" is added since the points (circles) in the scatter plots themselves represent mean amplitudes and mean frequencies for the individual segments so represented.

In order to convert the semilog plot of amplitude vs. frequency to the required log-log plot of amplitude vs. frequency, a smooth curve was drawn through the data points of figure 7.5; from the resulting curve, four sample points were then selected for replotting with log-log coordinates. The manual replotting was necesssary because the original computer processing of this series of EEGs (which was carried out for the purpose of EEG pattern classification) included plots of log amplitude vs. frequency but only a very few plots of log amplitude vs. log frequency. The results from one of the exceptions in which both types of plots were made are shown in figure 7.6, from which it is evident that the trend of the points of the plot of log amplitude vs. log frequency appears to be more nearly linear than that of the semilog plot.

The plot of log amplitude vs. log frequency for the four points on the line drawn through the data in figure 7.5 is shown in figure 7.7, from which it is evident that the sequence of points describes a straight line. (Actually, the line included in the figure has a slope of -1, which would characterize data points if amplitude were indeed inversely proportional to frequency.)

The same procedure was carried out for five additional slow-wave EEGs, and the results for all six EEGs are shown on a log-log plot in figure 7.8. The dashed line in the figure is the same as the one in figure 7.7; the remaining two lines are parallel to it and have been added to facilitate inspection of the results. It is evident that the sets of points for the individual EEGs exhibit much the same slope as the lines, differing largely only in their vertical position. (The latter would correspond to the constant of proportionality between amplitude and frequency.)

From figure 7.8 it is evident that the amplitude of the slow waves in these EEGs was inversely proportional to their frequency, or, equivalently expressed, the amplitude of the individual slow waves (more exactly, the slow waves in a given segment) was directly proportional to their duration or period. This is equivalent to stating that the irregular slowing in these six EEGs was of the constant-slope type—i.e., that these EEGs can be modeled by Type 1 waves of the oscillator-modulator.

MIXED RANDOM AND RHYTHMIC SLOWING: EPILEPTIFORM SLOW-WAVE ACTIVITY

In the results shown in figure 7.8, the constant-slope feature was evident throughout the entire range of amplitudes and frequencies; i.e., the slope of the data points for a given EEG was almost always parallel to a line corresponding to a reciprocal relationship between amplitude and frequency. In another, smaller group of EEGs, this feature was evident for all but the lowest frequencies; for the latter, a different behavior was apparent. An illustrative example is shown in figure 7.9. For this EEG, the amplitude of the first derivative (trace 3) tends to parallel that of the EEG itself (trace 2), as do the respective running means (traces 5 and 4), especially during the high-voltage bursts at the right in figure 7.9. The Coefficient of Variation (trace 8) for the running mean slope, however, is generally less than that for the running mean amplitude (which suggests a tendency toward a constant-slope effect), except during the high-amplitude rhythmic bursts. During the latter (for which the mean running frequency, trace 6, decreases somewhat), the two Coefficients of Variation are rather similar. Clearly, these high-voltage slow-wave paroxysms cannot be characterized as being random and having a constant slope; they are, in fact, rhythmic, or at least quasi-rhythmic, for the most part.

92 Chapter 7

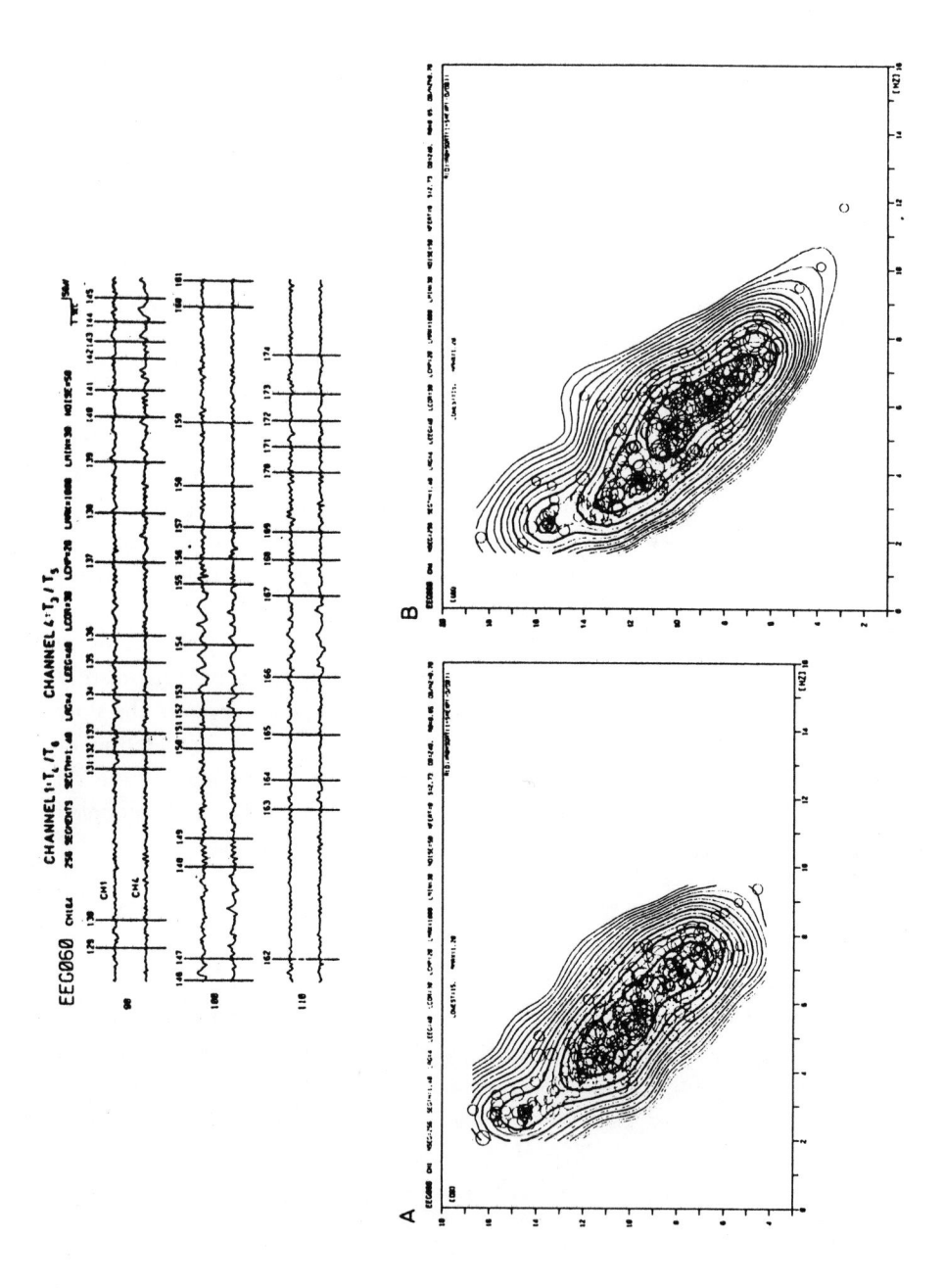

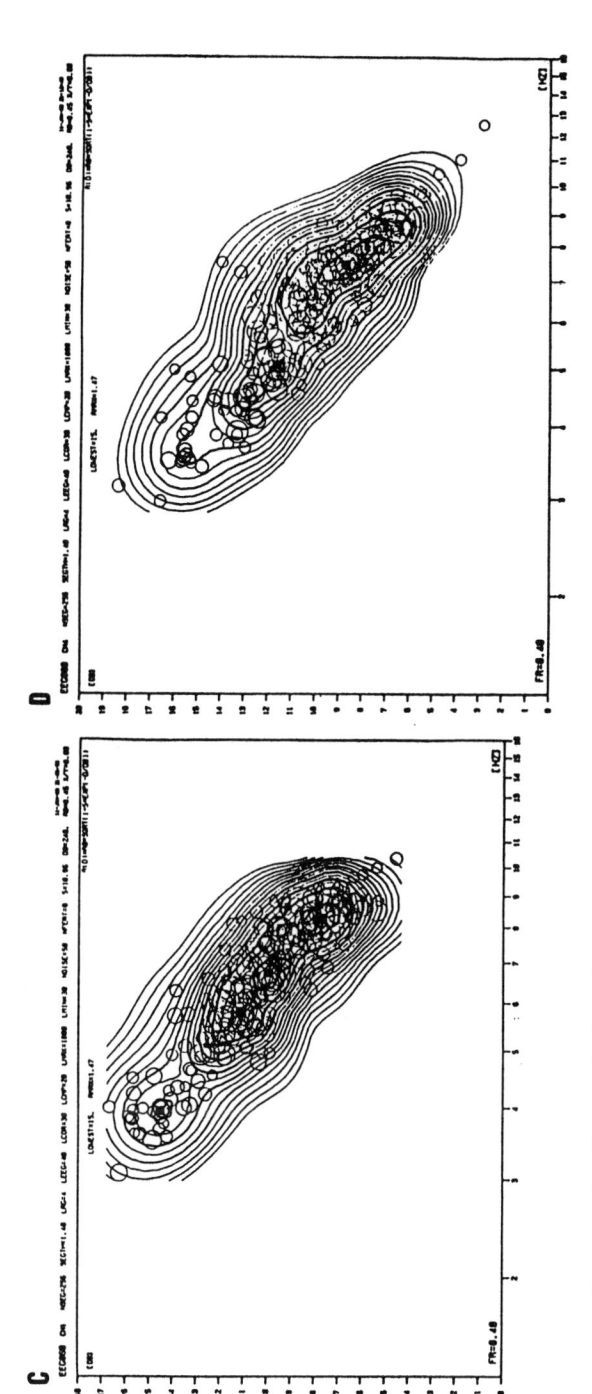

Figure 7.6 Computer plot of log amplitude vs. frequency (upper pair of probability-density contour plots) and log amplitude vs. log frequency (lower pair of contour plots) for an EEG (060) exhibiting irregular slowing, excerpts from which are shown at the top. Note that the trend of the data in the plot of log amplitude vs. log frequency appears to be more linear than that for the plot of log amplitude vs. frequency.

Random Slowing in the Waking State

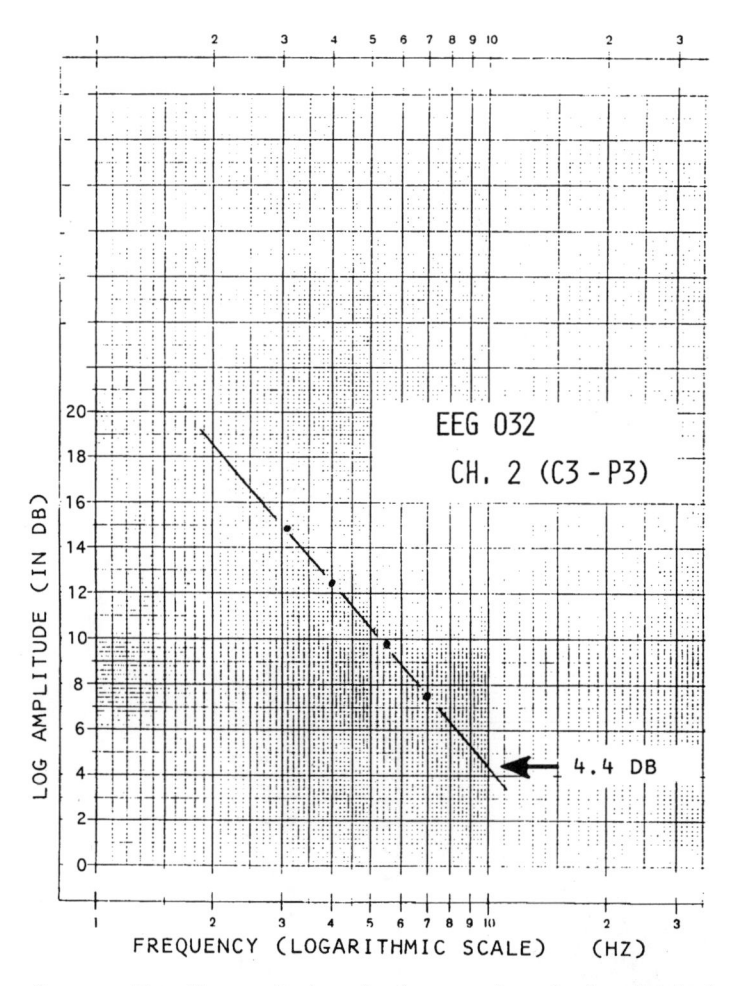

Figure 7.7 Plot of log amplitude vs. log frequency (i.e., a log-log plot) for four sample points selected from a smooth curve drawn through the data points of figure 7.5 (EEG 032). The straight line has a slope that would occur if amplitude were inversely proportional to frequency. (The amplitude at 10 Hz is seen to fall at 4.4 on the dB scale.)

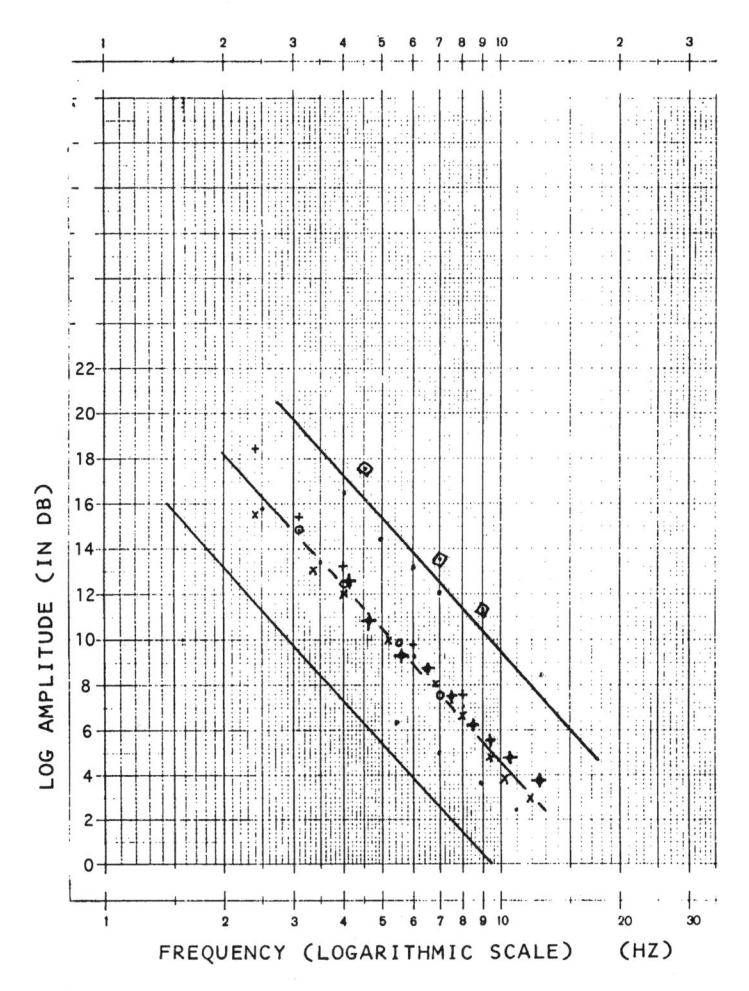

Figure 7.8 A plot of log amplitude vs. log frequency similar to that of figure 7.7 but for the EEG of figure 7.7 together with five additional EEGs. The dashed line is the same as the one in figure 7.7; the additional two lines, which are parallel to the first, are included to facilitate viewing the data points. Note that the data points for the individual EEGs are essentially parallel to the lines, indicating that amplitude and frequency were inversely related for these six EEGs.

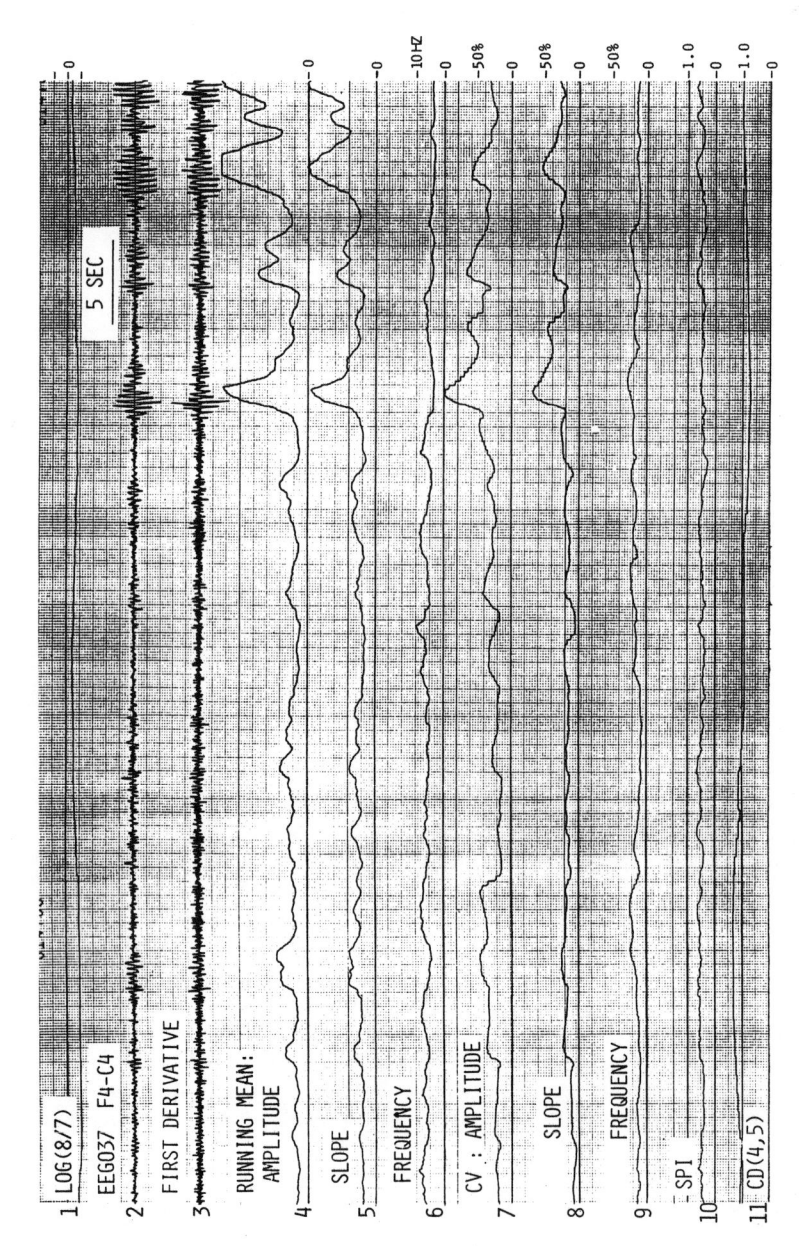

Figure 7.9 Analysis of an EEG (037) showing both a constant-slope effect (note the lower Coefficient of Variation for the running mean slope (trace 8) than for that of the running mean amplitude (trace 7)) and a constant-frequency effect (trace 6), the latter when there are high-voltage rhythmic waves. Note the relatively small change in the Coefficient of Variation (trace 8) for the running mean frequency (trace 6) during the transitions between the two patterns. (In this instance, the averaging times for the logarithm of the quotient of the Coefficients of Variation for slope and for amplitude (trace 1) and for the Coefficient of Determination for the running means of slope and amplitude (trace 11) were too long to reflect the transitions between the two patterns.)

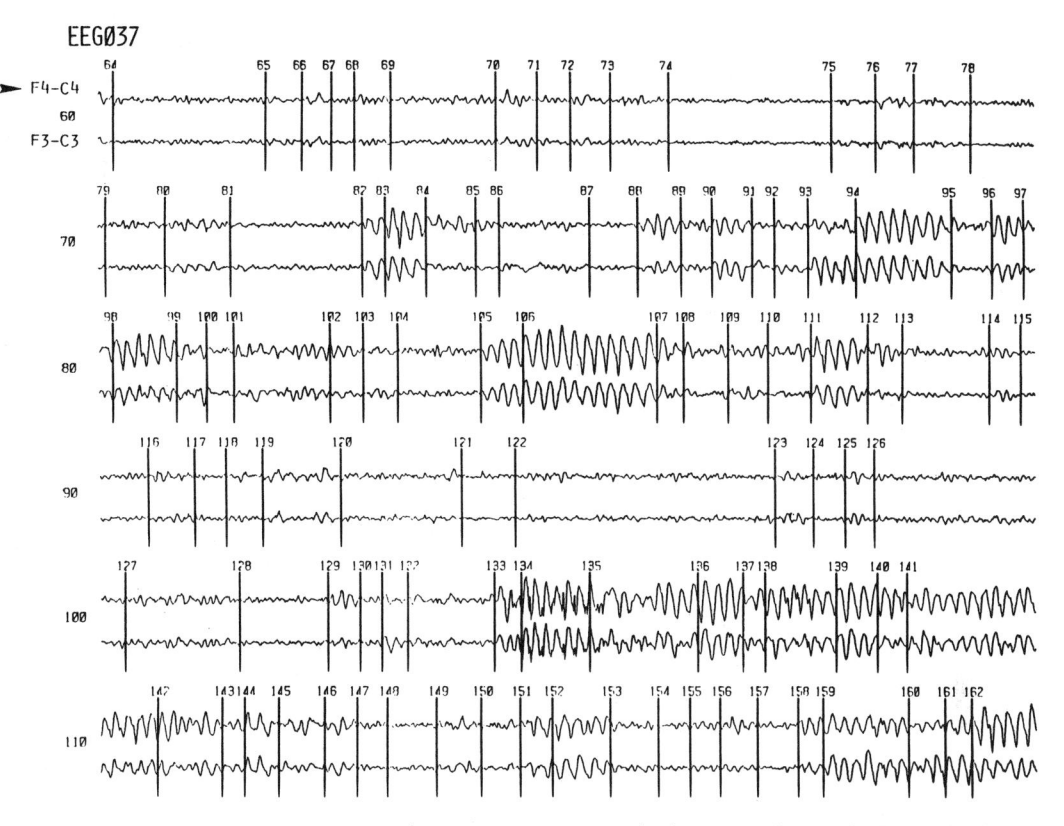

Figure 7.10 Segmented EEG (037, same EEG as for figure 7.9), showing both irregular slowing and high-voltage rhythmic bursts (segments 82 and 83 are the same as the first high-voltage burst on the right in figure 7.9). In segment 135, spike components are evident.

This same EEG (037), adaptively segmented, is shown in figure 7.10. The semilog plot of amplitude and frequency for all the segments from this recording is shown in figure 7.11, from which an extremely steep trend is apparent for the segments having the lower frequencies. Figure 7.12 shows a log-log plot of points selected along a smooth curve fitted to figure 7.11. From figure 7.12 it is evident that the trend of amplitude vs. frequencies for the higher frequencies is much the same as in figure 7.8 (the dashed line in figure 7.12 has the same slope as the one in figure 7.8); as the frequency decreases, however, the sample points diverge increasingly from the straight line. (This divergence is associated with the high-voltage slow waves in the EEG, not with spike components. (Segment 135 in figure 7.9, which is outlying in figure 7.11 (upper left) because of its spike components, is not included in the trend of the points in figure 7.10.)

The points for this EEG are shown in figure 7.13 together with those from three additional EEGs that also exhibited such a divergence at the lower frequencies. For each of the four patients from whom these EEGs were recorded, a clinical diagnosis of epilepsy had been made. From figure 7.13 it is apparent that the points cluster about a line corresponding to constant slope

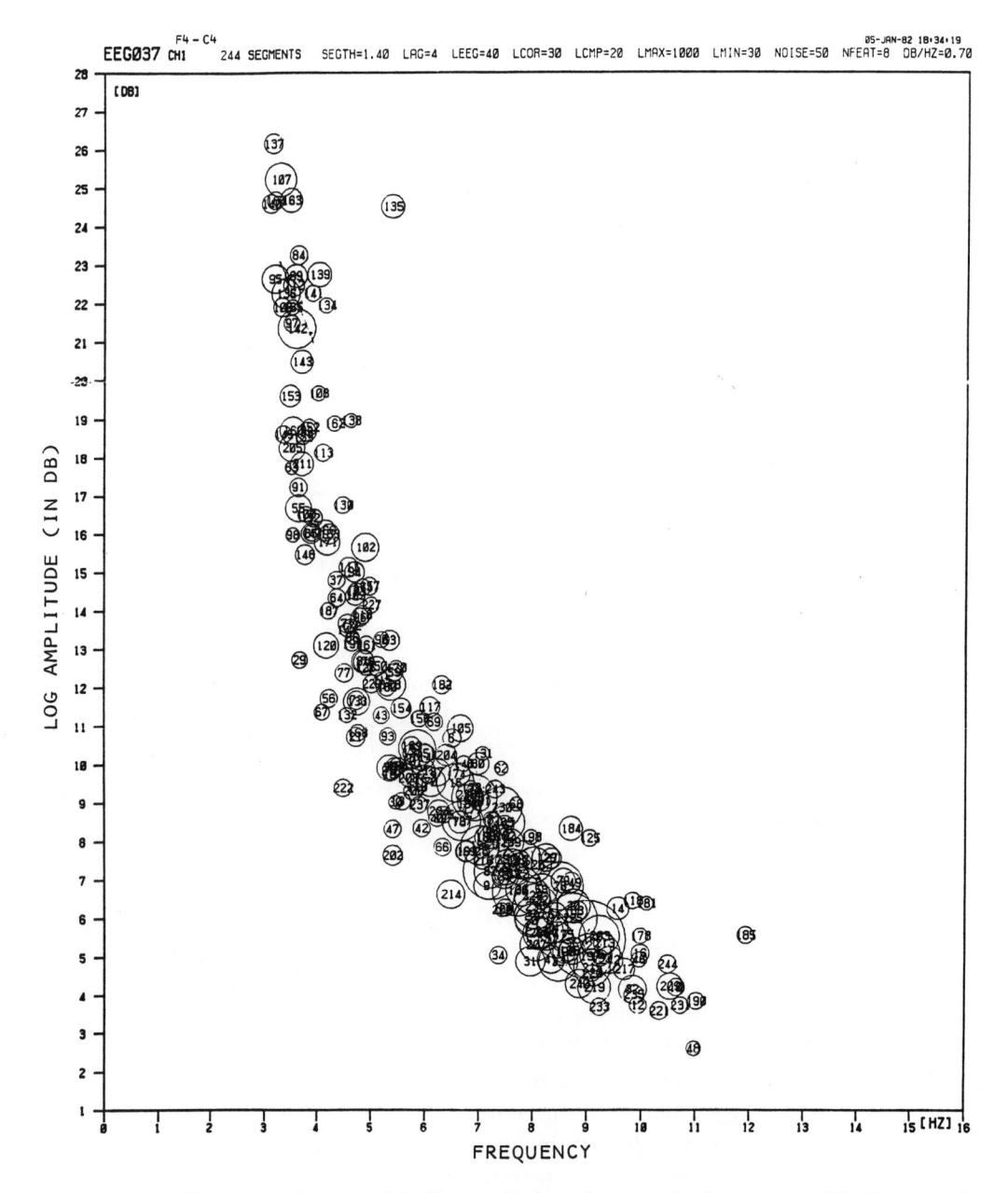

Figure 7.11 Computer plot of log amplitude vs. frequency for the segments of the first channel (F4–C4) of figure 7.10. Note the steep trend of the points at the upper left. Note also the outlying point for segment 135, in which there are spike components (lower middle of figure 7.10).

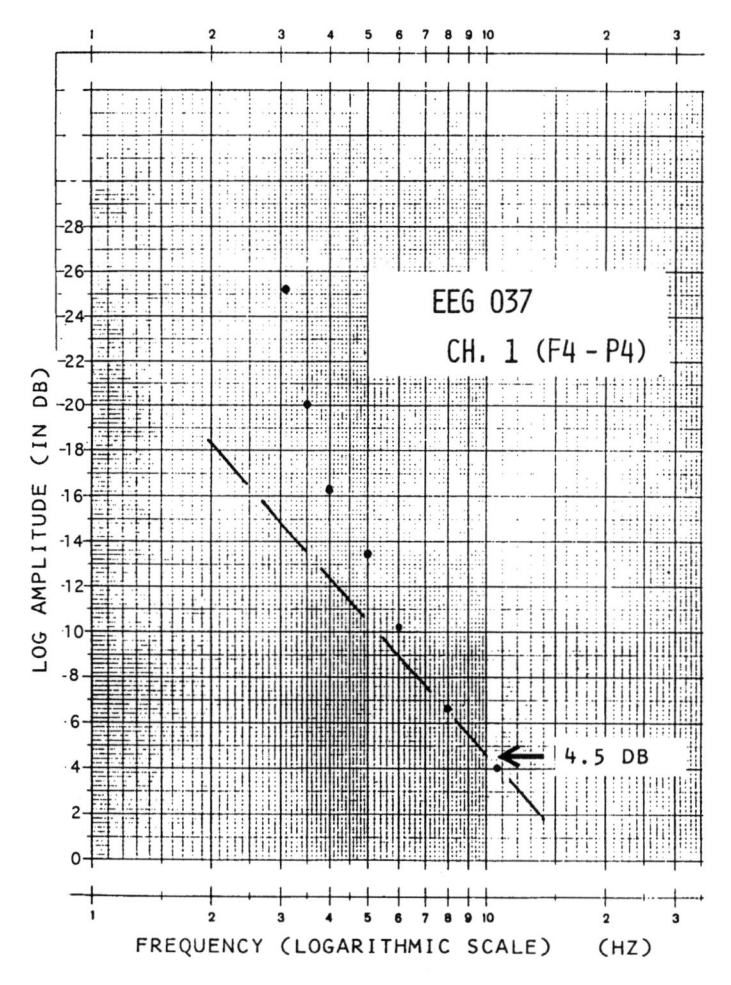

Figure 7.12 Plot of log amplitude vs. log frequency for seven sample points taken from a smooth curve drawn through the data points (excluding that for segment 135) of figure 7.11. The broken line has the same slope as in the previous log-log plots; it has a slope that would occur if amplitude were inversely proportional to frequency.

only for frequencies higher than about 5 Hz. For lower frequencies, the points appear to approach asymptotically a vertical line corresponding to a frequency of close to 3 Hz. (A vertical line on such a plot would indicate truly rhythmic activity, since in that case waves of different amplitude all have the same frequency.)

In summary: The prediction of constant slope for pathological random EEG slowing was tested on ten clinical EEGs. The analyses of six of these EEGs provided confirmatory evidence for the constant-slope prediction (i.e., that the waves in these EEGs could be modeled by Type 1 waves of the oscillator model). For four of the EEGs, however, all of which were from patients having a clinical diagnosis of epilepsy, the constant-slope characteristic was evident only for the lower amplitudes and the higher frequencies. As amplitude progressively increased, a transition from constant-slope to constant-frequency

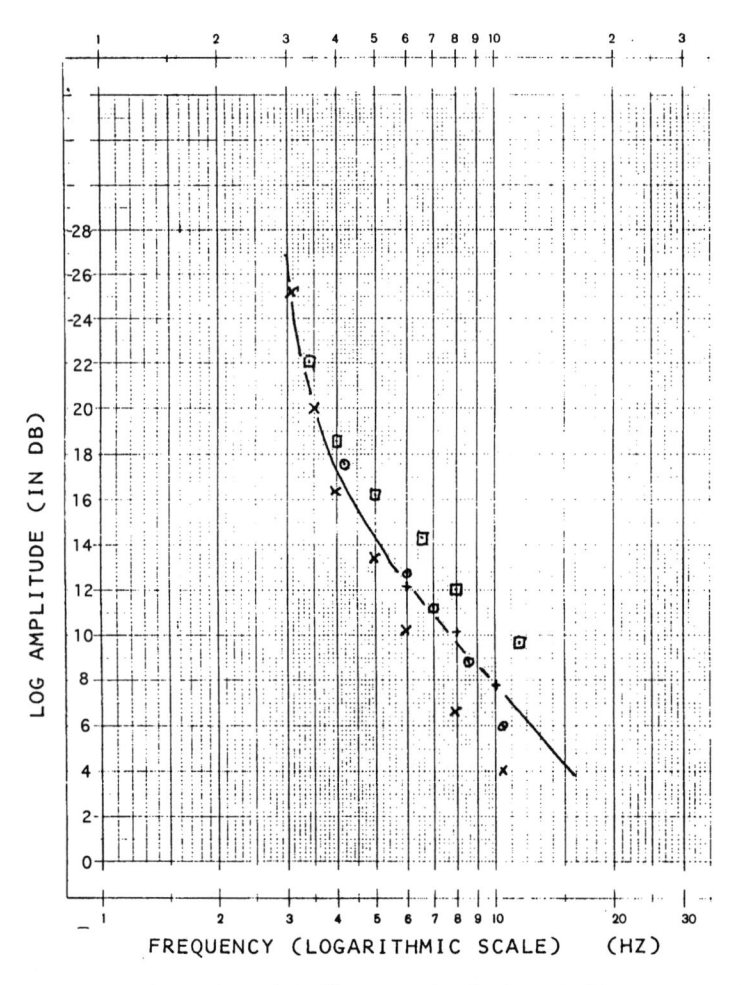

Figure 7.13 Plot similar to that of figure 7.12, but for the EEG of figure 7.12 together with three additional EEGs. Only the initial portion (lower right) of the inscribed curve has the same slope as in figure 7.12 (and in previous log-log plots); the remainder of the curve was drawn to fit the data points for the four EEGs.

waves (i.e., rhythmic activity) occurred, corresponding to a transition from Type 1 to Type 3 waves of the oscillator model. Whether this effect might serve as a possible indication of the presence of subtle EEG indications of a predisposition to epilepsy is discussed in chapter 17.

NORMAL HYPERVENTILATION-INDUCED SLOWING

Hyperventilation is an activating procedure used to induce abnormalities or to enhance existing (minimal) abnormalities, such as epileptiform activity or focal slowing; however, it can also result in generalized slowing of the EEG as a normal finding, particularly in children, adolescents, and young adults (Takahashi 1987; Kellaway 1990). In chapter 3 it was suggested that Type 1 waves (i.e., waves of constant slope) might be a model for the slow waves that

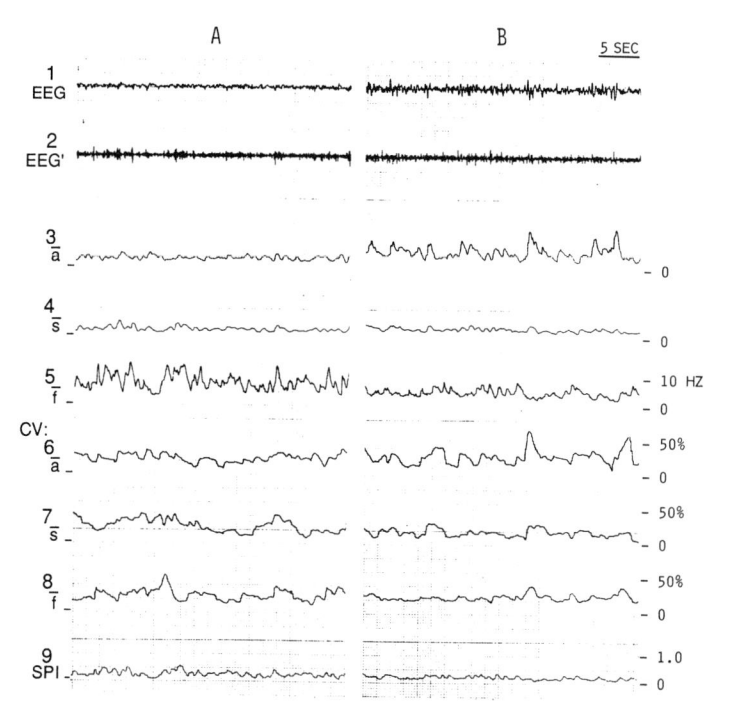

Figure 7.14 Analysis of the slowing induced by hyperventilation in a young adult (B). Results for the baseline recording are shown in A. With hyperventilation, relatively high-voltage slow waves appear (trace 1), but the first derivative of the EEG changes (trace 2) relatively little. The Coefficient of Variation for the running mean amplitude (trace 6) generally increases with hyperventilation, but that for the running mean slope (trace 7) remains much the same. As expected, the running mean frequency (trace 5) decreases (from about 8 Hz to about 3–5 Hz), amid appreciable fluctuations. The Spectral Purity Index (trace 9) decreases from about 0.35 to about 0.2.

may appear as a normal response to hyperventilation. The results of the analyses of two EEGs in which this prediction was examined are shown in figures 7.14 and 7.15.

In figure 7.14A, low-voltage irregular activity is evident at the beginning of hyperventilation (trace 1), and the running means of amplitude and slope (traces 3 and 4) are at about the same level on the arbitrary scale as their Coefficients of Variation (traces 6 and 7). The running mean frequency (trace 5) is rather variable (note the frequency calibration), and the Spectral Purity Index (trace 9) fluctuates between 0.2 and 0.5. During the third minute of hyperventilation (figure 14B), the amplitude of the EEG and its running mean (traces 1 and 3, respectively) have increased appreciably, as has the Coefficient of Variation of the running mean amplitude (trace 6). However, the first derivative of the EEG (trace 2) and its running mean (trace 4), and the Coefficient of Variation of the latter (trace 7), show relatively little change. There is also little change in the Spectral Purity Index (trace 9). These findings are consistent with a relatively constant slope of the EEG during hyperventilation for this EEG. Figure 7.15, for another EEG, shows much the same changes with

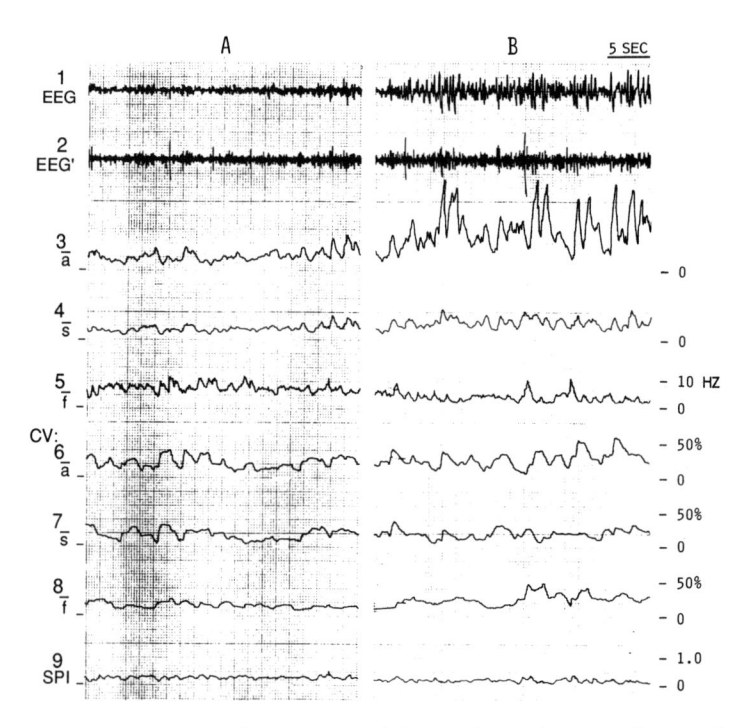

Figure 7.15 Hyperventilation-associated changes for another EEG, showing changes similar to those of figure 7.14.

hyperventilation as in figure 7.14 for the running mean amplitude and the running mean slope, and also for their Coefficients of Variation.

In summary: The analyses of these two EEGs, and of another not shown, provide corroborative evidence for the prediction that EEG slowing during hyperventilation is of the constant-slope type.

8 Epileptiform Patterns

Epileptiform patterns of two types will be considered here: the 3-Hz spike-wave pattern of primary generalized epilepsy and the spike-and-slow-wave complex of focal epilepsy.

In chapter 2 it was suggested that Type 2 waves of the oscillator model (i.e., waves of relatively constant amplitude but variable slope) might serve as a model for certain types of epileptiform patterns, specifically the 3-Hz spike-wave pattern.

THREE-HZ SPIKE-WAVE ACTIVITY AS A CONSTANT-AMPLITUDE VARIABLE-SLOPE PATTERN

As was pointed out in chapter 2, waves of constant extrema but variable slopes are equivalent to simple frequency modulation of the waves (as in the frequency-modulated output of a conventional voltage-controlled oscillator). If the input modulation is removed, such waves will continue to oscillate at the center or unmodulated frequency, which will ordinarily be at the midpoint of the extremes of the frequency swings. Thus, a wave having a frequency of 10 Hz when unmodulated could oscillate at frequencies ranging from, e.g., 5 Hz to 15 Hz.

As was mentioned in the introduction, one of the earliest observations in connection with the present work (i.e., during the testing of the electronic circuit for deriving the running mean frequency) was that the running mean frequency of the very first test EEG appeared to change rather little (figure 8.1), remaining within ± 2 Hz during brief bursts of 3-Hz spike-wave activity appearing amid a normal background of 9-Hz alpha activity. In contrast, the running mean amplitude and the running mean slope both increased appreciably. The results of a later reanalysis of this EEG are shown in figure 8.2. In that instance, the averaging window of 0.5 sec for the running mean frequency was longer than that of a single spike-wave event (of about 0.3 sec), the duration of the entire bursts being of the same order as the averaging window. This incidental finding suggested that the mean frequency during the spike-wave bursts was about the same as that of the background alpha activity. (It may at first sight appear surprising that the Spectral Purity Index in figure 8.2 (trace 9) remains relatively unchanged during the spike-wave event,

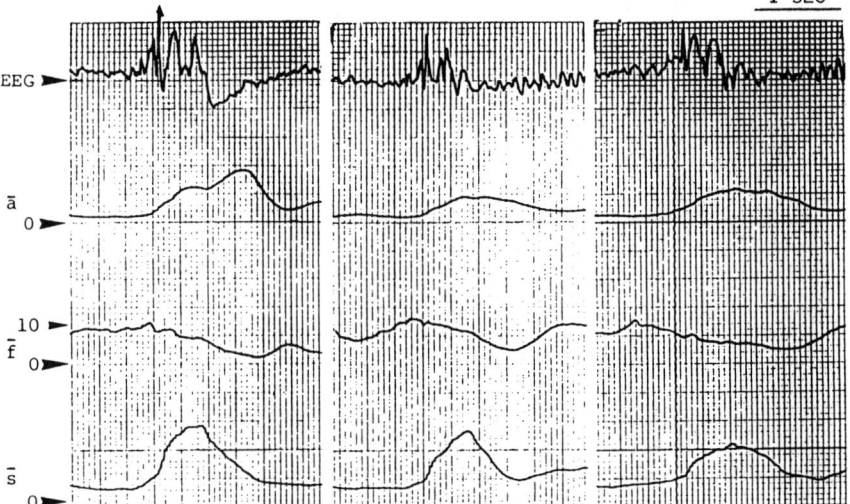

Figure 8.1 Analysis of an EEG showing brief 3-Hz spike-wave bursts, during which the running mean frequency changes rather little, in contrast to appreciable changes in the running mean amplitude and the running mean slope. In this early analysis, the running mean frequency (trace 3) was placed between the running mean amplitude (trace 2) and the running mean slope (trace 4). Time calibration: 1 sec. Averaging window for running means: 0.5 sec.

since the latter implies a wide swing of the instantaneous frequency (high for the spike, low for the wave). The Spectral Purity Index, however, reflects primarily frequencies that are *simultaneously* present, rather than those that are sequentially present, as is essentially the case for the spike-wave sequence (chapter 25).

The above-described finding that the mean frequency during a 3-Hz spike-wave burst may differ little from that of the background EEG was independently corroborated from a re-review of the results of analysis by adaptive segmentation of two recordings from the Göttingen library of clinical EEGs. A portion of one of these segmented EEGs is shown at the top in figure 8.3, and the plot of log amplitude vs. frequency for all the segments is shown below, for the two channels (right and left sides). The segment during which there is 3-Hz spike-wave activity is marked by the three arrows (segment 53); the mean frequencies on the two sides for this segment, denoted in the scatter diagrams below by the arrows, are seen to be approximately the same as the mean frequencies of the preponderance of the remaining segments.

Figure 8.4 shows the second example of the similarity of the mean frequency of the EEG during a segment (denoted by arrows above and below) having a spike-wave burst of mean frequency (about 8.5 Hz) that is similar to that of the background EEG (about 8.5 Hz).

These results indicate, by two entirely independent techniques, that the mean frequency during 3-Hz spike-wave activity remains largely unchanged from the mean frequency of the background EEG, i.e., before and after the spike-wave activity. This finding appears to corroborate the prediction that

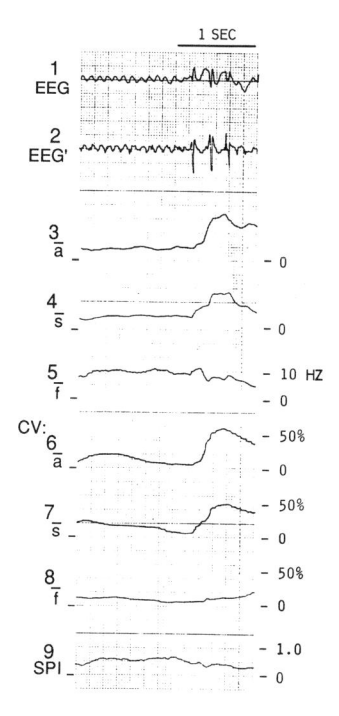

Figure 8.2 Re-analysis of the same EEG (trace 1) as shown in figure 8.1, but shown with its first derivative (trace 2) and with additional measures: running means of amplitude (trace 3), slope (trace 4—note that the spike components are enhanced), and frequency (trace 5), as well as the Coefficients of Variation of the latter (traces 6–8), and the Spectral Purity Index (trace 9). The relatively small change, during the spike-slow wave events, in the running mean frequency (as compared with the running means of amplitude and slope) is again apparent, a difference that is confirmed by the respective Coefficients of Variation (note the much smaller change in the CV for frequency than in the CV for amplitude and slope). Averaging window for the running means and for the SPI: 0.5 sec. For the Coefficients of Variation: 2 sec.

Type 2 waves of the oscillator model can serve as a model for 3-Hz spike-wave activity, or, conversely, that the 3-Hz spike-wave activity can be considered as having relatively constant amplitude but variable slope.

THE NATURE OF THE VARIATION OF THE INSTANTANEOUS ENVELOPE OF SLOPE IN THE 3-HZ SPIKE-WAVE PATTERN

In chapter 4, the 3-Hz spike-wave pattern was simulated by means of the oscillator model with output waves of constant amplitude and a simple and straightforward alternation of a high value of the slopes modulation during the spike component, changing abruptly to a low value of the slopes modulation during the wave component. Indeed, the supposed quite different mechanisms for the spike component and for the wave component (as reviewed in chapter 13) would be consistent with such a simulation. However, from close inspection of the 3-Hz spike-wave patterns of a number of clinical EEGs, the change of modulation of slopes from that for the spike to that for the wave appeared to be gradual rather than abrupt, possibly reflecting an exponential

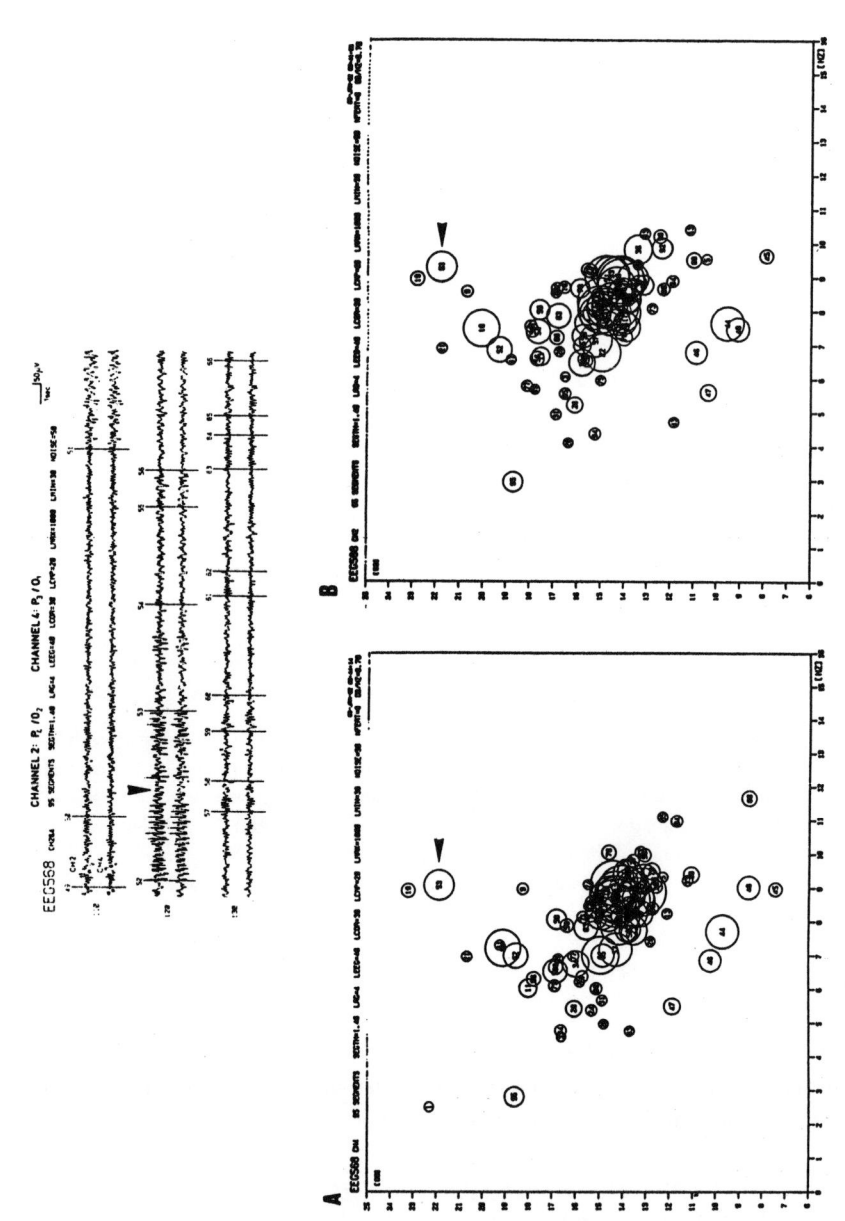

Figure 8.3 Top: portion of a segmented EEG that includes 3-Hz spike-wave activity (arrow) in one segment (No. 53). Bottom: amplitude (log power in dB) vs. frequency plots for the two sides of the scalp for all of the segments, showing that the mean frequency of the segment with the spike-wave activity (arrows) (about 9.0 Hz for the EEG on the left side of the scalp and about 9.5 for the right side) is approximately the same as the mean frequencies of the remaining segments (about 9.0 Hz on the left and about 8.5 Hz on the right, for the most dense concentration of segments). In this example, the amplitude of the spike component is somewhat greater than that of the wave component. (Bilateral parieto-occipital recordings.)

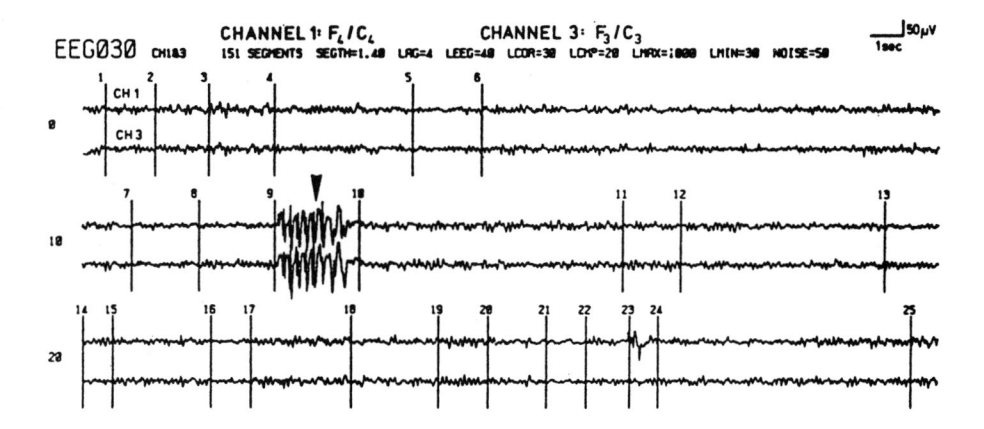

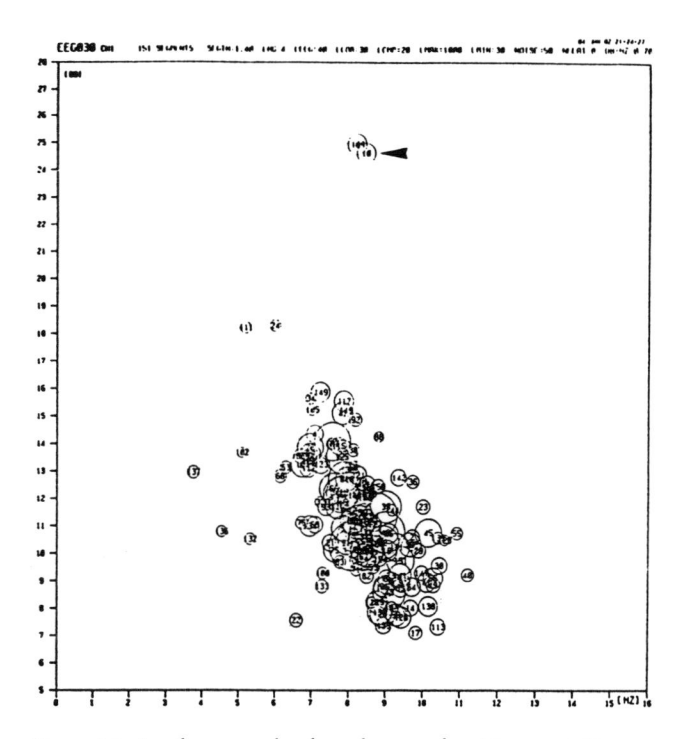

Figure 8.4 Another example of a spike-wave burst (segment 10; see arrows) having about the same mean frequency (about 8.5 Hz) as that of the background EEG activity (about 8.5 Hz). The spikes and the waves are approximately the same amplitude. (Bilateral fronto-central recordings.)

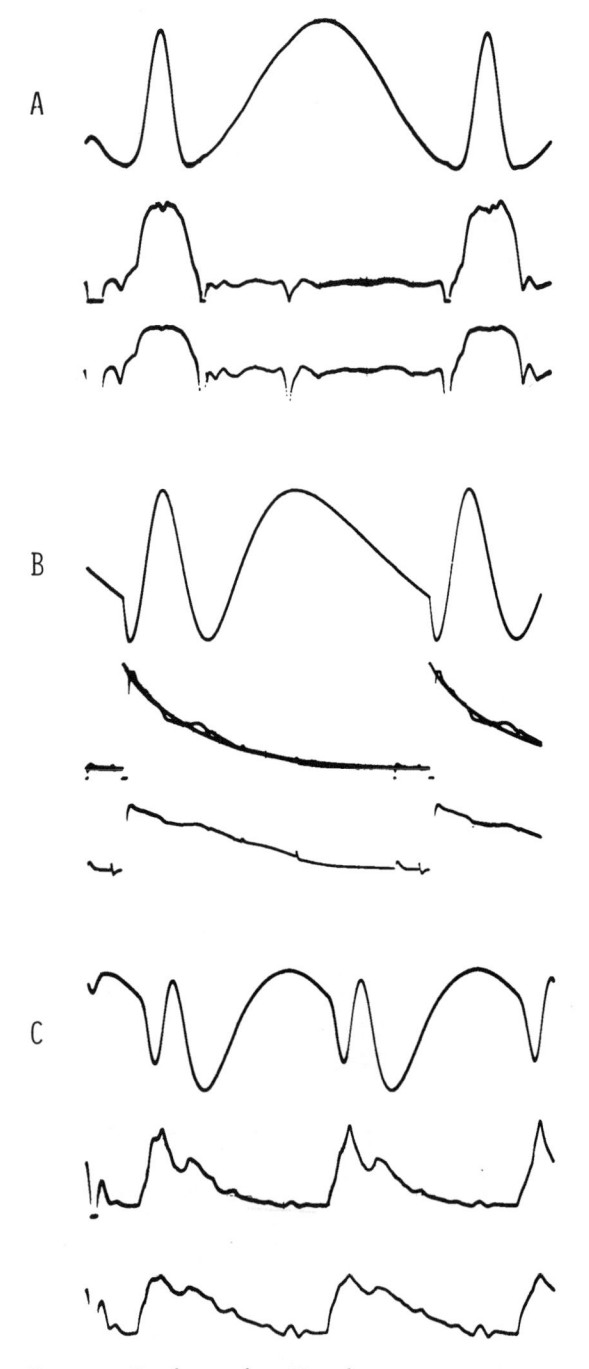

Figure 8.5 Simulation of a 3-Hz spike-wave pattern (top traces) having two different instantaneous slope characteristics: (A) a constant high instantaneous slope during the spike component, changing abruptly to a constant low instantaneous slope at the beginning of the slow-wave component; and (B) an exponential decline in the envelope of the slopes, beginning at the onset of the spike component and continuing to decrease during the slow-wave component. The envelopes of the slopes are shown in the middle traces, their logarithms in the bottom traces. Note the exponential form of the middle trace in Part B, shown as the more irregular curve (the superimposed smooth curve is the original waveform for modulating the slopes of

decrease in the slopes modulation (in the terminology of the oscillator model), at least for scalp-recorded EEGs.

As a preliminary to the analysis of actual EEGs, the two types of behavior of the modulation of slopes—an abrupt decrease and an exponential decrease—were simulated. If indeed the amplitudes of the spike component and the wave component are approximately equal, and if the modulation of the slopes decreases abruptly (i.e., in a stepwise manner) rather than exponentially, then the waveforms shown in the top trace of figure 8.5A should result. On the other hand, if the modulation of the slopes decreases exponentially, a waveform such as that shown in the top trace in figure 8.5B should result.

These two alternatives can be tested by obtaining the instantaneous envelope of the slope of the waveforms in question. In the case of the abrupt change of the envelope of the slopes, a relatively constant high value of the envelope for the slope during the spike component should result, followed by an approximately stepwise decrease occurring at the junction between the spike and the wave component, followed in turn by a relatively constant low value during the remainder of the wave component. On the other hand, if there is an exponential decay of the envelope of the slopes, a continuous, exponentially decaying curve should result for the envelope of the slopes, beginning at the onset of the spike and continuing through at least a major portion of the wave component. Further, display of the latter curve on a semilogarithmic plot should approximate a straight line.

The instantaneous envelopes (chapter 29) of the slopes (i.e., the instantaneous envelope of the first derivative), computed for the waveforms at the top in figures 8.5A and 8.5B, respectively, are shown in the second traces of the two figures. In figure 8.5A, a relatively high value of the instantaneous envelope, and of its logarithm (third trace), is evident for the spike component, followed by an abrupt transition to the low, constant value during the wave component. In figure 8.5B, in contrast, a continuous exponential decline in the instantaneous slope is evident (trace 2), the logarithm of which approximates a straight line (trace 3), as expected from such an exponential decline. In figure 8.5C, the spike component begins at an earlier phase of the slow wave than in figure 8.5B, but the curves of the instantaneous slope (trace 2) and its logarithm (trace 3) show approximately an exponential and a linear decrease, respectively, as in figure 8.5B.

The results of carrying out these tests on actual EEG recordings of 3-Hz spike-wave events will now be considered. The procedure for delineating the slope in the course of a spike-wave event included retrieval of the pattern by photo-optical scanning at a slow paper speed (to increase temporal resolu-

---

the oscillator model). Note also the linear behavior of the logarithm of the latter (bottom trace in part B). In part C, the transition from slow wave to spike begins at an earlier phase of the slow wave, with essentially the same results (note the slightly different time base). (The instantaneous envelopes of the slopes were computed as the envelopes of the first derivative of the waveforms by the method described in chapter 29.)

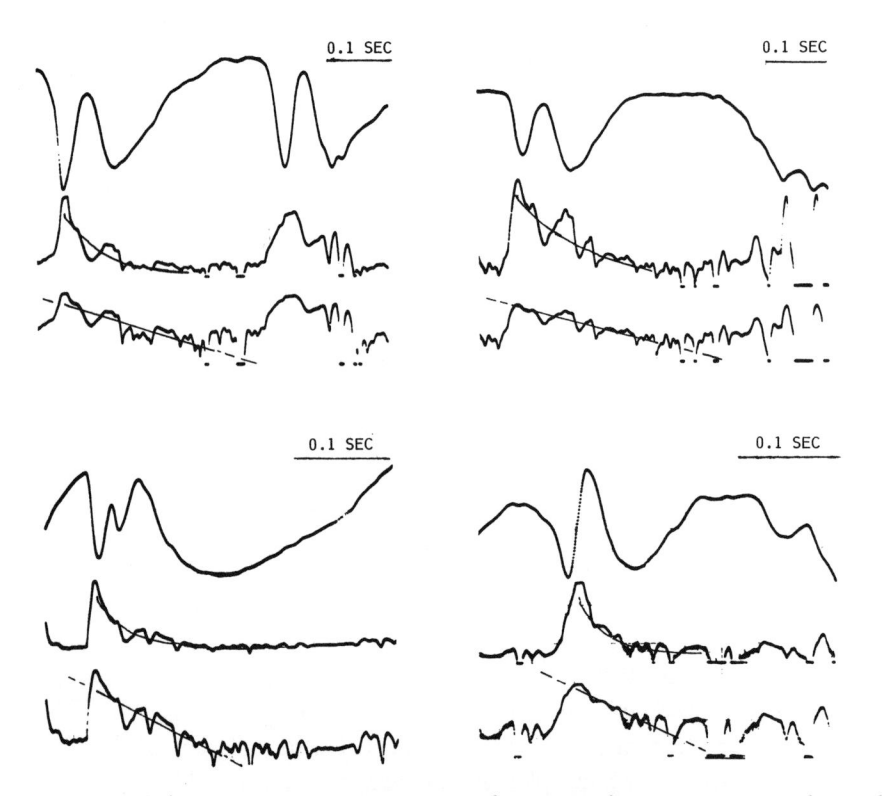

Figure 8.6 Spike-wave sequences (top trace in each instance), the instantaneous envelopes of their first derivative (middle trace), and logarithm of the latter (bottom trace), for four EEGs having 3-Hz spike-wave patterns. (The spike-wave event on the lower left is inverted in comparison with the remaining ones, but the inversion is irrelevant to the determination of the instantaneous envelope of the first derivative.) Despite some noise, the first part of each of the four instantaneous envelopes of the slope appears to decrease or decay exponentially, which, after logarithmic conversion, appears as a linear decrease. (Note that the time scale for the top two sets of curves is slightly different from that for the bottom two. The superimposed curves on the second and third traces for each of the spike-waves were drawn manually.)

tion), reading the output of the scanner into a temporary storage device, reading the latter out repetitively at a higher speed, and determining the instantaneous envelope of the first derivative of the stored waveform. (Technical details on the photo-optical scanner, the temporary (analog) storage device, and the method of deriving the instantaneous slope are given in chapters 26, 27, and 29.)

The single spike-wave sequences from four EEGs that were analyzed to test these predictions are shown in figure 8.6. In each case, there appears to be an exponential decrease of the instantaneous slope (second traces), with a corresponding linear decrease on the logarithmic plot of the instantaneous slope (third traces). Although not attempted, it seems probable that averaging of several spike-wave events in each instance would have resulted in a closer fit to the manually drawn superimposed smooth curves in each instance.

These findings suggest that in the case of 3-Hz spike-wave events recorded from the scalp—at least, for the four EEGs in figure 8.6—there is an exponential decrease in the instantaneous slope, beginning with a relatively high value at the onset of the spike component and progressively decreasing through at least the first part of the wave component. This result appears to be in contrast to the conventional view of a stepwise or abrupt decrease in instantaneous slope at the transition point between spike and slow waves.

A separate question is whether the instantaneous slopes of the different 3-Hz spike-wave patterns in figure 8.5 behave the same way—i.e., whether the inclinations (the angles relative to the x (time) axis) of the straight lines suggested by the semilogarithmic plots are all the same. In this connection, it is important to note that the inclination of any trend evident in the semilogarithmic plot is insensitive to a change in scale factor (e.g., the sensitivity setting of the original EEG recording); such a change merely shifts the semilogarithmic plots up or down on the ordinate but leaves the inclination of any resulting trend unchanged. In fact, the inclinations of the third traces in the top pair of curves appear to be approximately the same, as do the inclinations of the third traces in the bottom pair of curves. The inclinations of the third traces for the top pair of logarithmic curves appears to differ from those of the bottom pair, however, when the small difference in the time scales for the upper and lower sets of curves is taken into account.

The instantaneous frequency can be obtained as the quotient of the instantaneous envelope of the first derivative of the EEG and the instantaneous envelope of the EEG itself, and hence a separate question is that of whether the instantaneous frequency declines exponentially in the course of a 3-Hz spike-wave event. This determination, not carried out for the EEGs in figures 8.6 and 8.7 (for which only the slope parameter was examined), is considered further in chapters 17 and 29.

THE NATURE OF THE VARIATION IN THE INSTANTANEOUS ENVELOPE OF SLOPE FOR SPIKE-AND-SLOW-WAVE COMPLEXES

In contrast to the simulation (chapter 4) of the 3-Hz spike-wave pattern as an alternation of high and low values of the modulation of slopes, for the spike and the wave components, respectively, an exponential decay of the slopes modulation was used for simulating the interictal spike-and-slow-wave-complex pattern of focal epilepsy, since such a modulation had been found to be satisfactory empirically for the purposes of simulation. It seemed reasonable, therefore, to expect that the analysis of actual EEG spike-and-slow-wave complexes by the technique described above would yield an exponentially decaying curve as the waveform for the envelope of slope, i.e., as the envelope of the first derivative of the complexes.

Tests of the same type described above for the 3-Hz spike-wave pattern were therefore also applied to a number of spike-and-slow-wave complexes of focal epilepsy, but the results were more variable than for the 3-Hz pattern; i.e., the "noise level" in the analyses was greater than for the latter pattern. It appears probable that such greater variability for the spike-and-slow-wave complexes resulted from the presence of independent ongoing background

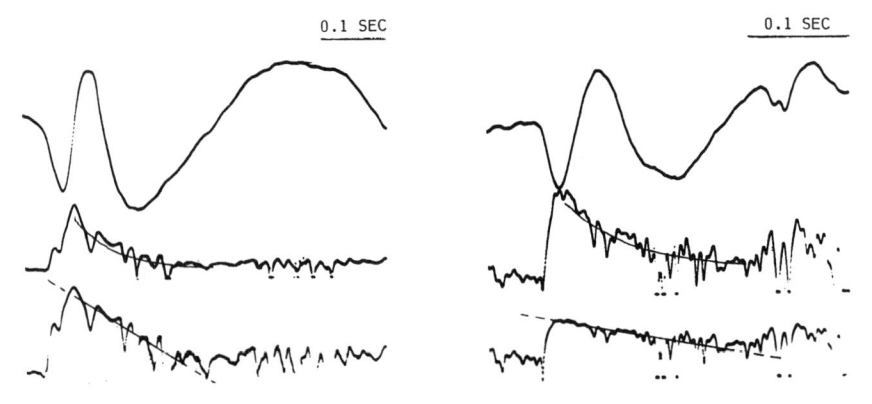

Figure 8.7 Instantaneous envelope of the first derivative (slope) (second traces) and its logarithm (third traces) for two EEGs showing focal spike-and-slow-wave-complex epileptiform patterns (first traces). The results for both cases suggest an exponential decrease of the instantaneous envelope of slope (second trace) and a linear decrease in its logarithm (third trace). (The superimposed curves in the second and third traces were drawn manually.)

EEG activity, an interference that is less likely to occur for the 3-Hz pattern. Two instances in which the behavior of the instantaneous envelope of slope was relatively well defined are shown in figure 8.7. In these two cases, the rate of decrease of the instantaneous envelope of slope appears to be exponential (second traces), and the logarithm of the instantaneous slope appears to exhibit a linear behavior (third traces).

SUMMARY

Analyses of a limited number of examples of the 3-Hz spike-wave EEG pattern by two independent methods indicate that the mean frequency during such events approximates that of the background EEG before or after the slow-wave event. This finding is consistent with the view that during such events the instantaneous frequency of the EEG varies between a high value during the spike component and a low value during the wave component, in comparison with its preictal and postictal values for the background EEG.

Further, analyses of a small series of additional 3-Hz spike-wave patterns of primary generalized epilepsy suggest that the envelope of the slopes of these two patterns (i.e., the instantaneous envelope of the first derivative of the EEG) decreases progressively as the spike component gives way to the wave component, rather than abruptly as the spike component ends and the slow-wave component begins. In addition, the decline in the envelope of slope appears to be an exponential one, as evidenced by an approximately linear behavior of the time course of a semi-logarithmic plot of the envelope of the slope.

Similar analyses of the instantaneous envelope of the slope for several examples of the spike-and-slow-wave complexes of focal epilepsy also suggest an exponential decay, but the resulting curves are generally more irregular. The latter effect probably results from interference with this pattern by the ongoing background EEG appearing at the same recording site (electrode).

Since slope is scale-factor dependent (i.e., dependent on the sensitivity setting on the EEG machine, etc.), whether the slope is similar for spike-wave patterns in different EEGs cannot be determined. The question could, however, be asked of the normalized envelope of the slope (i.e., the slope envelope divided by the envelope of the spike-wave pattern), which in the present context is just the instantaneous frequency. The latter determination was not, however, carried out in the analyses just described, which were concerned only with the behavior of the slope.

9 Reconstitution of EEGs from Extrema and Slopes

In chapter 3 the third method of testing the extrema-slopes hypothesis of the EEG was described as that of reconstituting an EEG on the basis of its extrema and slopes and comparing it quantitatively with the original (figure 3.1, Method 3). In contrast to the first method of testing the hypothesis (i.e., by simulating EEG patterns—see figure 3.1, Method 1), and also in contrast to the second method (i.e., testing EEGs for specific predictions made on the basis of the hypothesis—Method 2), the third method makes no assumptions about the nature of the EEG pattern in terms of one or more of the four basic types of waves of the oscillator model. The evolution of this third approach was as follows.

In chapter 3, for Method 2 of testing the extrema-slopes hypothesis, the running means of amplitude and slope, using an averaging window of 0.5 sec, were described as basic measures from which several descriptors of EEGs were obtained, including the running mean frequency, Spectral Purity Index, and Coefficients of Variation of the running means of amplitude, slope, and frequency. (Details of the techniques appear in chapters 24 and 25.) In chapter 4, on the other hand, and quite independently of these measures, EEG patterns were simulated by means of the oscillator model, using input modulating signals for extrema and for slopes generated by function generators, noise generators, etc., in connection with the first method of testing the hypothesis. The third approach to testing the hypothesis then suggested itself as a logical combination of the first two approaches.

RECONSTITUTION ON THE BASIS OF RUNNING MEAN AMPLITUDE AND RUNNING MEAN SLOPE—LIMITATIONS

In principle, it would be possible to reconstitute EEGs by using the running means of amplitude and frequency as a pair of input modulating signals, for extrema and for slopes, respectively, of the oscillator model, as indicated by the schema in figure 9.1A. Reconstitution of EEGs on the basis of the running means would, however, be feasible only for an EEG for which the rate of change of the respective running means is slow in comparison with an averaging window of, e.g., 0.5 sec for determining the running means—i.e., for very rhythmic alpha activity occurring in relatively long spindles. On the other

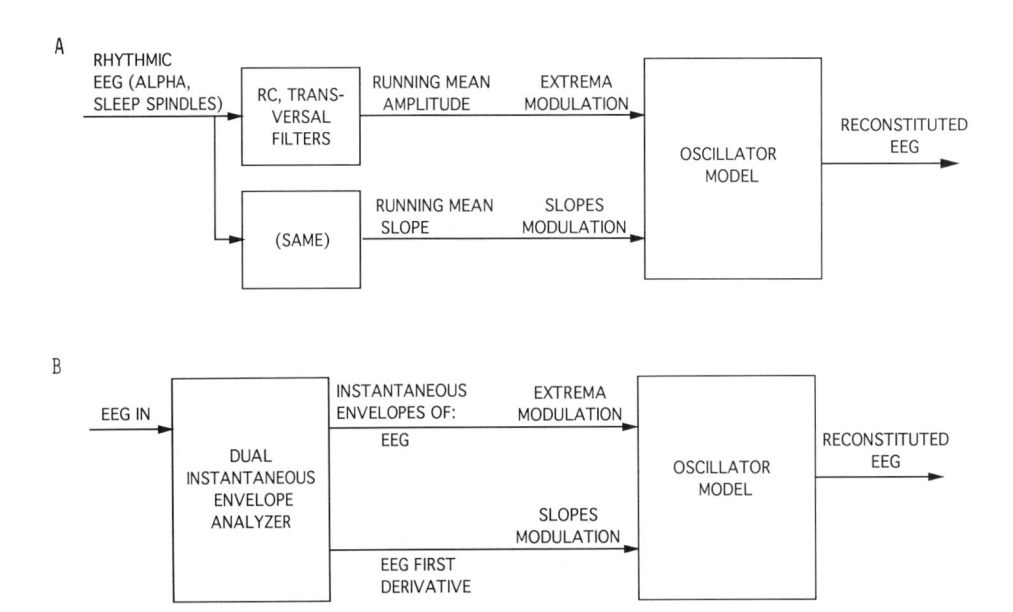

Figure 9.1 Schema of reconstitution of an EEG having an alpha rhythm: (A) from its running mean amplitude and running mean slope, by means of the oscillator model, and (B) from the instantaneous envelope of the EEG and of its first derivative. In part A, for reasonably faithful reconstitution, the alpha activity must be nearly sinusoidal and in relatively long spindles, in view of the duration of the averaging window (0.5 sec).

hand, decreasing the duration of the averaging window would ultimately introduce unacceptable "noise" in the averaging process. (In such a reconstitution process, running *means* are not the appropriate signals as input for modulating the *extrema* of the waves of the oscillator model; however, for quasi-sinusoidal alpha activity having well-developed spindles, the two differ essentially only by a constant of proportionality. For more complex EEG waveforms, this assumption would not in general hold.)

The problem of loss of a higher frequency response as a result of effectively low-pass filtering by the running-mean technique would be ameliorated if, instead of the running mean amplitude of the EEG and its running mean slope (i.e., the running mean of its first derivative), the envelope of the EEG and that of its first derivative were available. As indicated in chapter 29, however, the customary techniques for obtaining the envelopes of EEG signals (e.g., full-wave or multi-phase rectification followed by peak detection followed by smoothing) have their own limitations with respect to their effective smoothing windows or averaging times.

RECONSTITUTION ON THE BASIS OF INSTANTANEOUS ENVELOPES OF THE EEG AND OF ITS FIRST DERIVATIVE

An alternative approach to obtaining smoothed envelopes as just described is that of determining the instantaneous envelope of the EEG and that of its first

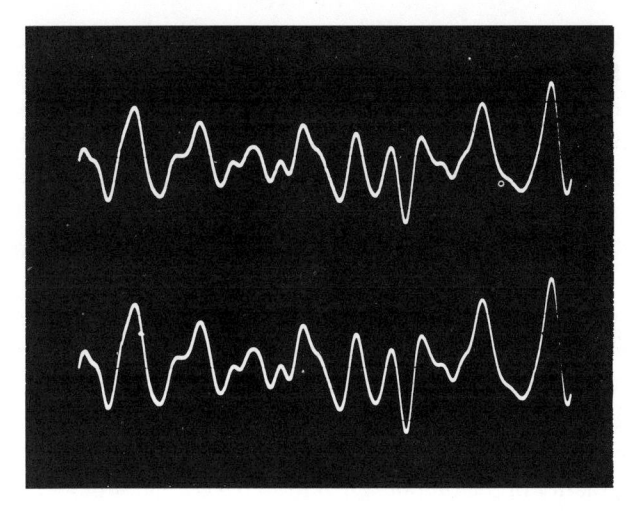

Figure 9.2 Demonstration that the successive processes of integration and differentiation yield a signal (lower trace) that is indistinguishable from the original (upper trace). Ideally, reconstitution of EEGs on the basis of their instantaneous envelopes and the instantaneous envelopes of their first derivative would be as faithful to the originals. (Operational amplifiers were used for the integrator and the differentiator. Original signal: 0.2–100-Hz random noise.)

derivative; in the instantaneous envelope, there is in principle no smoothing or time averaging, by definition. The technical details of the different methods of obtaining the instantaneous envelopes are detailed in chapter 29. (I am indebted to William M. Siebert of the Department of Electrical Engineering and Computer Science at the Massachusetts Institute of Technology for the suggestion of exploring the possible use of instantaneous envelopes instead of the above-mentioned technique of full-wave rectification with smoothing.) In turn, the pair of signals consisting of the instantaneous envelope of the EEG and the instantaneous envelope of its first derivative could then be used as input modulating signals for the extrema and for the slopes, respectively, of the oscillator model. An inherent characteristic of this approach is that the polarity of the reconstituted signal is arbitrary; it may be the same as, or, opposite to that of the original signal (see chapter 29).

ACCURACY OF THE RECONSTITUTION

Ideally, the reconstituted EEG would be indistinguishable from the original, as is a signal that has been passed through a differentiator and a (DC-stabilized) integrator in succession (figure 9.2). The original and the output traces in figure 9.2 are seen to be identical, as expected.

To evaluate the question of whether the original and the reconstituted EEGs have the same statistical properties (e.g., averages or expectations), spectra (obtained either by Fourier analysis (Dumermuth and Molinari 1987) or by the autoregressive technique (Lopes da Silva and Mars 1987)), or autocorrelation functions (Gevins 1987), could be compared. Although these methods can be used to evaluate statistical similarity, they cannot be used to evaluate the degree of wave-by-wave similarity, since in none of them is phase information retained. Therefore, it was originally planned to use the Coefficient of Determination, the square of the Pearson Product-Moment Correlation Coefficient (Sokal and Rohlf 1973), for evaluating the degree of wave-by-wave similarity of the reconstituted EEGs as compared with the originals. As indicated in chapter 25, a value of 1.0 indicates perfect agreement between the two, whereas a value near 0 indicates a near-chance relationship. The Coefficient of Determination, which ranges in value from 0 to +1.0, is more suitable for the present purpose than its square root, the Pearson Product-Moment Correlation Coefficient, which ranges in value from −1.0 to +1.0, because the Coefficient of Determination is insensitive to the relative polarity or sign of the two signals being compared. The difference is an important one, since the polarity of the output signal from the oscillator model relative to the original EEG is, as was mentioned above and as will be discussed further below, necessarily arbitrary (i.e., in the reconstitution process there is a 180° ambiguity in phase), and the Coefficient of Determination is independent of any such polarity difference.

In actual practice, however, evaluation of the Coefficient of Determination for the overall wave-by-wave similarity of the reconstituted EEGs as compared with the originals (as contrasted with the similarity of envelopes) disclosed an appreciable greater variability of phase of individual waves of reconstituted EEGs as compared with the original EEGs; in short, the phase differences were not simply a matter of polarity inversion. This approach to the evaluation of the accuracy of the reconstitution process was therefore abandoned. An alternative, although less desirable, possibility is that of applying the same test (i.e., evaluating the Coefficient of Determination) to the envelopes of the reconstituted and the original EEGs, and to the envelopes of their first derivatives.

RECONSTITUTED EEGS

Figure 9.3 shows the reconstitution of an EEG that had been subjected to narrow-band filtering at the alpha frequency of about 9 Hz, so as to obtain very smooth alpha waves and spindles. The interval of much lower amplitude corresponds to an interval of drowsiness or Stage 1 non-REM sleep. The reconstituted EEG appears as the bottom trace (trace 10) and was obtained as the output of the oscillator model using the instantaneous envelope of the original EEG (trace 7) and the instantaneous envelope of its first derivative (trace 8). The Coefficient of Determination (trace 9) in this instance was computed for the two instantaneous envelopes of the original EEG, not for the original and the reconstituted EEGs; it fluctuates near 1.0, reflecting that the two instantaneous envelopes are virtually identical for this very rhythmic signal. The pronounced difference between the running means and the respective instantaneous envelopes indicates the impracticality of an adequate recon-

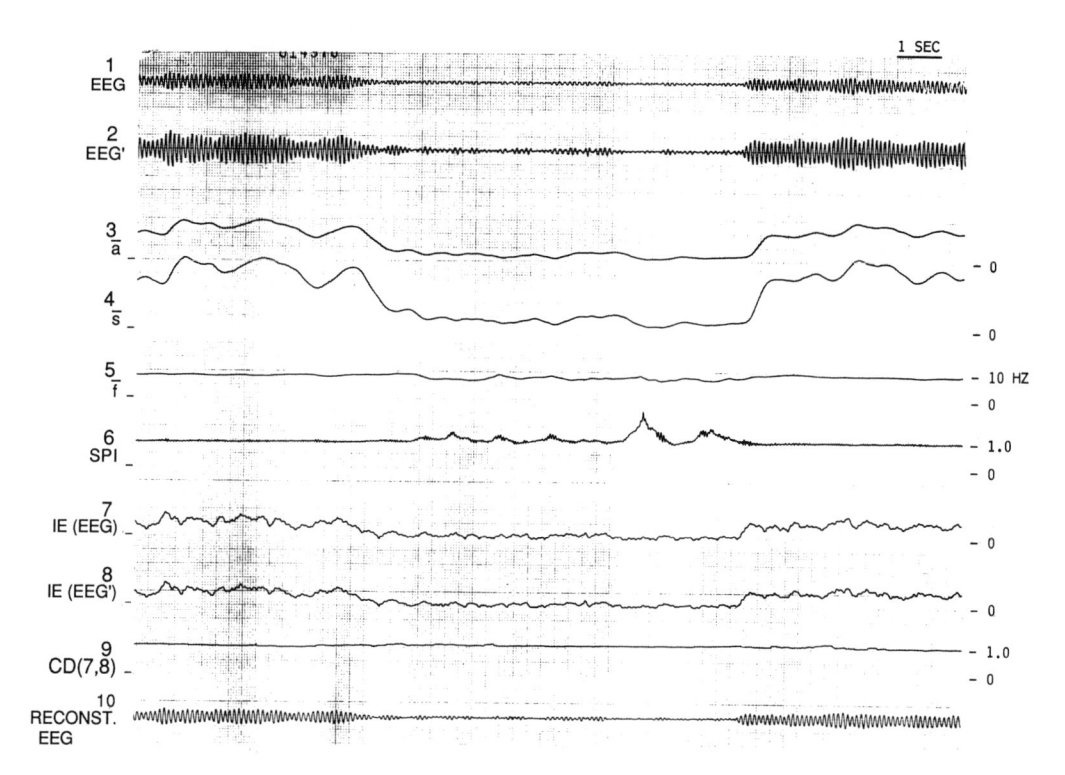

Figure 9.3 Original (trace 1) and reconstitution (trace 10) of an EEG that had been filtered in the 7–11-Hz range (24 dB attenuation per octave outside the pass band), so that only the alpha activity, at about 9 Hz, remains. The low-amplitude portion corresponds to a brief period of drowsiness. Other traces (the sequence is the same for the subsequent figures, except for figure 9.9): (2) first derivative of the EEG; (3–5) running means of amplitude, slope, and frequency, respectively; (6) Spectral Purity Index; (7 and 8) instantaneous envelopes of the EEG and its first derivative, respectively; (9) Coefficient of Determination for the two instantaneous envelopes. Note the much greater detail in the instantaneous envelopes (traces 7, 8) as compared with the running means (traces 3, 4). The running mean frequency (trace 5) decreases somewhat during drowsiness. The Spectral Purity Index (trace 6) remains at nearly 1.0 (indicating that the narrow-band filtered EEG is almost sinusoidal), except during the period of drowsiness, when the EEG amplitude intermittently becomes too low for accurate determination of the Spectral Purity Index (indicated by values greater than 1.0). The Coefficient of Determination (trace 9), calculated for the two instantaneous envelopes, remains close to 1.0 throughout; a high degree of similarity between the two instantaneous envelopes is a hallmark of rhythmic activity. (Bipolar posterior temporal to occipital recording. Averaging windows: 0.5 sec, except 4 sec for Coefficient of Determination.)

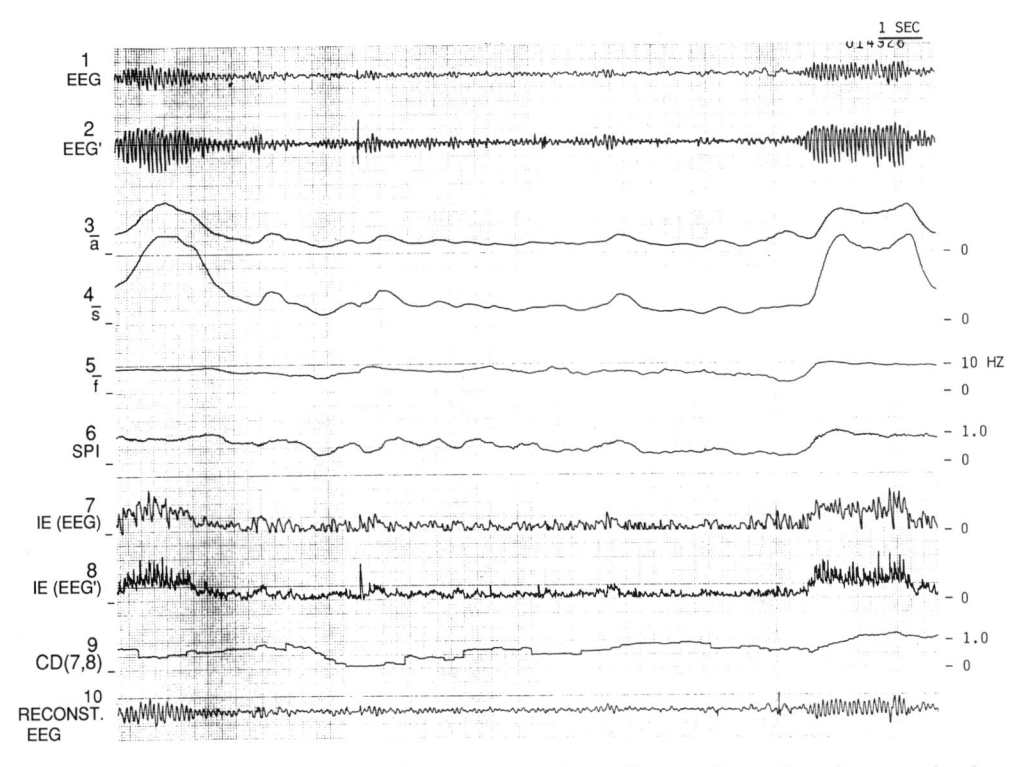

Figure 9.4 Another section of the same EEG as in figure 9.3 but without the narrow bandpass filtering at the alpha frequency. Note the resemblance between the reconstituted (trace 10) and the original EEG (trace 1), even during the period of low-voltage irregular activity during drowsiness. Note also the difference between the two instantaneous envelopes (traces 7 and 8). The Coefficient of Determination (trace 9) for the two instantaneous envelopes now fluctuates around 0.5 instead of around 1.0. The running mean frequency (trace 5) decreases more during drowsiness than in figure 9.3, as does the Spectral Purity Index (trace 6). (An artifact is present in the EEG (trace 1) toward the left.)

stitution of even this narrow-band-filtered EEG on the basis of the running means. The running mean frequency (at 9 Hz) and the Spectral Purity Index (at 0.9–1.0) remain rather constant despite the fluctuations in amplitude of the filtered alpha, except during drowsiness. Unlike Fourier analysis (chapter 17), these two determinations are by nature not sensitive to fluctuations in amplitude of a signal whose frequency remains essentially constant.

Another section of the same EEG but without the narrow bandpass filtering is shown in figure 9.4. The difference between the rhythmic alpha portion and the low-voltage irregular activity of drowsiness is now more striking, but the similarity of the reconstituted EEG (trace 10) and the original (trace 1) is evident for both types of activity. The two instantaneous envelopes (traces 7 and 8) are now rather different from one another (confirmed by the generally lower values of their Coefficient of Determination in trace 9), a reflection of the presence now of frequency components both below and above the alpha-frequency range. In particular, the effect of asymmetrically peaked alpha

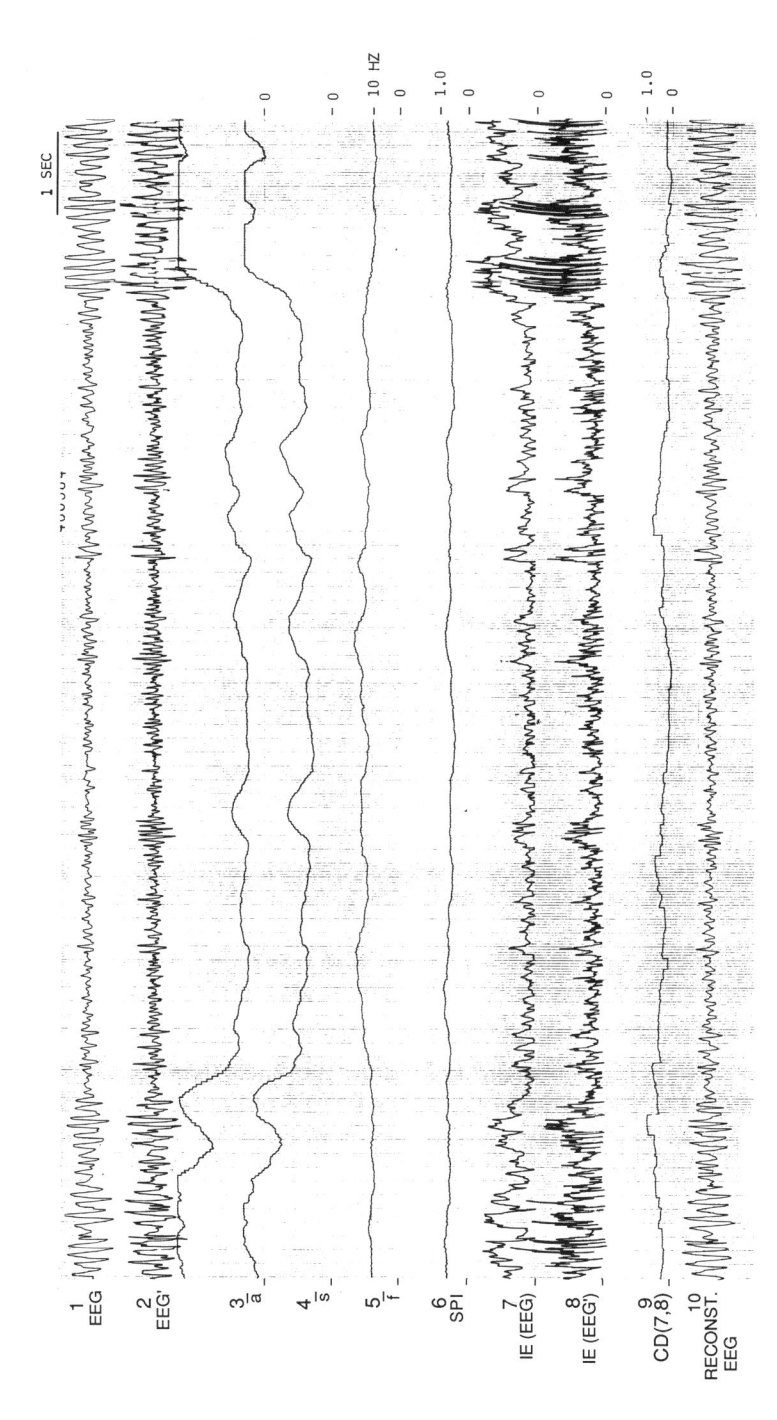

Figure 9.5 Reconstitution (trace 10) of an EEG (trace 1) showing blocking of relatively irregular alpha activity (at the left and at the right) when the eyes are open (middle section). During the eyes-open period, a "desynchronized EEG" pattern appears, for which the running mean frequency increases somewhat but the Spectral Purity Index and the Coefficient of Determination for the two instantaneous envelopes show little change in comparison with that for the relatively irregular alpha activity present when the eyes are closed. (Note the expanded time base.)

Reconstitution of EEGs from Extrema and Slopes

waves is evident in the first derivative of the EEG (trace 2) and in its instantaneous envelope (trace 8), and, in turn, in the reconstituted EEG (trace 10).

The reconstitution of an EEG showing blocking of a moderately irregular alpha rhythm with eye opening is shown on an expanded time scale in figure 9.5, during which period a "desynchronized" EEG pattern (i.e., an irregular low-voltage pattern) appears. The reconstituted EEG for the latter (trace 10) closely resembles the original (trace 1). (Two other examples of reconstituted "desynchronized" EEGs are shown in figure 5.6.) Three additional EEGs showing both regular (rhythmic) and somewhat irregular activity are shown in figures 9.6–9.8. The latter three EEGs, which were high-pass filtered to eliminate activity below 4 Hz, showed a pattern of frequencies in the alpha range, but the state is that of coma and the activity, which tends to be anteriorly rather than posteriorly predominant, is unresponsive to sensory stimulation—hence the term "alpha coma." These examples were selected to illustrate the accuracy of the reconstitution process despite appreciable variability of wave-to-wave amplitude.

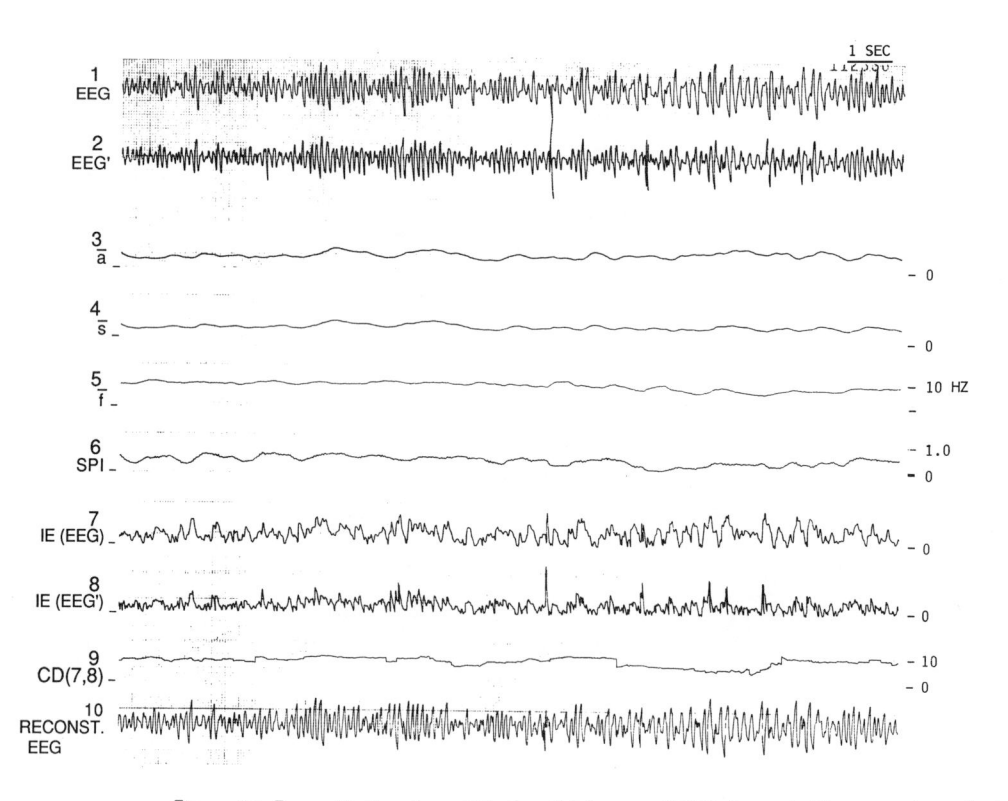

Figure 9.6 Reconstitution (trace 10) of an "alpha coma" EEG (trace 1). The original was high-pass filtered so as to eliminate activity below 4 Hz. Note the variability of amplitude from wave to wave, and also the decrease of frequency on the right. A spike-like artifact is present in the EEG (middle section); note its reappearance in the reconstituted EEG.

In figure 9.6, the wave-to-wave amplitude variability is particularly prominent, and correspondingly, the instantaneous envelope of the EEG (trace 7) and that of its first derivative (trace 8) are quite irregular. Nonetheless, the reconstituted version (trace 10) is very similar to the original (trace 1), except for the evident and expected ambiguity of polarity. The differences between these two instantaneous envelopes are also reflected in the Coefficient of Determination, which fluctuates around 0.7. Two additional examples of EEGs having prominent wave-to-wave amplitude variability are shown in figures 9.7 and 9.8.

The original and reconstituted versions of an EEG showing repetitive epileptiform discharges are shown adjacent to one another (note the difference in sequence of the traces from the previous figures) in figure 9.9. (The EEG voltage between the discharges is relatively low, so that the recording can be considered an example of a burst-suppression pattern; compare figures 4.6 and 4.7.) The ambiguity of the polarity of the reconstituted version is evident in that the polarity of some of the reconstituted epileptiform events is inverted.

Especially noteworthy in figure 9.9 is that for several of the epileptiform events the instantaneous envelopes of the EEG and of its first derivative show a rapid rise (the rise time for the latter being the shorter), which is followed by a decay that appears to be exponential in form (the decay of the instanta-

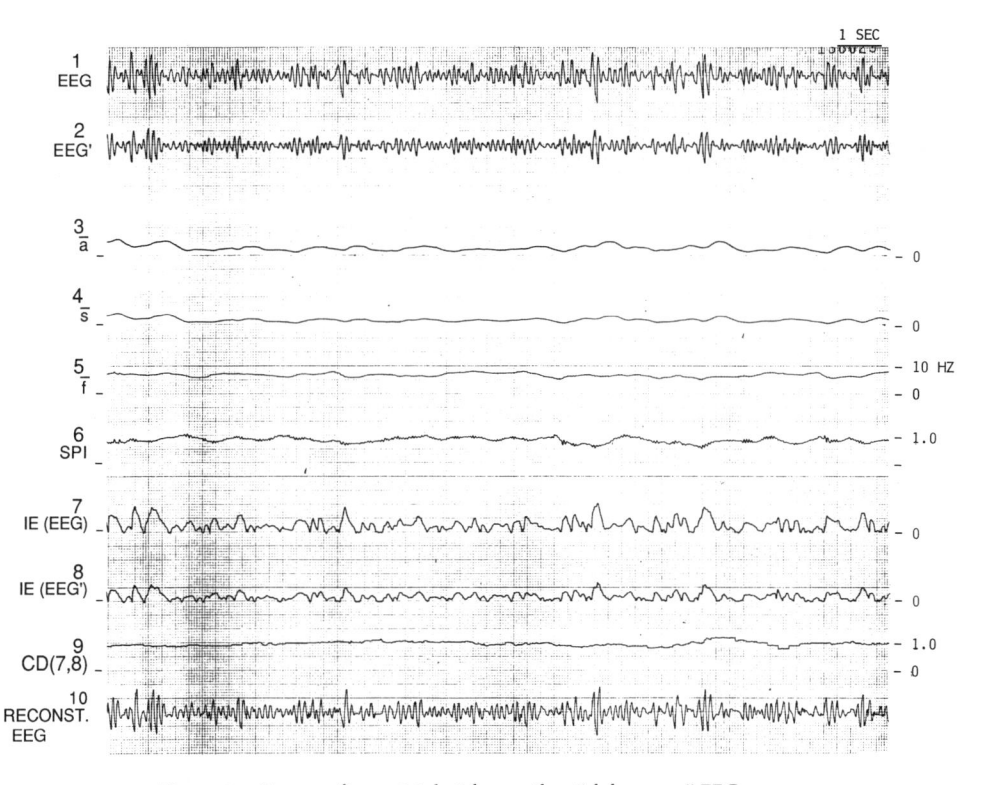

Figure 9.7 Same as figure 9.6, but for another "alpha-coma" EEG.

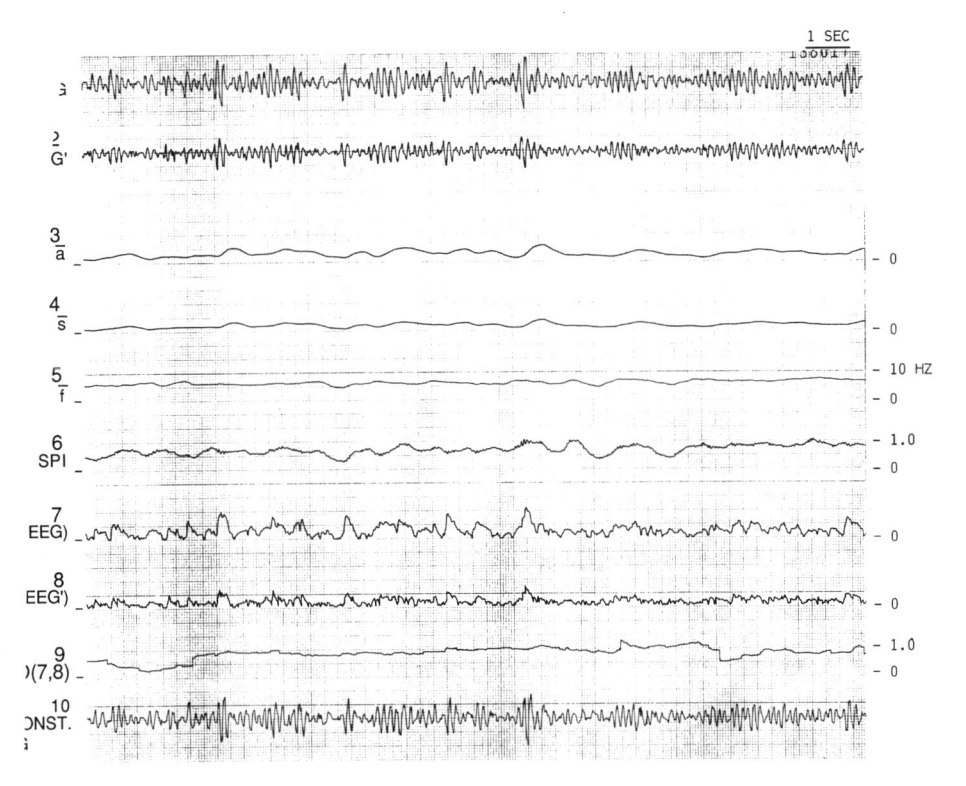

Figure 9.8 Same as figure 9.6, but for an additional "alpha-coma" EEG.

neous envelope of slope being the faster). This finding would be consistent with an exponential decrease of the instantaneous frequency; direct determination of the latter was attempted; however, the resulting trace proved to be extremely noisy, because of the fluctuations in the instantaneous envelopes (figure 9.9, traces 7 and 8). The total inadequacy of the running means of amplitude and of slope from which to reconstitute the EEG is also evident from figure 9.9 (traces 3 and 4). On the other hand, there is a suggestion of a progressive decrease in running mean frequency (trace 5), after an intial relatively more rapid rise, in the course of the epileptiform discharges (trace 5). In contrast, the rising and falling phases of the peaks of the Spectral Purity Index (trace 6), which are not perfectly correlated in time with the rising and falling phases of the running mean frequency (trace 5), appear to be about equal in duration.

The results from the epileptiform EEG pattern of figure 9.9 which were just described appear to be consistent with the findings of an exponential decay of the instantaneous envelope of slope for the epileptiform patterns depicted in figures 8.6 and 8.7, although the test of linearity of a logarithmic plot used in the latter figures was not applied to the events in figure 9.9.

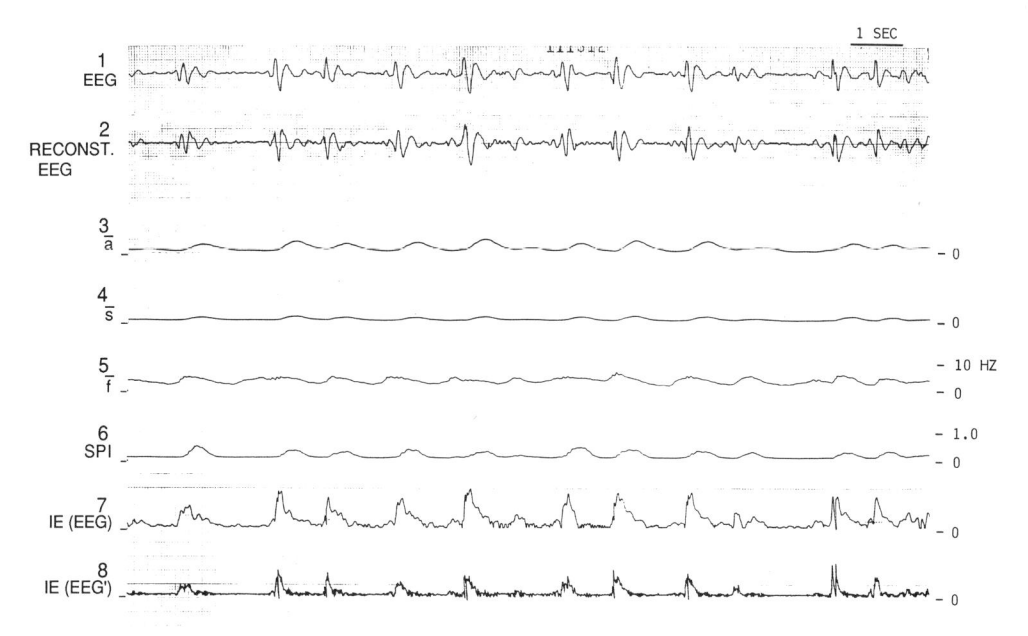

Figure 9.9 Original (trace 1) and reconstitution (trace 2; note the different order of traces from the previous figures) of an EEG showing a repetitive seizure discharge pattern. (Original EEG filtered to eliminate activity below 4 Hz.) The remaining traces show the running mean amplitude (trace 3), running mean slope (trace 4) and running mean frequency (trace 5), the Spectral Purity Index (trace 6), the instantaneous envelope of the EEG (trace 7), and the instantaneous envelope of the first derivative of the EEG (trace 8). Some of the epileptiform events are inverted in polarity in the reconstituted version. For several of the events, both the instantaneous envelope of the EEG and of its first derivative appear to exhibit an exponential decay following a rapid buildup, both the rise and decay times being shorter for the instantaneous envelope of slope.

COMMENT

Although in the end quantitative tests were not applied to evaluate the degree of similarity between the original EEGs and their reconstituted versions, it seems apparent from visual inspection of the figures that the reconstitutions closely resemble the originals, save for the previously mentioned ambiguity of polarity of the reconstructions. This feature of the reconstruction process appears to be of little consequence except when the EEG pattern is asymmetrical about the baseline—in particular, for epileptiform patterns (e.g., spikes and spike-wave patterns). It is characteristic, in clinical electroencephalography, that spikes have a particular polarity for a particular electrode combination (i.e., negative—and by EEG convention, an upward deflection—at the active electrode). However, polarity information is inherently not conserved in the present EEG-reconstruction process (as indeed it is also not conserved in power spectral analysis or autocorrelation), and hence the polarity of the reconstructed EEG is necessarily arbitrary. One possible scheme for ensuring that the reconstruction was always of the correct polarity, wave by wave, was explored, but it was found to be unsatisfactory. Since, as mentioned above, the polarity-ambiguity feature appears to be of little consequence except for EEG patterns that are asymmetrical about the baseline (e.g., epileptiform patterns), another scheme, not explored, would be to ensure that abrupt increases in the instantaneous envelope of the slope be reflected in the correct polarity—by forced polarity reversal of the reconstituted EEG output, if necessary. Such a scheme, however, could have difficulty in the case of the asymmetrical mu rhythm (figure 4.11) or the pattern of 14- and 6-Hz positive bursts (figure 4.13).

10 Appraisal and Revision of the Extrema-Slopes Hypothesis on the Basis of Tests

In this chapter, the extrema-slopes hypothesis as delineated in chapter 2 (i.e., that the EEG can be considered as though it were a signal the amplitude and slope of individual waves of which are separately modulated) will be appraised in relation to the results of the three different types of tests of it that were outlined in chapter 3, and the results of which have been detailed in chapters 4–9. The three basic types of tests of the hypothesis were (1) simulation of a selected set of EEG patterns by means of the oscillator model, using standard signals for its two input modulations; (2) tests of actual EEGs for predictions concerning features which had been predicted on the basis of the hypothesis; and (3) reconstitution of actual EEGs on the basis of their instantaneous envelopes and the instantaneous envelopes of their first derivatives.

The appraisal of the extrema-slopes hypothesis in this chapter will be in relation to the EEG purely as a signal, without regard to its underlying physiological and pathophysiological mechanisms; in short, the evaluation will be phenomenological, in the sense that the EEG is considered to originate from a "black box," since only after such a validation of the basic hypothesis is it sensible and appropriate to proceed with the evaluation of it from a broader perspective.

Results from the three methods of testing the hypothesis will now be reviewed, in the order of the three basic approaches to testing.

SIMULATION OF EEG PATTERNS BY MEANS OF THE OSCILLATOR MODEL (Chapter 4)

If the extrema of the output waves of the oscillator model are modulated with a random signal, the slopes of the waves being kept constant (i.e., Mode 1 of the oscillator model), the resulting Type 1 (constant-slope) waves approximately resembled the irregular pattern of Stages 3 and 4 of non-REM sleep (sometimes termed slow-wave sleep), and also resembled the abnormal random EEG slowing termed irregular or polymorphic delta activity.

Modulation of only the slopes of the waves of the oscillator model (i.e., Mode 2 of the model) in combination with a baseline shift, on the other hand, resulted in waves (Type 2 waves) that have some resemblance, on the one hand, to the classical 3-Hz spike-wave pattern, and, on the other hand, to certain normal and normal-variant EEG patterns—i.e., the patterns of the mu rhythm, 6-Hz spike waves, and 14- and 6-Hz positive spikes. That a baseline shift was necessary to simulate the 3-Hz spike-wave pattern is of particular interest in view of the fact that such a baseline shift is a characteristic feature of the actual EEG pattern (Cohn 1954, 1964; Chatrian et al. 1968).

Congruent or identical modulation of both the extrema and the slopes of the waves of the oscillator model (Mode 3) resulted in waves of constant frequency but variable amplitude (Type 3 waves) that resembled rhythmic EEG patterns such as spindles of alpha waves or sleep spindles. Small amplitude differences between the two modulations resulted in a small dependence of frequency on amplitude of the output waves of the oscillator model.

Independent modulation of extrema and slopes (Mode 4 of the oscillator model) resulted in an irregular pattern that appeared to have some resemblance to the "desynchronized" or "activated" EEG pattern of the alert, eyes-open state, or, for some individuals, the low-voltage irregular pattern of the awake eyes-closed state. By simultaneous modulation of extrema and slopes with selected paired waveforms, a pattern could be obtained from the oscillator model that resembled the epileptiform pattern of the spike-and-slow-wave complex encountered in focal epilepsy.

From this summary of the results of the first type of test of the extrema-slopes hypothesis, it is evident that a relatively wide variety of waveforms can be simulated by the oscillator model which, upon visual inspection, resemble actual EEG patterns, attesting to the versatility of this device as an EEG pattern simulator. Since the design of the oscillator model is specifically based on the extrema-slopes hypothesis, the aforementioned simulation results can be considered to provide corroborative evidence for the hypothesis itself. Thus, the four primary patterns of waveforms from the oscillator model appear to match four major categories of EEG patterns: random slowing, epileptiform, rhythmic, and irregular (mixed frequencies). It is to be emphasized, however, that the resemblances that have been mentioned between simulated and actual EEG patterns are based on visual comparisons.

TESTING OF EEGS FOR CHARACTERISTIC FEATURES PREDICTED ON THE BASIS OF THE EXTREMA-SLOPES HYPOTHESIS (Chapters 5–7)

In the second type of test of the hypothesis, EEGs were analyzed to determine whether they exhibited certain specific characteristics predicted on the basis of the hypothesis, i.e., predicted from the behavior of one or another of the four basic types of waves available from the oscillator model, as follows. Several methods of analysis were used (as detailed in chapter 3), including determinations of running mean EEG amplitude and running mean slope (i.e., running mean of the first derivative of the EEG), running mean frequency (as the quotient of running mean slope to running mean amplitude), Spectral Purity

Index (as a quantitative measure of rhythmicity), running Coefficients of Variation (the quotient of the standard deviation to the mean), the logarithm of the quotient of the Coefficients of Variation of running mean slope and running mean amplitude (as a linear measure of their relative variability), and the Pearson Product-Moment Correlation Coefficient and its square, the Coefficient of Determination (as measures of the similarity between, e.g., running envelopes of amplitude and of slopes).

The results of testing the specific predictions can be summarized as follows.

Prediction 1: that the EEGs of non-REM sleep, i.e., Stages 1–4, are of the constant-slope type (Type 1 waves, generated in Mode 1 of the oscillator model). In practice, this prediction implies that the short-term (seconds) variability of the running mean slope of an EEG should be relatively small, and that its long-term (minutes) trend should be relatively flat, as compared with the same measures of amplitude. The prediction was confirmed (chapter 6) for Stages 3 and 4 of non-REM sleep, and intermittently for a minority of subjects for Stage 1; it was not confirmed for the EEG of Stage 2 sleep. An unexpected finding in the latter was that the apparent frequency of vertex sharp transients appears about the same as the running mean frequency of the background EEG, which in turn was about half that of the waking alpha rhythm for the same subject. Indeed, the disappearance of this effect in the analysis marked the transition from Stage 2 to Stage 3 sleep. In connection with the fact that constant-slope waves have the characteristic that amplitude and frequency vary inversely, or, amplitude and duration of such waves vary directly with one another, it is relevant to note that Knott and Travis (1937) found a correlation of 0.4 ± 0.04 between amplitude and duration for normal EEG waves ranging in duration from 0.04 to 0.4 sec (2.5 to 25 Hz); it was not indicated whether the subjects were awake or asleep.

In addition, it was predicted that abnormal irregular or random (polymorphic) EEG slowing is also of the constant-slope type, corresponding to Type 1 waves of the oscillator model. Confirmatory evidence for this prediction appeared both directly and indirectly, as a reciprocal relationship between amplitude and frequency (chapter 7).

In chapter 2, it was suggested that hyperventilation-induced normal slowing in the EEG would correspond to Type 1 (constant-slope) waves. This prediction appears to have been confirmed by the data analyzed (chapter 7).

The characterization of this category of EEG waves as being of relatively constant slope (or, equivalently expressed, as having amplitude and duration directly proportional to one another) places on a quantitative basis a feature of some EEG patterns that has long been familiar in electroencephalography: that, at least in sleep and in pathological slowing, waves of higher amplitude often appear to be longer in duration.

In contrast to the relatively constant mean or DC level of the running mean of the first derivative of the EEG during Stage 3 and Stage 4 sleep, the running mean of the EEG itself appears to rise progressively as sleep deepens. (The possible physiological significance of this contrasting behavior will be considered in chapter 17.)

Prediction 2: that at least some forms of epileptiform patterns correspond to the constant-amplitude variable-slope Type 2 waves of Mode 2 of the oscillator model. This prediction was tested primarily by examining the behavior of the slope in epileptiform patterns. As detailed in chapter 9, the prediction was confirmed with EEGs showing the 3-Hz spike-wave pattern, but with a result different from the one originally anticipated. Originally, it had been assumed (figure 4.10B) that there would be a stepwise alternation between a relatively high slope for the spike component and a relatively low slope for the wave component. In fact, the slope was found to decrease gradually, as a decaying exponential, from the beginning of the spike toward the end of the wave component.

An additional finding that is consistent with the prediction was that the mean frequency during a 3-Hz spike-wave burst was approximately the same as that of the background activity before or after the burst.

Although the pattern of the spike-and-slow-wave complex cannot be considered as an example of Type 2 waves (since the amplitude of the slow-wave component progressively diminishes), the aforementioned decremental slope behavior was also found for interictal spike-and-slow-wave complexes, although an exponential behavior was much less well defined than in the spike-wave pattern (perhaps because of the absence of background EEG components in the latter).

Prediction 2 can therefore be said to have been basically confirmed for the 3-Hz spike-wave pattern.

Prediction 3: that alpha activity can be modeled by Type 3 waves and therefore should be of relatively constant frequency (a reflection of a close parallel between the running means of amplitude and of slope). Results of tests (chapter 5) of this "prediction," which are hardly surprising, confirmed that the running mean frequency of alpha activity is indeed relatively constant, as indicated by very low values of the Coefficient of Variation—a finding that was corroborated by values of the Spectral Purity Index of close to 1.0. A corollary of this prediction, namely that a slight difference in the amplitudes of the identical waveforms used to modulate the extrema and the slopes of the oscillator-model output waves would result in a small dependence of frequency on amplitude, was also confirmed by the behavior of the alpha activity in the EEGs of several subjects (chapter 5).

Prediction 4: that the "desynchronized" EEG (i.e., low-voltage irregular activity) of the eyes-open waking state (in some individuals, also with eyes closed), and also the EEG during REM sleep, could be modeled by Type 4 waves of the oscillator model (i.e., waves in which amplitude and slope are independently variable). However, both for the "desynchronized" EEG and for the EEG in REM sleep, tests of this prediction (chapters 5 and 6), carried out primarily by means of comparisons of the running mean amplitude and the running mean slope with the aid of the Coefficient of Determination, disclosed partial interdependence rather than complete independence of these two variables. Thus, the resulting Coefficients of Determination were not, as predicted, close to 0; they were in the vicinity of 0.5. (An interesting incidental but inconstant finding was that the "sawtooth waves" of REM sleep appeared to have some resemblance to the constant-slope Type 1 waves of the oscillator model.) In their original report, Dement and Kleitman (1957) considered the EEG during REM sleep to be the same as that for Stage 1 non-REM sleep, and the two patterns are still considered to be indistinguishable on the basis of power spectra alone (Johnson et al. 1969).

From the above discussion, it is evident that the first three predictions were confirmed, but the fourth one only partially.

RECONSTITUTION OF EEGS FROM THEIR INSTANTANEOUS ENVELOPES (Chapter 9)

As was mentioned in chapter 3, this third method of testing the extrema-slopes hypothesis is carried out quite without reference to the four principal types of waves in the hypothesis and the corresponding four principal modes of the oscillator model, since the instantaneous envelope of the EEG and the instantaneous envelope of the first derivative of the EEG are fed directly to the two respective modulating inputs of the oscillator model (chapter 9). Except for the ambiguity of polarity of the output of the oscillator, which as mentioned previously is inherent in the reconstitution process, the reconstituted EEGs bear a quite reasonable resemblance to the originals.

COMMENT AND REVISIONS TO THE HYPOTHESIS AND THE OSCILLATOR MODEL

The results summarized above appear basically to confirm the extrema-slope hypothesis and its embodiment as the oscillator model. That the prediction that Type 4 waves (complete independence of amplitudes and slopes) could be a model for the irregular low-voltage pattern of the "desynchronized" EEG and also the EEG of REM sleep was not confirmed can really be considered an error in the original prediction, on the author's part, rather than a failure to confirm the hypothesis itself, since EEG patterns of the desynchronized type are readily reconstituted (figures 5.6 and 9.5). In fact, for these EEG patterns a partial (if not a complete) independence of amplitudes and slopes exists, as indicated by values of the Coefficient of Determination in the range of 0.5. Thus, in relation to the oscillator model itself, a partial mixing of the two modulating inputs (for extrema and for slopes) appears indicated (figure 10.1B) rather than the originally postulated schema (figure 10.1A)—at least, for the "desynchronized" EEG.

In retrospect, and as previously indicated, a less-than-complete independence, for non-epileptiform activity, of the running mean absolute amplitude and the running mean absolute slope could perhaps reasonably have been expected, in view of the central limit theorem. As was mentioned in chapter 5, the latter theorem states that the amplitude distribution function of an

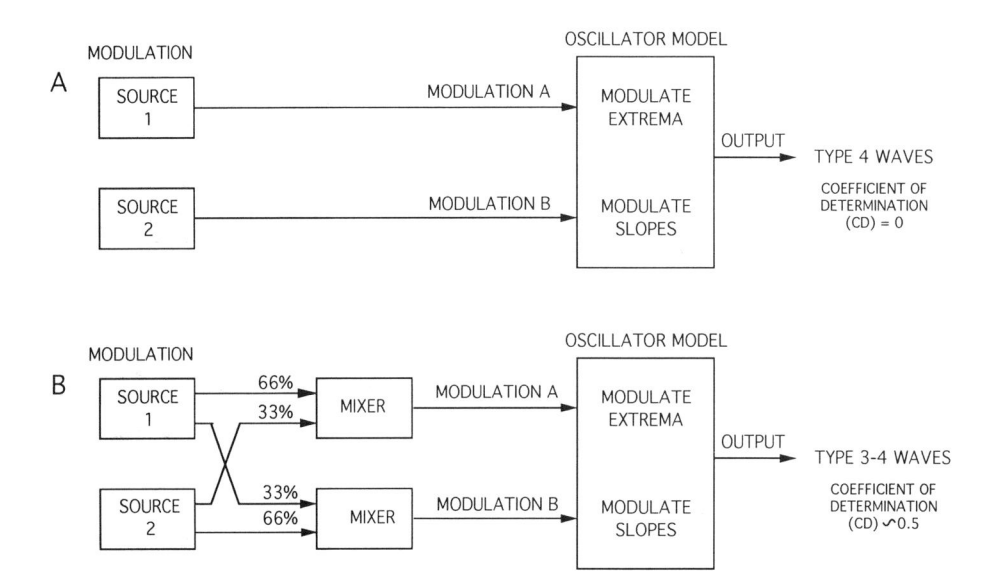

Figure 10.1 Original (A) and revised (B) schemas of the oscillator model. In part A, Type 4 waves are generated by completely independent modulation of extrema and slopes, whereas in part B the output waves are intermediate between mode 3 and mode 4, because of the partial mixing of the two modulations shown at the left. For the percentage contributions indicated in part B, a Coefficient of Determination (CD) of about 0.5 was found, rather than a value of close to 0 as for the arrangement depicted in part A. A value of the CD of approximately 0.5 was the one usually found for the paired running means, or for the paired instantaneous envelopes, of the EEG and its first derivative, for "desynchronized" EEGs and for the EEG of REM sleep.

increasingly large ensemble of processes (in the present instance, elementary neuronal oscillators) having any arbitrary amplitude distribution function will tend toward a Gaussian distribution. Thus, for a signal having a Gaussian amplitude distribution function, there will be a correlation between the two running means (reflected in a coefficient of Determination greater than 0 but less than 1.0), the narrower the bandwidth of the Gaussian or random signal, the greater the Coefficient of Determination. Thus, for a narrow-band Gaussian signal, the first derivative is very similar to the original, save for a 90° phase shift.

If a pair of independent random signals having a rectangular rather than a Gaussian amplitude distribution function (the Coefficient of Determination for the rectangular pair is close to 0) are used as modulating signals for extrema and slopes of the oscillator model, the resultant spectrum has the unusual feature of being relatively uniform from some lower limit (e.g., 1–2 Hz) up to the intrinsic frequency of the oscillator model, and declines moderately rapidly for still higher frequencies (figure 5.10). As detailed in chapter 5, the spectra of "desynchronized" EEGs during reading exhibited a similar behavior in relation to the resting alpha frequency of the same subject, thus providing some supporting evidence for at least a partial independence of the running means of amplitude and slope for this group of "desynchronized" EEGs.

It is to be stressed, however, that despite the revision indicated in figure 10.1 of the input modulations to the oscillator model as a consequence of the results of the analysis of amplitude and slope characteristics of actual EEGs, the basic extrema-slopes model and its hardware embodiment as the oscillator model, with its separate modulations of extrema and of slopes, remains unaltered. Indeed, the reconstitutions of EEGs on the basis of the instantaneous envelope of the original and the instantaneous envelope of the first derivative of the original EEG (chapter 9) for a variety of types of EEGs were carried out without any mixing of the two instantaneous envelopes, i.e, the two modulating inputs to the oscillator model.

CONCLUDING REMARKS

The consideration of the experimental evidence concerning the extrema-slopes hypothesis, considered phenomenologically—i.e., with the EEG treated purely as a "signal from a black box" (the brain)—is now complete, and in many respects the hypothesis has been corroborated. The question can be raised whether to some extent the argument has employed "circular reasoning"—i.e., if the EEG is decomposed into its instantaneous envelope and the instantaneous envelope of its first derivative, then it is perhaps not surprising that, with appropriate selection of an oscillator capable of being modulated in two different ways, the original EEG could readily be reconstituted. Could not then the process of decomposition of an EEG into a pair of instantaneous envelopes, followed by reconstitution, be a trivial one, not unlike the resynthesis of a short section of an EEG by inverse Fourier transformation of the Fourier components (sine and cosine) of the original (see for example, figure 11 in Walter et al. 1972a), which sheds no light on possible generating mechanisms? Perhaps, but it seems remarkable that the extrema-slopes hypothesis can account for such a large variety of EEG patterns by only two parameters and, at the same time, account for subtle and even unanticipated features of the behavior of certain EEG patterns. The latter features include the amplitude-frequency dependence of alpha activity (figure 5.5), the particular spectral features of the "desynchronized" EEG during reading (figures 5.9–5.11). The hypothesis also suggests the possibility of a new approach to the study of epileptiform events in the form of the behavior of the instantaneous envelope of the first derivative of the EEG, particularly in view of the implication, from these findings, that EEG spikes may give way gradually, rather than abruptly, to the following slow wave (figures 8.6–8.7).

From the perspective of the "successes" just enumerated, it may be useful to recall that the design features of the oscillator model (i.e., the extrema-slopes dual modulation of what is basically a nonlinear oscillator) were prescribed or mandated by specific EEG features themselves (beginning with the constant-slope phenomenon). These design features may thus carry specific implications concerning basic EEG-generating mechanisms—for example, a physiological counterpart of the process of modulation of extrema, and some physiological mechanism for dual modulation. Neither of these phenomena in oscillatory mechanisms appears to have been described previously.

Before exploring the implications of the extrema-slopes hypotheseis for actual EEG-generating mechanisms (in chapter 16), it is appropriate to review some anatomical, physiological, and pathophysiological aspects of the EEG (chapters 11, 12, and 13, respectively), and also to consider other models of the EEG and related phenomena (chapter 14) and the relationship of the present model to the latter (chapter 15).

III Appraisal of the Hypothesis in Relation to Anatomy, Physiology, and Pathophysiology of the EEG; Other Models; Overall Appraisal

11 Some Aspects of Neocortical Anatomy

Of the vast amount of information currently available concerning the mammalian neocortex, this brief survey will touch upon only a few points that are relevant to the hypothesis being explored in this book. Many or most of the statements below should be understood to carry a qualification such as "Currently available evidence indicates that..." or "With few exceptions...."

The basic architecture of the six-layer neocortex, which is extremely complex, is the same throughout its extent; the cell types found in different areas are similar, and the cell content is remarkably similar in different regions of cortex (visual area 17 or V1 being an exception, having twice the usual cortical density) (Rockel et al. 1980; Gilbert et al. 1988). The variations, e.g. in size and laminar distribution of neurons, are determined principally by the connections of the different regions (Powell 1981; Braitenberg 1978; Creutzfeldt 1978; Hendry et al. 1987; Gilbert et al. 1988). Functionally, at least, cells of the major thalamic nuclear groups appear to have similar properties (Jahnsen and Llinás 1984a,b). Although much remains to be clarified in detail, the general organization of the neocortex has become relatively well established (Braitenberg 1977, 1978; Creutzfeldt 1977, 1978; Szentágothai 1978a,b, 1983; Brodal 1981; Feldman 1984; Jones and Peters 1984; Peters and Jones 1984; Gilbert et al. 1988).

TYPES OF NEURONS

Neocortical cells can be categorized in two partially overlapping ways: pyramidal and non-pyramidal, and spiny and non-spiny. The spiny cells, which are probably excitatory, form asymmetrical synapses as seen under the electron microscope, and include both pyramidal and spiny stellate cells. Non-spiny (or spine-free) cells are GABAergic or inhibitory, and form symmetrical synapses; these cells make up 25% of the total number of cortical neurons.

Of the approximately 10^{10} neurons in the human cerebral cortex, about 75% are pyramidal cells (Braitenberg 1977). The non-pyramidal cells or interneurons (which include both spiny and non-spiny neurons) constitute a heterogeneous group. Pyramidal cells (figure 11.1), named originally because of their shape (although *conical* would be a better characterization), have several characteristics. There is a dominant apical dendrite rising to layer I of

I
II
III
IV
V
VI

A

B

C

D

Thalamus[p.]
Corticocortical
Claustrum
(Callosal)

Spinal cord
Pons
Medulla
Tectum
Thalamus[n.s.]
Red nucleus
Striatum
(Cortical[x])

Callosal
Corticocortical

Corticocortical

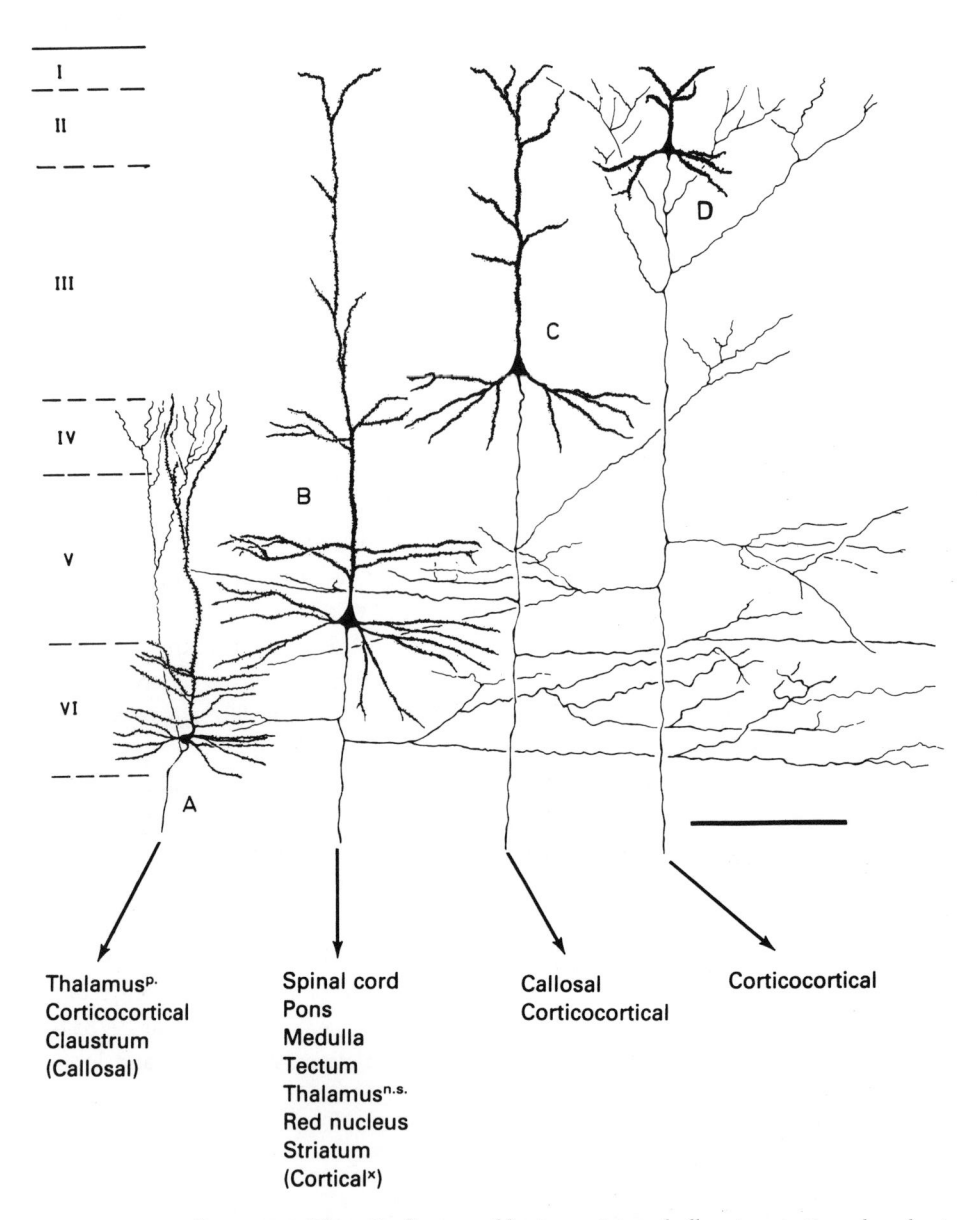

Figure 11.1 Schematic diagram of laminar origins of efferent projections, based primarily on data from monkeys. Parentheses indicate that a projection may not arise from the layer indicated in all species or all areas. (From Jones 1984.)

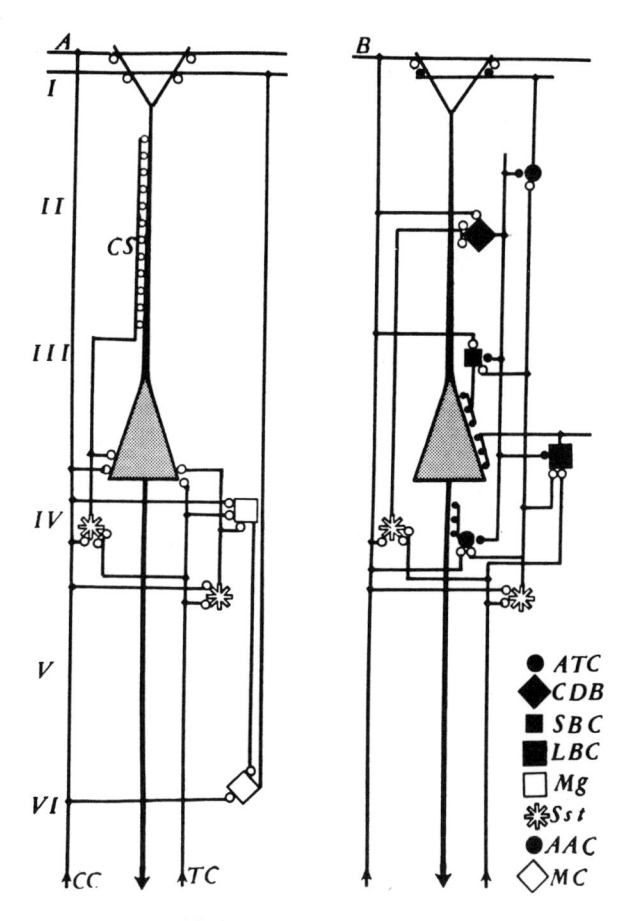

Figure 11.2 Simplified diagram of modular design in the association neocortex, the laminae being indicated on the left. In part A, the excitatory cells with their excitation by the cortico-cortical (CC) and thalamocortical (TC) inputs are shown. In part B, the synaptic connectivities for inhibitory cells are depicted. The stippled cells in the center of each diagram are pyramidal cells. The symbols for cell identifications to the lower right are arranged in the same depth order as the cells in the diagram: ATC, axonal tuft cell; CDB, cellule à double bouquet; SBC, small basket cell; LBC, large basket cell; Mg, neurogliaform cell; Sst, spiny stellate cell; AAC axoaxonic cell; MC, Martinotti cell. CS indicates cartridge synapse. All excitatory cells and synapses are in outline. All inhibitory cells and synapses are in solid black. (From Eccles 1984.)

the cortex (with the exception of the pyramidal cells of layer VI), where extensive branching occurs. There is also a basilar dendritic system that extends out roughly spherically from the cell body. Pyramidal cells also have an axon that arises from the cell body (soma) or from the initial portion of a basilar dendrite, and which, after giving off intracortical branches or collaterals that synapse onto the basal dendrites of nearby pyramidal cells, enters the subcortical white matter. The axons of all pyramidal cells terminate in excitatory synapses. The initial segment (trigger zone) of pyramidal cells is unmyelinated, as are their recurrent branches (Szentágothai, 1978b).

Non-pyramidal cells (figures 11.2, 11.3) comprise a heterogeneous group of spiny or excitatory neurons (spiny stellate, bipolar Martinotti, neurogliaform)

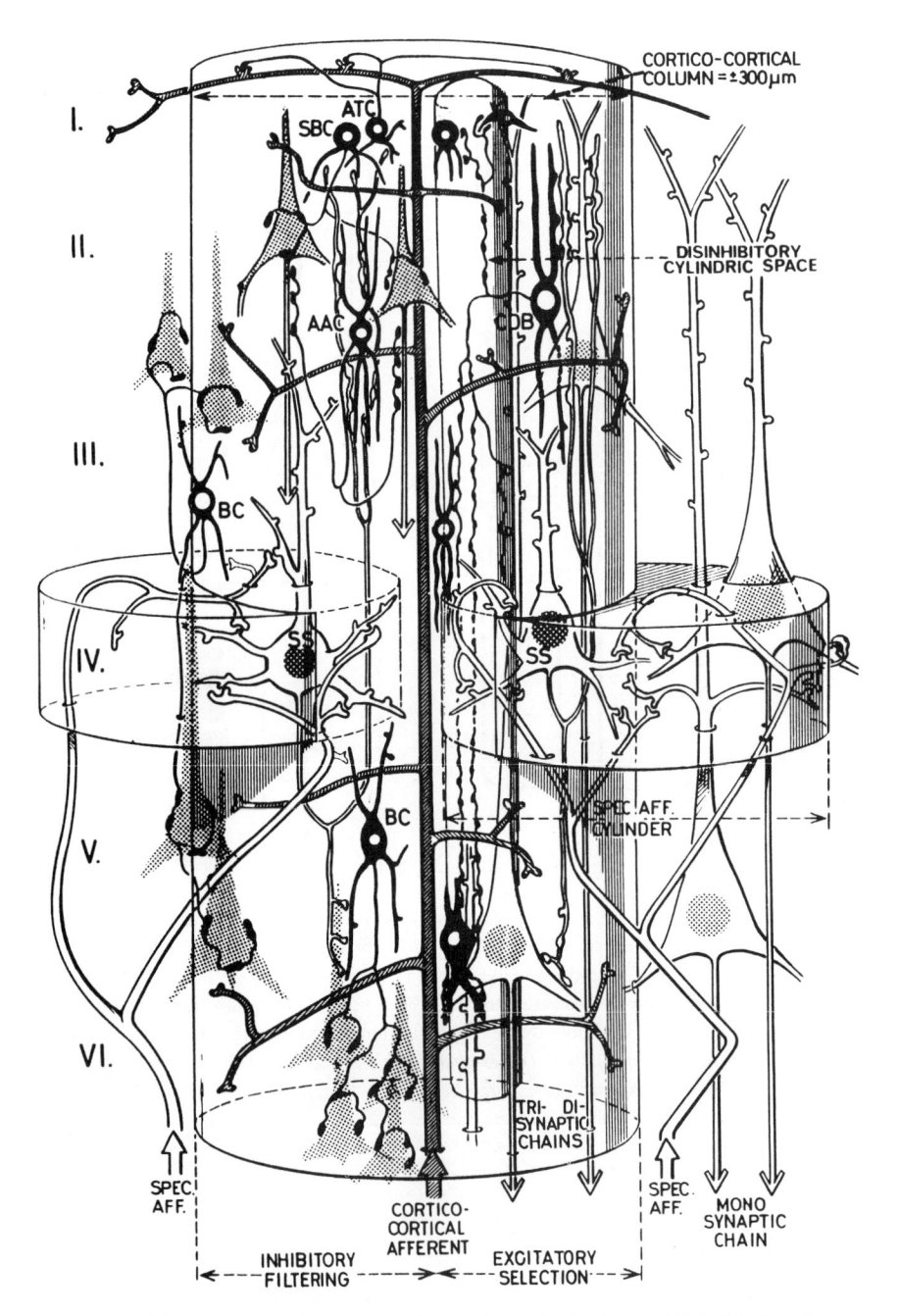

Figure 11.3 Neuron circuits of a representative corticocortical column. Cells in black are known or assumed to be inhibitory. ACT: axonal tuft cell. SC: small basket cell. AAC: axoaxonic (chandelier) cell. BC: basket cell. The following pyramidal cells and excitatory interneurons are drawn in outline: SS: spiny stellate cell. CDB: double bouquet cell, assumed to be predominantly disinhibitory, acting in a very narrow vertical cylindric space due to its narrow vertical axon strands. (From Szentágothai 1983.)

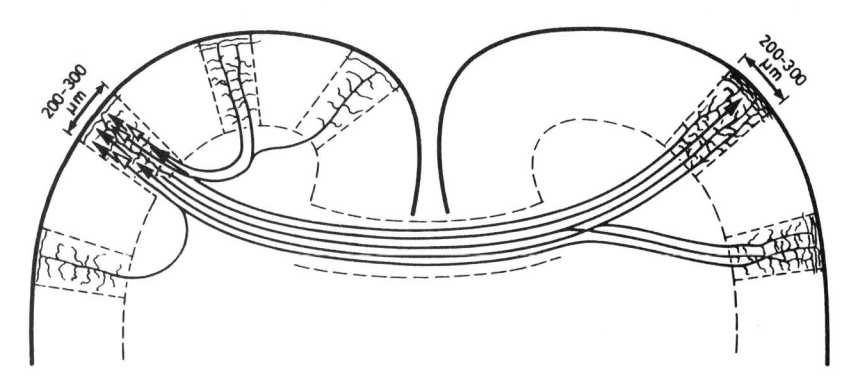

Figure 11.4 Corticocortical connectivity visualized as a mosaic of quasi-discrete columns 200–300 microns in diameter connected mainly by axons of pyramid cells in layer III ipsilaterally (outlined arrowheads) and contralaterally (solid arrowheads) from any layer. Connections may be reciprocal but are not necessarily so. (From Szentágothai 1978b.)

and non-spiny presumed inhibitory neurons (large and small basket cells, smooth and sparsely spinous stellate cells, double-bouquet cells of Cajal, axo-axonic cells, and axonal tuft cells). Since none of these non-pyramidal cells have axons that descend into the subcortical white matter, they are termed *intrinsic neurons*, *interneurons*, or *local-circuit neurons*. Since the non-spiny or inhibitory neurons are in this group, it follows that all inhibitory activity in the cortex is generated locally (i.e., within cortical columns—see below) (Creutzfeldt 1977, 1978; Fairén et al. 1984).

THE LAYERED STRUCTURE OF THE NEOCORTEX

Of the six layers of the cerebral cortex, layer I has very few neurons. Pyramidal cells (figure 11.1) and non-pyramidal cells are distributed throughout layers II–VI. The axon collaterals of pyramidal cells synapse onto the basal dendrites of nearby pyramidal cells, as mentioned above. Association fibers—connections with the cortex on the same (ipsilateral) side—arise from pyramidal cells mainly in layer III (figures 11.1, 11.4). Callosal fibers—fibers making connections with the cortex on the opposite (contralateral) side—arise from pyramidal cells in layers II–VI (figures 11.1, 11.4). Fibers projecting to subcortical structures arise from pyramidal cells in layers V and VI, corticothalamic fibers arising from the latter (figure 11.1).

In relation to the input to the cortex (figures 11.3–11.5), thalamocortical fibers terminate primarily in the middle layers, III and IV, but also in layer I, whereas corticocortical (i.e., association and callosal) fibers terminate in all layers. Callosal fibers, which have been estimated to number 180 million in the human brain (Brodal 1981), primarily interconnect corresponding (homotopic) points of the two hemispheres (Szentágothai 1983; Innocenti 1984). (The primary sensory cortical areas—visual, auditory, somesthetic—are not interconnected by callosal fibers.) Thalamocortical fibers, like association and callosal fibers, terminate in excitatory synapses.

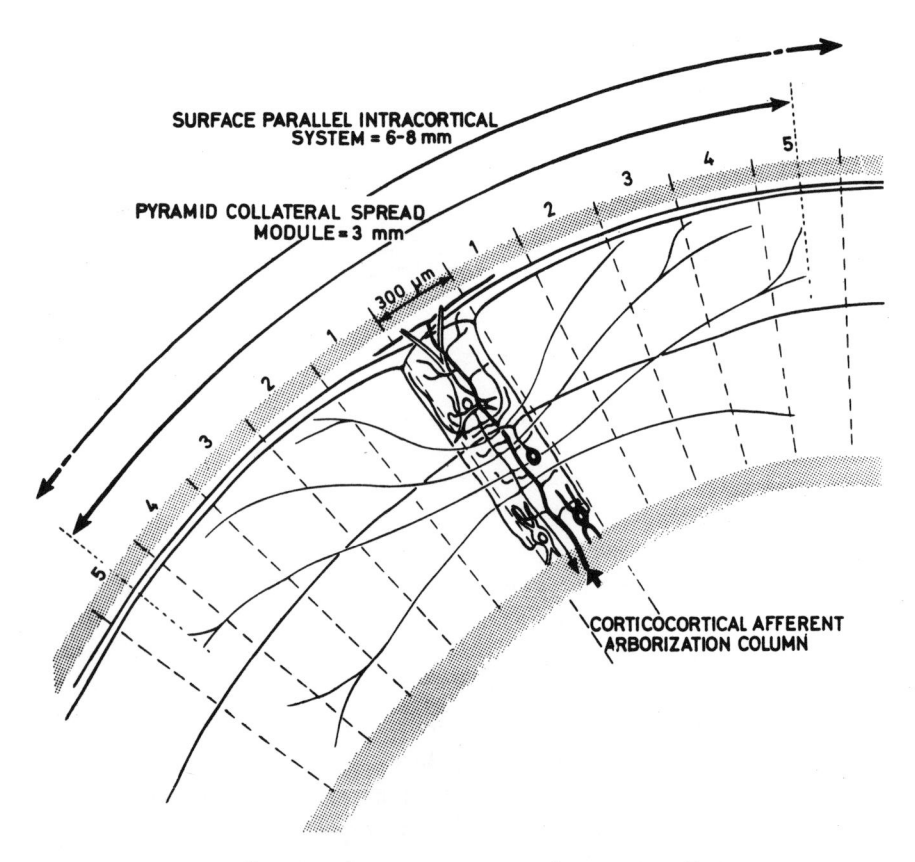

Figure 11.5 Diagram illustrating long-range intracortical connections. Excitatory neurons in outline, inhibitory interneurons in solid black. (From Szentágothai 1978a.)

Initially from physiological and later from anatomical evidence, the concept of a functional unit or module of the cortex, the cortical column, some 200–300 microns in diameter, has emerged (figures 11.2–11.5) (Hubel and Wiesel 1962, 1977; Mountcastle 1957, 1978; Goldman and Nauta 1977). Physiologically, it was the fact that neurons in all layers of the cortex may be excited by the same group of afferent fibers that led to the hypothesisis (Creutzfeldt 1978). (A possible model for part of the function of the cortical column is suggested in appendix B in the form of the adaptive signal processor.)

Anatomically, a phenomenon much the same in principle was observed in the transport of radioactive tracers to terminal branches of axons. Such units or modules, which appear to make up a mosaic encompassing the entire neocortical surface, are interconnected by association and callosal fibers. It is noteworthy that the latter greatly outnumber the corticothalamic and thalamocortical fibers—by perhaps 100:1, according to Braitenberg (1977, 1978). The cortical columns appear to be organized not around the thalamocortical fibers but rather around the corticocortical fibers, since the former occupy an eccentric whereas the latter occupy a central position in a given column (figure 11.3).

Interconnections among adjacent and nearby columns (figure 11.5) are effected by collaterals of axons of pyramidal cells, which may extend 6 mm from the soma (Gilbert et al. 1988), as well as by fibers coursing in layer I (and also in layer II); the latter connections, like the former, are excitatory.

The spontaneous firing rate of cortical neurons is much lower than that of thalamocortical projection neurons. Cortical neurons cease firing after deafferentation, according to Creutzfeldt (1977, 1978).

Eccles (1984) pointed out that, in contrast to the possibility of reentrant loops between cortex and thalamus (since thalamocortical connectivities are reciprocal), there appears to be no internal system of communication that could give reverberatory loop operation within a cortical module or column. On the other hand, Eccles (1984) suggested that there could be opportunities for reentrant loop operation for the ipsilateral cortex via association fibers and for the contralateral cortex via callosal fibers.

THE DISTRIBUTION OF SYNAPSES ON NEURONS

The distribution of excitatory and inhibitory synapses on pyramidal cells is not uniform. On the distal, more remote part of the apical dendritic tree, both types of synapses occur, but on the proximal portion of the apical dendrite, and especially on the cell body (soma), inhibitory synapses predominate. (Shepherd et al. (1985) have suggested that signal enhancement may occur in distal cortical dendrites as a result of interactions between active dendritic spines.) Indeed, the synapses on pyramidal cell bodies are evidently only inhibitory (Peters and Jones 1984; Houser et al. 1984). Such a dense inhibitory synaptic covering of the proximal dendrites and cell body is characteristic of all pyramidal cells, irrespective of their destination, whether to a different part of the cortex, ipsilaterally or contralaterally, or to the thalamus, the brainstem, or the spinal cord (Houser et al. 1984).

By virtue of their location, inhibitory synapses on the cell body are more powerful than those on individual dendrites (figure 11.2), since an inhibitory synapse on one dendrite would have no effect on another dendrite. Martin (1984) has drawn attention to several lines of evidence that point to a divisive function of inhibitory synapses from basket cells on pyramidal cell bodies, in contrast to the subtractive inhibition that characterizes synapses onto more distal parts of the dendritic tree, including those located on the necks of dendritic spines. Inhibitory synapses at the latter sites could inhibit a specific excitatory input to a particular dendrite or dendritic spine.

Blomfield (1974), in modeling a simple neuron mathematically, found that inhibitory synapses produced large conductance changes, and that, being located primarily on the soma, they are ideally suited to carry out division by shunting synaptic currents through low-impedance pathways. (In this model, provided their conductance changes were sufficiently small, excitatory synapses were linearly additive and inhibitive synapses linearly subtractive, irrespective of location.) Confirmatory experimental evidence for such a divisive or scaling operation was found by Rose (1977) from a study of a two-variable experiment in which one variable was the rate of firing of a visual cortex neuron (which depended on the orientation of a bar of light moved through the cell's receptive field) and the other variable was the rate of iontophoresed GABA (gamma-amino butyric acid) near the cell's soma. Evidence of a divisive function was also reported by Dean et al. (1980), from a two-grating experiment with visual units, and by Morrone et al. (1982), whose two stimuli were a grating and a visual noise of various contrasts.

Martin (1984) suggested that such a divisive function for inhibitory synapses may be a function of the basket cell, which forms inhibitory synapses on cell bodies, as contrasted with the double-bouquet cell, which does not form synapses onto the soma of its target neurons. Martin (1984) also raised the question of a possible difference in the distribution on target neurons of GABA-A and GABA-B receptors, which have somewhat different properties (see also Crunelli and Leresche 1991). Thus, the properties of GABA-A receptors could suggest a preponderant distribution on the soma and the axon initial segment, whereas GABA-B may have a preponderantly dendritic localization (Martin 1984).

An even stronger inhibitory effect can be attributed to the axoaxonic or chandelier cell, the axons of which spiral around the initial segment (trigger zone) of pyramidal-cell axons. Axoaxonic cells, each of which may contact a number of pyramidal cells, could thus "choke off" or inhibit completely the firing of pyramidal cells (Szentágothai 1978b). This powerful axoaxonic inhibitory synaptic mechanism is largely restricted to the pyramidal cells of layers II and III, which give rise to corticocortical (association) projections, and is much less prominent in the deeper layers (V and VI) (Eccles 1984; Martin 1984).

The inhibitory control of pyramidal cells by basket cells is somewhat different from that by axoaxonic or chandelier cells: each basket cell contacts the cell body and proximal dendrites of numerous pyramidal neurons over a relatively considerable distance in the horizontal plane, whereas axoaxonal cells (concerning the input for which little is known (Peters 1984)) contact pyramidal cells in a vertical disk-like field in layers II and III (Houser et al. 1984). In turn, basket cells (and also neurogliaform cells) receive an excitatory input from thalamocortical fibers, which would form a basis for disynaptic inhibition of pyramidal cells (Houser et al. 1984). In addition, since the recurrent collaterals of pyramidal cells excite other pyramidal cells, a concurrent excitation of inhibitory cells could provide the basis for another kind of disynaptic inhibition of pyramidal cells (Houser et al. 1984)

On the other hand, the very narrow vertical column of the inhibition of double-bouquet cells (figures 11.2, 11.3), if acting upon cells that in turn inhibit pyramidal cells (i.e., disinhibiting the former), could form the basis of mini-columns perhaps 30 microns in diameter (figure 11.3)—much smaller than the aforementioned columns of some 300 microns in diameter (Eccles 1984).

Of the non-pyramidal neurons, only the spiny stellate cell (which, as an excitatory neuron, can perhaps be considered as a kind of local-circuit pyramidal cell) appears to have exclusively inhibitory synapses on its cell body; all other non-pyramidal cells have both excitatory and inhibitory synapses on their cell bodies (Lund 1984; Peters and Jones 1984).

Of all the putative transmitter and modulator substances, only gamma-butyric acid, as an inhibitory transmitter, appears to be firmly established—a situation made possible by the fact that its synthesizing enzyme, glutamic acid decarboxylase (GAD), which can be demonstrated immunocytochemically, is entirely confined to neurons (Houser et al. 1984).

Martin (1984) has pointed out that axoaxonic or chandelier cells have been found in all regions of the brain that are known to be capable of generating epileptic discharges: neocortex, hippocampus, and amygdala. Roberts (1976) has suggested that loss of (GABA-mediated) inhibitory control of pyramidal cell activity could be important in activating excessive pyramidal-cell activity, i.e., epilepsy.

Brief mention may be made of electrical ephaptic (non-synaptic or non-chemical) transmissions, but these appear more likely to be of significance in relation to pathological states, such as in epileptic discharges, rather than in normally functioning cortex (Dichter and Ayala 1987; Gilbert et al. 1988).

TERMINATIONS OF THALAMOCORTICAL FIBERS IN THE NEOCORTEX

Although thalamocortical fibers were traditionally considered to terminate in one or at most a few cortical areas, and in these areas, in Layer IV, a more diffuse termination, both in different cortical areas and in different cortical layers, now seems apparent (Steriade et al. 1990a). Thus, there is now anatomical evidence for thalamocortical synapses on spiny intrinsic neurons, on one or more non-spiny GABAergic neurons, as well as on corticocortical, callosal, corticothalamic, corticostriatal, corticospinal, and possibly other types of pyramidal neurons (Steriade et al. 1990a, p. 102).

The above brief overview, which does not include the corticostriatal projections that arise from virtually the entire neocortex (Goldman-Rakic and Selemon 1984), can be summarized as follows:

• The main (if not the entire) input to and output from the neocortex, including its own interconnections (i.e., association and callosal fibers), and to and from the thalamus, is excitatory, with the exception of the input from certain brain-stem nuclei (e.g., the locus ceruleus and the raphe nuclei; see chapter 12). The latter inputs may be considered to be relatively diffuse to the neocortex, in contrast to the more discrete or localized inputs of the former.

• All neocortical inhibitory activity of a localized or discrete nature is generated locally, by interneurons or local circuit neurons within cortical columns; there are no fibers with inhibitory synaptic terminals arriving from elsewhere in the cortex or from the thalamus.

- The interconnections among cortical columns greatly outnumber the interconnections between cortex and thalamus.

- In addition to the familiar subtractive inhibition that takes place on the distal dendritic tree, the basis of a divisive inhibition is afforded by inhibitory synapses on neuron cell bodies. The former would constitute linear interaction of excitatory and inhibitory synapses; the latter would imply non-linear (i.e., scaling) control of excitatory synaptic effects by inhibitory ones.

12 The Physiological Basis of the EEG

The physiological basis of the EEG has been the subject of several reviews (e.g., Creutzfeldt 1969, 1983; Elul 1972b; Creutzfeldt and Houchin 1974; Frost 1976; Dutertre 1977; Goldensohn 1979b; Bindman and Lippold 1981; Speckman and Elger 1987; Pedley and Traub 1990; Steriade et al. 1990b; Lopes da Silva 1991; Martin 1991). Although some newer aspects have been added in recent years (see below), the basic picture of the origin of EEG potentials has remained largely the same for some years. In this view, the EEG reflects primarily the summated fluctuations of excitatory and inhibitory postsynaptic potentials in the pyramidal cells of the upper layers of the cerebral cortex. More exactly, the EEG is considered to reflect the extracellular current flows associated with such postsynaptic activity (Martin 1991).

This view of the basis of the EEG originated with the suggestion by Eccles (1951), based on his experience with spinal motorneurons, that the EEG originated from synaptic (more exactly, postsynaptic) potentials in the superficial layers of the cortex. (Eccles' concept of the origin of the alpha rhythm represented a combination of the notion of circulation of impulses in closed neural chains and the idea of an inherent rhythmicity.) That inhibitory as well as excitatory postsynaptic potentials summated to make up the EEG was already well established by the late 1950s. (The early history of the development of concepts concerning the EEG can be found in Purpura 1959 and in Elul 1972b; the 1936 Cold Spring Harbor Symposium volume (volume 4) includes several contributions concerning the EEG (e.g., Jasper 1936b).) Verzeano (1972) pointed out that the summation of postsynaptic potentials alone would not, however, explain the origin of the EEG waves that can be recorded in white matter (for example, in the internal capsule, the pyramidal tract, or the optic tract).

Within the above-described general framework, the details of how specific human EEG patterns that are recordable from the cortex or from the scalp originate has remained less clear. For example, rhythmic activity such as alpha activity was originally considered to entail reverberating activity in corticocortical and corticothalamic circuits (Kubie 1930; Lorente de Nó 1933), low-voltage irregular activity (i.e., the "desynchronized" EEG) from more randomly recurring postsynaptic potentials, and the lower-frequency waves of non-REM sleep from a greater preponderance of inhibitory than excitatory postsynaptic potentials.

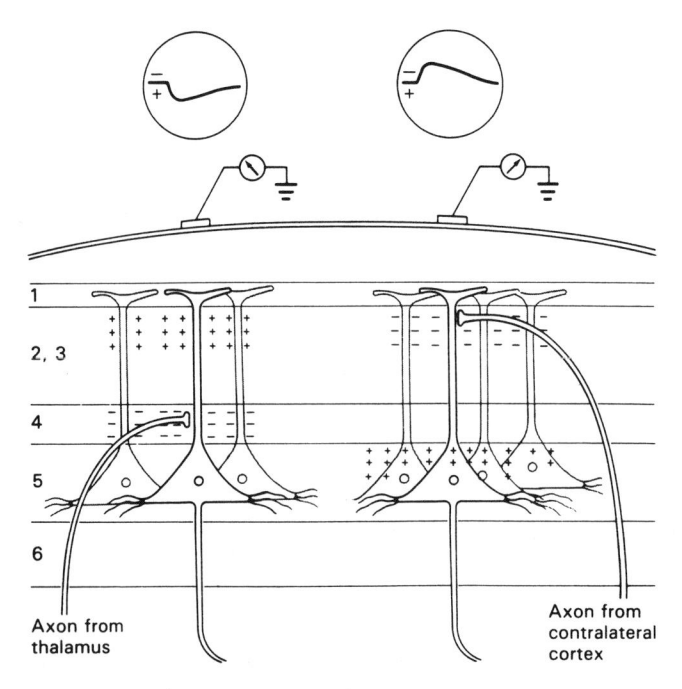

Figure 12.1 Left: positive potential at the scalp resulting from excitatory inputs to cortical neurons predominantly in layer IV of the cortex. Right: negative potential at the scalp resulting from excitatory inputs from callosal neurons in the contralateral cortex which terminate in the superficial cortical layers. (From Martin 1991.)

In general, and neglecting the effects of intracortical or local-circuit neurons, the postsynaptic excitatory potentials from fibers synapsing onto the apical dendrites of cortical pyramidal cells nearer the cell bodies of the latter (i.e., in layer IV) are reflected at the cortical surface (and in the EEG) as positive transients, as indicated on the left in figure 12.1. (For a recent review of neuronal excitability and synaptic transmission, see Rutecki 1992.) On the other hand, postsynaptic excitatory potentials from association and callosal fibers synapsing onto the more distal part of the apical dendritic tree (i.e., in layers II and III) of pyramidal cells are reflected as a negative transient, as indicated on the right in figure 12.1. Table 12.1 summarizes the effects of excitatory as well as inhibitory postsynaptic potentials.

If the relative contributions of postsynaptic excitatory potentials of corticocortical (association and callosal) fibers is in proportion to their relative

Table 12.1 Effects of postsynaptic excitatory and inhibitory potentials and their corresponding deflections. (From Martin 1991.)

Postsynaptic potential	Cellular response	Intracellular recording	Extracellular surface recording	
			Synapse in superficial layer	Synapse in deeper layer
Excitatory	Depolarization	Upward	Upward	Downward
Inhibitory	Hyperpolarization	Downward	Downward	Upward

numbers (of the order of 100:1; see Braitenberg 1977), then the EEG may represent preponderantly corticocortical postsynaptic excitatory activity. Adey (1988) has suggested that EEG-like events (more particularly, that portion of the EEG that is distributed in the extracellular space) may have a feedback effect on the domain in which the neurons are a part.

The EEG at the surface of the cortex and at the surface of the scalp is thus considered to reflect the extracellular current flow associated with summated postsynaptic potentials in synchronously activated, vertically oriented pyramidal cells; for reasons of geometry as well as because of the extreme extracellular attenuation, action potentials from firings of pyramidal cells contribute only minimally or not at all to the EEG (Martin 1991).

SOME CHARACTERISTICS OF THE NORMAL HUMAN ADULT EEG

As a preliminary to consideration of results from experimental studies in animals concerning EEG-generating mechanisms, a few fundamental aspects of normal adult EEG patterns will be summarized briefly.

The normal waking adult human EEG, generally speaking, can be classified into two principal patterns: the posterior rhythmic activity in the frequency range of 8–13 Hz that characterizes the relaxed, eyes-closed state in most subjects, and a lower-voltage, irregular pattern that is distributed diffusely over the scalp and occurs (at least transiently) with visual attention with eyes open or during active mental activity, such as attempted visualization of an image with eyes closed or mental arithmetic. (In some subjects, the latter pattern prevails posteriorly as well.)

In non-REM sleep, the adult human EEG exhibits a generally increasing content of slow waves (i.e., increasing in voltage and decreasing in frequency) with increasing depth of sleep from Stage 1 to Stage 4 (figures 6.1, 17.8). In REM sleep, the relatively high-voltage slow waves are not present (see below).

SOME ASPECTS OF TERMINOLOGY: THE "SYNCHRONIZED" VS. THE "DESYNCHRONIZED" EEG

Much of the experimental electrophysiology that has given rise to concepts and terminology of the EEG was carried out on animals (e.g., cats) that do not exhibit the full range of human EEG patterns (e.g., the alpha rhythm), although some early reports (e.g., Remple and Gibbs 1936) suggested a parallel. Closer approximations to the human alpha rhythm can be found in dogs (Lopes da Silva and Storm van Leeuwen 1978; Lopes da Silva et al. 1973a,b) and especially in the higher primates (Caveness 1962). Thus, the terms *desynchronization* and *synchronization* arose primarily from studies in animal physiology (see figure 12.2), referring to the waking alert state and the EEG during sleep—more exactly, slow-wave sleep, since the EEG in REM sleep in humans was not discovered until the latter half of the 1950s (Dement and Kleitman

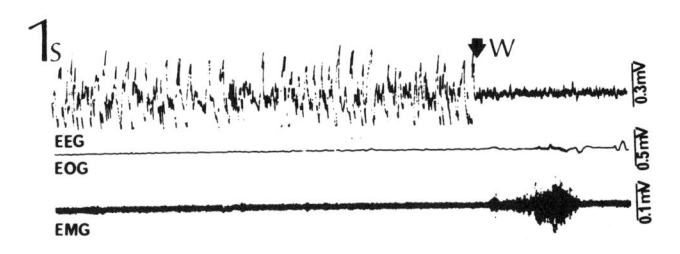

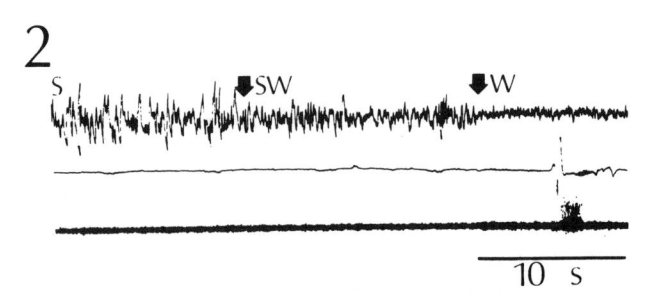

Figure 12.2 Abrupt (1) and progressive (2) transition from slow-wave sleep (S) to wakefulness (W). SW denotes a transitional state. (From Steriade et al. 1982.)

1957). Subsequently, the term *desynchronization* was applied to the EEG during REM sleep (see e.g., Hobson and Steriade 1986).

Actually, the term, *desynchronization* was originally introduced by Adrian and Mathews (1934), at a time when the EEG was considered to represent summated unit or action potentials of single cortical neurons, to imply asynchrony among such unit potentials (Schlag 1974). Jasper (1936b) introduced the term *activation* to indicate a change (i.e., an increase) in the cortical excitatory state. (Jasper indicated later (1981) that his original use of the term *activation* could also be considered to reflect inhibitory as well as excitatory processes.)

Jasper (1936b) characterized a sequence of progressive change in excitatory state in detail as follows:

The characteristic changes, both in man and in the cat, from a condition of high general excitation, such as the immediate effects of startle or extreme emotional tension, down to low levels of excitation, as in deep sleep, might be described by the following sequence of alternation in brain potential patterns.

1. Extreme excitation. No rhythmic brain potentials. This does not rule out changes in the level of polarization [i.e., DC potentials] whch are non-phasic in nature.

2. Moderate excitation. High frequency, low amplitude brain potentials. First irregular, then at a slightly lower level of excitation, more regular high frequency potentials.

3. Moderate relaxation. Fairly regular rhythms at a more or less constant frequency and somewhat increased in amplitude.

4. Further relaxation and drowsiness. Slower rhythms and beginning of irregularity; tendency for bursts, etc.

5. Sleep. Further decrease in frequency and regularity of brain potentials with definite increase in amplitude.

6. Very deep sleep. Very slow random potential swings.

(REM sleep, which as mentioned above was not discovered until much later, was not included in Jasper's designation of states.)

In time, *desynchronization* came to imply asynchronous occurrence of graded (as opposed to unit) potentials, presumably at least primarily of postsynaptic origin. Schlag (1958, 1974) reported that the most conspicuous change in the shift from "slow" to "fast" EEG activity is a shift from firing of single neurons in bursts or clusters to a more continuous mode of discharge—a quite prominent change in the cerebral cortex and the thalamus, but much less prominent in the brain stem. The term *arousal* refers to the behavioral change that typically accompanies "activation" in the waking state (compare O'Leary and Goldring 1976, p. 160). The term *activation* is sometimes used in an opposite sense to *inhibition*—i.e., as a synonym for *excitation*.

The parallel change between the progressive change of decreasing EEG amplitude and increasing frequency, on the one hand, and increasing activation in the organism from the comatose state to extreme arousal, on the other, has formed the basis of "arousal theory" (Freedman et al. 1966).

In the present discussion, *arousal* and *sleep* will be used in a behavioral sense, to indicate the level of alertness, whereas *activation* or *desynchronization*, and *spindling* or *synchronization*, will be used to refer to the EEG itself. (In REM sleep, the EEG has been considered to be activated, for which the term *activated sleep* is sometimes used.)

Some authors, including Verzeano (1972), use *synchronization* to refer primarily to rhythmic waves such as those that occur in the alpha rhythm or in sleep spindles, recognizing that the nature of the synchronized activity giving rise to such rhythmic waves is ill-defined. Verzeano (1972) defined synchronization as "a dynamic process characterized by a highly organized circulation of activity through the neuronal networks of the cortex and of the thalamus." In this context, the level of synchronization is taken to be the equivalent of the degree of rhythmicity in such circulating activity.

Jasper (1981) has pointed out that the amplitude of the EEG is "inversely related to the normally integrated activation of a given cortical area or to the 'arousal' of the brain as a whole." When a given cortical area becomes involved with integrative functions, with its "finely organized asynchronous pattern of neuronal activity," then "the surface slow waves disappear, resulting in the 'arousal,' alerting, or 'orienting response,' the pattern of desynchronized activation of which has been related to certain 'higher' brain functions" (Jasper 1981).

Hobson and Steriade (1986, p. 729) used the term *activation* to refer to "a balanced level of excitatory and inhibitory drives on sensory and motor neurons that provides for rapid responsiveness and accurate discrimination."

"Thus," they note, "an activated neuron, circuit, or brain is both sensitive and finely tuned for discriminative response."

The above-noted apparent similarity between the patterns of the desynchronized EEG of the alert eyes-open state and the EEG pattern during REM sleep in experimental animals could also be inferred for human subjects, from descriptions of the activity of both states (figure 6.1A, G) as of the "relatively low-voltage mixed-frequency" type (Carskadon and Rechtschaffen 1989; Radtke 1990). (This description that has also been applied to Stage 1 non-REM sleep (figure 6.1C) in the absence of theta activity (3–7 Hz) in Stage 1 (Carskadon and Rechtschaffen 1989).) Clinical experience, on the other hand, suggests that there is often a greater content of theta activity in the EEG during REM sleep (not unlike that during the later stages of Stage 1 sleep—see figure 17.8) than during the alert eyes-open state. At the same time, on the basis of the EEG alone it can be difficult to distinguish the desynchronized EEG of the alert eyes-open state from that during early Stage 1 sleep (minimal drowsiness). Further, the spectra of the EEG during REM sleep (excluding periods when sawtooth waves are present) have been reported to be indistinguishable from those of the EEG during Stage 1 sleep, thus necessitating the inclusion of other physiological measures (e.g., eye movements) for computerized discrimination between these two stages (Johnson 1972). Characterizing the EEG in different states may therefore be more complex in human subjects than in some experimental animals (e.g., cats).

THE ORIGINS OF ALPHA ACTIVITY

As was mentioned above, rhythmic EEG activity such as the alpha rhythm was originally attributed to corticocortical and corticothalamic circuits (Kubie 1930; Lorente de Nó 1933). Andersen and Andersson (1968, 1974) implicated the specific thalamic nuclei as a thalamic pacemaker for the human alpha rhythm, basing their argument strongly on an analogy between barbiturate spindles recorded from the cortex of the cat and the human alpha rhythm, a long-standing parallel (Jasper 1949).

However, the drawing of a parallel between the alpha rhythm and barbiturate spindles has been challenged by several workers (Elul 1972a,b). Important differences have been found, in recordings from dogs, with respect to spectra, topographic distribution, coherence, direction of propagation (i.e., thalamocortical vs. corticothalamaic), and with respect to the levels of behavioral arousal necessary for these two types of activity to appear (Lopes da Silva et al. 1973; Steriade et al. 1990b). These findings have been interpreted to indicate that the alpha rhythm is primarily cortical in origin (Steriade et al. 1990b). Finally, the inhibitory feedback loops in the form of recurrent collateral of thalamocortical axons, which were postulated by Andersen and Andersson (1968) as a basis for rhythmic activity, have not been demonstrated anatomically, nor has a mechanism been found for intrathalamic diffusion of spindles among the various thalamic nuclei having thalamocortical projections (Jones 1985; Steriade et al. 1990b).

DC ASPECTS OF THE EEG

That activation of the EEG is accompanied by a negative DC shift has long been known (Jasper 1936, 1981). In experimental animals, a DC shift toward a greater surface negativity is a well-established aspect of the experimental penicillin focus (Matsumoto and Ajmone-Marsan 1964b; Gumnit and Takahashi 1965) and has also been observed during the clonic bursts of seizures induced by pentylenetetrazol (Metrazol) (Creutzfeldt 1969). O'Leary and Goldring (1976) found that a DC (or steady potential (SP)) shift accompanied all seizure discharges recorded in the electrocorticogram, whether from animals or from human subjects. Cohn (1954, 1964) found such a DC shift from scalp EEG recordings in patients during seizures with the 3-Hz spike-wave pattern. Such DC shifts were subsequently studied in greater detail by Chatrian et al. (1968) (figure 4.16 above). It is relevant to note that repetitive electrical stimulation has been reported to result in a progressive negative DC shift for human epileptogenic neocortex, but not for non-epileptogenic neocortex (O'Leary and Goldring 1964).

NEWER DEVELOPMENTS

Much of the preceding discussion can be considered as the "classical" view of the physiological basis of the EEG, largely in place by the late 1950s and early 1960s, reflecting the fundamental electrogenesis in neurons in terms of excitatory and inhibitory postsynaptic potentials. Since about 1975, however, additional developments have appeared. A number of these developments, summarized in Steriade et al. 1990b, will now be considered.

Earlier experimental work had suggested that activation of the cerebral cortex—i.e., the emergence of low-voltage irregular activity (figure 12.2)—was a result of increased activity of the ascending reticular activating system of the brain stem (Moruzzi and Magoun 1949); contrariwise, a decrease in activity in the latter system was presumed to result in the presence of slow waves (i.e., "synchronization") in the cortex. However, Brodal (1981) pointed out that "the 'activating system' is a functional concept, the 'reticular formation' a morphological one, and it has been obvious for many years that these two do not correspond." (See also Jones 1985.) On the other hand, these earlier skeptical views have themselves been called into question by more recent developments (see Steriade et al. 1990a, p.55ff).

The role of the brain-stem reticular formation and the thalamic intralaminar nuclei as a part of the nonspecific thalamic system has become less clear than had been previously thought. The thalamic reticular nucleus (see below) does not project to the cortex at all (Macchi and Bentivoglio 1984, p. 385). It has been suggested that the most likely basis for "activation" (desynchronization) of the EEG is a direct projection from the thalamic intralaminar nuclei to the deep layers of the cortex, where axonal termination on the proximal dendrites of pyramidal cells could profoundly alter their threshold for excitation (Macchi and Bentivoglio 1984).

Recent work has indicated that the supplanting of slow waves in the cortex by the "activated" or "desynchronized" pattern results from a decrease of, or interference with, projections to the neocortex of basal forebrain cholinergic pathways. (A review of the changing perspective on the different neocortical EEG patterns appears in Buzsaki et al. 1988.) This perspective on the relationship between the neocortex and basal forebrain structures can be considered a variant of the deafferentiation hypothesis of sleep, which has had a long history (Moruzzi 1964).

Moruzzi and Magoun (1949) proposed that the EEG desynchronizing effect. is mediated at least in part by the diffuse or "nonspecific" thalamocortical projection system, which corresponds to the cortical projections of the midline and intralaminar thalamic nuclei (Jones 1985), which had been studied earlier beginning with Dempsey and Morison (1942) and Morison and Dempsey (1942). The cortical synaptology of these nonspecific afferents, has, however, apparently not been explored (Jones 1985). Thus, rostrally projecting brain-stem reticular axons reach the thalamus but not the cortex itself, save for a few fibers to the visual cortex (Steriade et al. 1990a, p. 303).

Of the "nonspecific" afferents that are distributed diffusely to the cortex but do not synapse in the thalamus, the best known are those that contain noradrenaline and arise primarily from the locus ceruleus of the pons, those that contain serotonin and arise primarily from the dorsal nucleus of the midbrain raphe, those that contain dopamine and arise primarily from the midbrain ventral tegmental area, and those that contain acetylcholine and arise primarily from the substantia innominata (in primates, the nucleus basalis of Meynert) of the forebrain (see Steriade et al. 1990a, p. 55, for references). The importance of these in relation to cortical desynchronization remains unclear, in part because of the proximities of the systems to one another. Furthermore, the question whether rostral reticular stimulation drives neurons in the basal forebrain (with consequent desynchronization of the cortex) has not been settled (Steriade et al. 1990a, p. 165). To compound the picture further, the cholinergic terminals in the cortex presumed to originate from the basal forebrain may be inhibitory (at least, the synapses are symmetrical by electronmicroscopy), in contrast to the expected excitatory role of cholinergic synapses (Steriade et al. 1990a, p. 303).

Steriade et al. (1990a) remarked that, with the exception of the theta rhythm arising in the septohippocampal system and the spindle rhythmicity originating in the thalamus (in the reticular nucleus), there are no systematic studies at a cellular level to indicate the sites of origin and the mechanisms of other EEG rhythms, such as alpha and slow waves.

Since some of the newer developments concerning the origins of the EEG relate to the structure and function of the thalamic reticular nucleus, some aspects of the anatomy and physiology of this nucleus will now be considered.

THE THALAMIC RETICULAR NUCLEUS

The reticular nucleus of the thalamus (or thalamic reticular complex (Jones 1985)) comprises a thin sheet-like layer of cells along almost the whole external (lateral) surface of the thalamus, and is separated from the main body of the thalamus by a thin layer of white matter, the external medullary lamina (Brodal 1981; Jones 1985; Ohara 1988). Because of its position, the reticular nucleus is traversed by virtually all fibers interconnecting the thalamus and the cerebral cortex, and both thalamocortical and corticothalamic fibers give off excitatory collaterals to dendrites in the reticular nucleus as they pass through it (these are indicated schematically in figure 12.3). The thalamic reticular nucleus gives off inhibitory (GABAergic) fibers to the thalamic nuclei of origin of the respective thalamocortical fibers, but does not itself project to the cerebral cortex as a part of the "nonspecific" or "diffuse" thalamic system

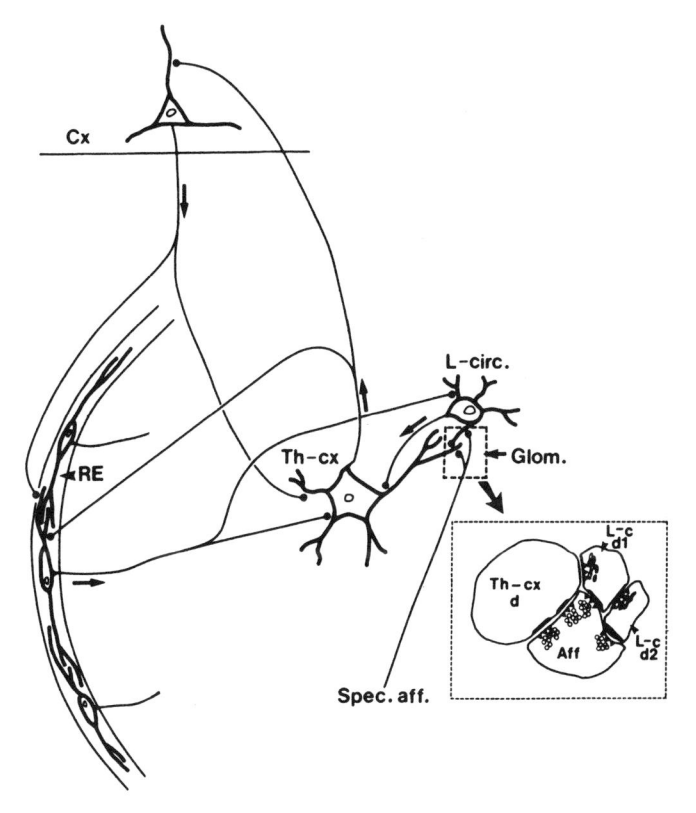

Figure 12.3 Schema indicating the input and output connections of the thalamic reticular nucleus (thalamic reticular complex). Excitatory collaterals are given off to the reticular nucleus by excitatory fibers from both corticothalamic (Cx) and thalamocortical (Th-cx) cells, as the latter fibers pass through the shell-like structure of the reticular nucleus. Cells in the reticular nucleus (RE) give off inhibitory fibers terminating on both thalamocortical neurons and on local-circuit (L-circ.) neurons, thus providing the basis of a complex multiple-loop negative feedback arrangement. The inset indicates the contacts between an ascending specific afferent fiber (Spec. aff; aff), and dendrites of a thalamocortical neuron and two local-circuit dendrites (L-c d1, L-c d2). See also figure 1 in Steriade et al. 1990b. (From Steriade and Llinás 1988.)

The Physiological Basis of the EEG

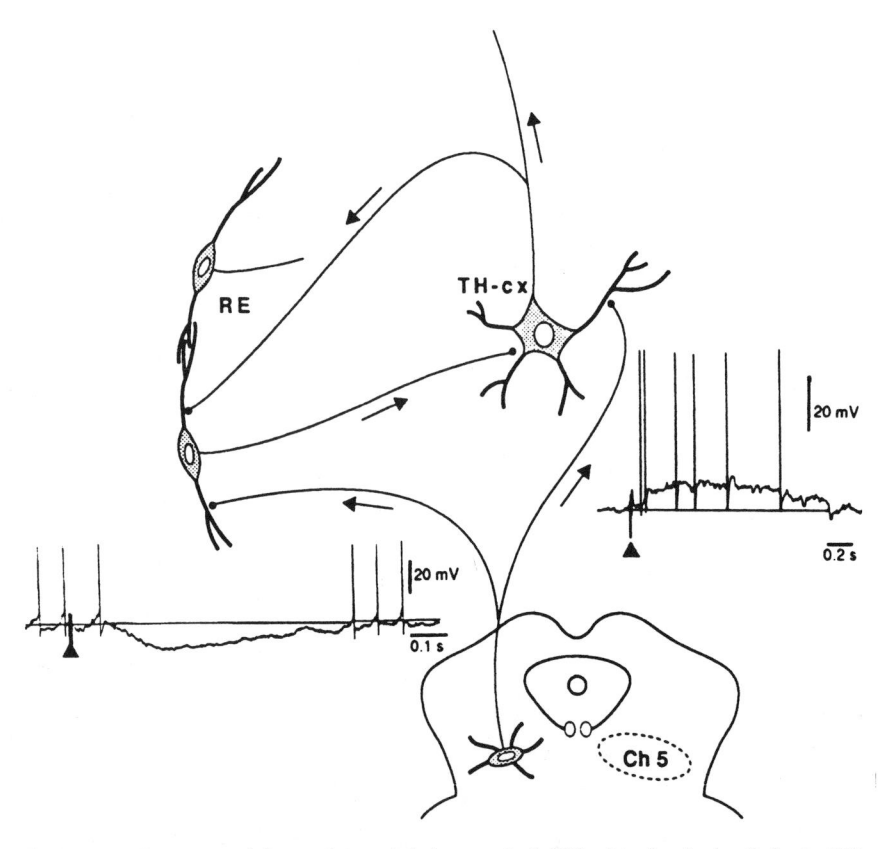

Figure 12.4 Recurrent inhibitory loop of thalamocortical (TH-cx) and reticular thalamic (RE) neurons, and side loop (via RE neurons by mesopontine cholinergic afferents (only the Ch5 group of pedunculopontine tegmental neurons is depicted). Since the latter hyperpolarize RE thalamic neurons, a disinhibition of TH-cx neurons occurs, thus potentiating the effect of the main mesopontine cholinergic afferent terminating on TH-cx cells. (From Steriade et al. 1990b.)

(Brodal 1981), as had been thought earlier. The thalamic reticular nucleus is thus in a position to exert a negative feedback control on thalamocortical neurons (Ohara 1988).

There are also collateral inputs to the thalamic reticular nucleus from the brain stem (Jones 1985; Ohara 1988); these form a side loop for thalamocortical neurons, as indicated in figure 12.4. Additional details on the complex synaptic organization within most thalamic nuclei (excluding the reticular nucleus itself) are shown in figure 12.5; these are included here because their complexities may be less familiar than those of neocortical synaptic organization, and because of the strategically important role that the thalamic reticular nucleus must have in corticothalamic and thalamocortical interactions. The essential elements of these large aggregations of synaptic terminals (or glomeruli) are a postsynaptic dendritic component and two presynaptic components (Jones 1985). The one or two dendrites present are usually the primary branches of one or more relay cells close to their parent cell somata and, if present, one or more of their dendritic appendages (figure 12.5). Of the two

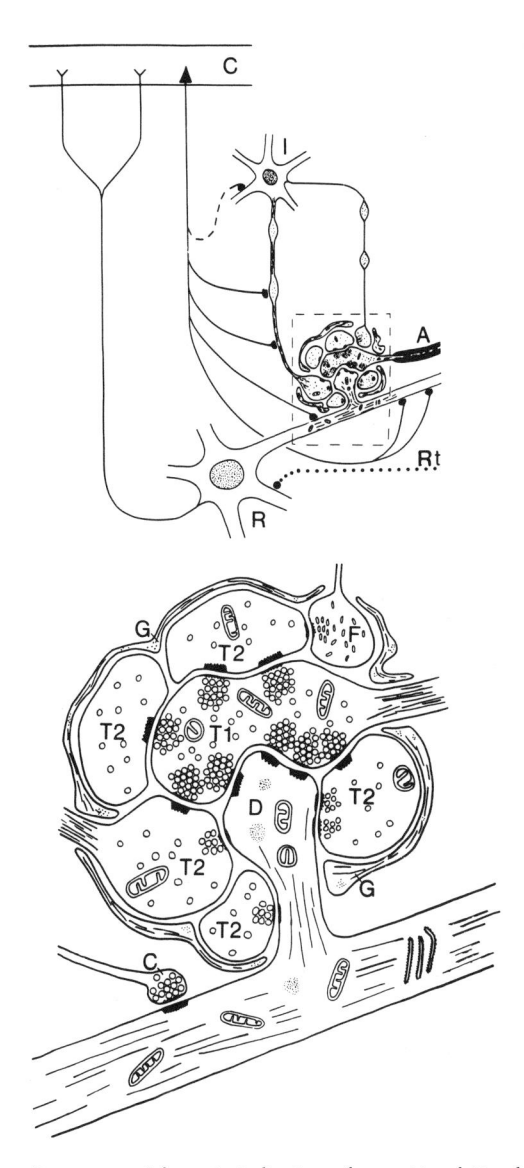

Figure 12.5 Schematic indication of synaptic relationships typical of the majority of thalamic nuclei. Dendritic protrusions (D) of thalamocortical relay cells (R) receive terminals (T1) of ascending afferent fibers (A) and presynaptic dendrites (T2) of interneurons (I). Presynaptic dendrites and probably conventional dendrites of interneurons are also postsynaptic to the afferent fiber terminals (and sometimes to one another). Axons of interneurons also terminate (F) mainly on the presynaptic dendrites. The complex synaptic aggregation tends to be ensheathed in astrocytic processes (G). Outside this, corticothalamic terminals (C) end on relay cell dendrites and on presynaptic dendrites of interneurons. In the case of the relay cell, most cortical terminals are distally situated. Terminals of reticular nucleus axons (Rt) also terminate on or close to somata of relay neurons. (From Jones 1985.)

types of presynaptic elements, the first (the minority type) is a conventional axon terminal derived from the principal ascending afferent fiber system to the nucleus. The second component, outnumbering the first by three or four times, is a presynaptic dendrite from thalamic interneurons (T2 in figure 12.5), but resembles an axon terminal in that it contains synaptic vesicles of symmetrical (i.e., presumably inhibitory) shape, and makes conventional synaptic contacts on the dendritic elements of the aggregation and sometimes on one another. These presynaptic dendrites are at the same time postsynaptic, with asymmetrical synaptic contacts (i.e., presumably excitatory) to the subcortical afferent terminals (T1 in figure 12.5). Finally, at the periphery of a glomerulus a further type of presynaptic terminal may be seen: a conventional axon terminal with symmetrical synaptic contacts (i.e., presumably inhibitory) onto one or more presynaptic dendrites, which is thought to originate from thalamic interneurons.

Recapitulating: The thalamocortical and corticothalamic collaterals terminating in the thalamic reticular nucleus are excitatory; the fibers given off by the reticular nucleus itself to other thalamic nuclei are exclusively inhibitory (GABAergic); the nucleus is thus in a position to exert a negative feedback control on thalamocortical neurons (Ohara 1988). Although the precise mechanism is unclear, a role for the thalamic reticular nucleus as a thalamic pacemaker has been suggested (Mulle et al. 1986); this topic is considered in greater detail below.

Steriade et al. (1987) have reported that the surgically isolated thalamic reticular nucleus can generate spindle rhythmicity in ketamine-anesthetized cats in response to very low doses of a short-acting barbiturate (Brevital), as well as in chronically implanted animals during natural sleep (Steriade et al. 1986). In contrast, cortical spindle activity was not present after isolation of the thalamic reticular nucleus, although irregular slow waves persisted. (The latter finding is consistent with the previously cited results, reported by Kellaway et al. (1966), concerning irregular slow cortical activity after cortical isolation.)

The barbiturate-induced spindling activity in the thalamic reticular nucleus was accompanied by a bursting pattern in single neurons, which the above-mentioned authors attributed to dendrodendritic interaction (i.e., presynaptic to dendritic shafts and spines but postsynaptic to other terminals (Ohara 1988)), dendritic hyperpolarization, inactivation of a low-threshold calcium spike, and GABA secretion at a dendrodendritic synapse, to complete the chain (Steriade et al. 1987).

In their study of unit activity in the human thalamic reticular nucleus, Raeva et al. (1991) found three types of cellular discharge patterns: irregular low-frequency (0–10 Hz), bursting in short trains (10–30 msec) with unstable rhythmic patterns (2–5 Hz), and long-duration (0.1–2 sec) high-frequency bursts with relatively constant interburst silences (80–150 msec).

Recent experimental evidence indicates that cortical spindling activity (at least in cats with light doses of barbiturates) originates indirectly, from the thalamic reticular nucleus via other thalamic nuclei, rather than directly. As previously mentioned, there are no direct cortical projections from the thalamic reticular nucleus; it does, however, project to other thalamic nuclei, with exclusively inhibitory fibers. Also, as has been noted, the thalamic reticular nucleus receives excitatory collaterals from thalamocortical fibers and from corticothalamic fibers, and projects with inhibitory fibers back to the corticothalamic cells (figure 12.3).

The thalamic reticular nucleus also receives inhibitory (cholinergic) projections from the nucleus basalis of Meynert and from pedunculopontine tegmental neurons in the mesopontine area. The nucleus basalis also projects to the noeocortex, where, as previously indicated, it subserves "activation" of the neocortex and desynchronization of the EEG. The basal nucleus of Meynert thus activates the cortex directly as well as by inhibiting cortical spindling originating indirectly from the thalamic reticular nucleus. (Further aspects of the pharmacology of the nucleus basalis of Meynert in relation to the EEG are considered below.)

To reiterate: With behavioral arousal, cholinergic projections from the brain stem to the thalamus, and also cholinergic (and GABAergic) projections from the forebrain nucleus basalis to the thalamic reticular nucleus, result in a cessation of spindling in the latter nucleus and a consequent cessation of cortical spindling. Hence, a tonic instead of a rhythmic thalamocortical discharge results, with consequent cortical activation (Steriade et al. 1990b). (In addition, there is a cholinergic projection onto thalamic relay nuclei cells from the pontomesencephalic reticular formation, the effect of which is to enhance the response of thalamic relay neurons to afferent stimulation (Steriade et al. 1990b).)

INTRINSIC RHYTHMIC PROPERTIES OF SINGLE NEURONS

There have also been recent developments concerning intrinsic properties of single neurons; these have been reviewed by Llinás (1988), with particular reference to the ionic conductances that can give rise to such "autorhythmic" properties. For example, *in vitro* and *in vivo* studies have shown that, in addition to the familiar sodium and potassium conductances that generate the fast action potentials, thalamic cells exhibit a series of conductances which, taken together, lead to the possibility of two distinct firing rates: 6 and 10 Hz, according to the specific conditions (Jahnsen and Llinás 1984a,b). Such behavior of individual neurons (which may be modifiable by synaptic influences) obviates the previously presumed necessity of network properties (entailing, for example, recurrent excitation and inhibition) as a basis for rhythmic firing of a given neuron (Llinás and Jahnsen 1982; Jahnsen and Llinás 1984a,b). But in addition to such autorhythmic capabilities, these authors point out that the same neurons are capable of functioning as relay elements for neuronal information.

Among thalamic neurons, those of the reticular nucleus have a greater capability of intrinsic oscillation because of their particular constellation of conductances (Steriade et al. 1990b). Thus, as previously mentioned, the neuronally isolated thalamic reticular nucleus can generate spindle rhythmicity in response to very low doses of a short-acting barbiturate (Brevital), as well as in chronically implanted animals during natural sleep (Steriade et al. 1986). (Steriade et al. 1987). During light sleep, this nucleus promotes oscillatory activity in a chain that includes thalamocortical neurons in other thalamic nuclei that have feedback to the reticular nucleus via collaterals of their thalamocortical projections (see figure 12.3), as was indicated above.

EEG-GENERATING MECHANISMS FOR SPINDLES AND FOR SLOW-WAVE SLEEP

It has been shown in experimental animals that the change from EEG desynchronization to EEG synchronization—i.e., the spindling (7–14 Hz) stage of light sleep—is characterized by a change in the firing patterns of thalamocortical neurons from a tonic or continuous firing to a burst mode that is associated with a hyperpolarization of the cell membrane. The latter consists of a few spikes at 250–400 Hz, recurring with the waxing-and-waning spindles (Steriade et al. 1990a, p. 167ff; see also Verzeano and Negishi 1960).

A similar pattern of increased discharge rates and increased excitability of neurons in the intralaminar thalamic nuclei (i.e., centralis lateralis-paracentralis) that project widely to the cortex (and which relay midbrain reticular formation activity during the desynchronized EEG during the waking and REM sleep states) was reported in Glenn and Steriade 1982. (See also Hobson and Steriade 1986.) Contrariwise, Glenn and Steriade attributed the bursting pattern (e.g., 300–400 spikes/sec during the bursts) of the thalamic neurons, which generally occurs during synchronized or slow-wave sleep, to a sustained hyperpolarization. One effect of the latter is to provide a mechanism for closing sensory channels during slow-wave sleep.

DESYNCHRONIZED VS. SYNCHRONIZED EEG: RECENT CONTRIBUTIONS

Steriade and Llinás (1988; see also Steriade and Deschênes 1984, and Steriade et al. 1990a,b) listed the following factors as accounting for the onset of spindles in thalamocortical systems during EEG-synchronized states: the intrinsic (membrane) properties of thalamic neurons, an intrinsic rhythmic capability of the thalamic reticular nucleus and the consequent effect of this on thalamocortical neurons, and a dampening of the activity of rostral brain-stem reticular neurons having thalamic projections. (The inverse effect can be mimicked by stimulating cholinergic pathways originating in rostral brain-stem reticular neurons (Steriade and Llinás 1988).)

The above-described multi-modal functioning of thalamic neurons can be modeled by a set of nonlinear differential equations (Rose and Hindmarsh 1985; see also Goldbeter and Moran 1988 and Rinzel and Ermentrout 1989). This approach can be considered as a logical sequence to Fitzhugh's (1961) model of the action potential, the latter model itself being a generalization of van der Pol's (1926) equation for a relaxation oscillator (see also chapter 14 below).

Since the deafferented reticular nucleus generates spindle rhythmicity, it has been suggested that the pacemaker for thalamic (and, in turn, cortical) spindles is the thalamic reticular nucleus (Steriade et al. 1987, Steriade et al. 1990a, p. 196). The intrinsic spindling in the thalamic reticular nucleus has been attributed to the presence of dendrodendritic synapses (evident in electronmicroscopic images) that form a local inhibitory (GABAergic) network (Deschênes et al. 1985). These dendrodendritic synapses have also been considered to have an important role in the spread and synchronization of spindles within pools of neurons in the thalamic reticular nucleus (Mulle et al. 1986; Steriade et al. 1990a, p. 210).

Such a thalamocortical relationship has recently been extended down into the delta frequency range (0.5–4 Hz), i.e., the frequency range of EEG activity in the deeper stages of sleep (Steriade et al. 1991). The delta waves resulted from slow oscillations among hyperpolarized, rhythmically bursting, thalamocortical neurons in conjunction with GABAergic reticular and local-circuit neurons, the oscillations becoming sustained and synchronized under cortical control via thalamocorticothalamic loops. Under brain-stem and thalamic cholinergic modulation acting diffusely on thalamocortical systems, suppression of the delta oscillations occurred with transition from such slow-wave (delta) sleep either to arousal or to REM sleep with EEG activation (including 40-Hz waves) (Steriade et al. 1991). A possible origin of delta waves in the cerebellar nuclei has been raised (Steriade et al. 1990a, p. 177).

Delta waves can be of cortical origin, however, since they are recordable after thalamectomy. It has already been pointed out that the human alpha rhythm may be of neocortical origin, and it appears that the desynchronized low-voltage "fast" EEG is also of neocortical origin (see below).

THE IMPACT OF EXPERIMENTAL STUDIES ON THE UNDERSTANDING OF THE HUMAN EEG

Steriade et al. (1987) have indicated that the thalamic reticular nucleus is an essential structure for the generation of thalamic and therefore cortical spindles, but the relevance of such spindles to human sleep spindles and the alpha rhythm remains unclear. Pedley and Traub (1990) consider the establishment of a definite theory of such rhythmic activity premature, since they consider some essential neurophysiological details still to be lacking.

In a short review of the history of the development of concepts of origin of the EEG, Pedley and Traub (1990) suggest that little has changed since the early 1950s, when the spontaneous EEG was linked primarily to postsynaptic potentials and when the EEG as recorded from the surface of the cortex or from the scalp was considered to represent summated excitatory and inhibitory postsynaptic potentials generated within the cortex itself. In addition to the above-mentioned synaptic electrogenesis as a basis for EEG activity,

Pedley and Traub (1990) indicated that the following mechanisms may contribute to the genesis of the EEG:

active dendritic responses, including the so-called d-spike generated by low-threshold Hodgkin-Huxley sodium and potassium conductance changes, and the regenerative high-threshold calcium permeability change that produces graded depolarizing potentials

the afterhyperpolarization potential produced by a calcium-activated potassium current.

Although synchronization has traditionally been understood to imply the simultaneous and synchronized activation of a large number of neurons in a relatively small area, the summed postsynaptic events of which are reflected in rhythmic oscillations (Steriade and Llinás 1988), an alternative view could be that such rhythmic waves result from a relatively widespread synchronization (or mutual entrainment) of cortical areas mutually interconnected by association fibers, and, in the case of both hemispheres, by callosal fibers (but see below). Correspondingly, desynchronization of the EEG, with irregular low-voltage irregular potentials, has traditionally been attributed to increased cortical "activation" resulting from increased cellular excitability in thalamocortical systems (Steriade and Llinás 1988); however, an alternative view could be that the apparent activation results from the breakup of the relatively widespread mutual entrainment mentioned above.

CORTICAL VS. SUBCORTICAL DRIVING MECHANISMS OF EEG RHYTHMIC ACTIVITY

As previously mentioned, rhythmic neocortical activity (e.g., spindle waves, alpha waves) has traditionally been taken as an expression of a rhythmic drive of the cortex via its thalamic afferents rather than as of intrinsic cortical origin; during nonspecific activation (e.g., by electrical stimulation of the brain-stem reticular formation), the thalamic rhythmic generators were presumed to be desynchronized (Creutzfeldt and Houchin 1974).

On the other hand, studies of the EEG of the undercut cortex (chapter 13), as well as studies of corticocortical vs. corticothalamic coherence, suggest an intrinsic cortical origin of both arhythmic and rhythmic EEG activity (Lopes da Silva et al. 1980a). Lopes da Silva and Storm van Leeuwen (1978) concluded that in the dog alpha rhythms of the visual cortex are generated by an equivalent dipole layer centered at the level of the cell bodies and basal dendrites of neurons of layers 4 and 5. Further, the results from a study of the effects of vertical incisions in the nonfissured or lissencephalic rabbit cortex (on the degree of similarity of epileptiform patterns) indicated a primary role of the cortex in maintaining synchronization of such activity (Petsche and Rappelsberger 1970). In this connection, a study by Frost et al. (1966) of EEG-intracellular relationships in the isolated cerebral cortex provided evidence for intracortical neuronal synchronizing mechanisms, active particularly at the time of neuronal discharge.

Lopes da Silva et al. (1973a) found that, in general, corticocortical coherences were significantly larger than thalamocortical coherences; these authors concluded that important cortical mechanisms are responsible for the spread of alpha activity over relatively large domains of cerebral cortex. Further, the fact that delta waves are present in the EEG after subcortical lesions or after undercutting of the cortex (chapter 13) also suggest that the thalamus is not essential for the generation of EEG activity, although clearly the activity is altered in form in the absence of corticothalamic and thalamocortical connections. If, indeed, corticocortical fibers greatly outnumber thalamocortical ones (Braitenberg 1977, 1978), it is not surprising that spontaneous EEG activity should survive undercutting of the cortex—at least if only thalamocortical and corticothalamic interconnections are interrupted by this procedure.

However, despite such evidence indicating the cortex as the primary generator of EEG activity, the corpus callosum does not appear to have any major role in the synchronization of the alpha rhythm at homotopic points of the two hemispheres (Hoovey et al. 1972).

Lopes da Silva et al. (1973a) found that the above-mentioned relatively high coherences among cortical recording points for the alpha rhythm of dogs could not satisfactorily be accounted for by common thalamic driving sources. This finding led to the suggestion that the alpha rhythm is a natural consequence of the structural pattern of intercommunication between cortical modules or columns, i.e., the surface-parallel intracortical fiber system (Lopes da Silva et al. 1980b). To the extent that input to local modules originates from other neocortical modules via association and callosal fibers, a structural basis could exist for the intercortical relationships indicated by cross-correlation and other techniques (Gavrilova and Aslanov 1968; Gevins 1987). The possibility of intracortical positive and negative feedback activity as a basis of rhythmic cortical activity has been raised, and supporting experimental evidence has been adduced (Rinaldi et al. 1977).

It is relevant, in relation to the question of cortical vs. subcortical mechanisms, that Ingvar et al. (1976) found a strong correlation between EEG frequency and cerebral oxygen uptake by gray matter (i.e., cerebral cortex) but a weak correlation with oxygen uptake by white matter.

It might be supposed that the lower frequencies and higher amplitudes of the EEG in non-REM sleep would tend to exhibit a slower rate of decrease of coherence with distance from a given point on the cortex than would the higher frequencies and lower amplitudes of the waking alert state. However, in their study of lateral coherence in the rabbit, Bullock and McClune (1989) found no such difference, and they questioned the adequacy of the view that the EEG represents solely a summation of postsynaptic potentials.

DELTA WAVES IN THE EEG

It was supposed by Steriade et al. (1990b) that the statistical association between cortical surface-positive waves and an increased firing probability of single cortical neurons, and the association between cortical surface-negative waves and a decreased firing probability consequent to white-matter lesions reported by Ball et al. (1977), indicated that delta waves, whether of pathological origin (chapter 13) or arising in normal delta-wave sleep (chapter 12), indicated sequences of excitatory and inhibitory processes in cortical neurons. Steriade et al. (1990b) also suggested that, in addition to synaptic activity, slow waves may reflect intrinsic properties of cortical neurons, such as a long-lasting (200–500 msec) calcium-mediated potassium conductance—perhaps especially since this conductance is markedly attenuated by acetylcholine. It was further suggested that lesions of white matter may produce cortical delta activity by interrupting cortically projecting cholinergic fibers from the basal forebrain nucleus of Meynert (Steriade et al. 1990b). (The latter question is discussed further below.)

SOME OTHER TYPES OF NORMAL EEG ACTIVITY

Low-Voltage Irregular Activity

Low-voltage irregular activity can appear in the occipital EEG in response to eye opening ("alpha blocking"); it also appears, not infrequently, in the EEG anteriorly on the scalp (even in bipolar recordings). The EEGs of some normal individuals exhibit a low-voltage irregular pattern posteriorly (even under relaxed, eyes-closed conditions) as well as anteriorly. In such cases there may be little or no change in the EEG posteriorly with eye opening.

The nature of such low-voltage activity is somewhat unclear. The term *low-voltage* has often been used synonymously with *low-voltage fast* (Goncharova and Barlow 1990). On the other hand, Chatrian et al. (1974), in their glossary of EEG terms, indicated that the "low-voltage EEG can be shown to be composed primarily of beta, theta, and to a lesser degree, delta waves, without alpha activity, over the posterior areas."

The Mu Rhythm and Related EEG Rhythms

The mu rhythm, encountered in recordings from the central (vertex) area of the scalp, has an arcuate or picket-fence-like waveform (as suggested by the form of the Greek letter μ) and a frequency in the alpha-frequency range of 8–13 Hz (figure 4.11). The mu rhythm, which behaves independently of the alpha rhythm, characteristically blocks not with eye opening but with movement or intended movement of the opposite upper extremity, such as clenching of the fist or passive movement of the arm (Niedermeyer 1987a; Kellaway 1990). Its "wicket" waveform has been taken to indicate a strong component at double the basic frequency.

In addition to the well-known blocking of the mu rhythm by actual or intended movement (Chatrian et al. 1959), Pfurtscheller (1981) has reported a desynchronization of central beta rhythms (12–22 Hz) during movement independent of, as well as simultaneous with, blocking of the mu rhythm. Kuhlman (1978) has shown that the mu rhythm can be systematically enhanced by feedback training.

Fast Rhythms

An apparent counterpart of the human mu rhythm has been reported in the monkey during conditions of high vigilance and focused visual attention; it appears in the sensory hand area (Brodmann's fields 1 and 2) and independently in the posterior parietal area (Area 5). These rhythms, at about 18 Hz, are blocked by body movement (Rougeul et al. 1979). This rhythm is at about twice the frequency of the above-mentioned human mu rhythm, which, as already noted, generally lies in the range 8–13 Hz. (Actually, the human mu rhythm may be asssociated with bursts of beta waves that are often, although not constantly, of a frequency twice that of the mu rhythm itself (Chatrian et al. 1959).) A rhythm comparable to that described above in the monkey, but at higher frequencies (35–45 Hz), has been described in the cat, in which the rhythm appears in cortical areas where giant pyramidal cells are found (Bouyer et al. 1981, 1987; Rougeul-Buser et al. 1983).

Activity in the 40-Hz Range

Recently, intracortically generated frequencies in the range of 40 Hz (lying in the "gamma" band of frequencies) have received some attention. (See, e.g., Başar and Bullock 1992.) (The question of the presence in the EEG of frequencies higher than the usual range of 1–35 Hz has long been of interest; see, e.g., Trabka 1962.) In the human, such rhythmic activity appeared as quasi-sinusoidal waves time-locked to stimuli (clicks) arising from the auditory cortex and having a maximum response at about 40 Hz (Galambos et al. 1981; Spydell et al. 1985; Mäkelä and Hari 1987; DeFrance and Sheer 1988; Johnson et al. 1988; Pantev et al. 1991). In the visual cortex in cats, intrinsic oscillations in the range of 40 Hz have been observed within single and (coherently) among multiple cortical columns during the presentation of simple stimuli, i.e., appropriately oriented moving bars of light (Eckhorn et al. 1988; Gray et al. 1989; Gray and Singer 1989; Baringa 1990; Engel et al. 1990). Somewhat lower frequencies, in the vicinity of 30 Hz, have been found in the monkey visual cortex by Freeman and van Dijk (1987), who used a visual conditioning paradigm and an array of subdural electrodes. Odor-specific responses appearing as distributed high-frequency oscillatory bursts (55–75 Hz in the rabbit, 35–55 Hz in the cat) in the olfactory system had been noted earlier (Freeman and Skarda 1985). Such "coherent stimulus-evoked resonances" have been taken to be indicative of a mechanism linking or temporally coordinating the distributed cortical representation of stimuli (Freeman and van Dyjk 1987; Eckhorn et al. 1988; Gray and Singer 1989; Engel et al. 1990; Pantev et al.

1991). A theoretical basis for such synchronization had been proposed by von der Malsburg and Schneider (1986).

Very-high-frequency rhythmic activity (>50 Hz) appearing with EEG amplitude suppression in frontal-lobe intracerebral recordings at seizure onset has recently been reported (Allen et al. 1992). The activity, which ranged up to 120 Hz in frequency, suggested to these authors the possibility of sequential involvement of elements of a neuronal network.

From *in vitro* intracellular recordings from layer 4 of guinea pig frontal cortex, Llinás et al. (1991) recently reported finding two neurons that showed different types of subthreshold (i.e., in the absence of neuronal firing) oscillations of amplitude in the range of several millivolts. In the first type of neuron, the oscillations increased in frequency from about 10 to 45 Hz with increasing membrane depolarization; action potentials for this type of cell showed clear afterhyperpolarizations. In the second type of neuron, a more limited range of frequency of oscillations in the range of 35–50 Hz was found, the frequencies being independent of the level of membrane depolarization. In both types of cells, the subthreshold oscillations could trigger spikes at the oscillatory frequency if the membrane was sufficiently depolarized. Neurons having the narrower frequency range of oscillations appeared to be sparsely spinous cortical interneurons (i.e., probably inhibitory). A "conjunctive" role of the narrow-band rhythmic activity for the cortex and between the cortex and the thalamus was postulated (Llinás et al. 1991).

THE EEG DURING REM SLEEP

A recent review of the origin and nature of the EEG during REM sleep and the similarities and differences between it and the waking desynchronized EEG in animals can be found in Steriade et al. 1990a. Some apparent differences between the human EEG during REM sleep and the EEG during REM sleep in the cat (the usual experimental animal for such studies) should be pointed out. In the cat, there appear to be few differences between the desynchronized EEG of the waking alert state and the EEG during REM sleep. In the human, on the other hand, the EEG during REM sleep characteristically resembles that during Stage 1 of non-REM sleep (i.e., drowsiness), the pattern being one of irregular low-voltage activity, often primarily in the theta frequency range of 4–7 Hz, rather than the even lower voltage pattern of the alerted (e.g., attentive, eyes open) stage, in which higher frequencies in the alpha (8–13 Hz) and beta ranges (14–35 Hz) are also well represented. It is usually considered impossible to distinguish the spectra of the EEG during REM sleep from those during Stage 1 non-REM sleep (Johnson et al. 1969), at least if the particular pattern of "sawtooth waves" (of 2–3 Hz, appearing in brief runs of a few seconds in REM sleep; see Carskadon and Rechtschaffen 1989) are not present. (Indeed, in clinical electroencephalography it can at times be difficult to distinguish the alert "desynchronized" EEG from that during Stage 1 sleep, as both show low-voltage irregular activity.)

TOPOGRAPHY OF ALPHA VS. LOW-VOLTAGE FAST ACTIVITY: THE EEG AND CORTICAL ARCHITECTONICS

Characteristically, but with exceptions, rhythmic alpha activity in the range of 8–13 Hz (if present) is evident in the normal adult human EEG recorded from the posterior regions of the scalp, whereas low-voltage irregular "faster" activity (in the range 14–40 Hz, approximately) predominates anteriorly, at times with some admixed activity in the alpha and theta frequency ranges. The exceptions include those subjects whose EEGs are characterized by low-voltage, predominantly fast activity both anteriorly and posteriorly, as mentioned previously. (If electrodes on the earlobes are used as references in referential (as opposed to bipolar) EEG recordings, alpha activity can appear to arise from frontal leads as a result of actual alpha activity originating from the ear-reference electrode. Nonetheless, in their report of recordings directly from the cortical surface, Jasper and Penfield (1949) noted "occasional bursts of regular alpha waves at 8–10 per second" from the more anterior frontal regions.) Broughton (1987) and Santamaria and Chiappa (1987) (the latter authors using a noncephalic neck-chest reference) reiterated and confirmed earlier reports of frontal alpha waves (of slightly slower frequency—by 0.5 to 1.5 Hz—than the posterior waking alpha) appearing in a transitional state between wakefulness and drowsiness, termed Stage 1A by Broughton (1987). An anterior alpha pattern can also be seen during general anesthesia (Sharbrough 1987).

On the basis of observations of the extent of responses recorded from the intact skull in dogs and cats, Kornmüller (1933, 1935) concluded that there was a correlation between type of electrical activity and cortical architechtonics—for example, relatively slower waves in the sensory areas and relatively faster ones in the motor areas. On the other hand, inspection of Brodmann's cytoarchitectural map of the human brain (Brodal 1981, p. 791) does not suggest a close correlation of the familiar distribution of the resting eyes-closed adult's waking EEG patterns (i.e., low-voltage irregular activity anteriorly and alpha activity posteriorly). From recordings of the exposed neocortex, alpha activity is of highest voltage in the posterior temporal, parietal, and peristriate occipital cortex (Jasper 1949). Inspection of cytoarchitectural maps (Brodal 1981, pp. 791, 792) suggests that the primary sensory receiving areas of the cerebral cortex make up a relatively small part of the posterior cerebral cortex that would be reflected in the EEG. (As previously mentioned, low-voltage irregular activity predominates posteriorly as well as anteriorly in some individuals.)

As was pointed out in chapter 11, the structure of the neocortex is essentially uniform, and the apparent differences in cortical architectonics lie in differences in connectivity with other parts of the neocortex and with subcortical structures. Thus, Creutzfeldt (1978) maintained that the morphological differences of the different cortical areas are not essential and that the functional distinctions among the various cortical areas are their differing connections with afferent projection systems and with efferent target structures, rather than to fundamental differences in their functional structures. As an example of this view, the greater density of neurons in the binocular part of the primary visual cortex (Area 17) can be viewed as a reflection of its special connectivity (Powell 1981).

In this connection, it is relevant that the prefrontal (anterior frontal) cortex is reciprocally connected with the medial dorsal nucleus of the thalamus (Creutzfeldt 1978); it is in this area of the cortex, among others, that low-voltage irregular EEG activity is characteristically seen. In contrast, much of the posterior region from which alpha activity can be recorded, namely the parieto-temporal-occipital association cortex, is reciprocally connected primarily with the pulvinar nucleus of the thalamus (Brodal 1981). On the other hand, interconnections between particular thalamic nuclei and cortical regions are not as specific as was once thought (Jones 1985). Further, as important or more important than corticothalamic interconnections are corticocortical interconnections, which, for the prefrontal cortex, are more extensive and appear to be organized in a fundamentally different way from those for the posterior cortex (i.e., posterior to the Rolandic fissure) (Goldman-Rakic 1988a,b; Goldman-Rakic and Selemon 1984; Mesulam 1986, 1990; Gevins and Illes 1991).

If this difference is indeed of primary importance in relation to the topography of EEG patterns, then the following formulation could be advanced for the waking state: Low-voltage irregular activity anteriorly can be taken to reflect a continuously "active" prefrontal cortex, with extensive interconnections with other cortical areas. Rhythmic alpha activity posteriorly may be taken to be a reflection of an "idling" posterior cortex (Barlow 1985a), reflecting a relatively low level of functional interconnection with the constantly active prefrontal cortex. On the other hand, low-voltage irregular activity posteriorly (as well as anteriorly) is taken to be a reflection of an "active" cortex posteriorly because of a relatively high level of functional interconnection with prefrontal cortical areas. Thus, in this formulation alpha activity posteriorly in the waking state in the human would reflect "functional disconnection" or dissociation of posterior association areas from the anterior association areas of the prefrontal cortex. As a possible corollary, waves of alpha frequency during drowsiness could appear anteriorly (Santamaria and Chiappa 1987) as a reflection of a less "active" frontal cortex.

OTHER TYPES OF NORMAL AND ABNORMAL EEG ACTIVITY

Several recent reviews have been devoted to alpha rhythms (Markand 1990b), beta and mu rhythms (Kozelka and Pedley 1990), unusual normal and normal-variant EEG patterns (Westmoreland 1990; Westmoreland and Klass 1990), abnormal non-epileptiform slow EEG rhythms (Schaul 1990), and periodic (repetitive) primarily epileptiform EEG patterns (Brenner and Schaul 1990). Of these, there has been relatively little work concerning fundamental mechanisms of unusual normal (normal-variant) patterns.

MODIFICATIONS OF THE EEG BY THE SCALP AND OTHER TISSUES

The electrical activity of the brain as recorded from the scalp is, as a rule, different from that recorded from the cortical surface itself, not only because the degree of coherence or similarity of activity at two points on the cortex itself can vary with distance and with frequency, but also because the various tissues intervening between the cortex and the surface of the scalp (i.e., meninges, cerebrospinal fluid, bone, vascular channels, muscles, etc.) act as a spatial filter or averager (Abraham and Ajmone-Marsan 1958; Geissler and Gerstein 1961; DeLucchi et al. 1962; Cooper et al. 1965). Alpha amplitude can vary with skull thickness, for example (Leissner et al. 1970). Thus, a very localized spike on the cortex can be very attenuated in the scalp recording (Abraham and Ajmone Marsan 1958). Cooper et al. (1965) stated that the attenuation in such a case could be as high as 5000 to 1, but for coherent activity over a wide area the attenuation may be only 2 to 1. Pedley and Traub (1990) mentioned a range of attenuation factors from less than 10 to 300. Cooper et al. (1965) estimated that a cortical area of at least 6 cm^2 must be synchronously or near synchronously active to be observed in the scalp EEG at standard sensitivities (7 mV/mm). An additional complicating factor is that of the geometry of gyri, i.e., the infolding of the cortex (Woodbury 1965; Gloor 1985, 1987; Nunez and Pilgreen 1991).

Summarizing these effects, Pedley (1984) indicated that, of the several factors determining whether an event at the cortex will be reflected at the level of the scalp, the most important factors appear to be the voltage of the event, the area involved in synchronous activity, and the location of the area of the cortex in relation to the cortical convolutions.

Additionally, Pfurtscheller and Cooper (1975) stressed frequency as a factor. These authors found that the cortex-to-scalp attenuation for activity of frequencies between 15 and 30 Hz is appreciably greater (e.g., by a factor of 100) than that for frequencies lower than 15 Hz, and they modeled the effect by a low-pass filter. However, since the various tissue layers between the cortex and the surface of the scalp act at most as passive conductors acting as a spatial filter, it is usually assumed that the higher attenuation factors for such frequencies reflect their smaller degree of synchronization. Conversely, it is presumably because of relatively wide synchronization that beta rhythms in the range of approximately 17–25 Hz can be relatively prominent anteriorly as a result of barbiturates and the benzodiazepine drugs (e.g., Valium, Librium).

NEUROACTIVE AGENTS (NEUROTRANSMITTERS, NEUROMODULATORS, AND NEUROPHARMACOLOGICAL SUBSTANCES)

The complex and rapidly evolving subject of neurotransmitters and neuromodulators (neuropeptides), collectively termed *neuroactive substances*, has been reviewed by Jones (1986, 1987), Siggins and Gruol (1986), Kandel et al. (1991), and McCormick (1992a,b), among others. The subject is made even more complex by recent findings (see e.g., McCormick and Williamson 1989) indicating that, in human cerebral cortex *in vitro*, both convergence and divergence among the actions of putative transmitters occurs—i.e., that several neurotransmitters can result in the same postsynaptic response, and, conversely, application of a single putative transmitter can result in more than one postsynaptic response in the same neuron. Further, recent evidence indicates that nitric oxide (a gas) acts as an unorthodox messenger molecule in cell-to-cell signaling in the central nervous system (Garthwaite 1991).

Only a very few aspects of this extensive field will be touch upon here, primarily those related to the EEG.

Acetylcholine

Acetylcholine (ACh) is known to have a relatively slow and prolonged excitatory effect on cortical neurons. Such an effect could be particularly effective in enhancing repetitive firing, thus constituting an essentially facilitatory mechanism (Krnjević 1980; Krnjević and Phillis 1963a,b). This effect would clearly be relevant to mechanisms of cortical arousal evoked by pathways ascending from the brain stem and deeper regions of the forebrain, i.e., the basal forebrain nuclei (Krnjević 1980), and indeed Kanai and Szerb (1965), Sie et al. (1965), and Celesia and Jasper (1966) found rates of release of acetylcholine from the cortical surface that were consistent with the hypothesis that ascending activation of the EEG of brain-stem origin is mediated in part by acetylcholine released from afferent terminals in the cortex.

On the other hand, isolation of an area of cortex leads to a loss of cholinergic input as well as to the development of a tendency toward electrical seizure activity; there is also evidence that seizures are inhibited by acetylcholine-potentiating drugs, but the mechanism of this action is unclear (Krnjević 1980).

Glutamate and Aspartate

Whereas acetylcholine has a relatively prolonged action, the putative excitatory transmitters glutamate and aspartate act relatively rapidly; hence, their excessive release or impaired re-uptake mechanisms could well be expected to be associated with excessive neuronal activity and possibly seizures (Krnjević 1980). In addition to such an effect of glutamate via the classical "ionotropic" receptors, glutamate "metabotropic" receptors have recently been shown to have a much longer effect (up to 30 sec); McCormick and von Krosigk (1992) attributed corticothalamic control (modulation) of the firing mode and the excitability of thalamic relay cells to activation of the glutamate "metabotropic" subclass of receptors in the relay cells and the consequent decrease in resting K^+ conductance.

GABA and Glycine

Of the two inhibitory transmitters gamma-aminobutyric acid (GABA) and glycine, it appears that the longer inhibitory postsynaptic potentials (IPSPs) are probably mediated by GABA whereas the brief IPSPs seen in the spinal cord (and in the brain stem) are probably mediated by glycine. The action of GABA is antagonized by bicuculline and picrotoxin (although by different mechanisms), and the action of glycine is antagonized by strychnine (Krnjević 1980; Crunelli and Leresche 1991). All these antagonists are thus convulsants. Potentiators of GABA, whether by depression of its re-uptake or by sensitizing GABA receptors, include barbiturates, benzodiazepines, and phenytoin (Krnjević 1980).

The Catecholamines and Serotonin

Other possible neurotransmitters include catecholamines (epinephrine, norepinephrine, dopamine) and serotonin (5-hydroxytryptamine), which have been considered to be more often inhibitors than excitants but which may not play a major role in synaptic activity in the brain (Krnjević 1980).

Noradrenaline's effect on cortical neurons appears to be similar to its effect on thalamic neurons: a slow depolarization, associated with blocking of a resting potassium conductance. There is also evidence of a dual effect, in which noradrenaline inhibits spontaneous discharges of cortical cells while simultaneously enhancing the response to specific synaptic inputs; this would have the effect of increasing the signal-to-noise ratio (Steriade et al. 1990b).

These effects of noradrenaline on thalamic neurons are considered to parallel those of acetylcholine in shifting the mode of operation of thalamic neurons from one of burst-firing during sleep to tonic firing during wakefulness, with consequent enhanced responsiveness of the neurons (Steriade et al. 1990b, figure 7).

The origins of the various "state-setting" substances that act upon the thalamus and the cerebral cortex (Mesulam 1990) are indicated in figure 12.6. Powell (1981) has pointed out that the aminergic fibers from the brain stem, which are distributed to widespread regions of the cerebral cortex, enter the cortex near the rostral or anterior end of the hemisphere and pass posteriorly to the occipital poles at right angles to the columnar organization of the cortex.

Other Possible Transmitters: Neuromodulators (Neuropeptides)

The list of neuromodulators or neuropeptides is an increasingly long one (Schwartz 1991; McCormick 1992a,b). A consideration of these substances is outside the scope of this book. In contrast to the "classical" transmitters, which operate directly (i.e., by changing the cell membrane conductance), neuromodulators appear to have an indirect effect, modulating the responses evoked by the more conventional synaptic transmitters (Krnjević 1980).

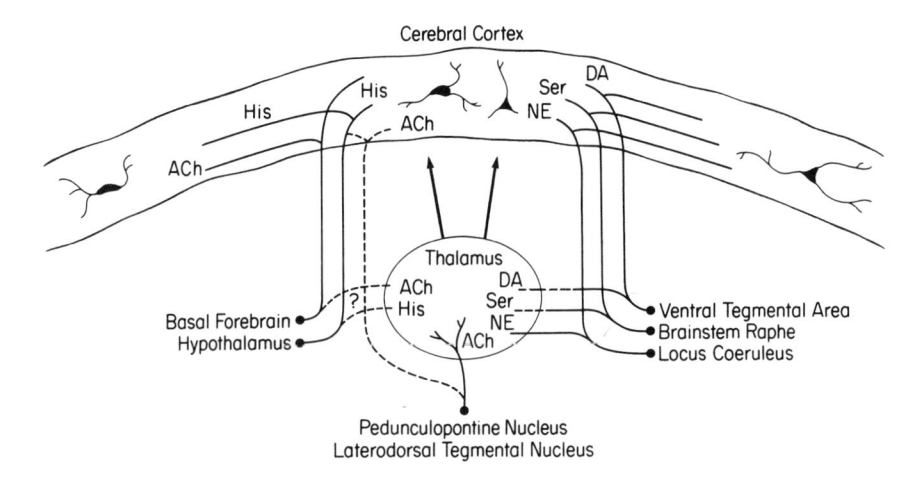

Figure 12.6 State-setting, chemically addressed connections of thalamus and cortex. Interrupted lines indicate minor connections. A question mark indicates that the existence of the pathway is not yet firmly established. Ach: acetylcholine. DA: dopamine. His: histamine. NE: norepinephrine. Ser: serotonin. (From Mesulam 1990.)

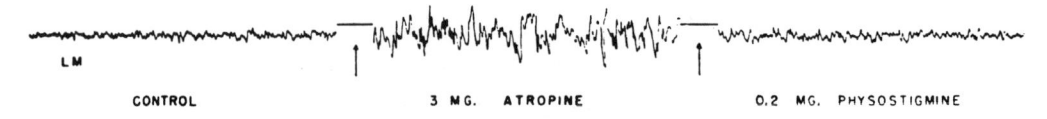

Figure 12.7 Effect on rabbit cortex of atropine followed by physostigmine. The atropine results in synchronous (low-frequency, high-amplitude) waves; the physostigmine counteracts the effect of atropine, restoring the activated or "desynchronized" EEG. (Left motor cortex recording, from White and Boyajy 1960.)

PHARMACOLOGICAL AGENTS

Atropine, an anticholinergic agent (i.e., an antagonist of actylcholine), induces slow (delta) waves in animals (figure 12.7) and in human subjects resembling those in sleep, but with relatively little apparent decrease in the level of alertness (Bradley 1953; Bradley and Elkes 1957; White and Boyajy 1960; Jasper 1969; Stewart et al. 1984). True EEG-behavioral dissociation in human subjects after administration of atropine has, however, been questioned, since some behavioral alterations have been reported, and the resulting EEGs have more fast (beta) activity, less high-voltage slow activity, and fewer sleep-spindle bursts than in normal non-REM sleep. In addition, confusion, disorientation, altered speech patterns, and fluctuations in consciousness have been noted, even though simple commands could still be carried out (Glaze 1990).

On the other hand, physostygmine, a cholinesterase inhibitor (and therefore an acetylcholine potentiator), results in a low-voltage fast or "activated" EEG (figure 12.7) consistent with, but not actually accompanied by, an alert behavioral state (Bradley 1953; Bradley and Elkes 1957; White and Boyajy

1960). In contrast, amphetamine resulted in both an activated EEG pattern and an altered behavioral state (Bradley and Elkes 1957).

Di-isopropyl flurophosphate (DFP), which inactivates the cholinesterase enzymes, thus allowing acetylcholine to accumulate, results in an increase in frequency and a decrease in voltage of the EEG, a change that is reversible by atropine; the latter alone results in a decrease in frequency and an increase in amplitude (Wescoe et al. 1948).

Results such as those just summarized were considered to be consistent with a basic cholinergic nature (White and Boyajy 1960) of the ascending reticular activating system (Starzl and Magoun 1951). More recent studies, though confirming that the mechanism for activating the EEG is fundamentally cholinergic, have implicated that the substantia innominata (or nucleus basalis of Meynert, as it is termed in humans) of the forebrain is of key importance (Stewart et al. 1984; Détári and Vanderwolf 1987). Thus, after lesions in this area, an activation pattern (i.e., low-voltage fast activity) is no longer possible; further, the rhythm- (spindle-) generating mechanism of the thalamic reticular nucleus is suppressed, as previously mentioned, since the latter nucleus receives an input from the nucleus basalis (Buzsaki et al. 1988). The latter authors have proposed that acetylcholine, known to act as a slow excitatory neurotransmitter in the neocortex, provides in effect a tonic facilitatory effect for other excitatory effects, in short, an "activating" effect (Buzsaki et al. 1988). These authors further suggested that the neocortical slow (delta) waves may arise, at least in part, from long-lasting afterhyperpolarizations in deep neocortical pyramidal cells (layer V), rather than reflecting synaptic activity. Since this effect is considerably attenuated by local application of acetylcholine, neocortical activation could in principle result from acetylcholine-induced attenuation of such afterhyperpolarization, resulting in neocortical activation (Buszaki et al. 1988).

EFFECT OF TEMPERATURE ON THE EEG

It has long been known that the effect of temperature on the frequency of the alpha rhythm in the human EEG is apparently less than that of ordinary chemical processes, including metabolic ones, a characteristic that is relevant to the possibility of partial temperature-compensation features of the EEG model advanced in this book (chapter 16). The Q_{10} (the quotient or factor of increase in the rate of a process for a 10°C increase in temperature) is in the range of 2.5 for most chemical reactions (Ehret and Barlow 1960; Barlow 1962c; Michenfelder and Theye 1968). A Q_{10} of 1.0 would indicate no variation of rate with temperature. Michenfelder and Theye (1968) found a Q_{10} of 2.23 for the cerebral metabolic rates for oxygen, glucose, and lactate in dogs. From the data reported by Hoagland (1936a,b), the Q_{10} for the alpha frequency of normal subjects warmed by diathermy is in the range of 1.45 (e.g., from 10 Hz to 12.25 Hz for a 5°C increase in temperature), which suggests that the alpha frequency may be at least partially temperature compensated. Hoagland's data indicated a greater temperature effect with a more severe degree of general paresis (syphilis of the brain), possibly suggesting a less effective temperature compensation in this disease.

Walter (1962) considered that alpha-generating mechanisms are to some extent protected from the primary effects of temperature change. Gaenshirt et al. (1954) found that, for the cat electrocorticogram, frequency decreased exponentially with decreasing temperature between about 38 and 32°C, whereas amplitude increased exponentially over the same temperature range. These results indicate an inverse relationship between frequency and amplitude over this temperature range, which would be consistent with the constant-slope feature of the model described in this book. (Over a lower temperature range from 32 to 20°C (at which temperature the EEG became isoelectric), both frequency and amplitude progressively diminished; see Gaenshirt et al. 1954.)

In unanesthetized cats, Kawakami and Gellhorn (1963) found a quite marked variation of the frequency of waves in spontaneous spindle bursts, from 15 Hz at 40°C to 6 Hz at 26°C, with relatively little change in the amplitude of the spindles. During the periods of activity (which alternated with periods of silence) in large neuronally isolated slabs of cat cortex, Gidlöf and Söderberg (1964) found that the frequency of the waves was constant throughout a temperature range of 25 to 40°C, whereas the amplitude, although constant at temperatures above 32°C, was only a quarter of this level for a temperature of 25°C.

It is evident that these several studies have yielded mixed results concerning the temperature variation of EEG frequencies; some results suggest a partial temperature compensation of frequency, but other results indicate changes in opposite directions for frequency and amplitude. These results will be discussed further in chapter 16.

13 Pathophysiology of the EEG

Clinical studies and investigations in experimental animals on the pathophysiology of the EEG have largely been limited, on the one hand, to slow-wave abnormalities and on the other hand, to epileptiform patterns, of focal and generalized distribution. Both clinical studies and results from experimental animals have tended to implicate subcortical lesions (especially lesions of subcortical white matter) in irregular slow-wave abnormalities, and disease of the cortex in epileptiform patterns, but Alzheimer's disease appears to be an exception. These aspects of the pathophysiology of the EEG will now be considered.

SLOW WAVES IN THE THETA AND DELTA FREQUENCY RANGES

Both metabolic and structural lesions may lie at the basis of generalized theta activity (4–7 Hz) in the EEG, localized theta activity more likely indicating the latter (Steriade et al. 1990b). EEG patterns in the delta frequency range (1–4 Hz) have customarily been divided into two types: the irregular or polymorphic and the rhythmic (quasi-rhythmic) or monomorphic (Daly 1979). Jasper and van Buren (1953) reported that polymorphic delta waves (of 0.5–2.5 Hz) are usually associated with subcortical white-matter lesions, whereas bilaterally synchronous delta waves are usually found in cases of deep tumors near the floor of the third ventricle and the aqueduct of Sylvius.

From examining the EEG correlates of diffuse encephalopathies, Gloor et al. (1968) found that disease occurring at cortical and subcortical levels (e.g., Creutzfeldt-Jakob disease, subacute sclerosing panencephalitis) resulted in bilaterally synchronous paroxysmal (i.e., abrupt onset and abrupt termination) activity of either epileptiform or rhythmic-delta nature, whereas if the pathology were limited to the white matter (as in demyelinating disease), primarily polymorphic delta activity occurred, a finding that was reiterated by Goldensohn (1979a,b). On the other hand, if gray matter only were affected, slowing of the basic posterior rhythm and widespread irregular slow waves could be seen, as in Alzheimer's disease; alternatively, focal or multifocal epileptiform discharges could appear. Slowing was less prominent if the pathology were limited to the cortical gray matter than if white matter was involved. In this connection, Gloor (1975) pointed out that very-high-voltage delta activity appearing in the electrocorticogram after excision of an epileptogenic area should raise the question of an ischemic complication in the areas bordering the excision, or of a white-matter lesion underlying the cortex.

Some confirmatory results for these clinical findings have emerged from animal experiments (Gloor et al. 1977), in that discrete thermocoagulation lesions of subcortical white matter resulted in focal polymorphic delta waves, but lesions of the cortex resulted in decreasing voltages, particularly of the higher frequencies, but without focal slowing. Further, thalamic lesions resulted in ipsislateral polymorphic delta activity mixed with spindle waves. Bilateral lesions of the posterior hypothalamus and upper midbrain tegmentum resulted in bilateral generalized polymorphic delta activity, but unilateral lesions led either to no change or to ipsilateral slowing (Gloor et al. 1977).

In contrast to the above-described arhythmic, random, or irregular delta activity, frontal intermittent rhythmic delta activity (FIRDA), to which the term "generalized bilaterally synchronous slow burst" was applied by Schaul et al. (1981), may arise as a result of a dysfunction (as opposed to an interruption) of the thalamocortical connections, for example, in partial destruction of the dorsal medial nucleus of the thalamus (Gloor et al. 1977; Goldensohn 1979a,b). Schaul et al. (1981) found that patients with this EEG pattern had a significantly higher incidence of diffuse encephalopathy (e.g., of toxic or metabolic types) and a higher incidence of alterations of consciousness than did a control group (see also Zifkin and Cracco 1990). Some association between frontal intermittent rhythmic delta activity and encephalopathy of metabolic origin was also found by Fariello et al. (1982), but structural cerebral abnormalities were more frequently encountered in their series.

The finding that cortical lesions as such did not produce delta activity, but that interruptions of afferent inputs to the cortex were induced by lesions of subcortical white matter (and also by thalamic, hypothalamic, and brain-stem lesions), suggested to Gloor et al. (1977) (see also Daly 1979) that cortical delta activity results from some kind of (perhaps partial) cortical deafferentation, the delta activity itself being generated by primarily intracortical, recurrent neuronal circuits.

There have been few microelectrode studies of pathological slow-wave activity. A good correlation has been reported between surface-positive portions of slow waves and increased neural firing rate (Ball et al. 1977), pyramidal neurons in layer V being considered to be the origin of the delta waves. Since atropine, as an antagonist to acetylcholine, is known to induce delta waves in the EEG (Wescoe et al. 1948; Bradley 1953; Bradley and Elkes 1957; White and Boyajy 1960), Schaul et al. (1978) considered that cortical delta activity appearing as a consequence of subcortical lesions may result from a cholinergic deafferentation of the cerebral cortex, particularly since the microphysiological features of atropine-induced delta waves and those induced by subcortical lesions, as described above, were similar.

For the delta waves that are evident in hypoglycemia, a relationship between the discharge pattern rate of cortical neurons and the degree of slowing at the surface of the cortex was found (Creutzfeldt and Meisch 1963; Mergenhagen et al. 1968; Creutzfeldt and Houchin 1974); with decreasing levels of blood sugar, the more-or-less continuous neuronal firing became more grouped into bursts, the latter tending to be synchronized with some of the cortical slow waves.

Undercutting the Cortex

In contrast to earlier reports (e.g., Burns 1951) that the undercut cortex is electrically inactive, Kellaway et al. (1966) concluded that the surgically isolated cortex is always electrically active if circulation is adequately maintained. The latter authors found continuous or almost continuous high-voltage (up to 1 mV) aperiodic 0.5–4-Hz activity and a superimposed 25–70-Hz rhythm. On the other hand, the surgically isolated thalamus (e.g., the pulvinar nucleus) exhibited continuous rhythmic 6–9-Hz activity having a sinusoidal waveform. It was concluded that the aperiodic slow activity of the isolated cortex may reflect some characteristic peculiar to the cortex, for example, a dependence of certain neural elements upon subcortical influences for the development of organized rhythmic behavior (Kellaway et al. 1966). In this connection, Jasper (1949) had previously reported that a completely undercut cortical area, leaving only the pial circulation intact, could exhibit activity of normal frequencies and amplitudes after application of small amounts of acetylcholine preceded by local treatment with eserine.

In a related study, Frost et al. (1966) had found a reduction in the number of spontaneously active units in the isolated cortex as compared with normal cortex under similar experimental conditions, and unit discharges either ceased or decreased in rate during the brief periods of electrocortical silence. Occasional neurons tended to fire faster during electrocortical negative slow waves, and conversely for positive waves, but the association was weak. In general, neuronal discharges and EEG activity appeared to be largely independent of one another (Frost et al. 1966). However, in a subsequent study, in which the neuronal discharges were used as a trigger for averaging the EEG (Frost and Gol 1966), evidence was found for a nonrandom relationship between the two.

Slowing of the Posterior Rhythm

Bilateral slowing of the adult posterior rhythm (i.e., the alpha rhythm) from the alpha frequency range of 8–13 Hz to the theta range of 4–7 Hz can occur in metabolic disease (e.g., hypothyroidism, hypoglycemia, renal disease, hepatic disease), under toxic conditions (e.g., from drugs such as alcohol and excessive levels of some anticonvulsant medication) (Zifkin and Cracco 1990), and in degenerative encephalopathies (e.g., Alzheimer's disease—see below) (Markand 1990a). An increase in the frequency of the posterior rhythm can be seen in hyperthyroidism (Markand 1990b).

EPILEPTIFORM PATTERNS

Two principal categories of epileptiform EEG patterns will be considered: focal or partial epilepsy, the characteristic interictal manifestation of which is the spike or spike-and-slow-wave complex; and the generalized epilepsy of "absence" attacks, characteristically manifested in the 3-Hz spike-wave pattern. Other epileptiform EEG patterns, such as that in generalized tonic-clonic convulsions (in which rhythmic quasi-sinusoidal 10-Hz waves may appear) and that in Lennox-Gastaut Syndrome (in which repetitive spike-wave patterns of, e.g., 2–2.5 Hz are characteristically seen), will be considered more briefly. In this survey, information from both clinical studies and investigations with experimental animals will be considered, although it may be noted that Daly (1990) has suggested that the various models of epilepsy in experimental animals have been somewhat disappointing from the standpoint of clarification of human epilepsy.

Focal Epilepsy

Association with Cortical Lesions It was pointed out above that both clinical studies and studies with experimental animals indicate that irregular or polymorphic slow waves appear to be associated with lesions of subcortical white matter—more particularly, with a partial deafferentation of the cortex in relation to subcortical structures, primarily the thalamus. It is the cortex, however, that appears to be the site of the lesion in the case of focal epilepsy, rather than the subcortical white matter. Thus, in a study of 104 autopsy-proven cases of cerebral infarction and/or hemorrhage, Richardson and Dodge (1954) and Dodge et al. (1954) found an involvement of the cerebral cortex in all the patients who had had seizures, whereas if the lesions were confined to subcortical structures, no seizures had been reported in the case histories. The seizures themselves were primarily associated with infarction of thrombotic origin.

The hallmark of focal epilepsy is the spike, or, if there is an associated slow wave (as is often the case), the spike-and-slow-wave complex. Often, individual interictal spikes, for example, in temporal lobe epilepsy, vary in their waveform from one event to the next (Klass 1975; Barlow and Dubinsky 1976; Frost 1979, 1985; Pedley 1984).

At least in the case of temporal-lobe epilepsy, the interictal manifestation in the form of the focal spike or the focal spike-and-slow-wave complex is appreciably different from the ictal manifestation, which can be quite varied but which may begin, with rhythmic, almost sinusoidal waves of, e.g., 7 Hz, possibly originating in the hippocampus. Nor is the onset of the ictal manifestation reliably heralded by an increase in the rate of spiking (Katz et al. 1991). It is in part for this reason that the usefulness in relation to human focal epilepsy of the results from studies of focal epilepsy in experimental animals has been considered to be mixed (Daly 1990). It should also be mentioned, as pointed out by Daly (1990), that *epileptiform discharge* is not synonymous with *interictal discharge*; the former is a generic term for spikes and sharp waves (the somewhat arbitrary dividing point for duration for the two being 80 msec; see Chatrian et al. 1974), and can be seen in healthy individuals, whereas the latter term, by definition, implies that ictal (i.e., seizure) events occur at some time.

In discussions of the 3-Hz spike-wave pattern (see below) the wave component receives as much attention as the spike component, but in the case of the spike-slow-wave complex, the slow-wave component is often less emphasized. In this book, however, the slow-wave component of the spike-and-slow-wave complex is emphasized as much as the spike itself.

Experimental Studies in Animals   The characteristic epileptiform event in focal experimental epilepsy in animals, induced for example by local application of penicillin on the cerebral cortex, is the paroxysmal depolarizing shift (PDS), a sudden 20–50-mV depolarization of the membrane potential of a cell lasting 100 msec or longer and recurring spontaneously every 2–10 sec (Johnston and Brown 1984). The paroxysmal depolarizing shift, which triggers a burst of action potential discharges (Schwartzkroin 1987), was originally considered to entail both an extensive synaptic bombardment resulting in a large and long excitatory postsynaptic potential (EPSP) and also changes in the intrinsic properties of the neuronal membrane. It is followed by a long-lasting hyperpolarization (Goldensohn and Purpura 1963; Matsumoto and Ajmone-Marsan 1964a,b; Connors and Gutnick 1984). The exact nature of the paroxysmal depolarizing shift has remained unclear, as has the nature of the afterhyperpolarization, since the GABA blocking agents that induce PSDs would be expected to block such an inhibitory response. Some groups of cells, for which the burst of action potentials may be a manifestation of abnormal hyperexcitability and may represent the equivalent of a single discharge in a normal neuron, may act as a pacemaker region (Schwartzkroin 1987). More recent evidence speaks once again for the importance of both synaptic (i.e., loss of normal inhibition) and intrinsic (i.e., alteration of membrane properties) factors in focal epileptogenesis (Schwartzkroin 1987).

Prince and Connors (1984; see also Gutnick et al. 1982) stressed three factors concerning the interictal spike of focal epilepsy: (1) intrinsic neurons that generate bursts of spikes (i.e., intrinsic burst-generating neurons), (2) disinhibition, and (3) excitatory synaptic coupling. Correspondingly, these authors listed several possibilities that could underlie epileptogenesis in human focal epilepsy, including (1) selective vulnerability of inhibitory neurons to injury (e.g., hypoxia), (2) alteration of intrinsic properties leading to increased excitability (e.g., an increase in Na channels, depression of K conductances, increased Ca or Na conductances), and (3) increase in the number of excitatory synapses as a result of axonal sprouting, particularly if inhibitory synapses on cell bodies were displaced as a result. (In this context, one might ask why the cerebellar cortex appears to have such a low epileptogenic capacity. Prince and Connors (1984) suggested that the answer lies in the absence of recurrent excitatory connections among the cerebellar Purkinje cells, in contrast to the presence of recurrent excitatory connections among pyramidal cells in the neocortex.)

Pedley (1984) has suggested that an excitatory-inhibitory imbalance in favor of excitation in focal epilepsy, resulting from loss of inhibitory synapses, could be enhanced by an alteration of the density of different ion channels and by neuronal shrinkage resulting in a shorter electrotonic length constant, thus magnifying the effects of depolarizations on the distal dendritic tree.

Ribak et al. (1979, 1986) have demonstrated that in experimental epileptic foci there is a decrease of inhibitory (GABAergic) synapses onto the cell bodies of pyramidal neurons that is associated with a decrease in the number of inhibitory (GABAergic) neurons. A selective degeneration of neurons making symmetrical synapses, i.e., presumably inhibitory (GABAergic) interneurons, was observed by Sloper et al. (1980) in the motor cortex of infant monkeys after controlled hypoxia.

In general, there is a clear correlation between a decrease in GABA, intracortical inhibition, and a tendency to convulsive activity (Krnjević 1984) Further, substances that tend to block or antagonize the postsynaptic inhibitory effects of GABA, e.g., penicillin, picrotoxin, bicuculline, and pentylenetetrazol (Metrazol), also promote convulsive activity (Schwartzkroin 1987). Conversely, substances that potentiate inhibitory effects of GABA, such as barbiturates and benzodiazepines (e.g., Valium, Librium), tend to counteract epileptogenic tendencies.

Roberts (1980) proposed that a destruction or loss of efficacy of inhibitory GABA interneurons is the major defect predisposing humans to epilepsy resulting from traumatic injury, tumors, and interference with blood supply, and also in some hereditary metabolic disorders that predispose to seizures (figure 13.1).

Generalized Epilepsy: The 3-Hz Spike-Wave Pattern

Penicillin applied locally to the cortex in experimental animals is well known to induce epileptiform EEG activity, presumably as a result of interference with cortical inhibitory mechanisms. However, if injected intramuscularly in cats, penicillin induces generalized bilaterally synchronous spike-wave discharges, i.e., feline generalized penicillin epilepsy (FGPE), which has become an experimental model for the 3-Hz spike-wave discharge that is the EEG correlate of absence or petit-mal attacks in humans (Gloor 1984; Avoli 1987).

In feline generalized penicillin epilepsy, spike-wave discharges appear to emerge under an increased thalamocortical excitatory drive from a background of spindling or recruiting activity, appearing to begin in cortex and then to involve both cortex and thalamus (Gloor 1984; Gloor and Fariello 1988). It may be relevant that during spindling, cortical pyramidal neurons often show no inhibitory postsynaptic potentials (IPSPs) unless they discharge a brief cluster of action potentials (Creutzfeldt et al. 1966), which may suggest a threshold (nonlinear) effect for the appearance of IPSPs. Connors et al.

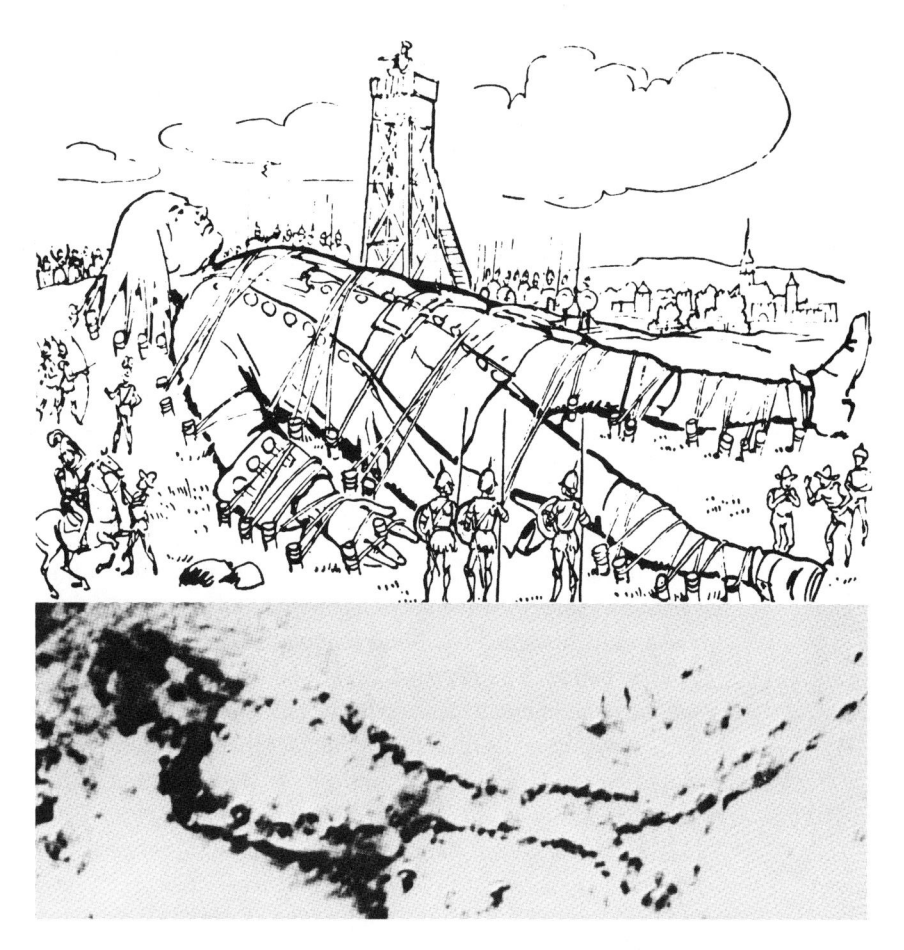

Figure 13.1 The inhibited nervous system. An unretouched photograph taken with Nomarski optics of a neuron in the rat interpositus (nucleus) studded with GAD (gamma-amino acid dehydrogenase)-positive terminals, presumably Purkinje cell axonal terminals, is placed below a picture of Gulliver, showing him when he awoke to find himself pinioned to the ground. The top picture is taken from the 1956 edition of *The Book of Knowledge* (Grolier Society, Inc.). (Figure prepared by Robert Barber; from Roberts 1980.)

(1982) observed spontaneous inhibitory events in only about 10 percent of guinea pig sensorimotor cells *in vitro*.

The cortex appears to be the essential component for feline generalized penicillin epilepsy. Thus, spike-wave discharges can be produced in the cortex by widespread application of a very dilute solution of penicillin restricted to the cortex itself, whereas intrathalamic injection of penicillin is ineffective (Gloor 1984; Gloor et al. 1977; Avoli and Gloor 1982a,b).

After intramuscular injection of penicillin, the sequence appears to be one in which the number of action or unit potentials in the neocortex (presumably from pyramidal cells) progressively increases as the spike component of the spike-wave discharge, the wave component evolving concomitantly as the recurrent (intracortical) inhibitory pathway with associated prolonged IPSPs become maximally excited, the wave component being accompanied by the absence of unit potentials (Gloor 1972, 1984). Thus, the "spike" appears to represent the sum of cortical excitatory postsynaptic potentials (EPSPs), whereas the "wave" component reflects a combination of hyperpolarizing (inhibitory) mechanisms (including Cl and probably also K outward currents (Avoli 1987)). Using an earlier model for producing the 3-Hz spike-wave pattern by stimulation of the midline intralaminar system of the thalamus in cats under light pentobarbital anesthesia (Jasper and Droogleever-Fortuyn 1947, Jasper 1949), Pollen (1964, 1968, 1969) found, from intracellular recordings, that the surface spike was associated with postsynaptic inhibitory activity, itself a consequence of the postsynaptic excitatory activity.

The successive alternation of strong excitatory drive (resulting in the spike) and strong inhibitory drive (resulting in the slow wave), which presumably also occurs in the human 3-Hz spike-wave pattern, contrasts with the situation in focal (partial) epilepsy as well as with that in generalized tonic-clonic seizures. In the latter, impairment of inhibitory drive is considered to lead to excessive excitatory drive and sustained depolarization of the neuronal membrane and to sustained cell firing (Gloor 1988).

The apparent paradox that penicillin disables inhibitory cortical mechanisms in experimental focal epilepsy but not in generalized feline penicillin epilepsy may be accounted for by the fact that the brain-tissue concentrations required to produce the latter are one or two magnitudes lower than those required to produce the former (Davenport et al. 1979; Gloor 1984; Avoli 1987). Such low concentrations of penicillin might increase the excitability of neocortical pyramidal cells by reducing tonic inhibition but leaving phasic inhibition unaltered (Gloor 1984), or by reducing some dendritic inhibitory (GABAergic) mechanisms but leaving the postsynaptic inhibition on the soma unaltered as in hippocampal pyramidal cells (Avoli 1984). Alternatively, penicillin could increase neuronal excitability directly (Gloor 1984, 1987) (see below). If, however, the spike-wave discharge begins to evolve into a generalized tonic-clonic seizure, the recurrent inhibition breaks down (Gloor 1984). The widespread synchronization—not always perfect, as pointed out by Petsche (1962)—was attributed by Gloor (1982, 1984) to cortical association and callosal fibers.

If such a mechanism gives rise to the spike component of the spike-wave discharge, then intracortical recurrent inhibitory pathways (themselves perhaps hyperactivated) can be supposed to give rise to a consequent long-lasting (e.g., 300 msec) inhibition, manifested as the slow-wave component, during which pyramidal cells do not fire (Gloor and Fariello 1988). A rhythmical repetition of this sequence constitutes the 3-Hz spike-wave pattern. Overall, this proposed mechanism is quite different from that of focal epileptogenesis, a principal component of which is an impairment of intracortical feedback mechanisms.

Weir (1965) has drawn attention to the inadequacy of "spike-wave" as a characterization of the 3-Hz spike-wave pattern in humans, pointing out that even in apparently simple 3-Hz complexes there are usually two negative spikes (the first, as the initial component of the complex, often of much smaller amplitude), a positive transient, and finally the usual negative slow wave.

Increased Cortical Excitability If feline generalized epilepsy suggests that the basis of the 3-Hz spike-wave pattern is not an impairment of cortical inhibitory mechanisms, then the question of an increased intracortical excitatory drive, i.e., a state of diffuse cortical hyperexcitability, arises (Gloor and Fariello 1988). One possibility is an increased leakage of glutamic acid from the intracellular into the extracellular compartment, which would expose neurons to its excitatory action, thus increasing the level of excitability responsible for transformation of spindles to spike-wave discharges (Gloor 1984, p. 129).

It is of interest, in this connection, that a probably genetically determined disturbance in amino acid metabolism has been reported in patients with absence (petit-mal) attacks and in some of their asysmptomatic first-degree relatives. This defect results in relatively high plasma levels of glutamic acid (van Gelder et al. 1980) and raises the question of cortical hyperexcitability in human 3-Hz spike-wave epilepsy.

Gloor and his colleagues have recently summarized their studies on the 3-Hz spike-wave EEG pattern (Gloor 1988; Gloor et al. 1990). In feline generalized penicillin epilepsy (FGPE), spike-wave discharges appear to evolve (by a mechanism that remains unclear) from spindles, a physiological mode of the thalamocortical relationship that is particularly evident during early slow-wave sleep. Gloor (1988) has offered the following explanation: Normally, during spindling (in drowsiness or light sleep), there is a low probability that a thalamocortical volley associated with a spindle wave will result in firing of a given cortical neuron. As a result, the recurrent cortical inhibitory pathway is either not activated or only weakly activated. Under the influence of penicillin, however, the probability of firing of cortical pyramidal cells is increased, with consequent maximal activation of the recurrent inhibitory pathway, with resulting pyramidal-cell silence. The burst of pyramidal-cell discharge coincides with the EEG spike (itself evolving from every other, or every third, spindle wave), and the pause in neuronal (i.e., pyramidal cell) firing corresponds to the EEG slow wave. Both cortex and thalamus are thus considered essential for the spike-wave pattern to develop.

In brief, it appears that the EEG spike represents summated cortical excitatory postsynaptic potentials (EPSPs) whereas the slow-wave component corresponds to summated intracortical inhibitory postsynaptic potentials (IPSPs) (Gloor 1988).

Consonant with the fact that feline generalized penicillin epilepsy (FGPE) tends to emerge as an altered spindling pattern, stimulation of the brain-stem reticular formation reduces or blocks the spike-wave discharge. Conversely, interference with the functioning of the ascending reticular activating system (e.g., by localized cooling) increases spike-wave activity, presumably via cortical cholinergic mechanisms (Gloor 1984, 1988). In this connection, Verzeano (1972) adduced experimental evidence that epileptogenic processes (of the generalized type) could result from overdriving of either of two systems that are normally in balance—the first being the pacemaker or synchronizing system of the nonspecific thalamic nuclei, which leads to relaxation, drowsiness, and sleep, and the second being the desynchronizing system that leads to arousal, wakefulness, and alertness.

Gloor (1988) has pointed out that neither in feline generalized penicillin epilepsy nor in human 3-Hz spike discharges has the abruptness of onset and termination in all cortical areas simultaneously been accounted for. In this connection, recall from chapter 12 that only the reticular nucleus of the thalamus projects to all other thalamic nuclei, has an inhibitory output, and participates in a negative (inhibitory) feedback system (i.e., receives collateral from both thalamocortical and corticothalamic fibers (Jones 1985). Further, the reticular nucleus appears to be of primary importance in the generation of spindles in cats under light barbiturate anesthesia (chapter 12). This raises the question of whether the thalamic reticular nucleus may have some role in the 3-Hz spike-wave pattern, especially in relation to its widespread distribution and its abrupt onset and termination.

In a recent retrospective, Jasper (1991) stressed the combined roles of cortical and subcortical structures, as opposed to the view of a predominance of cortical ones, in the generation of the 3-Hz spike-wave pattern, and raised some questions concerning the relevance of feline generalized penicillin epilepsy to human absence seizures.

Epileptiform Discharges and Sleep

Non-REM sleep characteristically activates both interictal (focal) discharge and generalized 3-Hz spike-wave discharges (Daly 1979; Pedley 1984). Pedley (1984) found that, for both focal and generalized epilepsy, transitions from wakefulness to Stage 1 non-REM sleep or from Stage 1 to Stage 2 sleep were especially activating. Kellaway et al. (1980) observed a "steplike increase" in the amount of 3-Hz spike-wave activity in the course of the first non-REM period of each night, and also during succeeding non-REM periods during the night. In a recent review, Daly (1990) also indicated that 3-Hz spike-wave discharges tended to become increasingly frequent as non-REM sleep deepened, but that focal discharges from the temporal lobe tended to occur maximally in Stages 1 and 2 of non-REM sleep, declining in frequency in Stages 3 and 4. Further, during non-REM sleep the regular 3-Hz spike-wave pattern of the waking state may be replaced by spikes or polyspikes without the slow-wave component (Pedley 1984).

During REM sleep, the incidence of 3-Hz spike-wave discharges drops markedly, to slightly below that for the waking state (Daly 1979; Pedley 1984). Focal spikes, however, particularly if from the temporal lobe, do not become less frequent, and may increase their frequency of occurrence during REM sleep (Pedley 1984).

The reported more frequent occurrence of 3-Hz spike-wave patterns in patients in the spindling stages of sleep (i.e., non-REM sleep) appears to parallel the emergence of the spike-wave pattern on a spindling background in feline generalized penicillin epilepsy (Gloor 1984).

Epilepsy and Brain Maturation

Schwartzkroin (1984) has suggested that an apparent intrinsic anti-epileptogenic mechanism may be evident in the immature brain, at least in experimental animals, in that there is an apparent lag in the development of excitatory postsynaptic potentials as compared with inhibitory ones, and in that the paroxysmal depolarizing shift (PSD) that is characteristic of neurons in adult animals is more difficult to induce in immature animals. (Such a maturational lagging of excitatory mechanisms behind excitatory ones may perhaps also find a reflection in the generally lower frequencies of the immature as compared with the adult EEG.)

DC Changes in Epilepsy

The negative DC or steady potential (SP) shift associated with the 3-Hz spike-wave pattern in the human EEG is well established (Cohn 1954, 1964; Chatrian et al. 1968; Gumnit 1974), as is a DC shift in association with focal epilepsy, in experimental animals (Gumnit 1974). A negative DC shift also occurs during ictal episodes in generalized seizures in experimental animals (Matsumoto and Ajmone-Marsan 1964b; O'Leary and Goldring 1976), including the generalized tonic-clinic seizures elicited by pentylenetetrazol (Metrazol) (Speckmann et al. 1972; Speckmann and Elger 1987). (Earlier studies concerning DC shifts during seizure discharges were reviewed in O'Leary and Goldring 1964.)

In their report on DC changes in the scalp EEG during 3-Hz spike-wave discharges in humans, Chatrian et al. (1968) characterized the initial DC potential change as a "paroxysmal negative shift," the topography of which was very similar to that of the slow-wave component. During non-REM sleep, when the spike-wave discharges occurred at generally lower rates (1.5–2 Hz), were of higher amplitude, and were often less regular than during wakefulness, the paroxysmal negative shift was greater. The paroxysmal negative shift appeared to be associated primarily with the wave rather than with the spike component of the discharge; for example, it was found that during paroxysms consisting only of repetitive spikes (as in generalized tonic seizures) there were only minimal DC shifts. Chatrian et al. (1968) concluded, following Pollen's (1964) experimental work on induced spike-wave discharges in cats, that the paroxysmal negative shift in humans was associated with summated current flows in apical dendrites acting as passive sinks for hyperpolarizing currents generated in the deeper cortical layers.

Basic Mechanisms of Focal and Generalized Epileptiform Discharges

Avoli et al. (1990) have recently contrasted the basic mechanisms at a cellular level in the cortex in feline generalized penicillin epilepsy with those of the interictal discharge of focal epilepsy, and also with those underlying generalized convulsive seizures. In feline generalized epilepsy, the recurrent cortical inhibitory (hyperpolarizing) mechanisms remain intact, thereby providing the basis of the alternating sequence of excitatory and inhibitory drive that is manifested as the 3-Hz (approximately) spike-wave pattern. In the epileptiform discharges associated with focal epilepsy, on the other hand, a giant excitatory postsynaptic potential (EPSP) presumably results from synchronous activation of recurrent excitatory pathways (reinforced, perhaps, by activation of "ectopic" spikes on the dendritic tree and, concomitantly, a marked decrease in recurrent inhibitory postsynaptic potentials in the area of the epileptic focus). During the paroxysmal depolarizing shift, there is a burst of action potentials, sometimes followed by hyperpolarization.

In generalized convulsive seizures (a term that, as Avoli et al. (1990) point out, is not necessarily synonymous with the term "tonic-clonic seizures") that evolve either directly from intramuscularly administered penicillin or from a focal lesion, the possible basic abnormalities include an increased cortical excitability associated with a penicillin-induced increase of extracellular glutamate and (more likely) an increased excitability resulting from impaired dendritic depolarizing inhibitory (GABAergic) potentials. The transition to the generalized convulsive seizure was considered to be associated with a breakdown of one or more of the hyperpolarizing inhibitory-potential systems (Avoli et al. 1990).

Gloor (1989) has suggested that the fact that transient (e.g., postictal EEG depression or slowing) or even permanent untoward consequences may occur in focal (partial) seizures and also in generalized tonic-clonic convulsive seizures, but not in 3-Hz spike-wave (absence) seizures, may relate to the fact that in 3-Hz spike-wave epilepsy (but not in focal or in generalized convulsions) the GABAergic inhibitory mechanisms remain intact. Gloor (1989) attributed the transient or permanent postictal effects of the latter two seizure types to the activation of N-methyl-D-aspartate (NMDA) receptors (Dichter and Ayala 1987) by the excitatory transmitter, glutamate (or aspartate) and to the consequent entry of appreciable amounts of calcium ion into neurons.

The EEG in Generalized Tonic-Clonic Conclusions

In generalized tonic-clonic seizures, or "grand-mal" epilepsy, the onset is characterized by uniform bilaterally synchronous rhythmic waves in the range of 10 Hz, persisting through the tonic phase; this pattern is preceded in some instances by a generalized spike-wave pattern having multiple instead of single spikes (Gloor 1984; Gloor and Fariello 1988).

The Slow Spike-Wave EEG Pattern of the Lennox-Gastaut Syndrome

The relatively characteristic EEG pattern in the Lennox-Gastaut Syndrome (the other two characteristics of which are severe seizures and mental retardation) is usually termed a "slow spike-wave" pattern; i.e., the repetition rate of the pattern is about 2 Hz rather than the 3 Hz of the classical spike-wave pattern discussed above (figure 4.17). The lower frequency results largely from a slower course of the wave component, especially its final part, which somewhat resembles a rounded sawtooth rather than the more nearly symmetrical form of the classical 3-Hz pattern.

An Overview of the Basic Disorders in Epilepsy

Symonds (1962) characterized the essence of epileptic seizures and the epileptic discharge as epiphenomena, i.e., as the occasional expressions of a fundamental and continuous disorder of function the essence of which is a loss of normal balance between excitation and inhibition at synaptic junctions (see also Schwartzkroin 1987 and Daly 1990). Subsequent work with experimental animals, as well as clinical studies, appear to be consistent with this formulation, and the basic hypothesis of the EEG presented in this book is consistent with it. A depiction of the essential and potentially powerful role of inhibitory activity in the nervous system from Roberts 1980 is reproduced in figure 13.1. Although the specific instance depicted in the illustration concerns inhibition in the nucleus interpositus by cerebellar Purkinje cells (e.g., in relation to movement control), inhibitory control (and, by inference, excitatory-inhibitory balance) is also of prime importance in the cerebral cortex in relation to epilepsy, at least the focal type.

CORTICAL PATHOLOGY WITHOUT EPILEPSY: ALZHEIMER'S DISEASE

It was mentioned above that slow-wave abnormalities in the EEG are characteristically associated with subcortical disease (in particular, with disease of subcortical white matter) rather than with disease of the neocortex. A number of diseases of the latter can give rise to epileptiform manifestations: trauma, infarction (particularly of thrombotic origin), tumor, viral infections (e.g., Creutzfeldt-Jakob disease, herpes encephalitis), autoimmune disease (e.g., acute postinfectious encephalomyelitis), and collagen diseases (e.g., lupus erythematosis) (personal communication, E. P. Richardson, Jr.). (On the other hand, it seems not unreasonable to suggest that the occasional manifestations of epilepsy that are seen in traditionally white-matter diseases such as multiple sclerosis or progressive multifocal leucoencephalopathy arise from localized extensions of the pathological process into the cortex that affect nerve fibers there—in particular, the axons of cortical inhibitory neurons.)

In Alzheimer's diease, however, although there is characteristically pathology of parts of the cerebral cortex, clinically seizures are relatively infrequent among patients, and epileptiform patterns are uncommon in the EEG. Instead, the EEG is typically characterized by slowing in the theta and delta frequency ranges (Soininen et al. 1982; Coben et al. 1983; Niedermeyer 1987d; Markand 1990a). The reason for the infrequency of epileptiform manifestations in the EEG in patients with this disease may be apparent from consideration of the details of the cellular neuropathology.

In those areas of the neocortex that are affected (namely, the association areas, as opposed to the sensory and motor areas), the pathology consists of so-called senile or neuritic plaques and neurofibrillary tangles, and it is the large pyramidal neurons (of layers II and III of the cortex) giving rise to the association fibers that are primarily affected in the disease (Roberts et al. 1985; Rogers and Morrison 1985; Duyckaerts et al. 1986; Hof et al. 1990). At the same time, a loss of neuron-to-neuron communication in the form of a decrease of neocortical synapses, correlating with cognitive impairment, has recently been reported (Terry et al. 1991). Contrariwise, smaller neurons, including those associated with intracortical inhibitory mechanisms, appear to remain relatively unaffected. In the face of relatively intact intracortical inhibitory mechanisms but impaired excitatory mechanisms (the latter being derived from the affected large pyramidal neurons via their recurrent collaterals), a tilt of the balance between excitatory and inhibitory mechanisms in favor of inhibitory ones would be expected, thus minimizing any tendency toward epileptogenesis in the affected neocortex.

In addition, the "corticocortical disconnection" resulting from the disease (Hof et al. 1990) would be expected to reduce further the excitatory input to a given small area of cortex, resulting in a still greater balance in favor of (local) inhibitory mechanisms. Yet another factor in favor of inhibitory mechanisms could be a decrease in the excitatory effects of cholinergic synapses in the neocortex as a result of loss of their cells of origin in the nucleus basalis of Meynert in the forebrain region (Roberts et al. 1985; Buzsaki et al. 1988; Davis and Robertson 1991; Riekkinen et al. 1991). EEG slowing as a consequence of both of these effects would not be surprising.

Levels of the inhibitory transmitter GABA and its synthesizing enzyme GAD (gamma-amino acid dehydrogenase) remain unchanged in Alzheimer's disease, whereas the binding of the putative excitatory transmitter glutamate is reduced (Jones 1988). These findings appear to be consistent with the previously mentioned findings that pyramidal cells of layers II and III are preferentially affected in the disease, and in turn to be consistent with the view that intracortical inhibitory mechanisms remain largely intact whereas excitatory mechanisms (including those associated with recurrent collaterals from pyramidal cells) are impaired.

The relatively unusual circumstance in which cortical pathology in Alzheimer's disease is not accompanied by epileptiform manifestations thus appears to be consistent with the known pathology of the disease. This point will be considered further, in relation to the possible physiological significance of the present model of the EEG, in chapter 16.

14 Other Models of the EEG, and Related Models

Models of the EEG can be classified in several different ways. One type of classification could be as to type: anatomical (i.e., according to the anatomical substrata of a generator system for the EEG), physiological, mathematical, or synthetic (i.e., with the EEG considered as a signal from a "black box"). (See also Lopes da Silva 1987a.) Another classification could be made according to perspective: derivative (in which an attempt is made to delineate from the EEG itself its basic generating mechanisms) or integrative (in which the EEG is sought as the summated activity of known or postulated neurophysiological processes—e.g., from postsynaptic potentials in the cerebral cortex). The present extrema-slopes model is derivative in type.

In turn, subclassifications can be made. Thus, some models are purely phenomenological, without any relevance to the content of the black box (i.e., the brain). Mathematical analysis in the form of Fourier analysis, or more exactly (in some applications) periodogram analysis, is such a method. The EEG is modeled as a series of sine and cosine waves, each of constant amplitude for the duration of the segment of signal analyzed. Such a model is clearly not a realistic physiological one, although very precise mathematically. As early as 1943, Bertrand and Lacape had distinguished between morphological analysis and physiological interpretation.

Alternatively, models of the EEG can be classified as either lumped (in which the ensemble of individual generators of similar or identical properties and connections is represented by a single summary process) or distributed (in which each element (e.g., neuron) is simulated, having its specific position in a "nerve net" or "local circuit") (Lopes da Silva 1987a). In both of these types of models, parameters (e.g., of transfer functions, interactions (synaptic strengths)) can be adjusted.

It is useful, at this point, to distinguish between a model and a theory. Dewan (1964) suggested that a model can be mathematical or "phenomenological," serving to display the underlying order and the uniformities in the data, and to guide further experiment; only after the latter then can a truly theoretical scheme be formulated. (See also Lopes da Silva 1987a.)

With this brief overview of the taxonomy of models, some aspects of EEG models themselves will now be considered in their historical perspective.

Perhaps the first attempt at modeling the EEG was that of Dietsch (1932), who, at the suggestion of Berger, carried out Fourier analysis of the EEG. But since Fourier analysis is a purely mathematical method, without any specific reference to the particular features of the EEG as a signal, it and related techniques (e.g., coherence, autocorrelation, and cross-correlation) will not be considered in detail in this chapter. (Some limitations of Fourier types of analysis are considered in chapter 15.)

THE RELAXATION OSCILLATOR

In one form of relaxation oscillator, the waveform is characteristically a sawtooth, representing the alternation of a relatively slow process in one direction and a relatively fast one in the other (such as the charging up of a condenser through a resistor, followed by a rapid discharge of the condenser when the voltage across it reaches a threshold value). Van der Pol took the name from the term "time of relaxation," which is a synonym for "time constant." The

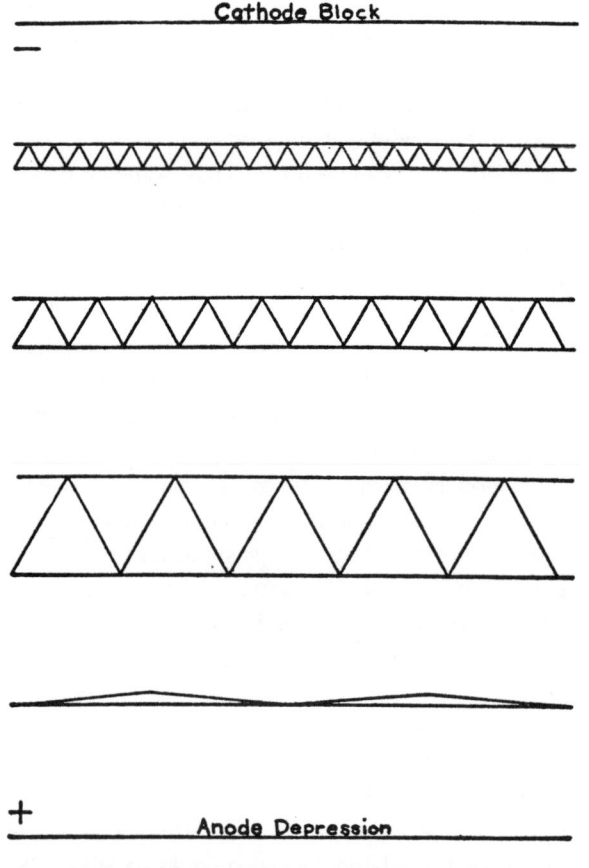

Figure 14.1 Schema (from Jasper 1936b) indicating waves of progressively increasing frequency and decreasing amplitude (in a sequence from anode depression to cathode block) as a model (e.g., from a relaxation oscillator) for the behavior of the EEG with increasing level of cortical excitatory state.

relaxation oscillator had been proposed as a model for the cardiac rhythm (van der Pol and van der Mark 1928).

Van der Pol (1926) had included, as a type of relaxation oscillator, the "multivibrator"—essentially a biphasic electronic relaxation oscillator, in which two relaxation oscillators operate back-to-back. Such an oscillator has two outputs: a triangular wave and an approximately square wave. (The term "multivibrator" referred to the high number of harmonics present in the output waveform of such a highly nonlinear device.)

By the time of the 1936 Cold Spring Harbor Symposium, an appreciable part of which was devoted to the EEG, the relaxation oscillator of van der Pol (1926) was being invoked as a model for the EEG (Hoagland 1936a,b,c; Jasper 1936a,b). (An excellent comparative discussion of the characteristics of relaxation and simple harmonic oscillators, with mechanical (a pendulum), hydraulic (a syphon-emptying tank), and electrical analogs, was given by Walter (1959), together with a comparison of the nonlinear (abruptly discontinuous) features of relaxation oscillators and those of linear (smoothly continuous) features of simple harmonic oscillators. (See also Hoagland 1936b.)

Jasper (1936a,b), in drawing attention to the trend from higher amplitudes and lower frequencies in sleep to lower amplitudes and higher frequencies in the awake alert state, used the term "cortical excitatory state" and drew a parallel with the relaxation oscillator and the trend that can be observed with the latter, namely a progressive trend from lower frequencies and higher amplitudes to higher frequencies and lower amplitudes. Jasper's schema is reproduced in figure 14.1, from which it is evident that the three sets of triangular waves have the same slope. This set of waveforms is equivalent to the constant-slope waves of the present oscillator model in Mode 1 of its

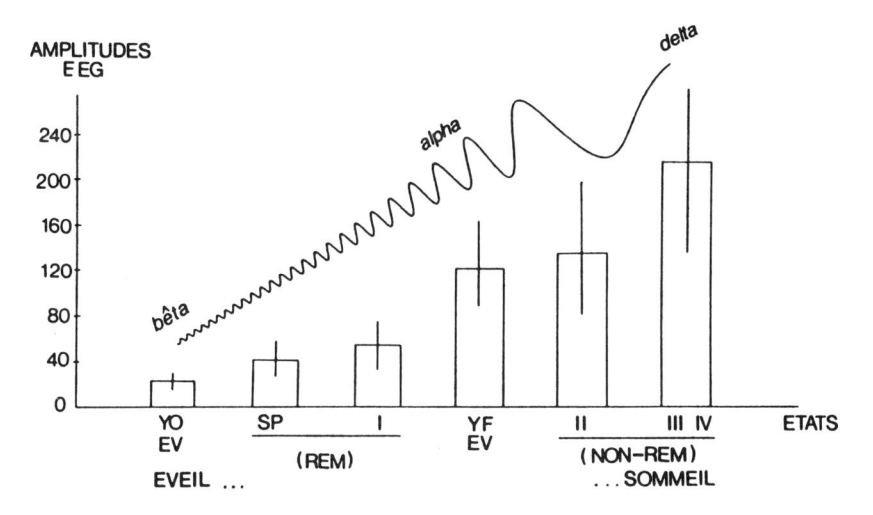

Figure 14.2 Schema of Étévenon (1987, p. 158) for classification of the EEG in states of wakefulness (EVEIL) and sleep (SOMMEIL) according to mean occipital EEG amplitude of each state. In this schema, REM sleep and Stage 1 sleep are interposed between the EEG for eyes-open awake (YO, EV) and eyes-closed awake (YF EV).

operation (see figure 2.1, upper left). Jasper's concept of the cortical excitatory state, which he subsequently considered to be sufficiently broadly defined to include inhibitory processes (Jasper 1981), will be considered again in chapter 15.

One representation of the general trend of a decrease in amplitude and an increase in frequency with an increase in the state of alertness or the level of consciousness is depicted in figure 14.2. (See also Étévenon and Guillou 1986.)

FILTERED-NOISE MODELS

As a preliminary to a consideration of models in which the EEG is simulated as the output of a linear system (i.e., a system in which superposition holds, or, alternatively expressed, in which doubling the input doubles the output), the question may be raised of whether the EEG itself is Gaussian or not (i.e., whether it has a Gaussian (normal) distribution of amplitudes). This question has been investigated by a number of workers, with generally affirmative answers (Lion and Winter 1953; Kozhevnikov 1958; Saunders 1963; Elul 1969, 1972a,b; Glass 1969; Dick and Vaughn 1970; McEwen and Anderson 1975; Siegel 1981). (However, Siegel (1981) has pointed out that the "desynchronized" EEG can be less Gaussian (random) than the "synchronized" EEG.) If the amplitude distribution of the EEG itself is Gaussian, then the envelope should have a Rayleigh distribution (Saunders 1963), which was confirmed by Dick and Vaughn (1970).

A Gaussian amplitude distribution function for a large number of individual oscillators does not necessarily imply that the individual elements also have a gaussian amplitude distribution function, since, according to the central limit theorem, a quantity that is the sum of N independent random variables (each individually negligible relative to the sum itself) has a probability density distribution that tends to be Gaussian for large values of N (Middleton 1960; Adey 1969; Dick and Vaughan 1970; Elul 1972a,b; Siegel 1981).

Perhaps the first proposal of a filtered-noise model of the EEG was that of Prast (1949), who suggested that the alpha rhythm represented the output of a narrow-band transmission system (i.e., filter) for an input of white noise (i.e., noise having a very wide flat spectrum), the latter the result of a "purely statistical summation of spontaneous cortical neuron spike discharges." In contrast, Prast (1949) considered non-alpha types of human and animal EEGs as the output of a relatively broad-band filter. Lowenberg (1959) reported on a circuit consisting of a gas-tube noise generator together with low-pass, high-pass, and band-pass filters (the latter in the alpha frequency range), for simulation of various types of EEG patterns (figure 14.3). Barlow (1962b) simulated alpha and abnormal slow-wave EEG patterns by means of trains of randomly recurring pulses (intended to simulate neuronal action potentials) in conjunction with band-pass and low-pass filters.

The filtered-noise model of Hendrix (1965) was based on randomly firing pulse sources (to simulate the discharge of neurons) and an assumed after-

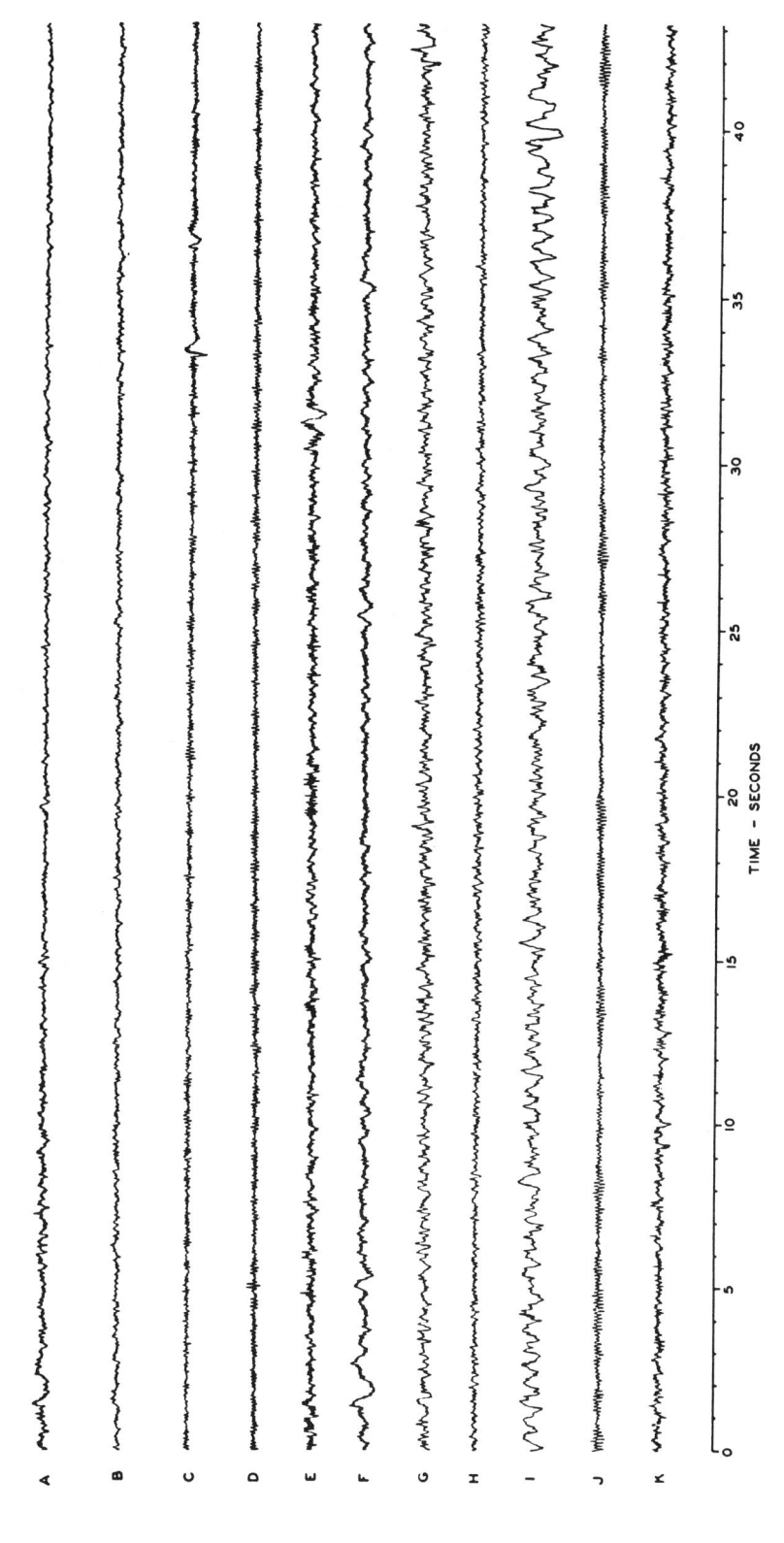

Figure 14.3 Actual and electronically simulated EEG patterns. The actual EEGs are traces A, D, E, J, and K. (From Lowenberg 1959.)

Other Models of the EEG, and Related Models

potential which, when imbedded in a diffuse medium of indefinite extent, had a single low-frequency peak in the alpha frequency range.

Dick and Vaughn (1970) simulated alpha activity by means of narrow-band Gaussian random noise, using two cascaded second-order band-pass filters. The EEG simulator described by Shaw (1971) employed a binary pulse sequence in conjunction with analog filters in the EEG frequency range to form repeatable patterns.

In conjunction with the modeling of EEGs by filtered noise and the characterization of EEGs by "spectral parameter analysis," Wennberg and Zetterberg (1971), Zetterberg (1973), and Zetterberg and Ahlin (1975) simulated EEG patterns and spectra resembling those of actual EEGs by means of four independent noise generators in combination with adjustable filters corresponding to each of the conventional EEG frequency bands (delta, theta, alpha, and beta). Narasimhan and Dutt (1985) described a digital-computer implementation of this approach.

In the filtered-noise model of alpha activity described by Kemp and Blom (1981), shown in figure 14.4 (see also Lopes da Silva 1987d), a white-noise source is used in conjunction with an alpha or no-alpha state (determined by the characteristics of a feedback loop consisting of a second-order band-pass filter) and a low-pass filter (simulating the cortex-to-scalp transfer characteristics reported by Pfurtscheller and Cooper (1975)).

In the filtered-noise model of the EEG described by Kemp et al. (1987) (which formed the basis of a sleep-staging system), alpha and sleep spindles (Kemp et al. 1985) were simulated by means of band-pass filters, and delta activity was simulated with a low-pass filter. In a subsequent modification (DaRosa et al. 1991), single random pulses were added to simulate vertex waves or K complexes, according to the particular background activity. The basic assumption of these authors was that these forms of EEG activity represent oscillations occurring in frequency-dependent feedback loops in noise-driven neuronal networks, and that, correspondingly, optimal detectors for such EEG patterns could be developed (Lopes da Silva and Mars 1987).

The generalized conceptual model for EEG activity advanced by Gasser (1977) included deterministic (periodic), random quasi-stationary (stochastic), and randomly triggered wavelets and other transients of deterministic waveform.

Freeman (1975) modeled the electrical activity of the three-layer olfactory cortex (a part of the allocortex, in contrast to the six-layer neocortex) with linear and nonlinear ordinary and partial differential equations, on the initial assumption that the resting, irregular, activity could be considered as filtered noise. In the latter sense, Freeman's earlier work could be considered a linear systems approach (see also Lopes da Silva 1987a).

In the mathematical model of Wright and Kydd (1984), which is basically a filtered-noise model, the EEG is considered to result from the linear superposition of the output (at the apical dendritic tree of pyramidal neurons) of an ensemble of linked corticosubcortical oscillators, under the control of (i.e.,

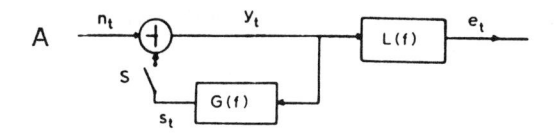

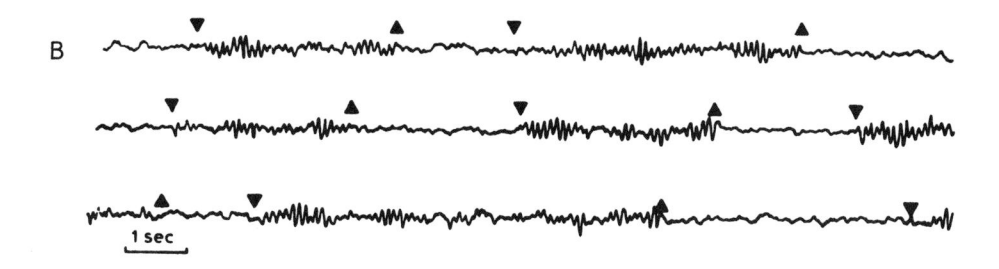

Figure 14.4 Model for generating occipital EEG showing intermittent alpha activity. (A) Block diagram with switch (S) for alpha state. L(f): low-pass filter simulating cortex-to-scalp transfer characteristics. (B) Simulated signals (upward triangles indicate switch open; downward, closed). (C) Frequency characteristic [G(f)] of the feedback loop; $f_0 = 10$ Hz, $B = 8$ Hz, $G_0 = 0.9$. G_0: gain at the center frequency. B: bandwidth at the peak frequency. (From Lopes da Silva and Mars 1987; after Kemp and Blom 1981.)

with damping characteristics determined by) the lateral hypothalamus, and driven by noise.

Although filtered-noise models of the EEG, particularly of alpha activity, have been quite popular, a fundamental limitation of this linear model should be kept in mind: the narrower the filter (i.e., the sharper the resonance), the longer its build-up and die-away times (Walter 1959). Nonlinear models do not suffer from this limitation. That the alpha rhythm can be a relatively pure sinsusoid, and yet attenuate very rapidly upon eye-opening, has long been known (Rohracher 1937, 1938).

AUTOREGRESSIVE MODELING OF THE EEG

In EEG modeling, an alternative to manual adjustment of filter parameters to obtain a pattern resembling a given EEG is autoregressive modeling (also known, in other fields, as the linear prediction or maximum-entropy method). An autoregressive representation of a signal (in the present case, an EEG) is obtained by regressing the signal on itself (Lopes da Silva and Mars 1987), thus yielding a set of autoregressive coefficients. This procedure is equivalent to considering the signal as having been generated by passing white noise through a linear filter (the autoregressive filter, constituted of the autoregressive coefficients). The output signal from the filter then has the same statistical properties as the original.

Fenwick et al. (1971) simulated specific stationary (i.e., statistically unchanging) EEG patterns in this way by using an autoregressive model of the original EEG as a filter having a random-noise input. Autoregressive modeling of nonstationary EEGs (i.e., EEGs in which the pattern varied with time) was carried out by Bohlin (1971, 1973, 1977), Duquesnoy (1976), and Isaksson and Wennberg (1976) using Kalman filtering, in which the autoregressive coefficients "track" the changing characteristics of the EEG. In these studies, the simulated EEGs resembled the originals and had similar statistical properties, but were not identical to the originals. An alternative to continuous tracking of the autoregressive parameters of an EEG is that of automatic adaptive segmentation, in which a change in the parameters of the autoregressive signals a segmentation (nonstationarity) in the EEG (Praetorius et al. 1977; Segen and Sanderson 1979; see Barlow 1985c for a review). In any event, it is self-evident that any satisfactory model of the EEG must take into account its nonstationary aspects (Barlow 1985c).

Starting from the modeling of the EEG as the output of a linear system (i.e., a filter) having white noise input, Franaszczuk and Blinowska (1985) derived the transfer function via the autoregressive method and then obtained the differential equations describing the system. The result was that the system, and thus the EEG, could be described as the sum of damped sinusoidal waves. The authors considered this representation of the EEG to be more realistic than the representation of the EEG as the sum of a large number of undamped (fixed-amplitude) sinusoids, as implied by fitting the model to the Fourier (FFT) spectrum as exemplified in the approach of, e.g., Wright and Kydd (1984).

MODULATION MODELS

The waxing-and-waning amplitude of the approximately constant-frequency alpha activity has given rise to models in which the envelope of alpha activity is modulated. Thus, Bertrand and Lacape (1943) proposed, in what Étévenon (1977) considered to be the first mathematical model of the EEG, a model of the alpha rhythm as a modulation of a sine wave of alpha frequency by a slower wave, in the first instance sinusoidal but then generalized to include an irregular modulation. As Étévenon has pointed out, the just-described model of Bertrand and Lacape (1943), entailing modulation, is basically multiplicative and is therefore nonlinear (in contrast to the linear models, considered in the previous section, in which the simulated EEGs were derived from linear systems or filters).

The model of Étévenon (1977; see also Étévenon et al. 1980), which can be considered a generalization of the model of Bertrand and Lacape, utilizes the generalized expression for a modulated carrier wave (Bernstein 1927; Middleton 1960):

$$y(t) = [m(t)] \cdot [\cos(2\pi f_0 t) + \phi(t)],$$

where $y(t)$ is the output, $m(t)$ is the amplitude modulation, f_0 is the carrier frequency (which can itself be varied), and $\phi(t)$ is the phase modulation. Étévenon pointed out that this is a dual-modulation model, with both amplitude and phase modulated. Alternatively, phase modulation can be viewed as frequency modulation, and hence Étévenon's model can be considered as incorporating combined amplitude and frequency modulation (Étévenon and Giannella 1980). Determinations of the instantaneous amplitude and instantaneous frequency of the rhythmic EEG during REM sleep of rats by these authors indicated an inverse relationship between the two modulations; i.e., when the amplitude modulation increased, the instantaneous frequency decreased (a variation of about ± 1 Hz around a mean of, e.g., 7.8 Hz).

Étévenon (1987) suggested that a continuum exists between the low-voltage higher-frequency (beta) waves of the alert, eyes-open state and the higher-voltage low-frequency (delta) waves of slow-wave sleep (figure 14.2). This could be taken to be consistent with the above-cited inverse relation between amplitude modulation and frequency modulation. However, Étévenon et al. (1980) pointed out that the above-mentioned modulation model was not without ambiguity, so that a 10.5-Hz sine wave modulated by a 1-Hz sine wave was equivalent to the superposition of 9.5-Hz and 11.5-Hz sine waves, i.e., the output of a linear model. (This ambiguity is discussed in chapter 17 below.)

The view of rhythmic EEG activity (e.g., alpha activity, sleep spindles) as a modulated signal (i.e., a relatively narrow-band process) has given rise to several techniques of obtaining the instantaneous envelope and phase (or frequency). These techniques, which include in-phase and in-quadrature filtering, complex demodulation, Hilbert transformation, and phase-locked loop demodulation, are considered in detail in chapter 29.

LUMPED AND DISTRIBUTED MODELS (NERVE NETS)

There have been a number of mathematical or computer-simulation models of the activity of masses or large assemblies of neurons. The models take into account excitatory and (usually also) inhibitory effects, and are based on a variety of assumptions and on assumed values for certain parameters that are difficult or impossible to obtain experimentally.

Beurle (1956) found that traveling waves of activity could occur in the spontaneous activity (i.e., oscillations) in an assembly of neuron-like cells in which only excitatory effects were present. Farley and Clark (1954) and Farley (1965) studied a computer-simulated neural network employing nonlinear elements with refractory periods and having only excitatory transmission. These workers found a number of similarities between the summated excitation in the network and electrophysiological slow potentials resembling alpha and also more irregular EEG activity, depending on the particular parameters of the neural network.

In the model of the EEG proposed by Lévy (1970), 1971a,b), spindles of alpha waves and alpha blocking (attenuation) in "macrocellular" ensembles of neurons with excitatory and inhibitory feedback loops were found to be related to different levels of the loop gain (itself a random variable), and also to the level of the external input. Under certain conditions, an asymmetry of the waveform (e.g., a comb-like appearance, resulting from the presence of a second harmonic component) or an asymmetry of the rising and falling phases of the waves could result (Lévy 1974).

Wilson and Cowan (1972, 1973) employed coupled nonlinear integro-differential equations to characterize the dynamics of populations of neurons (the thalamus being considered as a vertically downward extension of the cortex) that included both excitatory and inhibitory model neurons. With the aid of phase-plane methods and numerical solutions, these authors found that multiple steady states with hysteresis loops, as well as simple limit-cycle activity, would result (see also Dewan 1964). Several types of EEG-like phenomena were listed by Nogawa et al. (1977) in their further developments of the Wilson-Cowan model.

Using available anatomical and physiological data for a particular thalamic nucleus, the nucleus ventralis posterolateralis (a somatosensory relay nucleus), Lopes da Silva et al. (1974; see also Lopes da Silva 1987a) formulated a computer model of a neural network comprising two types of neurons: thalamocortical relay neurons (144 in number) and thalamic interneurons (numbering 36) interconnected by negative feedback. These authors found that rhythmic activity in the alpha frequency range could result for a random input,

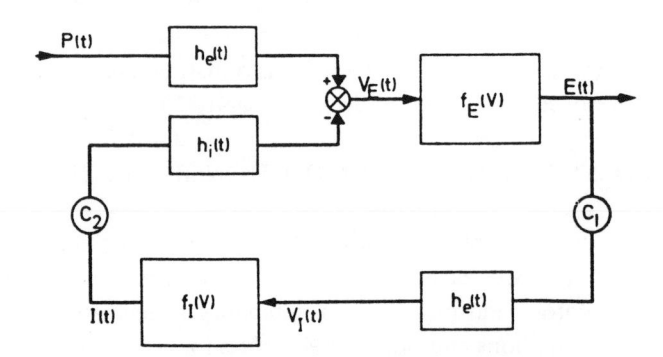

Figure 14.5 Block diagram of a lumped model for rhythmic activity of a simplified alpha-rhythm model. The upper part of the diagram represents thalamocortical relay neurons (assumed to be the primary source of the rhythmic activity), the lower part represents thalamic interneurons. P(t), E(t): input and output pulse density, respectively; $h_e(t)$ and $h_i(t)$: impulse responses of linear systems for generating excitatory and inhibitory postsynaptic responses, respectively, which summate to yield a membrane potential $V_E(t)$, which operates on a static nonlinearity $f_E(V)$ to generate the output spike train, E(t). In the feedback loop the output, E(t) is fed to some proportion (C_1) of interneurons, in which spikes are converted ($h_e(t)$) to excitatory postsynaptic potentials. In a given interneuron, the resulting membrane potential $V_I(t)$ generates ($f_I(V)$) a spike train I(t), which in turn is converted ($h_i(t)$) to inhibitory postsynaptic potentials on some proportion (C_2) of thalamocortical cells. (From Lopes da Silva et al. 1974; see also Lopes da Silva 1987a, figure 2.10.)

i.e., trains of pulses having a Poisson distribution. Linear systems analysis of a simplified lumped form of the model (figure 14.5) disclosed that, by changing the parameters of the model, a family of spectral curves were obtained which simulated maturational changes in the EEG, i.e., a progressive change from a broad low-frequency band to a narrow band in the alpha frequency range (figure 14.6). This change was principally associated with an increase in inhibitory feedback coupling (see also Lopes da Silva et al. 1976 and Lopes da Silva 1987a).

The model of Lopes da Silva et al. (1974, 1976) also confirmed their experimental results with dogs, in that thalamocortical coherences were smaller than cortico-cortical coherences—a result that was subsequently confirmed by a "theoretical thalamic deafferentiation," using partial coherence function analysis (Lopes da Silva et al. 1980a,b). Further, analysis of a "spatially distributed" neuronal chain version of the model, intended to model cortical alpha activity, showed propagation (traveling wave) properties that were in agreement with experimental results on the alpha rhythm of dogs (Lopes da Silva and Storm van Leeuwen 1978; Lopes da Silva et al. 1980a,b). The propagation properties were also concordant with anatomical data on

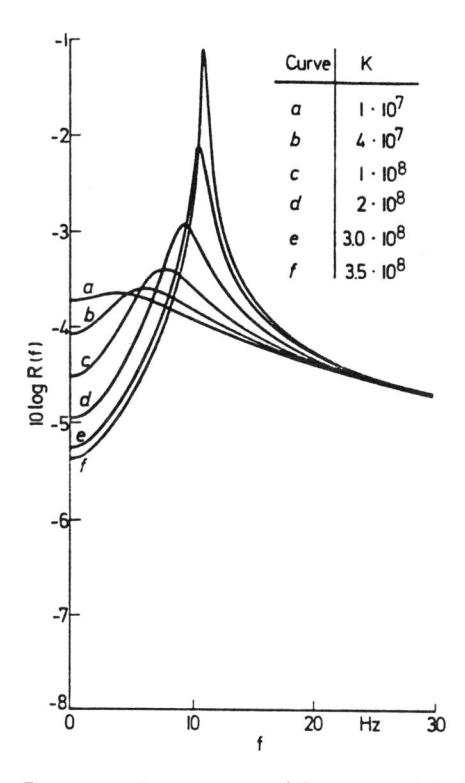

Figure 14.6 Power spectra of the output of the lumped alpha-rhythm model shown in figure 14.4, for different values of the feedback gain (K). The latter is determined mainly by the coupling constants representing the synaptic interactions within the neuronal set. As the synaptic interactions become stronger and K increases, the spectrum acquires a clear peak at the alpha frequency. (From Lopes da Silva et al. 1974.)

cortical columns (Lopes da Silva 1978). A review of these models can be found in Lopes da Silva 1987a.

In the computerized neural net model for the alpha rhythm described by Anninos and Zenone (1980), rhythmic activity was enhanced by restricting connectivity to a limited region around a given cell, i.e., by minimizing neuronal interactions between different regions of the network. Nakagawa and Ohashi (1980) suggested, from their mathematical spatio-temporal filter approach, that synchronous cortical activity may form some kind of delayed recurrent inhibition in layered structures, which, modified by neural nonlinearities, rhythmically interrupts neural activity, normal or epileptiform.

The mathematical and electronic filtered-noise model of Zetterberg (1977) and Zetterberg et al. (1978) includes two excitatory and one inhibitory subsets of neurons. Under stable conditions, oscillatory (alpha-like) waveforms resulted; however, with an input overload, instability resulted, the operation became that of a limit cycle, and paroxysmal (spike-like) waves emerged. The latter finding suggested to Zetterberg et al. that epileptic spikes may be generated by a population of neurons operating close to instability.

The first step in Zhadin's (1984, 1991) mathematical model is the derivation of an integro-differential equation to represent the summated postsynaptic potentials for a single neocortical pyramidal cell. An equation is then written for the EEG as a summation at the surface of the cortex of the ensemble of postsynaptic potentials of such pyramidal cells. Rhythmic activity is contingent upon recurrent inhibition. Zhadin (1984) found that an increase in afferent excitation (e.g., from the midbrain reticular formation) resulted in a shift in the EEG spectrum to higher frequencies, consistent with the "desynchronized" EEG. Conversely, a decrease in afferent excitation resulted in a shift of the EEG spectrum to lower (delta) frequencies, as in the EEG of slow-wave sleep. On the other hand, excessive afferent excitation would also result in a shift of the spectrum to lower frequencies, which, with a correlated increase in firing of cortical neurons, would result in epileptiform activity. Deafferentation of the cortex, leaving only intrinsic cortical excitatory processes, would shift the spectrum to lower frequencies.

In the mathematical model of the EEG proposed by Osovets et al. (1977, 1983), oscillators having various frequencies, formed by neurons in thalamic nuclei, act upon cortical elements that constitute a secondary oscillatory system having the properties of a passive, highly nonlinear oscillatory circuit, the free-running frequency of which (about 2 Hz) is much lower than the natural frequencies of the thalamic oscillators (pacemakers). The interaction between the nonspecific thalamus and cortex, as well as the effect of the reticular formation on the thalamus, was represented as a dynamic model involving a set of coupled nonlinear differential equations, the solutions of which would model the EEG in different states. As in the model of Wilson and Cowan (1972, 1973), excitatory and inhibitory influences were linearly combined. Certain epileptiform patterns were attributed to period-doubling phenomena. (See the section on chaos below.)

Frolov et al. (1984) simulated a nerve net of excitatory and inhibitory elements; the excitatory elements received recurrent and mutual excitation, and recurrent inhibition via an inhibitory element. No connections between inhibitory elements themselves were included. The authors found that the nature of the summated postsynaptic potentials depended more on the strength of the interconnections than on the excitability of the units or on the external input, which was applied only to the excitatory elements. Synchronization of activity resulted from increased inhibition, and also from an increase in reciprocal and mutual excitation. Contrariwise, a decrease of these two effects resulted in a desynchronized pattern of activity. If, in a synchronized pattern, recurrent inhibition was decreased further (by decreasing the effect of excitatory elements on inhibitory ones, or by increasing the threshold for activation of the inhibitory elements), a higher-voltage, lower-frequency "hypersynchronous" wave pattern suggestive of convulsive activity resulted. The "convulsive" pattern did not, however, include a spike component. Frolov et al. (1984) remarked that the presence of recurrent and reciprocal excitation in their model was the basis of such convulsive, hypersynchronous activity. In contrast, such activity was not seen in the model of Lopes da Silva et al. (1974).

The conditions for (e.g., synaptic strengths) and the characteristics of (e.g., period) oscillatory activity in a neural network incorporating recurrent inhibition were also explored by Tsutsumi and Matsumoto (1984).

In the model of EEG rhythms using a spatially uniform neuronal network consisting of interacting excitatory and inhibitory elements which was described by Frolov and Medvedev (1986), states approximating those of the desynchronized (low-voltage fast) and the synchronized (high-voltage slow) EEG were found, and transitions between the desynchronized and the synchronized states could be induced by decreasing the strengths of the connections between the excitatory elements in the network.

In the mathematical modeling of neocortical interactions by nonlinear nonequilibrium statistical mechanics described by Ingber (1982, 1984, 1985; see also Ingber and Nunez 1990), greater weight is given to inhibitory synapses because of their proximity to the soma (neuronal cell body).

Lagerlund and Sharbrough (1988, 1989) carried out an extensive series of computer simulations, employing a number of equations characterizing geometrical, anatomical, and physiological data. These authors found that local inhibitory feedback circuits were essential for the emergence of rhythmic EEG activity. The feedback circuits could be either thalamic (thus, "pacemaker") or cortical in location. Synchronization was the result of cortical association fibers. The frequencies of the cortical oscillations were primarily determined by local-circuit parameters, especially the durations and amplitudes of inhibitory postsynaptic potentials, rather than by global circuit parameters such as the range and velocities of long interconnecting axons. When Lagerlund and Sharbrough (1988, 1989) simulated the global EEG model of Nunez (1981), the expected sustained oscillations were not found (see below).

Traub et al. (1984) simulated intrinsic burst (epileptiform) discharges of hippocampal neurons by means of a computer model that incorporated both membrane properties (conductances) and network properties, using an assembly of elements randomly interconnected by excitatory synapses. The membrane properties included active regions ("hot spots") on the dendrites and on the soma (cell body).

Wiener (1958, 1961) advanced a model for the human alpha rhythm in the form of an ensemble of mutually entraining nonlinear oscillators, the nonlinearity being a prerequisite for entrainment (see also Dewan 1964 and Minorsky 1962). In these publications, Wiener (1958, 1961) indicated that the spectrum for such a mutually entrained ensemble of oscillator would have a peak with dips on either side, in comparison with a normal (gaussian) curve for the unentrained ensemble. Schetzen (1960, 1961) showed that the output of a large number of such mutually entrained oscillators, at least in the non-phase-locked case, tends toward a gaussian signal; i.e., the amplitude distribution function of the output is gaussian or normal. (Kreifeldt (1970) showed that a relatively simple mathematical model of a mutually entrained ensemble could account for the trimodal peak-dip spectral shape. (The determination of the stability of the alpha rhythm by Fourier methods is considered in chapter 19 below.)

The suggestion that EEG frequencies might be derived from microwave frequencies has arisen, on the one hand, from an approach to modeling of the current dipole moment of the extracellular field of the cortex (Tourenne 1985), and, on the other, as a reflection of the synchronization of microradiation from individual neurons,—a suggestion made by Norbert Wiener, according to Olson and Schadé (1965; see also Barlow 1985b).

Zeeman (1976) proposed the Duffing oscillator (which is similar to the van der Pol oscillator except that it can be driven by an external signal) as a basis for modeling the EEG as a collection of strongly coupled oscillators driving one another.

Kawahara (1980) showed that a system of coupled van der Pol equations can be derived from the Wilson-Cowan (1972, 1973) model, modified for a number of coupled excitatory and inhibitory neural subsets, so that the latter can be viewed as coupled van der Pol oscillators. Under certain conditions, interactions between excitatory and inhibitory subsets appear as linear, elastic (i.e., lossless) couplings, while those within and between excitatory and excitatory subsets appear as nonlinear frictional (i.e., with losses) couplings.

Rashevsky (1971) suggested that the alpha rhythm could be approximated by the undamped nonperiodic oscillations that represent solutions to a first-order linear system of ordinary differential equations of the Volterra type.

Petsche et al. (1984) have summarized several of these models, including those of Freeman (1975), Lopes da Silva et al. (1976), Nunez (1981), and Zetterberg et al. (1978) as models in which EEG activity is considered as resonance phenomena in large neuronal masses of interlocked excitatory and inhibitory populations that can be compared with spatio-temporal filters driven by inputs from midbrain structures.

A HYBRID OSCILLATOR: AN INFERIOR OLIVARY NEURON INTERCOUPLED WITH ELECTRONIC ANALOG OSCILLATORS

Yarom (1991) has recently described a hybrid generator of rhythmic patterns for which a single neuron from a slice preparation from the brain-stem inferior olivary nucleus was reciprocally connected with an analog simulator network made up of coupled oscillators. Neurons from this nucleus were selected for this purpose because of their known oscillatory properties as an ensemble (Llinás and Yarom 1986). The analog electronic units, of which there were four, each produced a damped sinusoidal oscillation in response to a trigger. But after mutual coupling, a trigger produced sustained oscillations so long as the mutual coupling remained intact. Incorporation of an inferior olivary neuron resulted in the same behavior, a low-threshold calcium spike in the neuron being the equivalent of a trigger to one of the analog electronic units, and activation of the low-threshold calcium conductance was considered to be essential for the generation of sustained oscillations. The results obtained were considered to substantiate the working hypothesis under test (i.e., that the subthreshold membrane potential fluctuations observed in inferior olivary neurons reflect both the unstable oscillations generated by each neuron and the electrotonic coupling between the neurons). The "preferred" frequency for the hybrid system, 5.2 Hz, was quite close to that observed in purely biological preparations.

Although this hybrid system highlights the role of electrotonic (nonsynaptic) connections in modeling the activity of neurons in the inferior olivary nucleus, Yarom (1991) foresaw an extension to synaptically coupled systems in which each unit would generate a synaptic current, the combination of which would be reintroduced into the biological part of the hybrid system.

THE ALPHA RHYTHM AS A STANDING-WAVE PATTERN

In a different mathematical approach, Nunez (1974) used an integral wave equation to describe the spatio-temporal variations of cortical potentials (which could include oscillations in the alpha frequency range). Assuming the cerebral cortex to be a closed planar surface, he then extended the development to include the possibility that rhythmic activity could reflect traveling waves on the cortical surface, coalescing to become standing waves somewhat analogous to those produced on a vibrating string of a stringed instrument (Nunez 1981, 1988). Katznelson (1981) extended the concept to include such standing waves on an (almost) closed spherical surface (to approximate the shape of the cortex). In this hypothesis, short-range (local-circuit) fibers and long-range (association) fibers play essential roles. The model, which included both excitatory and inhibitory effects, was based on the evident predominance of corticocortical (association) fibers in comparison with thalamocortical and callosal fibers, and on a propagation delay in the action potentials in association fibers. Resonant spatiotemporal patterns manifested as standing waves in the alpha frequency range were assumed to arise from random inputs to the cortex from subcortical (e.g., thalamic) structures. The decrease of EEG frequencies during general anesthesia was attributed to a decrease in propagation velocities in cortical association fibers, and epileptiform patterns were attributed to excessively long-range corticocortical connections.

In an experimental test of the hypothesis, Nunez et al. (1978) examined the relationship between head size and alpha frequency in 159 subjects. A significant correlation between the two was reported, larger heads being associated with lower alpha frequencies. (It should be noted, in connection with the Nunez hypothesis, that the frequency of the alpha rhythm in the smaller heads of monkeys approximates that in humans (Caveness 1962).)

Subsequently, Nunez (1989) combined the model of localized propagation of alpha waves described by van Rotterdam et al. (1982) with his own model of global (i.e., over the entire extent of the neocortex) standing waves (Nunez 1981). The localized propagation in the model of van Rotterdam and Lopes da Silva reflects properties of a neocortical column and includes such parameters as the rise and decay times of postsynaptic potentials, whereas Nunez's global-standing-wave model reflects primarily the velocity of propagation of action potentials along corticocortical fibers. More recently, Nunez and Ingber have joined forces to explore the latter's "statistical mechanics of neocortical interactions" (SMNI) as an approach to determining properties of neocortex over several widely disparate scales of resolution—e.g., to investigate relationships between activity in ensembles of cortical columns and EEG activity (i.e., "mesocolumnar vs. global macrocolumnar" properties) (Ingber and Nunez 1990).

LIMIT CYCLES, ATTRACTORS, NONLINEAR DYNAMICS (CHAOS), AND STRANGE ATTRACTORS

In recent years, a considerable literature has appeared on the topic of deterministic chaos. Earlier surveys can be found in Campbell and Rose 1983, Cvitanović 1984, Hao 1984, and Gleick 1987, and there have been number of publications in which this approach has been applied to the EEG.

As it has been applied to the EEG, nonlinear dynamics or chaos theory (the two terms are interchangeable) is not so much a method of modeling the EEG or specific EEG patterns as it is a method of characterizing the EEG (Mayer-Kress and Holzfuss 1987). Chaos, therefore, has pointed to analyses of phenomena that can be said to be rooted in modeling—more specifically, in oscillatory phenomena. The term *nonlinear* indicates simply that the argument (the EEG voltage in the case of the EEG) enters into the describing differential equation to the second power or some still higher power, rather than only to the first power (Minorsky 1962).

Perhaps the principal applicability of nonlinear dynamics to electroencephalography is to characterize a given EEG pattern by a single number (e.g., level of alertness, depth of sleep, depth of anesthesia). At one extreme would be a relatively stereotyped pattern, such as the 3-Hz spike-wave pattern; at the other end, an (apparently) completely random EEG pattern.

Deterministic chaos and aperiodic chaos have been used as synonyms, meaning nonperiodic or nonrepetitive behavior. Garfinkel (1983) has pointed out that, in contrast to stochastic or random (filtered) noise models, theories of nonlinear dynamics can offer a model for transitions between regular or periodic and irregular or aperiodic (i.e., deterministic) behavior within a single system. The oscillations of deterministic chaos, though irregular, are fully predictable (hence the term *deterministic*), but in their details they are extremely sensitive to the initial conditions. In this connection, the term *phase-plane portrait* refers to the set of phase-space (see below) trajectories for all possible initial conditions, for a given set of control parameter values (Roux et al. 1983). Actually, according to an der Heiden and Mackey (1987), deterministic and stochastic behavior, strictly speaking, are not necessarily mutually exclusive categories.

Several measures have been developed for characterizing the degree of chaos of a signal, including the dimensionality, the Lyapunov exponent, and the correlation dimension (see below). Low values of each of these are associated with stereotyped periodic EEG patterns, higher values being associated with activity that is more random in character. Some workers have attempted to evaluate the relative degrees of deterministic chaos as compared with truly random or stochastic chaos (e.g., random noise), but this is not an easy determination. For a recent tutorial review see Pritchard and Duke 1992.

Background of Chaos Theory: Simple Harmonic Oscillators, Nonlinear Oscillators, Phase Plane, and Phase Space

As Glass et al. (1986) pointed out, the difficulty of obtaining solutions for the sinusoidally forced or driven van der Pol (1926) differential equations lies at the basis of much of the current research in nonlinear dynamics.

The conventional display of an oscillatory phenomenon such as the EEG or any other signal is the voltage vs. time graph or y/t display. More convenient for discussing phenomena related to nonlinear dynamics is the y/x (or, more familiarly, x/y) display or plot, in which x is some variable that may or may not be related to y; in such a plot, the time variable has been eliminated explicitly (although it is still present implicitly). A familiar example is the oscilloscope display of the Lissajous pattern for two sine waves, $y(t)$ and $x(t)$. If the two sine waves are identical in amplitude and frequency and are in phase with one another, a 45° diagonal line results. If instead their phase differs by 90°, the resultant trajectory (as it is called) forms a circle.

If the second variable is the time derivative of the first, the resulting plot is said to be in the phase plane, or, in the case of more than two variables, in phase space. The phase-plane plot is particularly convenient for considering oscillators in nonlinear dynamics.

More generally, Poincaré had shown before the turn of the century that dynamical behavior could be characterized by analysis of trajectories in a multi-dimensional phase space in which a single point characterized the entire

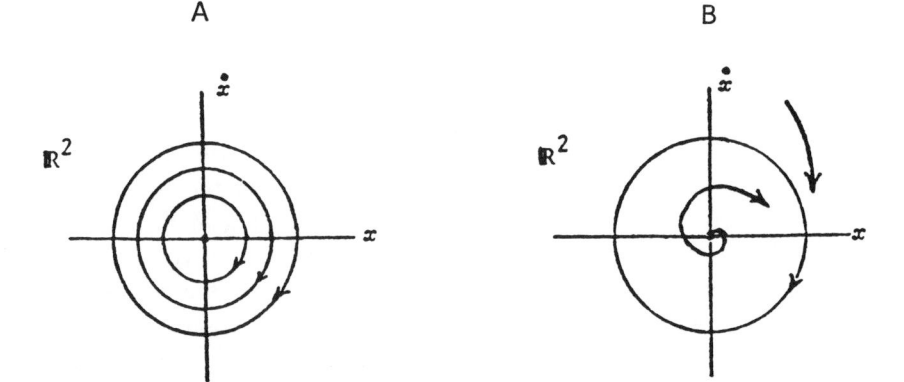

Figure 14.7 Phase-plane schema (R^2, a plot of x' (i.e., dx/dt) vs. x) for (A) simple harmonic motion (e.g., a frictionless pendulum) continuing to oscillate (in the absence of any perturbations), with one of three initial amplitudes, and (B) a van der Pol oscillator exhibiting a single limiting trajectory or limit cycle. The trajectories for the simple harmonic oscillator in A can be readily perturbed into new trajectories, however, and therefore they are considered to be unstable, whereas after a perturbation, the van der Pol oscillator returns eventually to the same trajectory or limit cycle. (From Zeeman 1976.)

system at a given instant in time. (A simpler alternative, obviating the need for multiple simultaneous determinations on a system, is that of a multidimensional phase portrait constructed from measurements of a single variable at successive fixed intervals of time (Swinney 1983).)

For a linear or simple harmonic oscillator, such as a simple pendulum, the phase-plane plot is a circle (more generally, an ellipse), since the derivative of the motion is 90° out of phase with the motion itself. Further, in the case of a pendulum the amplitude is, within limits, arbitrary. A pendulum, neglecting friction, will continue to oscillate at its initial amplitude (figure 14.7A). In fact, the phase-plane plot of any periodic phenomenon is a closed curve, or trajectory. On the other hand, a disturbance of the trajectory of a pendulum will result in a lasting change in the amplitude of oscillation; there is no return to the prior trajectory.

In contrast, the trajectory (and, correspondingly, the amplitude) of a van der Pol oscillator (a nonlinear oscillator, as previously mentioned) will tend to some limiting closed curve, irrespective of its initial trajectory and amplitude. The convergence of other trajectories to this "attracting" closed orbit, or attractor, is exemplified in figure 14.7B, The limiting trajectory, or orbit, is called a *limit cycle*, a term originated by Poincaré (see also Dewan 1964). The van der Pol oscillator can be viewed as having positive feedback if the amplitude is smaller than that of the limit cycle but negative feedback if the amplitude is larger than that of the limit cycle. The limit cycle is thus termed an *attractor* or, more precisely, a *simple attractor*. There are other possibilities than limit cycles; these include cases in which any arbitrary orbit will tend to zero, i.e., the oscillations die out sooner or later (this is the simplest attractor: a point at the origin in the phase plane).

Mathematically, the harmonic oscillator can be described by

$$\frac{d^2x}{dt^2} + x = 0$$

and the van der Pol oscillator by

$$\frac{d^2x}{dt^2} + \mu(x^2 - 1)\frac{dx}{dt} + x = 0,$$

where μ is a constant having a small value greater than zero (Zeeman 1976). The origin is a repeller (as opposed to an attractor), and hence the oscillation gradually builds up until an attractor region (having a radius of approximately 2) is reached, which is just the limit cycle or attracting closed orbit (figure 14.7B).

Such a phase-plane plot or profile of two variables against one another provides a ready means of determining, by inspection, whether there are one or more steady states (i.e., repetitive or stereotyped patterns) and whether some perturbation (stimulus) results in a shift between the steady states (Rinzel and Ermentrout 1989).

A second possibility, if there are three or more variables, is that of trajectories in three or more dimensions that become irregular or apparently random but remain within a bounded region of space, termed a *basin of attraction* (Babloyantz 1991). In such cases, the term *strange attractor* is used. A strange attractor can thus be characterized as a region in phase space to which nearby trajectories are attracted but, once attracted to the region, diverge from one another (Huberman and Zisook 1981). Thus, in the case of a strange attractor there are no such simple relationships, as there are for simple attractors.

Fractals

Although not directly relevant to EEG analysis, a final concept from nonlinear dynamics—that of fractals, or fractal dimensions—will be briefly considered, for completeness. Fractals can be viewed in the following way. In a phase-plane plot, a limit cycle can be considered as having a single dimension, as there is but one value of r, the radius of the circle (figure 14.7B). Adding more and more samples of the same phenomenon (signal) does not increase the number of dimensions required for the plot. There is only a single dimension: that of the angle in a polar or rotating plot. However, increasing the number of samples of a phase-plane plot of random noise will progressively increase the amount of space occupied in the plot, since in general there will be little or no duplication of points, at least for relatively short samples of the phenomenon.

The situation for a phase-plane plot of trajectories for strange attractors, on the other hand, is intermediate between that for a limit cycle and that for truly random (stochastic) noise. The plotted points or sample values occupy an area in the phase plane that is limited (i.e., the full two dimensions are not required); hence the term *fractal* (fractional) *dimension*.

Pavlidis (1965) pointed out that deterministic modeling of nerve nets could give rise to a multiplicity of trajectories, all lying in a certain limited region of phase space, as an intermediary between the extreme of a single trajectory (i.e., a limit cycle) and the extreme of trajectories in all regions (sectors) of phase space.

Quantitative Measures of Degree of Chaos

Several quantitative measures of the degree of complexity of chaos have been introduced. The Lyapunov exponent indicates the rate of divergence of two nearby trajectories of the strange or chaotic attractor; the higher the exponent, the more complex the trajectories, and the more likely are spontaneous transitions (Froehling et al. 1981; Mandell 1983; Babloyantz 1991).

The Kolmogorov entropy is a measure of the rate of loss of information about the state of a system in the course of time (Babloyantz 1991).

The Hausdorff dimension, D, has the value of 0 for a steady state (i.e., a point attractor) and the value 1.0 for a limit cycle. If D is a non-integer (i.e., is a fractal dimension), a chaotic attractor may be indicated (Grassberger 1983; Babloyantz and Destexhe 1986).

The correlation dimension, D_2 (Grassberger and Proccacia 1983), is easier to evaluate than the Hausdorff dimension, D, but has the same value as the latter for a steady state and for a limit cycle. It is a measure of the coherence of a signal with itself. Thus, for a point attractor or steady state, $D_2 = 0$; for a limit cycle, $D_2 = 1$. For a low-dimensional chaotic state, D_2 could have a value of 2.01 (Babloyantz 1991).

Başar et al. (1987) suggested that if the D_2 of a given EEG has a value from 4.0 to 6.0, then the EEG might be generated by a nonlinear dynamical system with 4 to 6 independent variables and differential equations. Başar et al. (1987) also suggested that if the neural population of the brain were regarded as a large number of independent oscillators that then became coupled, the correlation dimension would decrease.

Applications of Nonlinear Dynamics to the EEG

Several workers, including Başar et al. (1987), have pursued the question of the extent to which the EEG is truly random (stochastic, or noise-like), as opposed to a pseudo-random behavior of deterministic chaos, exhibiting some predictability. High values of the correlation dimension (e.g., 9.0) indicate the former, whereas lower values (e.g., 2.0–3.0) suggest the latter. (For white or truly random noise, D_2 is infinite.)

Babloyantz and Destexhe (1986, 1987) drew attention to a parallel between the value of the correlation dimension and the width of the power spectrum and the EEG amplitude, drawing on analyses of the normal waking and sleeping EEG (Babloyantz et al. 1985), spike-wave epileptiform patterns, and the EEG in Creutzfeldt-Jakob disease. Mayer-Kress and Holzfuss (1987) suggested that, while spectral methods can be particularly useful for studing regular periodic or quasi-periodic signals, these methods are less useful in cases in which the signal is very irregular, i.e., without sharp or well-defined frequency bands. On the other hand, such irregularity, in the form of deterministic (nonstochastic) chaos, is frequently encountered in nonlinear systems. Başar (1990) advocated the complementary use of spectra and the methods of nonlinear dynamics. There also appears to be some parallelism between the various indicators of the degree of chaos in an EEG and the extent to which its amplitude probability distribution function is Gaussian; a normal resting EEG tends to be strongly Gaussian whereas an EEG from an epileptic brain shows virtually no Gaussian tendency, according to Adey (1972).

It was mentioned above that the earlier work by Freeman (1975) on modeling the electrical activity of the olfactory cortex could be considered a linear systems approach, with the resting (basal) irregular activity considered as filtered noise. In more recent animal studies using methods of nonlinear dynamics, Freeman (1987, 1990) and Skarda and Freeman (1987) ascribed the above-mentioned irregular basal activity to a chaotic attractor, in contrast to the more regular patterns of rhythmic activity appearing during inhalation The latter pattern appeared superficially to be closer to a limit-cycle type of attractor. However, since the EEG patterns were different for different odors, they were attributed to different chaotic attractors, but of a lower order than for the irregular basal activity (Freeman 1987). The EEG patterns of the olfactory cortex were simulated as solutions of coupled nonlinear ordinary differential equations.

The change from the greater chaotic activity states and the quasi-limit cycle state (i.e., near-periodic activity) of a lesser chaotic state can be viewed as an example of a transition or bifurcation (also termed period doubling) that can occur in nonlinear dynamics (Freeman 1990); Ermentrout and Cowan 1980; Osovets et al. 1977, 1983).

Several authors have reported on the results of EEG analysis with nonlinear dynamics. Dvořák and Siska (1986) concluded from a study of different waking states that the EEG has a deterministic chaotic component but also has a significant random (stochastic) component. In the waking EEG states, Xu and Xu (1988) found relatively low correlation dimensions (D_2), which was suggestive of deterministic chaotic states; these authors also suggested that the correlation dimensions of the two hemispheres could differ during a mental task. Flytzanis et al. (1991) analyzed alpha activity recorded from eight electrodes on one side of the scalp by dimensional analysis (D_2); the results suggested a uniform attractor over the surface with small but consistent differences in the D_2 values. Friedrich et al. (1991), using synergetic analysis of the spatiotemporal behavior of the EEG, also found coherent spatial patterns, which undergo a complex temporal evolution in the case of alpha activity, and a more regular, time-periodic evolution in the case of seizure activity; a mathematical model was developed for the spatio-temporal behavior of alpha patterns.

A shift from low dimension values to appreciably higher ones has been reported to accompany eye opening, and higher values have been reported for Stage 4 sleep as compared with sleep onset and REM sleep (Mayer-Kress and Holzfuss 1987). These authors also suggested that dimension values of less than 3 may be associated with spectral rather than dimensional properties of the system.

A decrease in the level of chaos of the electrocorticogram near the seizure focus during temporal-lobe seizures, as evaluated by Lyapunov exponents, was reported by Iasemidis et al. (1990). Babloyantz and Destexhe (1986) reported a decrease in the correlation dimension (D_2) from 4.05 to 2.05 with the onset of 3-Hz spike waves in a patient. A correlation dimension of 3.8 was found for an EEG of a patient having Creutzfeldt-Jacob disease (Babloyantz 1991).

Using an improved test procedure for distinguishing between chaotic and random (stochastic) behavior with the aid of the correlation dimension (the procedure being to make the original EEG artificially more "random" by randomizing the phases of the Fourier transform and then resynthesizing the original EEG, so that the power spectrum remained unaltered), Pijn and Lopes da Silva (1991) and Pijn et al. (1991) found that, for recordings from rat limbic cortex, chaotic behavior of the EEG could not be distinguished from stochastic behavior during wakeful rest and locomotion. However, during an epileptic seizure, chaotic behavior was found, having correlation dimension values between 2 and 4.

Arle and Simon (1990) suggested using a running evaluation of the (fractal) dimension as a method of detecting transients in the EEG. Babloyantz (1991) has suggested that very slow periodic variations (e.g., of the order of 60 sec) may be detected by means of a technique termed the recurrence plot.

Appraisals of and Cautions about EEG Applications of Nonlinear Dynamics

After an initial period of some enthusiasm for applying the methods of nonlinear dynamics to the EEG, a period of caution and reevaluation has followed, with emphasis on closer attention to methodologies, selection of problems, selection of data, and choice of parameters (Babloyantz 1987; Xu and Xu 1988; Dvořák and Siska 1986). It has been pointed out that parameters in the estimation of correlation dimensions must be carefully selected (Babloyantz 1989). For example, despite the attractiveness, in principle, of dimensional analysis of the EEG in providing a single number instead of a function or a series of curves (e.g., spectra) for assessing depth of anesthesia, the procedure has been found not to be straightforward in practice, not only because of the difficulties with the methodology itself but also because of artifacts in the EEG (Mayer-Kress and Layne 1987).

Bullock (1988a,b; 1990), in particular, has raised a series of cogent questions concerning the methodologies and the implications of nonlinear dynamics (see also Mayer-Kress and Layne 1987 and Başar 1990). It has been pointed out, for example, that quasi-periodic signals contaminated by noise can resemble deterministic noise (i.e., exhibiting a chaotic or strange attractor); the number of dimensions can be the same for both (Rössler and Hudson 1989).

Perkel (1987) raised the question of whether, at least in some instances, some neurobiological applications of nonlinear dynamics may represent "a method in search of a problem," and Thom (1987) questioned the enduring viability of nonlinear dynamics as an approach.

Nonetheless, useful insights can emerge from chaos (nonlinear dynamics). Thus, Lopes da Silva (1991) recently advanced a proposal concerning EEG shifts between random patterns and oscillatory ones, from the several perspectives of chaos, intrinsic neuronal properties, and neuronal network properties. His proposal was that an oscillatory state in a neuronal network determines the mean level of membrane potential for an extensive neuronal population, resulting in a large and rapid change in the output characteristics of the network. He further suggested that the cholinergic system of the forebrain (see chapter 12) may be responsible for such a change.

There are two normal-variant spontaneous EEG patterns that may represent manifestations of a characteristic phenomenon in nonlinear dynamics and nonlinear oscillators known as *period-doubling* or *subharmonic bifurcations* (Ermentrout and Cowan 1980; Testa et al. 1982). Instead of successive waves being identical, so that successive cycles form the same repetitive closed trajectory, there is an alternation of the form of successive cycles, so that there are two cycles in phase space before the trajectory is repeated. This effect gives rise to a frequency component in the spectrum at half the mean frequency of the two cycles, or double the period (hence the term *period-doubling*). The EEG patterns are the slow and the fast alpha variant patterns, which typically consists of waves of approximately half and approximately twice the frequency of the ongoing alpha frequency, respectively (Kellaway 1990). In the first instance, the doubled period would correspond to half the alpha frequency; in the second, the doubled period would correspond to the alpha frequency itself, if indeed these EEG patterns correspond to the period-splitting phenomenon of nonlinear dynamics.

15 Comparisons with Some Other Models of the EEG

RELAXATION-OSCILLATOR MODELS

In view of its uniqueness in featuring a single oscillator having a dual modulation of extrema and of slopes, the present oscillator model and its associated extrema-slopes hypothesis cannot readily be compared with other models of the EEG. The dual-modulation oscillator model is of the nonlinear type, and can be considered as a generalized type of relaxation oscillator (Barlow 1962c). As was mentioned in chapter 14, the relaxation oscillator was a favorite early model for the EEG (Hoagland 1936a,c; Jasper 1936a,b), and, as was mentioned in chapter 13, the relaxation model suggested by Jasper (1936b) has the same type of waveforms as the triangular waves of Mode 1 (modulation of extrema only) of the present oscillator model. Thus, Jasper's relaxation model of the EEG also exhibits the constant-slope characteristic of Mode 1 of the present oscillator model. Jasper's model does not, however, include the other three modes of the present oscillator model.

FILTERED-NOISE MODELS

A favorite model for the EEG has been the linear one of filtered noise, with a narrow-band filter to simulate alpha and other types of rhythmic activity and a wider-band filter to simulate irregular EEG patterns of the waking state. Apart from the fact that the output of a 10-Hz narrow-band filter for a noise input is much smoother than the usual alpha rhythm from most human subjects, the response time of such a filter increases as the width (passband) of the filter decreases, so that a sudden increase in amplitude for the duration of a single wave becomes impossible. On the other hand, it has long been known that in some cases alpha waves can be essentially sinusoidal, as indicated by the absence of higher harmonics upon Fourier analysis (Rohracher 1937, 1938), and yet undergo abrupt change. Further, alpha activity of relatively constant amplitude can reappear with a delay of only a few tenths of a second after eye closure. Nor can asymmetrical patterns, such as the mu rhythm or a spike-wave complex, be simulated by filtering noise. Indeed, it can be argued that the presence of harmonically related components in the EEG, such as a slow or a fast alpha variant in the bispectrum (Lopes da Silva 1981; Dumermuth and Molinari 1987), necessarily indicates a nonlinear mechanism for the generation of such activity. There would, therefore, appear to be serious limitations to the conventional filtered-noise model of the EEG, or at least of the alpha rhythm, despite the long history of this model.

The dual-modulation oscillator model of the EEG does have in common with the filtered-noise model that low-frequency noise signals (a pair of them) are used in some instances to modulate the extremes and/or slopes of intrinsic oscillations as modulating signals for an intrinsic oscillator. But the use of the noise signals as modulations already implies a nonlinear model (cf. Étévenon et al. 1980), as does also the combination of the two independent modulations. It is this nonlinear feature of the extrema-slopes model, in combination with the modulation of extrema, that makes possible the simulation of a wide variety of types of EEG activity, including ones with asymmetrical waveforms such as the mu rhythm and epileptiform activity.

AMPLITUDE-FREQUENCY RELATIONSHIPS

Often a linear plot of EEG power vs. frequency will suggest an exponential decrease with increasing frequency (figure 15.1, top), with a corresponding linear decrease on a logarithmic plot of the power (figure 15.1, bottom). In their discussion of the constituent parts of power spectra of EEGs, Dumermuth and Molinari (1987), following Balestra et al. (1981; see also Matthis et al. 1981), listed three components: the white-noise part (of artifactual, e.g. muscle, origin, or arising from epileptiform spikes); the "pink"-noise component, which very often decreases exponentially with increasing frequency (or, on a plot of log power vs. frequency, decreases linearly as frequency increases); and the "colored"-noise component, i.e., the peaks corresponding to rhythmic activity (figure 15.2). Dumermuth and Molinari (1987; see also Dumermuth 1977) considered the "pink"-noise component to correspond to the "unstructured EEG component which is a natural feature of empirical data and often called amorphous or arhythmic activity." Balestra et al. (1981) considered this component to be intrinsic to the signal, and to be constant for individual subjects. Figure 15.3 illustrates a series of spectra showing such an exponential decrease in power with increasing frequency.

Using spectral parameter analysis as a basis for simulating EEG patterns, Zetterberg and his colleagues (Wennberg and Zetterberg 1971; Zetterberg 1973; Zetterberg and Ahlin 1975) used a first-order RC low-pass filter to simulate delta activity. For frequencies above the cutoff frequency of the filter, the power spectral curve for such a device also decreases exponentially with increasing frequency (or, on a plot of log power vs. frequency, the decrease is linear).

The exponential decrease of power depicted by the dashed line in figure 15.1A can be expressed by the relation

$$P = a^2 = A(e^{-Bf}), \tag{1}$$

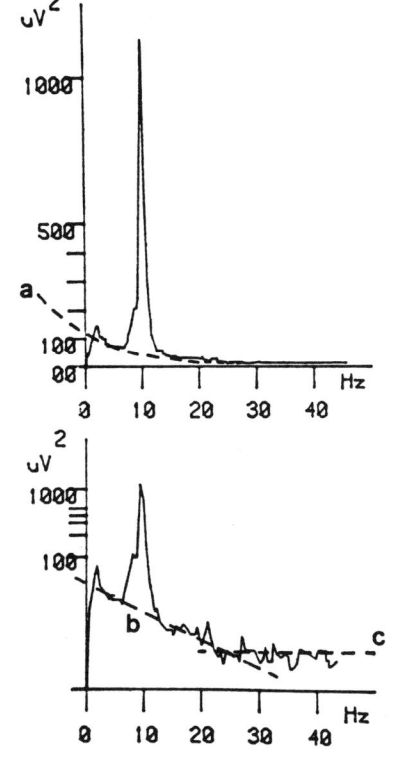

Figure 15.1 Power spectrum of a normal EEG plotted on a linear (top) and logarithmic (bottom) scale. The exponential function identified in the spectral profile is indicated by the dashed curve (a), and after logarithmic transformation as b. The uniform distribution of fast frequency components is indicated by c. (From Balestra et al. 1981.)

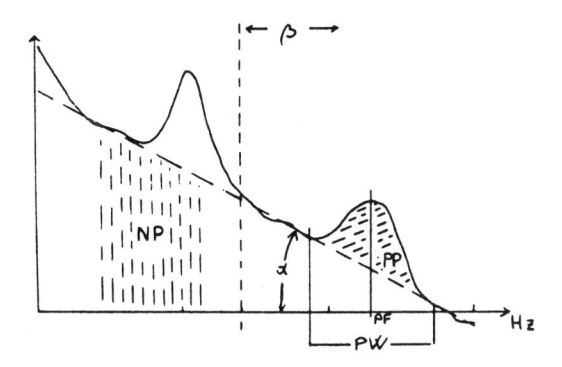

Figure 15.2 Schematic depiction of the "pink" noise component of an EEG, which, on a semilogarithmic plot, is a straight line with slope indicated by the angle, alpha. (The following peaks corresponding to rhythmic alpha and beta activity are also shown: NP: noise power. PP: peak power. PF: peak frequency. PW: peak width.) Dashed vertical line: junction of alpha and beta bands on the frequency scale. (From Dumermuth et al. 1983.)

215   Comparisons with Other Models of the EEG

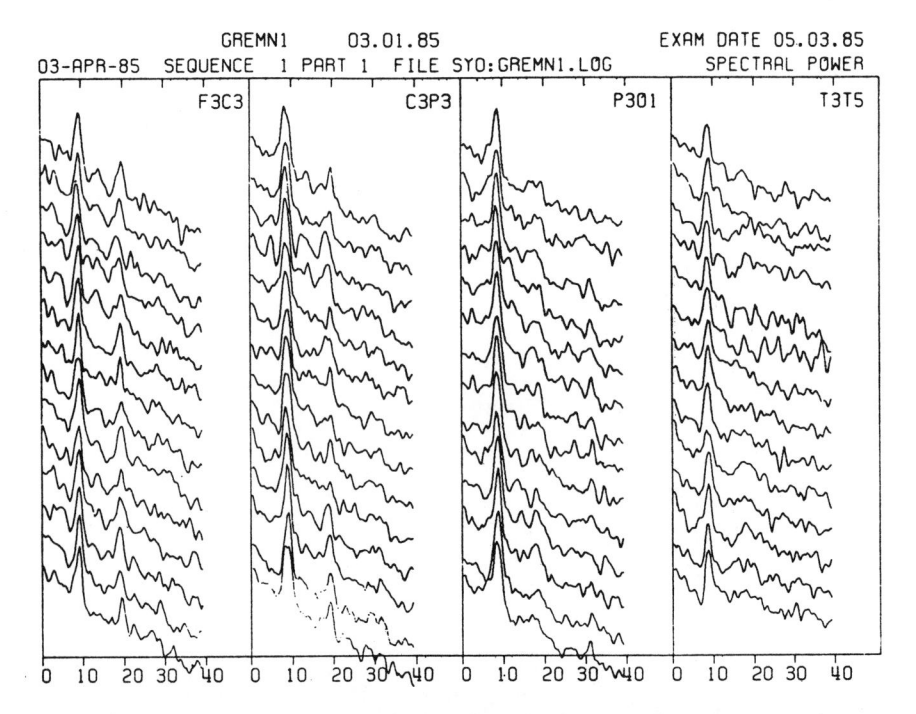

Figure 15.3 Log power vs. frequency for four channels of one EEG recording. Note the progressive downward trend with increasing frequency, with superimposed peaks at the alpha frequency and at twice the alpha frequency, in some channels. (From Dumermuth and Molinari 1987.)

in which a^2 is the power, or square of the amplitude, A and B are constants, and f is frequency. Taking the logarithm of both sides results in the expression for the dashed inclined line of figure 15.1B:

$$\log P = 2\log a = \log(A) - (B \cdot f), \tag{2}$$

or

$$\log a = [(A') - (B \cdot f)]/2. \tag{3}$$

Replacing $A'/2$ by A'' and $B/2$ by B' yields

$$\log a = A'' - B'(f), \tag{4}$$

in which the constant, $\log(A)$, has been replaced by another constant, A'. (On a logarithmic scale, amplitude (a) and power (P) differ only by a factor of 2. Thus, to change from a scale of power to a scale for amplitude one merely shifts the ordinate downward; i.e., A' is replaced by $A'' = A'/2$.)

For Type 1 (constant-slope) waves (chapter 2) of the extrema-slopes hypothesis, on the other hand, the amplitude of an individual wave is directly proportional to its duration or period (a characteristic that results in the constant-slope feature); equivalently expressed, amplitude and frequency are inversely or reciprocally related (chapter 2). This relationship can be expressed as

$$a = \frac{C}{f}, \tag{5}$$

which is the equation of a hyperbola (C is a constant).
Taking the logarithm of both sides yields

$$\log a = \log C - \log f, \tag{6}$$

and replacing $\log C$ by C' gives

$$\log a = C' - \log f. \tag{7}$$

From a comparison of equations 4 and 7, it is evident that the former expresses a linear relationship (with slope determined by the constant, B) between log amplitude and frequency, whereas the latter expresses a linear relationship (with slope −1) between log amplitude and log frequency.

It was pointed out in chapter 7 that EEG data on pathological slowing were better fitted by the latter (hyperbolic) relationship than by the former (exponential) one (figures 7.5, 7.7, 7.8). The "constant-slope" (Type 1 waves, chapter 2) finding for the physiological slowing during Stages 3 and 4 of non-REM sleep (figures 6.5–6.7) is also in accord with the latter relationship. The model of EEG patterns implied by Type 1 (constant-slope) waves of the present extrema-slopes model is therefore distinct from models of the EEG that characterize it (except for rhythmic activity) as having an exponentially decreasing power spectrum with increasing frequency.

The reciprocal relationship between amplitude and frequency of individual waves that characterized Type 1 (constant-slope) waves of the extrema-slopes model is also to be distinguished from certain types of noise for which power (not amplitude) varies inversely with frequency (e.g., the noise from DC amplifiers, from elevator motors, etc.). The reciprocal relationship between power (or, the squared amplitude, a^2) and frequency that characterizes the spectrum of such noise can be expressed as follows. (In equation 11, the constant K' replaces $(\log K)/2$.)

$$a^2 = K/f, \tag{8}$$

$$2 \log a = \log(K/f) \tag{9}$$

$$= \log K - \log f,$$

$$\log a = (\log K)/2 - (\log f)/2, \tag{10}$$

$$\log a = K' - (\log f)/2. \tag{11}$$

Equation 11 results in a straight line (of slope −1/2) in a plot of log amplitude vs. log frequency, the slope of the resulting curve being half as great (note the factor of 2 in the denominator on the right side of equation 10) as that in equation 7. To reiterate: For the extrema-slopes model, in the case of constant-slope waves (Type 1 waves, chapter 2), *amplitude* and frequency vary inversely—not *power* and frequency, as is the usual connotation of "$1/f$ noise."

The plots of log power vs. frequency and of log power vs. log frequency that appear in chapter 7 (figures 7.5, 7.7, and 7.8) are not spectral plots (i.e., a plot of total power at a given frequency vs. the frequency, as in figure 15.3) but rather scatter plots of log power vs the frequency (or log frequency) for waves of a given combination of power and frequency. Figures 7.7 and 7.8 thus depict the conjoint relationship between log power and log frequency in effect for each wave considered individually, rather than the relationship between power and frequency in which all waves of the same frequency are lumped together as in a conventional spectral plot. Alternatively expressed: Power spectral plots include information about the "percent time" (the portion of time that waves of a given frequency are present) and also about the summated power (i.e., the square of the amplitude) of the individual waves. The trend of a scatter plot of amplitude vs. frequency, in contrast, indicates only that one or more waves of a given power and frequency have occurred, but does not explictly indicate their number or the total power associated with them. (The latter information is, however, implied by the contour plots of the associated probability-density plots; see figure 7.6.)

It is this difference in the kind of information depicted in spectral plots (e.g., figure 15.3) as compared with that depicted in the scatter plots (e.g., Fig. 7.5) that accounts for the apparent discrepancy between the reports of a $1/f$ amplitude characteristic, which were based on observations of (FFT-derived) spectra, and the $1/f$ amplitude characteristic of the "constant-slope" mode of the present oscillator model.

MODULATION MODELS

As was noted in the preceding chapter, several models of the EEG have been based on a combination of amplitude modulation and phase modulation (or its equivalent, frequency modulation). The present model is referred to as employing extrema-slopes modulation, to distinguish it from conventional combined amplitude-slopes (or amplitude-frequency) modulation. A particular feature of extrema-slopes modulation that is not possible with conventional amplitude-frequency modulation is that of "constant-slope" waves, for which amplitude and frequency are inversely related; this feature cannot be obtained (at least, not without special compensating mechanisms) with conventional combined amplitude-frequency modulation, as was noted in chapter 2 (see figure 2.4).

In chapter 5, it was pointed out that, from simulation studies of EEG patterns, a relationship emerged between the spectrum for Type 3 waves of the oscillator model (corresponding to congruent modulation of extrema and slopes so as to simulate alpha activity) and the spectrum for Type 4 waves (i.e., in response to independent random modulation of extrema and slopes, so as to simulate the "desynchronized" EEG). Thus, the spectrum for Type 4 waves is essentially flat up to the frequency that corresponds to the peak of the spectrum for the Type 3 waves, but the power diminishes rapidly for higher frequencies. (As was also mentioned, corroborative evidence for this feature emerged from examination of EEG spectra.) Such a decrease in the spectrum above the "alpha" frequency is a specific characteristic of Type 3 and

4 waves according to the extrema-slopes hypothesis, and it cannot be obtained with conventional combined amplitude-frequency modulation. The reason for this particular spectral characteristic of Type 4 waves lies in that modulation of extremes of waves alters simultaneously their amplitudes and their durations and thus their frequencies (figure 5.11), whereas for conventional combined amplitude-frequency modulation the amplitudes and the frequencies of the resultant waves are completely independent.

NONLINEAR DYNAMICS (CHAOS)

As was indicated in the preceding chapter, it is not so much that nonlinear dynamics provides a model for the EEG as that if offers an approach or a method for characterizing EEG patterns. In this connection, it could be of interest to attempt to characterize, by the methods of nonlinear dynamics, EEGs that have been reconstituted according to the extrema-slopes hypothesis, using the oscillator model, and to compare the results with the characterizations of the respective original EEGs. It seems probable that the results of such a characterization, e.g., the correlation dimension, would be the same for the original and the reconstituted EEGs. No such attempt has been made, however.

CONCLUSIONS

Filtered-noise models have the limitation of being linear. Combined conventional amplitude and frequency modulation is unable to reproduce waves of relatively constant slope and certain nonlinear features of EEGs (e.g., asymmetrical rhythms such as the mu rhythm). Nonlinear dynamics provides more an approach to analysis than a model for a wide range of EEG activity.

In contrast, the oscillator model and the associated extrema-slopes hypothesis appear to have the capability of simulating a wide range of EEG patterns. The hypothesis leads to a series of predictions concerning specific features of EEG patterns, the testing of which appears to offer corroborative evidence for the hypothesis and, within certain limits (i.e., an ambiguity of phase), to provide the basis of an approach by which EEG patterns can be reconstituted on the basis of their extrema and slope features to yield a rather faithful replica of the original.

16 The Significance of the Extrema-Slopes Hypothesis: A Formulation

As a preliminary to consideration of the possible physiological and pathophysiological significance of the extrema-slopes hypothesis, a summary formulation of possible mechanisms of EEG generation will be advanced on the basis of the reviews in chapters 11–13 of the anatomy, physiology, and pathophysiology of the EEG. It is assumed that the EEG represents, at least primarily, the fluctuating postsynaptic potentials of cortical pyramidal neurons; possible roles of neuromodulators (as contrasted to neurotransmitters) and electrical transmission are not explicitly considered, nor is a possible role of neurons having quasi-bistable states (Marder 1991).

BACKGROUND POINTS

(1) From the review of neocortical anatomy and physiology in chapters 11 and 12, it appears that the input to a local area of the cortex (e.g., a cortical column approximately 0.3 mm in diameter)—i.e., from other cortical areas (including contralateral ones) and from subcortical sites (including the thalamus), and the cholinergic influence from the basal forebrain—is predominantly or exclusively excitatory, with the possible exception of some putative transmitters originating in the brain stem (e.g., noradrenaline, serotonin, and dopamine). The corresponding terminal fibers for the latter are relatively diffusely distributed in the cortex.

(2) From (1), it follows that inhibitory mechanisms are predominantly or perhaps exclusively intracortical, i.e., there is no inhibitory input to a given small cortical area.

(3) If the input to the cortex (as well as its output) is predominantly or entirely excitatory, and if inhibitory mechanisms are entirely intracortical (i.e., generated within a cortical column or module), then it follows that the effective action of intracortical inhibitory mechanisms is essential in preventing epileptiform activity, i.e., hyperactivity of neocortical pyramidal cells.

(4) From the review of the pathophysiology of the EEG in chapter 13, it appears that lesions of the subcortical white matter, both in humans and in experimental animals, typically result in random (irregular or polymorphic) delta slowing, and only rarely, if ever, in epileptiform manifestations.

(5) As a counterpart of (4), focal lesions limited to the cerebral cortex typically do not result in random delta slowing of the EEG, but rather in focal epileptiform manifestations, because of impairment of intracortical inhibitory mechanisms (e.g., in Creutzfeldt-Jakob disease). (Excessive activity of excitatory mechanisms, rather than impairment of inhibitory mechanisms, may underlie the generalized 3-Hz spike-wave pattern—see below.)

(6) As an exception to (5), epileptiform EEG manifestations typically do not appear if cortical pyramidal cells are primarily affected, as in Alzheimer's disease.

From the above statements, the following corollary emerges:

(7) The general level and the variability of intracortical inhibitory activity are determined, at least in part, by the general level of excitatory cortical input (as delineated in (1) above) and by its variability, and by the general level of cortical pyramidal-cell (excitatory) activity (in view of the intracortical recurrent collaterals of the latter).

From the review chapters on the physiology and pathophysiology of the EEG (chapters 12 and 13), it also appears that:

(8) Basic mechanisms for generation of EEG activity are an intrinsic feature of the cortex, independent of subcortical structures (in particular, the thalamus), since white-matter lesions characteristically result in random delta slowing but not in cessation of the EEG.

From the preceding statements, the following postulates are suggested in relation to the extrema-slopes hypothesis:

(9) With the exception of focal epileptiform activity, the instantaneous envelope of the EEG is inversely related to the amount of excitatory input to the area of the cortex reflected at the overlying recording electrode. In the case of focal epileptiform activity, the intracortical excitatory drive (primarily from pyramidal neurons) becomes predominant in determining the envelope of the EEG.

(10) The envelope of the first (time) derivative of the EEG is inversely proportional to the overall level of intracortically generated inhibitory activity in the region of the cortex reflected at the overlying recording electrode.

Figure 16.1, which is based in part on figure 10.1B, depicts the two relationships discussed in (9) and (10). The actual neurophysiological mechanisms resulting in the two inverse relationships in (9) and (10) are left unspecified. One possibility, in the case of excitatory activity, is simply that a greater level of activity of excitatory postsynaptic potentials and/or a greater dispersion of their occurrence would result in the appearance of a decreased level of the envelope of the EEG itself. The inverse relationship between the envelope of the first derivative of the EEG and inhibitory activity would appear to be less problematic, since decreased cortical inhibitory activity is well known to result in EEG activity of increased slope, at least for the spike component of epileptiform activity.

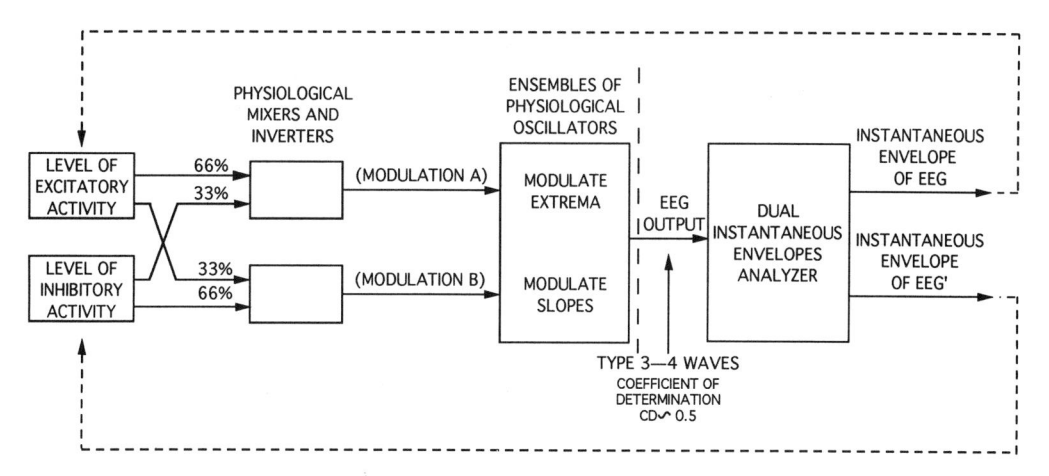

Figure 16.1 Schema, based in part on figure 10.1, of inferences (short-dashed lines) of an inverse relationship between level of excitation and instantaneous envelope of an EEG, and of a inverse relationship between the level of inhibition and the instantaneous envelope of the first derivative of the EEG, the inferences being based on observed characteristics of the instantaneous envelopes for different types of EEGs. The vertical long-dashed line indicates the interface between actually observed phenomena (to the right), and inferred brain mechanisms (to the left). The degrees of mixing at the left correspond to the observed Coefficient of Determination of about 0.5 between the two instantaneous envelopes for the "desynchronized" EEG, corresponding to Type 4 (Type 3–4) waves. (In an alternate schema, the "physiological mixers" and the "inverters" would be depicted separately from one another, allowing flexibility in the polarity of mixing of the components.)

(11) The frequency of the normal posterior resting eyes-closed background rhythm, i.e., the alpha rhythm (when present), reflects the frequency of primarily neocortical oscillators, functioning in concert with other areas of the cortex and with subcortical structures, including the thalamus. The mechanisms of this basic intrinsic intracortical oscillatory mechanism are also left unspecified, other than to indicate that combinations of intrinsic excitatory and inhibitory mechanisms in a feedback arrangement appear more than adequate for the purpose.

The phenomenon of the shift to constant-frequency waves (e.g., alpha activity) from constant-slope, constant-amplitude, or irregular waves, for which the two input modulations according to the extrema-slopes hypothesis become essentially identical, implies either a complete switch to one or the other of the two modulations or a complete mixing of two independent modulations. (The fact that, for a given EEG, the Coefficient of Determination for the instantaneous envelopes of the EEG and of its first derivative was never as large as 1.0 already suggests some degree of mixing for apparently irregular waves (figure 10.1B).)

In considering the question of how EEG-generating mechanisms of the brain might be constituted, if the principles are the same as those of the oscillator model (although obviously not the implementation), it should first be kept in mind that the oscillator model is a model of the EEG in the first instance as a signal recorded from the surface of the scalp. The latter signal, as indicated in chapter 12, can be quite different from the signal (or, more exactly, the constituent signals) as they appear in recordings from the surface of the cortex itself. Nonetheless, it may be useful to examine the characteristics of the oscillator model for possible clues to specifications for the actual physiological mechanisms.

CHARACTERISTICS OF THE OSCILLATOR MODEL IN RELATION TO PHYSIOLOGICAL MECHANISMS OF THE EEG

The primary features of the oscillator model are that it is an intrinsically oscillatory system and that it can be modulated in two different ways, independently: by extrema and by slopes. The dual modulations implicitly require a nonlinear oscillator system, since the existence of two independent modulations mandates a multiplicative (as opposed to a linear or additive) system.

Statements (9) and (10) can be formalized as follows:

$$\text{I.E.(EEG)} \propto \frac{1}{\text{Excitation}}, \tag{1}$$

$$\text{I.E.(EEG')} \propto \frac{1}{\text{Inhibition}}. \tag{2}$$

Here I.E.(EEG) and I.E.(EEG') are the instantaneous envelopes (see chapters 9 and 10) of the EEG and of its first time derivative, respectively.

From expressions 1 and 2, the quotient of excitation to inhibition is

$$\frac{\text{Excitation}}{\text{Inhibition}} \propto \frac{\text{I.E.(EEG')}}{\text{I.E.(EEG)}}. \tag{3}$$

But the right side of (3) is just the instantaneous frequency, f_i (chapter 29), and with a constant of proportionality (K) inserted we have

$$\frac{\text{Excitation}}{\text{Inhibition}} = K \frac{\text{I.E.(EEG')}}{\text{I.E.(EEG)}} = K(f_i).$$

Thus, the instantaneous EEG frequency, f_i, is seen to give an indication of the relative proportions of excitation and inhibition in that portion of the cerebral cortex sampled by the recording electrode(s).

The instantaneous frequency is independent of EEG voltage, in the same way as the running mean frequency (as the quotient of the running mean slope to the running mean amplitude) is independent of EEG voltage (chapters 3 and 24). The units of Envelope (EEG') are microvolts per second, and the units of Envelope (EEG) are microvolts; the units of their quotient are $\sec^{-1}$, or Hz.

POSSIBLE PHYSIOLOGICAL COUNTERPARTS OF THE OSCILLATOR MODEL

In the present formulation, the detailed nature of the basic neocortical oscillator mechanisms is necessarily left unspecified; it is assumed that the neocortex has inherent oscillatory capabilities, presumably representing the activity of very large ensembles of cortical columns and their interactions, via multiple feedback loops. (An elementary model for the latter is offered in appendix B in the form of an adaptive signal processor which was originally built for a quite different purpose but which has some remarkable properties.) As appears to be the case in the thalamus (chapter 12), intracellular (intrinsic) oscillatory mechanisms may also have a role in the cerebral cortex. Indeed, intrinsic oscillations of the relaxation type, capable of being modulated by chemical and electrical coupling, are possible for ensembles (in crustacea) consisting of very few neurons (Marder and Meyrand 1989; Kepler et al. 1990; Abbott et al. 1991; Marder 1991). What the extrema-slopes hypothesis does specify is that the basic oscillator be of such a nature that its waves can be modulated essentially independently in their extrema and in their slopes.

The possibility of specifying the details of the generating mechanisms for the respective modulating signals for extrema and slopes that are envisaged in the extrema-slopes hypothesis appears to be even more remote, in view of the enormous complexities of the cortex. Indeed, these "signals" may appear only intrinsically (as "hidden variables"), in some diffusely distributed manner, rather than explicitly. The generating mechanisms of the modulating signals thus must be left more poorly defined than the possible physiological basis of the oscillator mechanisms themselves, as sketched above. It may be that oscillator mechanisms and modulating mechanisms are so inextricably intertwined in the cortex as not to be separable. By the same token, it is difficult at best to relate oscillator and modulator mechanisms of the extrema-slopes hypothesis to volume-conductor approaches to large ensembles of generators (Zhadin 1984, 1991).

INSTANTANEOUS FREQUENCY OF THE EEG IN RELATION TO RELATIVE PREPONDERANCE OF EXCITATION AND INHIBITION

Expression 4 has several interesting implications:

(1) For rhythmic activity, such as alpha activity, the instantaneous frequency (which in the present formulation provides a measure of the relative amounts of excitation and inhibition) is essentially constant, irrespective of the instantaneous envelope of the EEG (i.e., EEG voltage).

(2) For instantaneous frequencies above the alpha frequency, excitation predominates over inhibition.

(3) For instantaneous frequencies below the alpha frequency, inhibition predominates over excitation.

(4) In the case of the 3-Hz spike-wave pattern, the ratio of excitation to inhibition varies over a wide range within a single full cycle of the pattern. During the spike component, excitation predominates; during the wave, inhibition predominates. This formulation conforms to the usual view. Detailed analysis of the spike-wave pattern (chapter 8) suggests that, at least for scalp recordings, this transition is continuous rather than abrupt.

(5) For the interictal spike-and-slow-wave complex of focal epilepsy, the same sequence as in (4) occurs, except that the pattern generally does not repeat and the wave component becomes attenuated in amplitude, in contrast to the wave component of the repetitive 3-Hz spike-wave pattern (at least, until the latter pattern, after decreasing somewhat in frequency, becomes no longer self-sustaining).

The preceding implications and the earlier statements will now be considered in relation to selected types or patterns of EEG activity, and also in relation to the types of waves from the oscillator model.

To recapitulate: The four basic EEG patterns that are inferred from the four types of waves of the oscillator model can be characterized as follows:

(1) In random delta slowing, in which the amplitude of waves is approximately proportional to their duration (i.e., waves of relatively constant slope, or Type 1 waves of the oscillator model), the excitatory activity is diminished as a result of subcortical lesions, but there is relatively little change in inhibitory activity, which is of intracortical origin.

(2) In the 3-Hz spike-wave pattern of epilepsy, in which there is appreciable change of the instantaneous envelope of the slope of the waves (i.e., the instantaneous envelope of the first derivative of the EEG) but less change of the instantaneous envelope of the EEG itself, there is a marked increase in the relative amounts of excitation and inhibition at the beginning of the spike component, which is followed by a progressive decrease in this ratio (and, correspondingly, in the instantaneous frequency) as the spike component gives way to the slow-wave component. This variation, which is thus primarily of the instantaneous envelope of the slope of the EEG, corresponds to waves of relatively constant amplitude—i.e., Type 2 waves of the oscillator model.

(3) For rhythmic activity (Type 3 waves of the oscillator model), excitation and inhibition vary similarly or congruently in the course of a spindle; thus, their ratio remains essentially constant, being determined by the type of activity (e.g, alpha activity or sleep spindles). In the case of alpha activity, the extrema-slopes hypothesis can be considered as consistent with the view of alpha activity as reflecting an idling state (cf. Barlow 1985a), in which the instantaneous envelope of the EEG and that of its first derivative are very similar in form, the Coefficient of Determination for the two approaching 1.0. Correspondingly, the resulting modulated signal reflects a relatively low information content, since the (instantaneous) frequency is relatively constant, and information is largely carried in the relatively slowly varying (instantaneous) envelopes.

(4) For the low-voltage activity of the "desynchronized" EEG, both excitation and inhibition are at a relatively high level, varying independently of one another to a considerable degree but not entirely (at least, as reflected in the scalp EEG). These waves correspond to waves intermediate between Type 3 and Type 4 of the oscillator model (chapter 10).

In addition to the conditions just described for a small area of cortex, it is evident that, within limits, the larger the area of the cortex that is synchronously active, the larger will be the EEG voltage at the scalp. For example, voltages in the generalized 3-Hz spike-wave pattern can be as high as several hundred microvolts.

The original description of the effect of stimulation of the brain-stem reticular formation on the EEG—namely, the change from the "synchronized" pattern of relatively high-voltage slow waves to the "activated" pattern of low-voltage fast activity (Moruzzi and Magoun 1949)—is qualitatively consistent with a reciprocal relationship between amplitude and frequency that characterizes waves of relatively constant slope (corresponding to Type 1 waves of the oscillator model). (See figures 12.2 and 14.1.)

From background point 8 it follows that a decrease of excitatory drive to a given small area of cortex (as a result of a white-matter lesion, for example) would be expected to result in an increase in the instantaneous envelope of the EEG and correspondingly in EEG waves of increased amplitude. On the other hand, little or no change in the intracortically generated inhibitory activity and, correspondingly, little change in the envelope of the first derivative of the EEG and hence of the slopes of the waves, would be expected. This combination would lead to waves of higher amplitude and longer duration, corresponding to Type 1 waves of the oscillator model, which would be consistent with the experimental and clinical findings reviewed in chapters 12 and 13. Further, according to expression 4 the instantaneous frequency and the running mean frequency would fluctuate about a level lower than normal.

The Spike-and-Slow-Wave Complex

In the case of focal epilepsy, a disorder of the cortex itself, the pathophysiology (chapter 13) can be briefly summarized as follows: With impairment of intracortically generated inhibitory drive, whether from damage to inhibitory cells themselves or to their synaptic terminations by GABA antagonists (e.g., penicillin, picrotoxin, bicuculline), the probability of excessive firing of pyramidal cells is increased in association with the paroxysmal depolarizing shift, with consequent interictal epileptiform discharges that are reflected in the scalp EEG as a spike. Such a discharge will often be followed by an inhibitory reaction, the EEG counterpart of which is the slow wave of the spike-and-slow-wave complex.

In terms of the extrema-slopes hypothesis and its associated oscillator model, the sharp increase in the instantaneous envelope of the first derivative of the EEG indicates a disproportionately greater intracortical excitatory synaptic drive as compared with inhibitory synaptic drive, marking the onset of the spike component. The synchronous discharge of pyramidal cells, by virtue of their recurrent collaterals, results in a subsequent increase in the overall level of intracortical excitatory synaptic drive (as compared with the excitatory drive arriving from elsewhere in the cortex and from subcortical structures); correspondingly, in the extrema-slopes model, the instantaneous envelope of the EEG itself is increased. The expected net result, therefore, is not only an increase in the instantaneous envelope of the slope of the EEG but also an increase in the instantaneous envelope of the EEG, so that often the spike stands out against the background EEG.

An increased intracortical inhibitory drive then occurs, presumably triggered by the masssively synchronized pyramidal-cell discharges, and is reflected in the EEG as the slow-wave part of the spike-and-slow-wave complex. In the extrema-slopes hypothesis, this effect is reflected as a rapid (exponential) decrease in the preponderance of intracortical excitatory drive relative to intracortical excitatory drive. At the same time, the decrease in intracortical excitatory drive results in a decrease in the envelope of the EEG, so that the slow-wave part of the spike-and-slow-wave complex is generally of lower amplitude than the spike component (see the second part of statement 9 above).

The 3-Hz Spike-Wave Pattern

In the 3-Hz spike-wave pattern, in contrast, there appears to be no impairment of cortical inhibitory mechanisms; rather, there may be overactivity of intracortical excitatory mechanisms, resulting in alternations between a relative preponderance of excitatory drive during the spike component and a relative preponderance of inhibitory drive during the slow-wave component (both being generally, although not invariably, higher in voltage than the focal spike-and-slow-wave complex). An important difference is that the 3-Hz spike-wave pattern tends to be repetitive—perhaps because of a rebound, preponderantly excitatory drive following the massive inhibitory drive.

THE NATURE OF THE TRANSITION BETWEEN THE SPIKE AND WAVE COMPONENTS IN THE 3-HZ SPIKE-WAVE PATTERN

Using the instantaneous envelope of the slope or the first derivative of the 3-Hz spike-wave patterns, and using the spike-and-slow-wave complexes (instead of the running mean slope averaged over a 0.5-sec moving window) to determine the variation in slope in the course of such events through a much shorter time window, yielded unexpected results, as was mentioned in chapter 8. Thus, it has been anticipated that the instantaneous value of the slope would be relatively high during the spike component, decreasing abruptly to a relatively low value during the slow-wave component. Instead, a progressive decrease was encountered in the cases examined; no clear demarcation appeared that would correspond to a sharp transition between spike and slow-wave. This finding suggests that, at least for the scalp EEG, the spike-wave event can be characterized as a single, continuously evolving event, despite the experimental evidence indicating that the two are generated by quite separate processes (chapter 13). The difference between an abrupt transition and a gradual one was pointed up by the results from simulation experiments in comparison with those from actual EEGs (figures 8.5 and 8.6).

An exponential decrement of the instantaneous slope also appeared to be the case for spike-and-slow-wave complexes, but the logarithmic plots for the latter were more irregular, suggesting a "noise" effect of the ongoing background EEG (figure 8.7). Since such background noise should presumably be uncorrelated with the spike-wave event, it should in principle be possible to diminish the "noise component" by averaging a number of such events, using a trigger derived from the onset of the spike component (i.e., from the leading edge of the instantaneous envelope of the first derivative of the EEG). This possibility of increasing the signal-to-noise ratio was not explored.

DIFFERENCES BETWEEN SPIKE-AND-SLOW-WAVE COMPLEXES AND 3-HZ SPIKE-WAVE PATTERNS

Presumably the smaller variability of the (exponential) decrement of the instantaneous envelope of the first derivative of the EEG in the case of the 3-Hz spike-wave pattern as compared with that for the spike-and-slow-wave complex is associated with the more widespread distribution as well as the absence of EEG background in the latter as compared with the former. Thus, in the case of the 3-Hz spike-wave pattern, the background activity may be completely preempted, whereas in the case of the spike-and-slow-wave complex the background EEG activity may be incompletely preempted.

This comparison of the instantaneous envelopes of the EEG and of its first derivative, which were carried out for spike-and-slow-wave complexes and for 3-Hz spike-wave patterns, suggests that the former could perhaps be viewed as a highly damped event, consisting of a single spike and a single slow wave, whereas the latter may be viewed as a repetitive, undamped train of spikes and waves (at least, until the pattern terminates, usually after some decrease in the repetition rate).

Then how and why are the two different in their respective patterns? One possible answer may be as follows: The spike of the 3-Hz spike-wave event is generally appreciably higher in voltage, which no doubt reflects in part its generalized distribution on the scalp, although with predominance in the frontal regions. Second, in the 3-Hz spike-wave pattern, the spike and the wave components are generally of about the same voltage. In contrast, the lower-voltage focal (interictal) spike, being of more localized origin, might be expected to be associated with a smaller amount of inhibition immediately after the spike, with the result that its associated slow wave would be of smaller voltage, as is indeed usually the case. Further, the probability of spike-and-slow-wave complexes appears to be greatest in Stages 1 and 2 of non-REM sleep, whereas the probability of a 3-Hz spike-wave discharge (though actually of somewhat irregular frequency) appears to be greatest in Stages 3 and 4 of non-REM sleep, during which stages the background activity is slowest and highest in voltage. In relation to the present extrema-slopes hypothesis, the question might be raised of whether existing high-voltage slow waves in the background tend to facilitate the 3-Hz spike-wave pattern, perhaps by a rebound excitary drive after the preponderantly inhibitory drive during the slow wave. The same question might be raised with respect to the induction of 3-Hz spike waves in the waking EEG on a background of high-voltage slow waves resulting from hyperventilation (chapter 7), and in some cases in response to stimulation with repetitive flashes.

In focal epilepsy, a predominant factor appears to be a localized or focal impairment of intracortical inhibitory mechanisms (chapter 13), whereas in the generalized epilepsy of the 3-Hz spike-wave type a diffuse increase in cortical excitability has been suggested. In relation to the present model, and for a given small area of cortex, the two can in some sense be considered equivalent—epileptogenesis arising in the one from increased excitation (more exactly, increased excitability) and in the other from a decrease in inhibition. Thus, since the ratio of the envelope of the first derivative of the EEG to the envelope of the EEG itself is taken to represent a measure of the relative strengths of excitation and inhibition, it is apparent from this standpoint that there is an increase in excitation relative to inhibition in both focal and generalized epilepsy. On the other hand, no suggestion arises from these consideration as to the factors immediately responsible for provoking a given epileptiform event.

Nonetheless, there are obvious differences between the two patterns. Perhaps because it is from the outset characteristically a generalized or widespread phenomenon on the scalp, the 3-Hz spike-wave pattern is self-sustained, and perhaps self-triggering. The spike-and-slow-wave complex, on the other hand, being focal, is generally limited to a single event (although multiple spikes can occur), though in some cases the discharge can become generalized.

STAGES 1 AND 2 OF NON-REM SLEEP AS TRANSITIONAL STATES IN RELATION TO EPILEPTIFORM PATTERNS

As was mentioned above in relation to the extrema-slopes hypothesis, the EEG of Stages 1 and 2 of non-REM sleep can be considered as transitional between the EEG of the waking state, manifested either as alpha activity (Type 3 waves of the oscillator model) posteriorly or as a "desynchronized" pattern both anteriorly and posteriorly (mixed Type 3 and Type 4 waves), and the EEG of Stages 3 and 4 of non-REM sleep (Type 1 waves). The EEG of Stages 1 and 2 is less well defined in relation to the four types of waves of the oscillator model. Thus, Stage 1 shows some elements of constant slope (Type 1 waves), but at best only intermittently, and Stage 2 shows some elements of "constant-frequency" waves (in the form of vertex sharp transients). However, as noted in chapter 6, the change in the EEG from Stage 2 to the much more clearly defined constant-slope waves of Stages 3 and 4 is relatively clear.

In this connection, it is of interest (see chapter 13) that it is during Stages 1 and 2 that focal epileptiform manifestations (i.e., spike-and-slow-wave complexes), as well as several normal variant patterns or benign patterns with an "epileptiform morphology"—i.e., 14- and 6-Hz positive bursts, "small sharp spikes" or "benign sporadic spikes of sleep," the 6-Hz spike-wave pattern, and wicket spikes (Westmoreland 1990)—tend to occur. (In contrast, as was noted above, the 3-Hz spike-wave pattern tends to occur more frequently during Stages 3 and 4 than during Stages 1 and 2.)

If epilepsy is viewed as an imbalance between excitatory and inhibitory activity in the cortex in favor of excitatory activity, then it may be appropriate to search for pathophysiological mechanisms underlying the imbalance in the different stages of non-REM sleep, in relation to the extrema-slopes hypothesis, as follows.

It is often the case that the transition between the waking state and drowsiness (Stage 1 sleep) is marked by a greater irregularity, a decrease in voltage, and some slowing of the alpha rhythm, and its replacement by irregular lower-voltage activity, or by irregular or rhythmic activity at about half the alpha frequency (see also Santamaria and Chiappa 1987). In terms of the extrema-slopes hypothesis and the associated oscillator model, this is a change from Type 3 (constant-frequency waves) and Mode 3 of the oscillator (congruent or identical modulation of extrema and slopes) to some mixture of Type 3 and Type 4 waves. (Occasionally, Type 1 or constant-slope waves appear in the transition for some subjects.) In any case, the running mean frequency decreases to about half the alpha frequency, and the Spectral Purity Index decreases from close to 1.0 for alpha activity to a smaller value. In contrast, during spontaneous alpha blocking in the waking state the running mean frequency remains relatively unchanged whereas the Spectral Purity Index decreases (Goncharova and Barlow 1990).

From the above considerations, it appears that the tendency of focal epileptiform activity (the spike-and-slow-wave complex) and of benign patterns with an "epileptiform morphology" (Westmoreland 1990) to occur during Stages 1 and 2 of sleep but not during Stages 3 and 4 may be reflected in, or associated with, the greater lability (variability) of the slopes of the EEG during Stages 1 and 2.

For the 3-Hz spike-wave pattern, however, a quite different mechanism may be operating, with the result that the probability of this pattern is greater in Stages 3 and 4 than in Stages 1 or 2 and is related, not to decreased variability of inhibitory effects (as reflected in relatively constant-slope waves of Stages 3 and 4), but to enhanced excitatory mechanisms. According to the relationship suggested earlier in this chapter, however, an increased excitatory drive results in a decrease in EEG voltage, not an increase such as is observed in Stages 3 and 4 of non-REM sleep. It does not appear, therefore, that the extrema-slopes hypothesis can account for the more frequent 3-Hz spike-wave bursts in the deeper stages of non-REM sleep.

GENERATING MECHANISMS FOR AND SIGNIFICANCE OF EXTREMA AND SLOPES MODULATIONS

The details of the physiological counterpart of the basic oscillatory mechanisms of the oscillator model have, of necessity, been left ill-defined, beyond a somewhat vague implication of intrinsic oscillatory capabilities of ensembles of neurons having excitatory and inhibitory interconnections. In an analogous manner, the details of the physiological counterparts for the generation of the modulating signals that form the inputs for the oscillator model are necessarily left ill-defined. The hypothesis does suggest, however, that the modulating mechanisms may be separate from the basic oscillatory ones; certainly this is the case in the oscillator model itself.

Perhaps the modulating signals themselves are inaccessible and only leave their traces or imprint on the modulated EEG (that is, they take the form of intrinsic or phantom variables rather than extrinsic ones). In this sense, it is perhaps remarkable that characterization of different EEG patterns in terms of the differences in the behavior of the two modulations (i.e, the respective instantaneous envelopes) has as much orderliness and self-consistency as it does, irrespective of the correctness or incorrectness of the suggestion that they reflect excitatory and inhibitory effects averaged over some area of cortex.

It has been noted that the instantaneous frequency, as the quotient of the envelopes of the EEG and of its first derivative, is "noisy." This is particularly the case for the "desynchronized" EEG of the alert, eyes-open state. On the other hand, the variability of the instantaneous frequency (reflecting rapidly varying relative amounts of excitation and inhibition) may be an indication of the level or the intensity of information processing in the neocortex. This question has not been pursued (e.g., by examining the variability of the instantaneous frequency in the different stages of wakefulness and sleep, with controls for possible non-EEG sources of noise).

NEUROTRANSMITTERS, NEUROMODULATORS, AND THE EXTREMA-SLOPES HYPOTHESIS

It seems reasonable to suppose that the total excitatory influence to a given small area of the cortex, at least from elsewhere in the neocortex and from the thalamus (as reflected in the extrema-slopes hypothesis as the inverse of the envelope of the EEG), could be ascribed primarily to some combination of acetylcholine (considered as a neuromodulator or slow-acting excitatory substance) and a rapidly acting excitatory neurotransmitter such as glutamine (if indeed glutamine is a neurotransmitter). The level of inhibition in a given small area of cortex is on firmer ground, and relates to the level of GABA and of its synthesizing enzyme, GAD (gamma-amino butyric acid dehydrogenase).

NORMAL VARIANT PATTERNS IN RELATION TO EPILEPTIFORM (EPILEPTOGENIC) PATTERNS

From the above discussion, it is evident that a frequent if not invariable characteristic of true epileptiform patterns, the 3-Hz spike-wave pattern and the spike-and-slow-wave pattern, is a biphasic excursion of the ratio of excitatory to inhibitory activity in the course of the spike-and-slow-wave sequence, reflected in the extrema-slopes hypothesis in a bidirectional swing of the instantaneous frequency. (Such a postulated swing is not illustrated in this book.) In relation to the mean frequency before the epileptiform event, the instantaneous frequency rises rapidly at the beginning of the spike component, then decreases with an overshoot that reaches its maximum during the slow-wave component; then the sequence is repeated (in the case of the 3-Hz spike-wave pattern) or ends, the instantaneous frequency returning to the pre-event level in the case of the spike-and-slow-wave complex.

Such excursions in instantaneous frequency also occur in several normal-variant patterns that have some resemblance to true epileptiform patterns, although the excursions are not as extreme. It is of interest to consider such normal variant patterns in this respect.

The normal-variant patterns in question are 14- and 6-Hz positive spiking, 6-Hz spike-wave, notched theta of drowsiness (psychomotor variant pattern), benign epileptiform transients or small sharp spikes, and wicket rhythm and wicket spikes. (The first four are illustrated in chapter 4.)

Although the question has not been specifically examined, it appears likely that in all these normal variant patterns the swings of the instantaneous frequency are less than that in the case of true epileptiform patterns. At the same time, it is perhaps not surprising that some of these normal variant patterns have been considered to be epileptiform in the past, because of their qualitative similarities to the true epileptogenic patterns.

These normal-variant patterns tend to occur during Stages 1 and 2 of non-REM sleep, as do spike-and-slow-wave complexes of focal epilepsy. (As mentioned above, the 3-Hz spike-wave pattern tends to be more frequent in the deeper stages of non-REM sleep, although often in a more irregular form and at a somewhat slower repetition rate.) The question can perhaps be raised of whether these normal variant patterns have some common features in their respective generating mechanisms; however, they are not associated with clinical epilepsy.

NONLINEAR INTERACTIONS

The specification of independent modulations of extrema and of slopes, required by the extrema-slopes hypothesis, is consistent with indications from anatomical studies (chapter 11) that inhibitory synapses on the proximal dendrites, the cell body, and the initial segment of the axon act more in a multiplicative (or, equivalently, shunting, divisive) manner, as compared with the more nearly linear (additive, summating) effects of excitatory and inhibitory synapses on the apical dendrites. Such a two-input nonlinear multiplicative effect is also supported by the parallel physiological evidence cited in chapter 12. However, if the level of inhibitory activity is at least partially dependent on the level of excitatory activity (e.g., inhibitory activity associated with recurrent collaterals of pyramidal-cell axons), as suggested earlier in the present chapter, then the two will not be completely independent. Indeed, the argument could be made that this is the normal condition, in which case the Coefficient of Determination of the instantaneous envelopes of the EEG and of its first derivative, in the case of an irregular EEG pattern (e.g., the "desynchronized" EEG), would have a value higher than near 0, perhaps in the range of the actually observed values of about 0.5. Such a formulation could be considered an extension of the concept of cortical excitation originally proposed by Jasper (1936b) (see chapter 14) to include cortical inhibition, but in a nonlinear (multiplicative or divisive) manner rather than an additive or subtractive manner.

THE EXTREMA-SLOPES HYPOTHESIS IN RELATION TO CLASSIFICATION OF EEG PATTERNS—NON-REM SLEEP

The finding that relatively constant slope characterizes the stages of non-REM sleep deeper than Stage 2 (chapter 6) is consonant with the view that Stages 3 and 4 of non-REM sleep represent a single physiological state (Martin et al. 1972). Further, the finding of a sharp demarcation between Stage 2 and Stages 3 and 4 (i.e., the onset of "constant-slope" sleep) may suggest consideration of the latter as an alternative definition of Stages 3 and 4 (i.e., slow-wave sleep)—i.e., an alternative to the standard definition as delta activity of 2 Hz or less and greater than 75 microvolts for more than 20% of the time (chapter 6). Alternatively, a threshold for the envelope of the EEG might distinguish between the EEG of Stage 3 and that of Stage 4, if such a distinction is desirable. (In this connection, a major difficulty in sleep staging in the past has been human versus computerized classification into Stages 3 and 4. There have also been difficulties in differentiating Stage W (waking) for low-alpha subjects, Stage 1 (drowsiness), and Stage REM, if eye movement (particularly) and/or EMG information is not included in the decision tree (Johnson 1977).)

It is of interest that the running mean frequency during Stage 1 sleep (about 5 Hz) does not change when vertex sharp transients occur, as though the quasi-frequency of these waves were much the same as that of the ongoing EEG. (Perhaps because of their relatively low amplitudes in the EEGs that were analyzed in this study, sleep spindles at about 14 Hz appeared to have little effect on the running mean frequency.)

TEMPERATURE COMPENSATION FOR THE FREQUENCY OF RHYTHMIC EEG ACTIVITY

The present model has the capability of at least partial temperature compensation for simulated rhythmic activity, such as alpha activity (Type 3 waves of the oscillator model). The frequency of simulated rhythmic activity (e.g., alpha waves) in the oscillator model is determined by the intrinsic frequency of the basic oscillator (i.e., for a pair of standard (test) DC modulating inputs) and by the ratio of the voltages of the two modulating signals (for Type 3 waves, the two are identical save for their relative amplitudes). Thus, if the basic oscillator has a positive temperature coefficient (e.g., a Q_{10} of 2.5) and the ratio of the modulating signals has a negative temperature coefficient (e.g., -1.0), an overall temperature coefficient or Q_{10} of about 1.5 would result.

As was summarized in chapter 12, there is some evidence that the frequency of the human alpha rhythm may be at least partially temperature-compensated, since the increase in alpha frequency with increasing body temperatures above normal levels results in a smaller change in frequency than would be expected from the increased metabolic rate. There was also some evidence of an impairment of the temperature compensation in cerebral disease. Although the physiological mechanisms for minimizing the effects of temperature variations on the frequency of the alpha rhythm are at best unclear, the extrema-slopes model has the capability of simulating temperature compensation of the frequency of rhythmic activity.

17 Implications for, and Applications to, Computerized EEG Analysis

In this chapter, the methods of EEG analysis developed for testing the extrema-slopes hypothesis are compared with some conventional methods of EEG analysis. Some of the limitations of the latter are also pointed out. A number of possible applications of the present methods to EEG problems are outlined, and some are illustrated; the latter are intended as examples of the methodology rather than as additional evidence to corroborate the extrema-slopes hypothesis.

As was detailed in chapter 3, a number of methods have been developed and used for characterizing the EEG (i.e., for feature extraction) and for testing the extrema-slopes hypothesis. These techniques include running means of (absolute) (1) amplitude, (2) slope, and (3) sharpness (curvature) of the EEG, (4) running mean frequency (as the quotient of (2) and (1)), (5) running Spectral Purity Index (which has a maximum value of 1.0, for a pure sine wave), and (6) running Coefficient of Variation (defined as the quotient of the standard deviation to the mean) for (1), (2), and (4). For comparison of two measures, the following were implemented: (7) the running Pearson Product-Moment Correlation Coefficient and its square, (8) the Coefficient of Determination. These measures are all made with moving windows—nominally 0.5 sec for (1)–(5), and 2.0 sec or longer for (6)–(8).

In addition to the above-listed "windowed" or smoothed (i.e., averaged over a short time interval) determinations, the following determinations were made: (9) the instantaneous envelope of the EEG, (10) the instantaneous envelope of the first derivative of the EEG, and (11) the instantaneous frequency of the EEG as the quotient of (10) and (9). In the latter group of measures, the averaging window mentioned above is diminished to essentially zero width. (Reconstitution of EEGs was accomplished using (9) and (10) as input modulations for extrema and slopes, respectively, for the oscillator model, the "hardware" implementation of the basic extrema-slopes hypothesis.)

SOME CONVENTIONAL METHODS OF EEG ANALYSIS

Extensive reviews of methods of analysis of the EEG and of their clinical applications can be found in Gevins and Rémond 1987 and Lopes da Silva et al. 1986, respectively. Shorter surveys can be found in Lopes da Silva 1987b,c and in Gotman 1990b. The principal methods can be classified for the purposes of the present discussion into spectral analysis (Dumermuth 1977; Dumermuth and Molinari 1987); autocorrelation and cross-correlation (Gevins 1987); parametric analysis in the form of autoregressive analysis (modeling), in which a model with a certain relatively small number of computer-evaluated parameters is fitted to a given EEG (Lopes da Silva and Mars 1987); and mimetic analysis, which attempts to mimic, quantify, and extend human analysis (Frost 1987). In addition, there are methods for analysis of nonstationary EEGs (i.e., those with changing statistical characteristics) (Barlow 1985c; Gersch 1987), including adaptive segmentation, in which changes in EEG patterns are automatically detected and the resulting segments are clustered into a small number of groups having similar statistical properties (e.g., mean amplitude, mean frequency). Special methods have been developed for the detection of fast transients of epileptiform activity, i.e., spikes and sharp waves (Ktonas 1987). Nonlinear methods of analysis of EEGs from different sites are considered in Lopes da Silva et al. 1989. Details of these and other methods can be found in the reviews cited above.

Spectral (Fourier-Based) Methods and Their Limitations

In several of the above-mentioned techniques of EEG analysis (some of which have been taken over from other fields, e.g. signal analysis—not always with adequate consideration of their appropriateness for EEG analysis), amplitude and frequency are considered to be the prime features (see also Lopes da Silva et al. 1989). This is explictly the case for spectral analysis (and its derivative techniques, such as coherence), in which amplitude or power is displayed as a function of frequency. The same is intrinsically true for correlation analysis, since the correlation function and spectra are merely inverse Fourier transforms of one another. Further, the autoregressive (predictor) coefficients resulting from autoregressive coefficients can be considered eqivalent to a spectral representation, since spectra can be derived from them (Gersch 1970; Lopes da Silva and Mars 1987).

Spectral methods have several limitations when used for analysis of EEGs (Walter et al. 1972a; Dumermuth and Molinari 1987; Walter 1987). In the first instance, spectral methods are in the strict sense applicable only for analysis of a "stationary" signal (i.e., a statistically unchanging signal, such as a relatively unchanging background EEG pattern). Unless special measures (such as adaptive segmentation—see below) are taken to ensure that sections of EEGs being subjected to spectral analysis are relatively uniform in their statistical characteristics (e.g., distribution of amplitudes), errors can result. Walter (1972) cites the example of finding that spectra of alternating periods of high-voltage bursts of delta activity and periods of very-low-voltage delta activity in sleeping infants (i.e., the *tracé alternant* pattern) were indistinguishable from the spectra of periods of fairly continuous delta activity of intermediate voltage. (See Barlow 1985d for analysis of *tracé alternant* recordings by adaptive segmentation.) Second, spectral analysis is a linear method of analysis (Middleton 1960); i.e., its answers are provided basically in the form of sums, as described in further detail below.

Even for stationary signals, the question can be raised of what spectra really represent—or, as the question is sometimes expressed, "Are the frequency components indicated by spectral analysis really there?" This question was considered by Walter (1987), who pointed out some of the pitfalls of spectral analysis and, at the same time, questioned the utility of spectra. Walter (1987) expressed the view that spectral analysis (or *Fourier-based methods*, to use his term) has not resulted in deep insights into the EEG. Pitfalls and ambiguities in spectral analysis and examples of resynthesis of waveforms from their Fourier sine and cosine components are also given in Walter et al. 1972a.

Walter (1987) considered the example of the spectrum of a 9-Hz sine wave varying in amplitude sinusoidally with a period of 1 sec (i.e., a 9-Hz sine wave amplitude modulated (more exact, multiplied) by a 1-Hz sine wave), which is technically equivalent to so-called suppressed carrier modulation. The spectrum of this waxing and waning wave has a pair of peaks of equal height, one at 8 and one at 10 Hz, but the point on the spectrum at 9 Hz has a value of 0. The reason for this behavior, which at first seems mysterious, is that the question asked of Fourier analysis is "What combination of constant-amplitude sine waves will summate to yield the original?" The answer is: a summation of 8-Hz and 10-Hz sine waves of equal amplitudes.

Mathematically, as Walter (1987) pointed out, the apparent contradiction is eliminated by considering the trigonometric identity

$$\cos x + \cos y = 2\cos[\tfrac{1}{2}(x+y)] \cdot \cos[\tfrac{1}{2}(x-y)].$$

Exchanging sides of the identity yields

$$2\cos[\tfrac{1}{2}(x+y)] \cdot \cos[\tfrac{1}{2}(x-y)] = \cos x + \cos y,$$

or, in terms of frequencies,

$$2\cos[\tfrac{1}{2}(2\pi f_1 + 2\pi f_2)] \cdot \cos[\tfrac{1}{2}(2\pi f_1 - 2\pi f_2)] = \cos 2\pi f_1 + \cos 2\pi f_2.$$

Inserting the frequencies 10 and 8 Hz for f_1 and f_2, respectively, yields

$$2\cos[\tfrac{1}{2}(2\pi 10 + 2\pi 8)] \cdot \cos[\tfrac{1}{2}(2\pi 10 - 2\pi 8)] = \cos 2\pi 10 + \cos 2\pi 8.$$

Simplifying, we get

$$2\cos[\tfrac{1}{2}(2\pi 18] \cdot \cos[\tfrac{1}{2}(2\pi 2)] = \cos 2\pi 10 + 2\pi 8,$$

or,

$$2\cos[2\pi 9] \cdot \cos 2\pi 1 = \cos 2\pi 10 + 2\pi 8,$$

where the left side indicates the 9-Hz wave of which the amplitude is being varied (i.e., modulated) by the 1-Hz sine wave and the right side indicates the same result as the summation of constant-amplitude (unmodulated) 8-Hz and 10-Hz sine waves. The left side can be viewed as a mathematical representation of a *nonlinear* process, entailing multiplication (indicated by the dot), of obtaining the sine wave that waxes and wanes whereas the right side is a mathematical representation of a *linear* process (entailing simple addition) of obtaining the same result (see figure 17.1). Spectral analysis, which is implicitly based on the summation of a series of sine (and cosine) waves of fixed amplitude to approximate a given waveform, is inherently a linear method.

Walter et al. (1972a) pointed out the spectral broadening that can result from amplitude variations (modulation) of a pure sine wave as a serious qualification to be considered in interpreting spectra. These authors also indicated both that two quite different waveforms could have the same power spectra and that two apparently similar waveforms could have rather different spectra. The latter circumstance is shown in figures 17.2 and 17.3. In the first case (figure 17.2), a wave that waxes and wanes in amplitude was obtained by amplitude modulation of a 10.5-Hz sine wave by a 1.0-Hz sine wave; its power spectrum has components at 9.5 and 11.5 Hz as well as at 10.5 Hz. In the second case (figure 17.3), the power spectrum of a waxing-and-wanning wave resulting from summation of 10.5- and 11.5-Hz sine waves has components at 10.5 and 11.5 Hz, but no component corresponding to the frequency of the resultant waxing-and-waning wave (i.e., 11.0 Hz). This difference in the spectra for the two types of waves can be understood by reference to figures 17.4–17.6 and their legends. In brief, the two waves in figures 17.2 and 17.3 are actually quite different from one another, with consequent differences in their spectra.

To reiterate the case depicted in figure 17.1: spectral (Fourier) analysis of a 9-Hz sine wave multiplied by a 1-Hz sine wave will result in a spectrum with peaks at 8 and at 10 Hz, but no peak at 9 Hz (compare figure 17.3). The mean frequency, if determined from the spectrum, would indeed be 9 Hz, but the spectral width is approximately 2 Hz. As given by the present technique, the mean frequency in this case, as the quotient of the mean slope and the mean amplitude (assuming preliminary calibration), would also be 9 Hz, in agreement with the results from the spectrum. However, the Spectral Purity Index would have a value of 1.0, rather than a value less than 1.0, since the SPI is normalized for amplitude and for variations in amplitude (figure 19.2). Whereas spectral analysis assumes a linear model of the signal (i.e., it is considered as though it were made up of pure sine waves of fixed amplitude), such an assumption is not a part of the determination of mean frequency by the slopes/amplitude method, nor of the degree of rhythmicity as measured by the Spectral Purity Index.

Although the above discussion has been limited to spectral (frequency, Fourier) analysis, the same points are relevant to other linear methods of analysis of the EEG, such as autocorrelation and cross-correlation, and to autoregressive analysis.

The following question arises: Is Fourier or spectral analysis, which fits a linear model (i.e., a series of sine and cosine waves) to a signal, an appropriate way to analyze the EEG, a very typical waveform (the alpha rhythm) of which is a waxing-and-waning quasi-sinusoid similar to the above-described

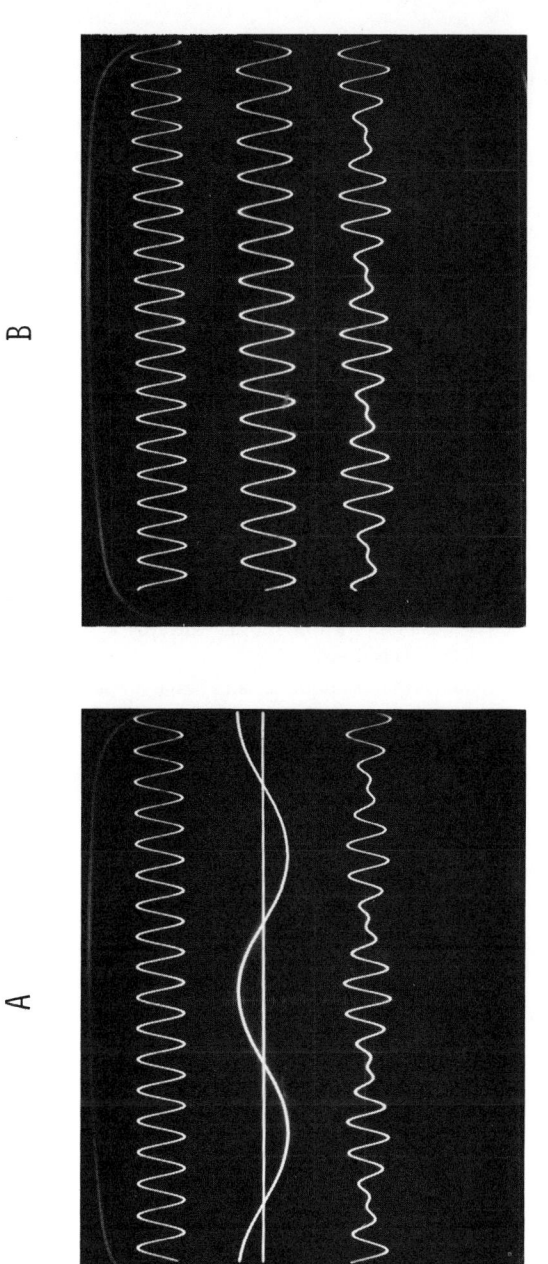

Figure 17.1 Multiplication of a 9-Hz sine wave (A, top trace) by a 1-Hz sine wave (A, middle trace) yields a result (A, bottom trace) that is the same as the summation of equal-amplitude 8-Hz and 10-Hz sine waves (B). (The amplitude scale for third trace is half that for the top two traces.)

Computerized EEG Analysis

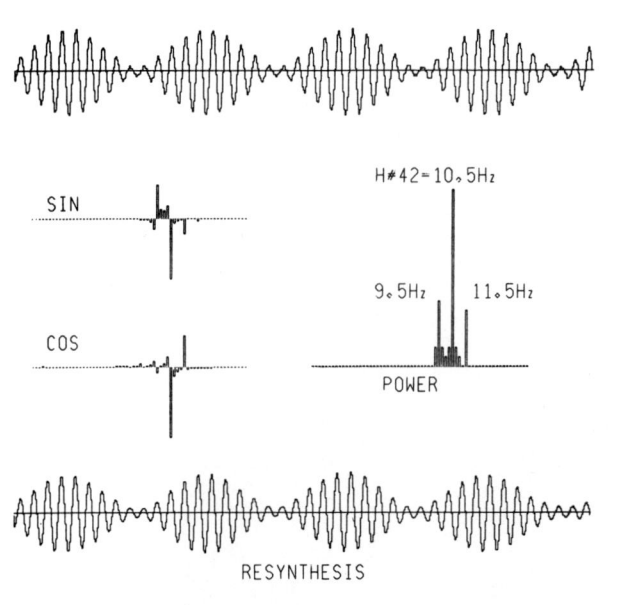

Figure 17.2 Amplitude modulation of a 10.5-Hz sine wave by a 1-Hz sine wave (top trace) yields a power spectrum having side bands at 9.5 Hz and 11.5 in addition to the component at 10.5 Hz. The power spectrum is the sum of the squares of the sine and cosine spectra; note that the latter can take on negative as well as positive values. The bottom trace is resynthesized from the sine and cosine spectra. (From Walter et al. 1972a.)

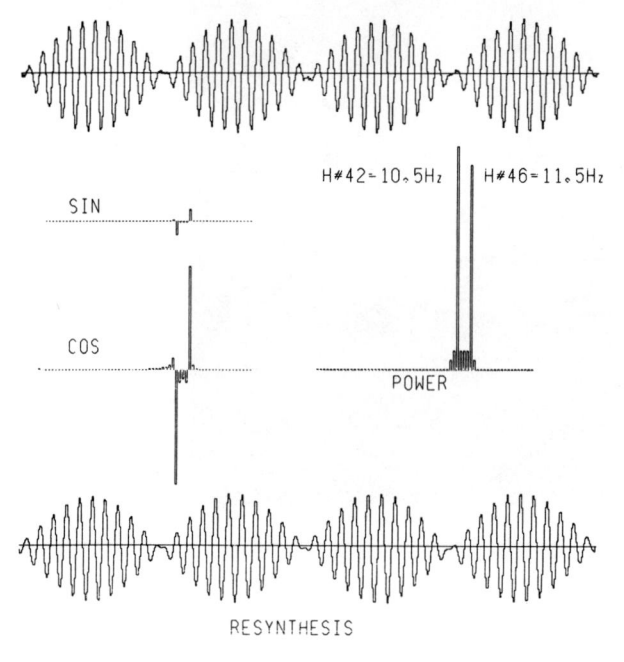

Figure 17.3 Summation (beating) of a 10.5-Hz sine wave and a 11.5-Hz sine wave of the same amplitude yields a waveform that apparently resembles that of figure 17.2, but has only two spectral components, (at 10.5 Hz and at 11.5 Hz); there is no component at 11.0 Hz. (From Walter et al. 1972a.)

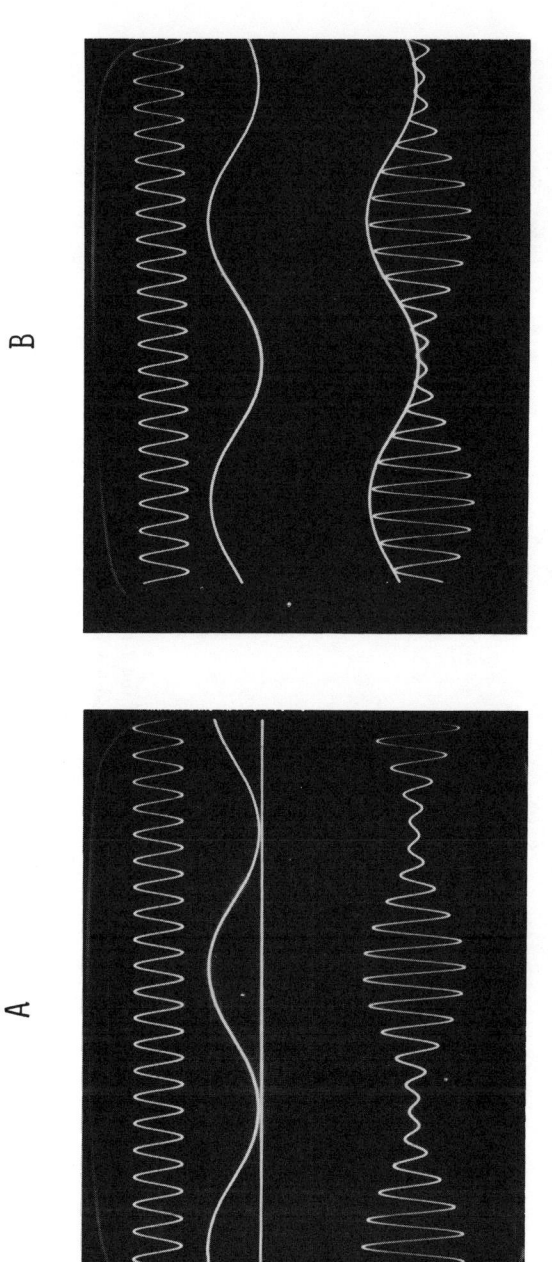

Figure 17.4 (A) Generation of the waveform of figure 17.2 by multiplication of a 10.5-Hz sine wave by a 1-Hz sine wave having a DC offset (note the baseline; depth of modulation, 100%). (B) Same, except that the envelope of the modulated wave is shown (bottom trace). Note that there are no phase reversals of the modulated wave.

Computerized EEG Analysis

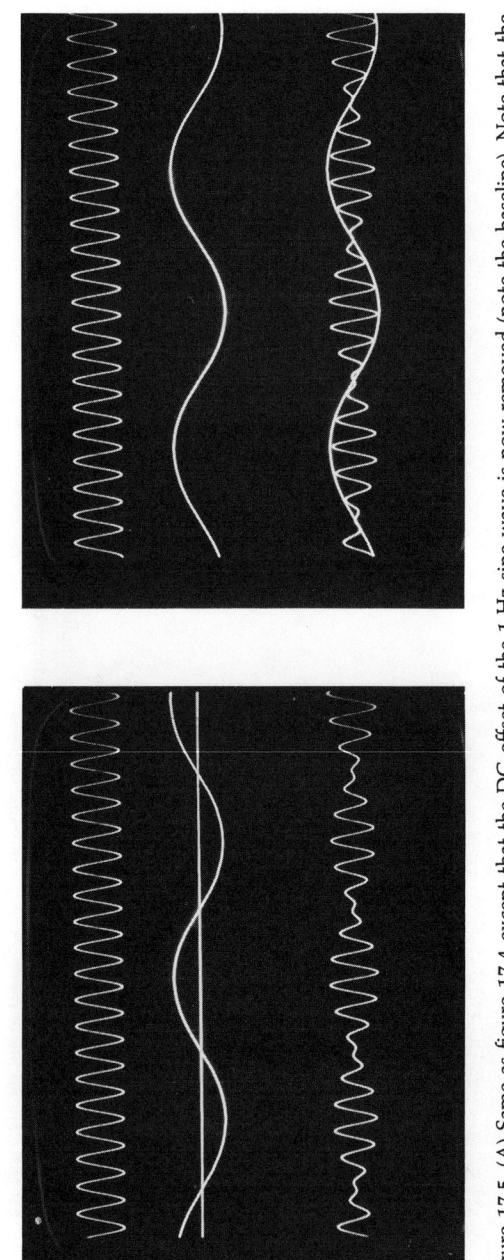

Figure 17.5 (A) Same as figure 17.4 except that the DC offset of the 1-Hz sine wave is now removed (note the baseline). Note that the phase of the modulated 10-Hz wave (bottom trace) is inverted during successive half cycles of the 1-Hz modulating wave, the change occurring at the null points of the latter; the phase reversals are shown more clearly in the bottom trace of B, in which the envelope is superimposed on the modulated wave. Amplitude scale is the same for the bottom traces of figures 17.1, 17.4, and 17.5.

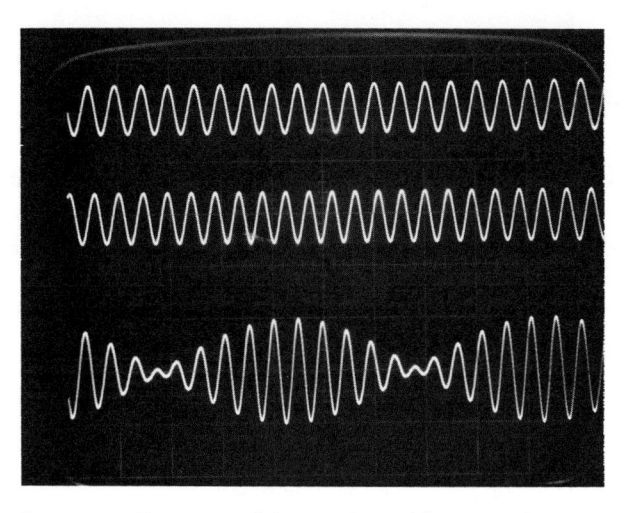

Figure 17.6 Generation of the waveform of figure 17.3 by summation of equal-amplitude sine waves of 10.5 and 11.5 Hz. (Amplitude scale for the bottom trace is twice that for the bottom traces of figures 17.1, 17.4, and 17.5.) The same result could have been obtained by multiplying a 11-Hz sine wave by a 0.5-Hz sine wave (cf. figure 17.1).

example? If a nonlinear model of the EEG is being considered, which is the case in the present extrema-slopes hypothesis, then spectral analysis, as a linear method, is inappropriate and results in a linear depiction of a nonlinear process—in the case of a waxing-and-waning rhythm, in a spurious broadening of the representation of frequencies (e.g., from 9 Hz to 8 and 10 Hz, as in the example given above). (This question is considered again in chapter 19.)

Another instance of the possibility of erroneous inferences that can arise from spectral and related methods of analysis is that of inferences of harmonic relationships among frequency components of an EEG. As an example, the arcuate form of the mu rhythm (figure 4.11) suggests a fundamental frequency in the range of 10 Hz to which a 20-Hz component has been added; such an apparent relationship, in the frequency domain, can indeed be confirmed by bispectral analysis (Lopes da Silva 1981; Dumermuth and Molinari 1987). On the other hand, the extrema-slopes model suggests a quite different nature of the mu rhythm arising from nonlinear processes (figure 4.10).

In summary: In spectral or Fourier-based analysis, the question being asked is "What combination of pure sine (and cosine) waves will add up to yield the section of the EEG in question?" Spectral analysis, and the above-mentioned methods related to it, are therefore considered to be linear methods of analysis, and (strictly speaking) implicit in their use for the EEG is a linear model of its generator mechanisms. (The filtered-noise model discussed in chapter 14 can also be considered a linear model.) It is thus important to keep in mind that Fourier methods provide a mathematical but not a biological model of the EEG (cf. Lopes da Silva 1987b). Nonetheless, these methods can be very useful in the characterization of EEG phenomena (see, e.g., figures 5.9 and 17.3).

Quasi-Linear Methods

Hjorth's Parameters (Normalized Slope Descriptors) The present measures of running mean amplitude, running mean frequency, and running Spectral Purity Index can be compared with Hjorth's "normalized slope descriptors" of Activity, Mobility, and Complexity, respectively, which provide measures of mean power, root-mean-square frequency, and root-mean-square frequency spread (Hjorth 1970, 1973, 1975).

Hjorth (1970, 1973, 1975) defined the normalized slope descriptors, in notation employed by Lopes da Silva (1987), as follows:

activity: $A = a_0$,

mobility: $M = [a_2/a_0]^{1/2}$,

complexity: $C = [(a_4/a_2)/(a_2/a_0)]^{1/2} = [a_4/a_0]^{1/2}$,

where a_0 is the variance (square of the standard deviation) or mean power of the signal, a_2 is the variance of the first derivative, and a_4 is the variance of the second derivative of the signal. These are equivalent to the zero-order, second-order, and fourth-order moments, respectively, of the power spectrum (more exactly termed the *power density spectrum*). Hjorth's three parameters can be referred to respectively as the average power in the epoch under measurement, the average power of the normalized derivative in the epoch, and the average power of the normalized second derivative in the epoch (Saltzberg and Burch 1971). The latter authors pointed out that Hjorth's parameters of mobility and complexity can be estimated from baseline-crossing data of a signal and of its first derivative over the epoch of interest. A formulation of Hjorth's descriptors for limited observation periods is given in Walmsley 1984.

Hjorth's parameters were applied to EEG studies by several authors (Lloyd and Binnie 1972; Chavance 1976; Berglund and Elmqvist 1975; Caille and Bassano 1975; Tolonen and Sulg 1981; Pronk and Simons 1982; Jonkman et al. 1986; Pronk 1986), some of whom compared several techniques.

The present measures are simpler to compute than Hjorth's parameters, and they are more closely related to conventional EEG measures of amplitude, average frequency, and regularity or rhythmicity (degree of sinusoidality). The Spectral Purity Index has a value of 1.0 (its maximum) for a pure sine wave. In comparison, Hjorth's Complexity parameter has a value of 0 (its minimum) for a pure sine wave.

On the other hand, the present measures of mean frequency and Spectral Purity Index are subject to the same limitations as Hjorths's parameters: strictly speaking, they are applicable only to signals having a single spectral peak, and high precision is required for the calculations (Denoth 1975; Lopes da Silva 1987a). Despite these limitations, Hjorth's method has been employed by a number of workers, as the above-cited references indicate. Actually, in a comparative determination of the mean frequency of 32 EEG recordings each of 5 sec duration by the present slope/amplitude method and by formal spectra (obtained by Fourier transformation of the autocorrelation functions), close agreement (i.e., within 1.4 Hz) was found, and for 27 of the 32 EEGs the agreement was within 1.0 Hz (Goncharova and Barlow 1990). Perhaps such a close agreement is not too surprising, in view of the fact that the mean frequency for an equal-amplitude mixture of sine waves of 1 and 10 Hz (a "worst case") was found to be 7 Hz instead of the correct 5.5 Hz—an error of only 1.5 Hz.

The advantages of running mean frequency and of frequency spread (i.e., the Spectral Purity Index) thus appear to outweigh their limitations.

Adaptive Segmentation and Clustering of Segments In this technique, boundaries are automatically indicated for changes of the type of activity within one channel or two (e.g., episodic high-voltage slow activity vs. normal background activity) and the resultant segments are automatically clustered according to their average features (mean amplitude, mean frequency). For this purpose, the autocorrelation function of five lags computed for the EEG "viewed" through a window (nominally 1.2 sec) that moves along the EEG is compared with an autocorrelation function of the intial 1.2 sec of the current segment (figure 17.7), a segment boundary being signaled when a preestablished difference has been exceeded (Bodenstein and Praetorius 1977; Michael and Houchin 1979; Barlow et al. 1981; Barlow 1984, 1985d; Bodenstein et al. 1985; Creutzfeldt et al. 1985).

Even in its most refined form (Bodenstein et al. 1985), adaptive segmentation with associated clustering and classification (by probability density function) was found to be satisfactory from a clinical standpoint in only about 65 percent of a series of 63 normal and abnormal EEGs (Creutzfeldt et al. 1985)—excluding artifacts, which were rather well detected as "singular" events.

Conventional Methods for Detection of Epileptiform EEG Activity

It has long been recognized that power spectra are not very useful for the study of epileptiform EEG patterns (see, for example, Walter 1987), in part because of the wide dispersion of frequencies in the spectra of such transients and in part because epileptiform phenomena are often of shorter duration (e.g., less than 1 sec) than the usual minimum duration of the computing window for the spectral analysis (e.g., by the Fast Fourier Transform method).

It is perhaps not very surprising that spectral techniques have not been found to be very satisfactory for the detection and identification of epileptiform transients in the EEG, and hence empirical methods, primarily based on waveform features, have been developed for this purpose, both for interictal events (Frost 1985; Gotman 1985; Ktonas 1987) and for ictal patterns (Gotman 1986, 1990a,b). With the possible exception of the combination of autoregressive modeling and inverse autoregressive filtering (Bodenstein and Praetorius 1977; Lopes da Silva and Mars 1987), a kind of dichotomy has developed between methods of analysis of ongoing background EEG activity

METHOD - SCHEMATIC

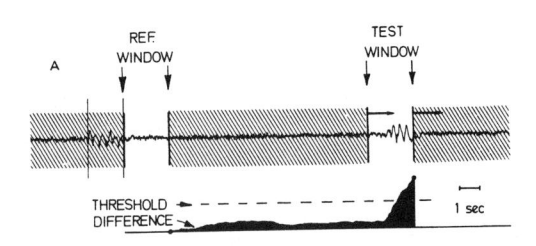

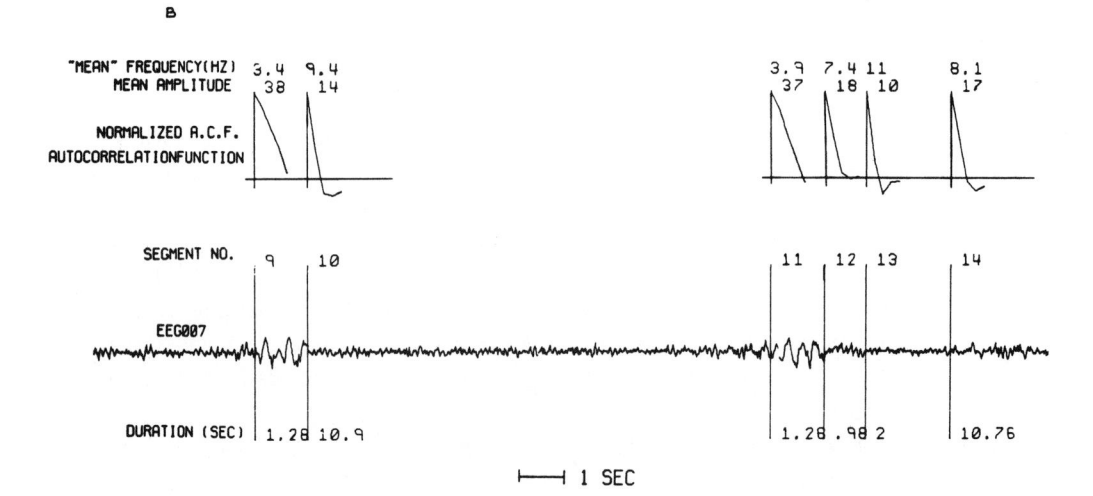

Figure 17.7 (A) Schema of method of adaptive segmentation according to Michael and Houchin (1979). The original EEG is shown at the top; the lighter vertical lines at the left enclose a just-segmented paroxysm. The new reference (fixed) window is at the left, the moving (test) window at the right. The difference measure (for amplitude and frequency combined) is shown below, together with the threshold level for segmentation (horizontal dashed line). (In actuality, separate thresholds are set for amplitude and for frequency.) Note that the point at which the threshold is exceeded lags the actual beginning of the change; a separate algorithm is therefore used to determine the latter point in time. Note also that the small spike component hardly affects the difference measure. (B) Segmented EEG, with normalized autocorrelation function of five points, mean amplitude in microvolts (for a sine wave, the peak-to-peak value would be 2.8 times the indicated mean (actually, root-mean-square) values), and an approximation to the mean frequency, for each segment. The latter are numbered in sequence. (From Barlow et al. 1981.)

(including those methods, such as adaptive segmentation, that take into account its changing patterns) and methods for analysis of brief epileptiform transients.

METHODS BASED ON THE EXTREMA-SLOPES HYPOTHESIS

The methods that have been developed for the analysis of EEGs in relation to the extrema-slopes hypothesis (chapter 3), on the other hand, were essentially based on features of the EEG itself. Hence they should, in principle, be more nearly free of the arbitrary and perhaps even at times misleading results that can ensue from the application to EEG analysis of methods brought in from other fields. In particular, the present methods are based on a model of the EEG that is nonlinear at the outset.

In the methods developed for testing the extrema-slopes hypothesis, amplitude (or, more exactly, extrema) and slope are the two prime features, in contrast to the primacy of amplitude and frequency in spectral analysis. Correspondingly, in the present methods, frequency is a derived or secondary measure, obtained from measures of amplitude and slope.

The present methods, like the model, encompass both ongoing background activity and brief transients (spikes, sharp waves) in the EEG. Further, the present approach encompasses an EEG phenomenon that is not explicitly included in either the conventional approaches to background activity or the conventional approaches to transient activity: the slow-wave component of the spike-and-slow-wave complex (or sharp-and-slow-wave complex). (In contrast, the wave component of bursts of 3-Hz spike-wave activity and similar patterns can be taken into account by conventional methods because of their repetitive nature and their generally longer duration.)

The combined use of the running mean frequency and the Spectral Purity Index, as described in chapters 3 and 25, although subject to certain limitations, does not entail the ambiguous and perhaps misleading results from analysis of a waxing and waning rhythm that is inherent in spectral analysis. Thus, the running mean frequency of such a waxing-and-waning rhythm (e.g., an alpha rhythm) remains essentially constant irrespective of the nature of the modulation (sinusoidal or irregular) of its amplitude. Likewise, its Spectral Purity Index will remain at essentially 1.0 irrespective of the modulation. These characteristics are evident from inspection of the analyses of EEGs in chapter 5 showing alpha activity. Because of these features, and because of their ease of evaluation, running mean frequency and Spectral Purity Index may be preferable, at least in some instances, to spectra—for example, in EEG monitoring in intensive care units. In the following section, an example of such applications is considered.

The feature of the present approach that permits a common or combined approach to the analysis of both background and transient EEG activity is the capability of evaluating the running means of various parameters (over time intervals of a minute or longer) as well as the capability of deriving instantaneous values of selected parameters (i.e., instantaneous envelopes of the EEG and of its first derivative, and, as the quotient of these two, the instantaneous frequency). The latter determinations are made possible by a new approach to on-line real-time determination of the envelopes for a variety of EEG patterns, not merely rhythmic (narrow-band) ones (chapter 29).

POSSIBLE APPLICATIONS OF THE PRESENT METHODS TO EEG ANALYSIS

In some respects, the methods developed in connection with the extrema-slopes hypothesis are more suited for following or monitoring EEGs than for evaluating features over fixed successive epochs, although the latter determinations are quite possible. In this respect, they can be compared with other methods of monitoring, especially those based on Hjorth's normalized slope parameters (Hjorth 1970, 1973; Binnie 1986; Pronk 1986; Smith 1986; see also chapter 25 for a comparison of the present methods of running means of amplitude, frequency, and the Spectral Purity Index with Hjorth's parameters).

Thus, a combination of the running mean frequency (a parameter that has long been of interest (Darrow et al. 1960) and the running Spectral Purity Index, or the former alone, may be useful in monitoring the EEG in the Intensive Care Unit, or during carotid endarterectomy procedures (Barlow 1984; see below), or during cardiac surgery (Pronk and Simons 1984). The running mean frequency is considerably easier to compute as the quotient of the running mean slope to the running mean amplitude than by the conventional method of determining the second moment of the power spectrum (Saltzberg and Burch 1971; Saltzberg et al. 1985; Goncharova and Barlow 1990).

Actually, evaluation of a mean from the power spectrum yields the root-mean-square frequency, which is not necessarily identical with the mean frequency itself. (A comparison can be made with the root-mean-square voltage and the mean voltage, respectively.) For example, if there is a dependence of alpha frequency on amplitude (see chapter 5), e.g., a slightly higher frequency than the mean frequency (of, e.g., 10 Hz) of the higher-amplitude waves than the lower-amplitude ones, the mean frequency as derived from power spectra will be slightly biased toward the frequency of the waves of larger amplitude. Such skewing or distortion does not result when the mean frequency is derived by the present method. These differences are doubtless of little consequence, however, in the actual practice of EEG monitoring.

Similarly, the Spectral Purity Index is appreciably easier to evaluate than is the measure of spectral width given by the fourth moment of the power spectrum (Saltzberg and Burch 1971).

Changes in mean frequency and Spectral Purity Index provide relatively sensitive indications of a change of state as reflected in the EEG, for example, the onset of drowsiness, or alpha blocking upon eye opening), or during brief spontaneous alpha blocking (Goncharova and Barlow 1990).

The Coefficient of Variation provides a convenient indication of a change in (e.g.) amplitude or frequency, and of its magnitude (increase or decrease), occurring with a change of state, provided that the change occurs within the computational window width (figure 5.1). A gradual change is unlikely to be so signaled.

Use of the Envelope of the EEG and Its Coefficient of Variation to Characterize Alpha Blocking and Other Changes in EEG Patterns

The phenomenon of alpha blocking in human subjects, i.e., the attenuation of the alpha rhythm, has long been of interest (see, e.g., Knott 1939). Wilson and Wilson (1959) and Berlyne and McDonald (1965) used as a criterion for an "arousal response" a suppression of alpha rhythm following a single flash as a decrease (at the end of a normal latency period) of at least 50 percent in the voltage and/or an increase in the frequency beyond the upper limit (13 Hz) of the alpha frequency range. This definition is consonant with the findings of Creutzfeldt et al. (1969), in a series of mental and visuomotor tasks, that complete "blocking" of alpha activity was never observed; the term "alpha reduction" was suggested instead. In the present context, the running mean of the amplitude of the EEG could provide an indication of the changes of voltage, the running mean frequency of any changes in mean frequency, the Spectral Purity Index of changes in the degree of rhythmicity or relative absence thereof, and the Coefficient of Variation of the extent (as a percentage or a decimal fraction) of any change in any of these measures.

Measures of the "Regulation" of the EEG

Regulation is a descriptive term used in clinical EEG reporting to indicate the variability of frequency and/or amplitude of alpha activity (Kellaway 1990). The Coefficient of Variation of the running mean frequency, or that of the running mean amplitude, could provide a quantitative measure of regulation. The Spectral Purity Index could provide a measure of the extent to which different frequencies are simultaneously present (i.e., of the bandwidth of the EEG).

Extrema-Slopes Analysis vs. Spectral Analysis of the EEG in Non-REM Sleep

Spectral analysis, with particular attention to the delta-frequency components, has perhaps been the most widely used method for computerized characterization and classification of sleep—i.e., sleep staging (Smith 1986)—although additional physiological monitors (e.g., eye movement, EKG, EMG) have generally been found necessary for distinguishing the waking state, REM sleep, and Stage 1 non-REM sleep. Further, some investigators propose combining Stages 3 and 4 of non-REM sleep (the combination sometimes being termed *slow-wave sleep*) for purposes of analysis (Martin et al. 1972), although by the usual definition Stage 4 non-REM sleep contains more delta activity than

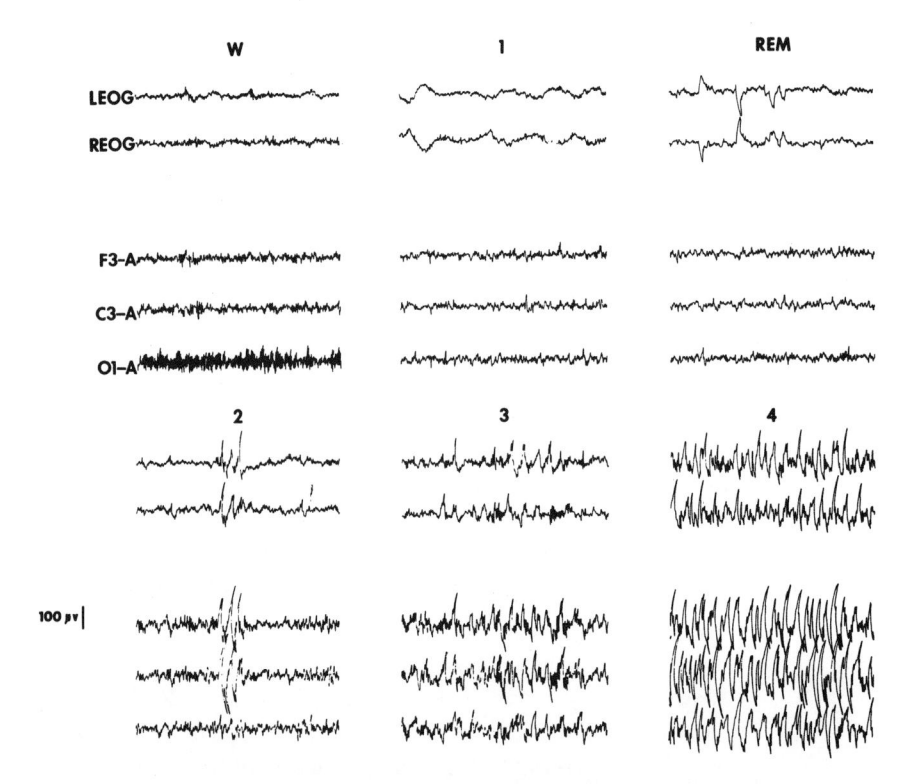

Figure 17.8 Samples of EEGs and EOGS (30-sec excerpts) in the waking state (Stage W) and during the different stages of sleep (REM and non-REM Stages 1–4), for comparison with the respective spectra in figure 17.3. Electrodes: F3, left midfrontal; C3, left midcentral; O1, left occipital; A, ear; LEOG, REOG, left and right electro-oculograms. (From Johnson 1977.)

Stage 3 (figure 6.1) (Carskadon and Rechtschaffen 1989). At best, however, there are difficulties in using spectra for sleep staging in adults (Johnson 1972, p. 288; Smith 1972) as well as in children (Walter 1972). Smith (1972) reported having abandoned Fourier analysis of the EEG in favor of nonlinear detection techniques for sleep staging as well as for refined analysis of sleep data.

For comparison with the results, reported in chapter 6, of the analyses of EEG sleep recordings carried out according to the extrema-slopes hypothesis, it is of interest to examine spectra for the different stages of sleep.

The progressive change from low-voltage, irregular, relatively faster activity in the alert eyes-open waking state to the high-voltage delta activity of Stage 4 non-REM sleep (the EEG in Stage REM being quite similar to that of Stage 1 non-REM) is illustrated in figure 17.8, and the corresponding spectra are shown in figure 17.9. The similarity between the spectra for Stage 1 and Stage REM is evident. In comparison with Stage 1, Stage 2 shows the expected peak for sleep spindles at about 14 Hz, peaks at this frequency also being evident for Stages 3 and 4. In comparison with Stage W (the waking state), which shows an alpha peak, Stage REM, and Stage 1, all of which show about the same level and trend of a decrease with increasing frequency, the spectrum for Stage 2 is shifted up and is somewhat steeper, particularly for

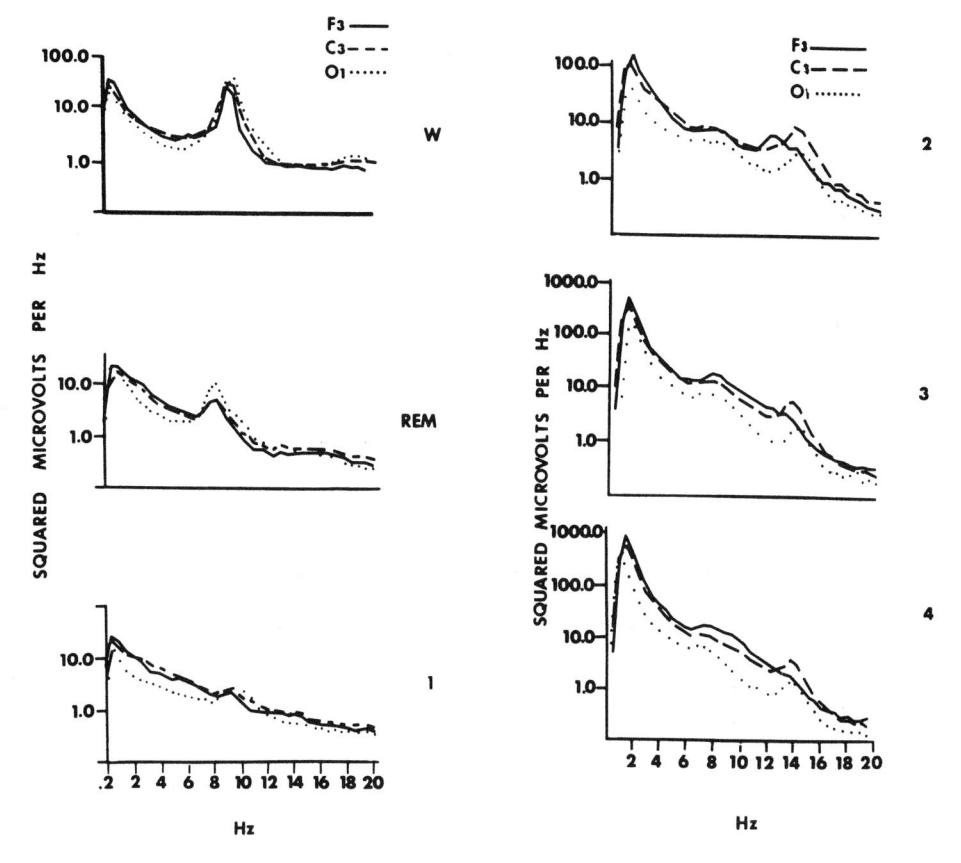

Figure 17.9 Power spectra (in microvolts squared) on a semi-logarithmic scale for 1-min EEG recordings corresponding to the EEG patterns excerpted in figure 17.2. (From Johnson 1972.)

the lower frequencies. This change is more prominent for Stage 3 and even more prominent for Stage 4, in which a distinct nonlinearity in the trend is apparent for the lowest frequencies. Johnson (1977) found that the power of delta activity increased monotonically from the waking state through Stage 1, Stage 2, Stage 3, and Stage 4, the quantity of delta activity being nearly the same in Stage 1 and Stage REM. (Distinction between the latter two states is greatly facilitated by analysis of the electro-oculogram). Separating Stage W (waking) from Stage 1 can pose a problem, especially for low-alpha subjects (Johnson 1977). The highest rate of occurrence of sleep spindles has been found in Stage 2; the rates are lower for Stages 3 and 4 (Johnson 1977).

The progressive upward trend (especially of the lower-frequency components) in the sequence of Stages 1 through 4 in figure 17.8 corresponds to the progressive increase in running mean amplitude with increasing depth of non-REM sleep that is evident in the figures in chapter 6. (Average amplitudes relative to that in Stage 1 were found by Dumermuth et al. (1983) to be 1.6, 2.0, and 2.42, for Stages 2, 3, and 4, respectively.) However, the constant-slope feature which is evident for Stages 3 and 4 in the latter figures is not at all evident from the sequence of spectra shown in figure 17.9. In brief, it can be said that spectra tend to obscure rather than bring out any constant-slope feature that may be present in an EEG.

The question then arises of whether measures developed in connection with the extrema-slopes hypothesis may be useful in sleep staging. The results from analyses of sleep recordings indicate the presence of Stages 3 and 4 of non-REM sleep by a relatively constant running mean slope, and the transition from Stage 2 to Stage 3 is marked by the onset of this feature. (The running mean amplitude, as previously mentioned, tends to increase progressively with increasing depth of sleep during Stages 1–4.)

In the results presented in chapter 6, Stages 1 and 2 and Stage REM were less well characterized by the extrema-slopes measures. If an alpha rhythm were present, the waking state was of course characterized by constant frequency (i.e., the alpha frequency). Stage 1 for some subjects was intermittently characterized by constant slope, but this finding was an inconsistent one. Stage 2, somewhat surprisingly, tended to show relatively constant frequency, at about half the alpha frequency, but with a wider range of frequencies (as reflected by values of the Spectral Purity Index rather less than the 1.0 that characterizes waxing-and-waning alpha activity). No characteristic feature of the EEG in Stage REM emerged, although constant slope was intermittently observed, (as in Stage 1 non-REM sleep), especially if "sawtooth waves" were present.

In relation to non-REM sleep, it appears that the most useful of the measures of the EEG that have emerged from the extrema-slopes hypothesis are the running mean slope and the running mean amplitude (particularly the former), which are useful for identifying Stages 3 and 4 sleep and for identifying the transition between Stage 2 and Stages 3 and 4. If alpha activity is present, the decrease in the Spectral Purity Index from a value near 1.0 can indicate the onset of Stage 1, as can, of course, the decrease in running mean amplitude.

A Possible Continuous Depth-of-Sleep Indicator for Non-REM Sleep

The definitions of the various stages of non-REM sleep are given in chapter 6. Stages 3 and 4 of non-REM sleep (sometimes termed slow-wave sleep) are defined not as a continuum but in terms of a percentage of time (i.e., whether greater or less than 25%) of activity of a given amplitude (75 mV) and a given frequency (1 Hz). Such a definition hardly permits a continuous quantitative evaluation of the depth of sleep in these two stages. On the other hand, in computerized evaluation of the EEG during sleep, the objective is usually that of automatic sleep staging, the results of which are considered to be good if they are in agreement with the results of scoring by trained human observers. That is, a stepwise rather than a continuous evaluation of the EEG in sleep is attempted.

In contrast to the aforementioned stepwise evaluation of Stages 3 and 4 of non-REM sleep, the extrema-slopes hypothesis offers the possibility of a continuous evaluation, as follows.

In chapter 2, the constant-slope characteristic of Type 1 waves of the oscillator model was shown to be equivalent to a reciprocal relationship between amplitude and frequency, or, alternatively, a direct relationship between period (duration) and amplitude. It is further evident that a single number combining the increase of amplitude and the decrease of frequency of constant-slope waves (more exactly, waves of relatively constant mean slope) could be provided by the quotient of running mean amplitude to running mean frequency. Thus, the depth of slow-wave sleep can be expressed as

$$D_{sws} = \frac{\bar{a}}{\bar{f}} = \frac{\bar{a}}{\bar{s}/\bar{a}} = \frac{\bar{a}^2}{\bar{s}}.$$

But s is a constant for constant-slope waves; hence

$$D_{sws} = k(\bar{a}^2),$$

where k is a constant. The inconvenience of the nonlinear relationship can be eliminated by taking the logarithms of both sides:

$$\log D_{sws} = k + 2\log(\bar{a}).$$

Such a progressively increasing number with depth of sleep can be compared with the more complex information contained in the upward shift of the spectra of Stages 1–4 of non-REM sleep (figure 17.3). Stages 1 and 2 of non-REM sleep are not characterized by relatively constant slope (at least, in the case of Stage 1, relatively constant slope is intermittent at best, and in a minority of individuals), and hence such an index of depth of sleep cannot be applied to these stages of non-REM sleep.

Alternatively, the running mean frequency may itself be used as an indication of the depth of sleep, since it tends to decrease progressively from the waking state to Stage 4. The nature of the relationship is, however, not immediately apparent; it seems possible that a logarithmic scale may be more suitable than a linear scale. Frequency, of course, has the advantage of being normalized for amplitude of the EEG; amplitude is not.

Detection of Paroxysmal Slow Waves

In chapter 7 it was pointed out that irregular (random, polymorphic) delta slowing could be characterized as having relatively constant slope. In turn, this characteristic could be used as the basis of a slow-wave detection scheme using as a criterion a decreased variability (as measured by the Coefficient of Variation) of slope.

An important parameter in detecting brief slow-wave abnormalities is the width of the computational window. The running mean frequency, computed over a moving window of (e.g.) 0.5 sec, should in principle be more sensitive to transient or intermittent slow-wave abnormalities, which may be missed by the longer analysis windows (e.g., 2 or 4 sec) of conventional computerized EEG spectral analysis (e.g., compressed spectral arrays obtained by the fast Fourier transform, particularly after averaging of the latter (Oken et al. 1989).

Perioperative EEG Monitoring with Running Mean Frequency and the Spectral Purity Index: Carotid Endarterectomy

The development of methods for obtaining running means of amplitude, slope, frequency, and the (running) Spectral Purity Index, and also the Coefficient of Variation of these measures, is relevant to the general problem of EEG monitoring (Binnie 1986, Pronk 1986). As an example of such an application of these measures, monitoring the EEG as an indicator of adequacy of cerebral perfusion during carotid endarterectomy procedures will be considered. In such procedures, the EEG may be monitored for changes during test clamping of the carotid artery system, as a possible indication for bypassing the portion of the blood vessel being operated on by means of a shunt, during the endarterectomy procedure itself. (In an earlier study in which three methods of analysis of EEGs previously recorded during monitoring were compara-

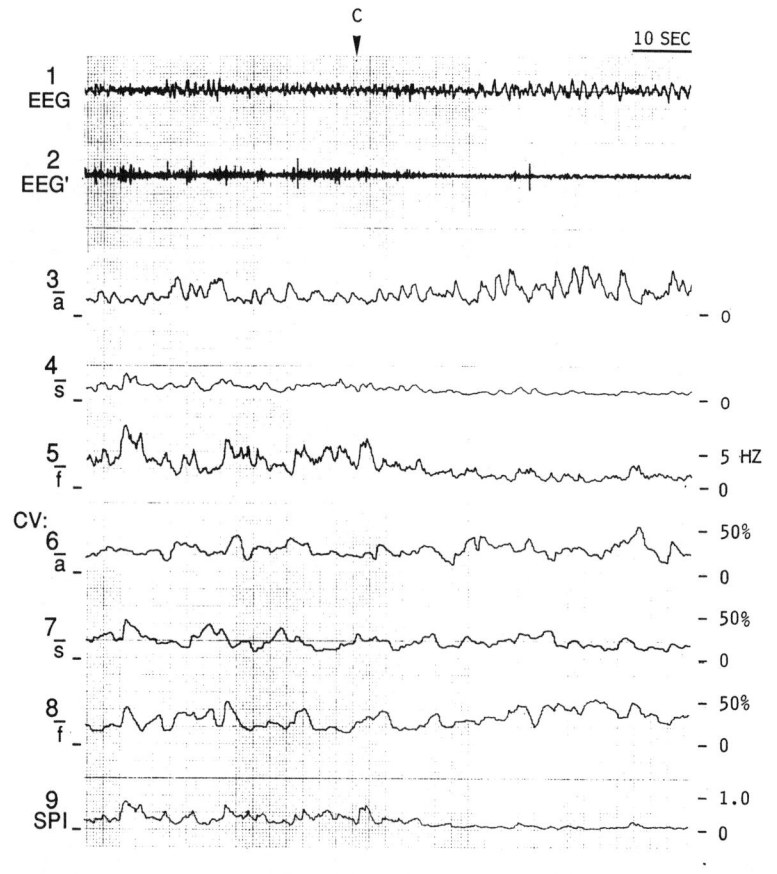

Figure 17.10 Original EEG and its analyses showing increased slow (0.8–1.0 Hz) and decreased fast activity (4–20 Hz) in response to arterial clamping during carotid endarterectomy. Traces in this and in figures 17.11–17.16 as follows: (1) original EEG, (2) its first derivative, (3) running mean amplitude, (4) running mean slope, (5) running mean frequency, (6–8) Coefficients of Variation for running mean amplitude, slope, and frequency, respectively, (9) Spectral Purity Index (SPI). C indicates clamping.

tively evaluated (Barlow 1984), the method of adaptive segmentation mentioned in chapter 7 above was found to be superior to inverse digital filtering and also to selective analog filtering in lower and higher frequency ranges, for detecting EEG changes.)

In the above-cited study, four types of EEG responses to carotid clamping were found: increased slow (0.8–1.0 Hz) activity and decreased fast (4–30 Hz) activity; no change of slow but decreased fast; decreased slow and decreased fast; and no change in slow and no change in fast. In the reanalysis of those EEG recordings by the present methods, an additional type of response was found: increased slow with no change of fast. The analyses of the original representative examples of responses of the original four types (in reordered sequence) are shown together with the analysis of an example of the fifth type in figures 17.10–17.16. In the present analyses, an increased running mean amplitude can be taken to be the approximate equivalent of the earlier "slow" activity, and an increased running mean slope (which, for a given amplitude, increases linearly with increasing frequency) can be taken to be the approximate equivalent of the earlier "fast" activity. Additionally, the running mean

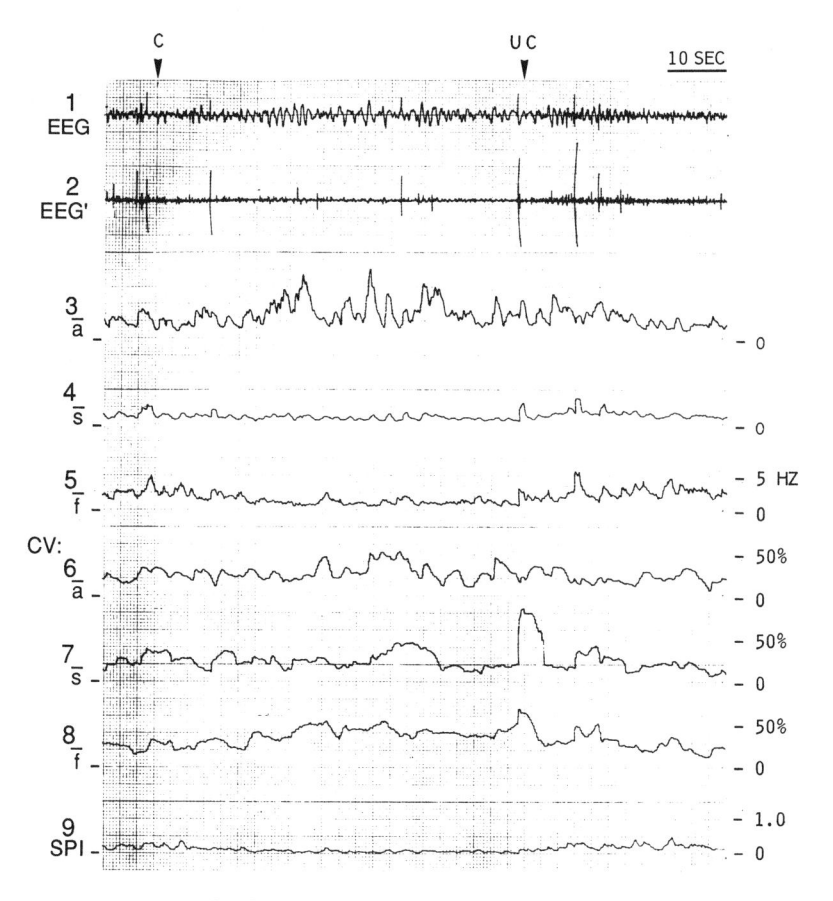

Figure 17.11 Carotid endarterectomy EEG showing no change in slow activity but decreased fast activity. Several artifacts are apparent in the EEG (trace 1).

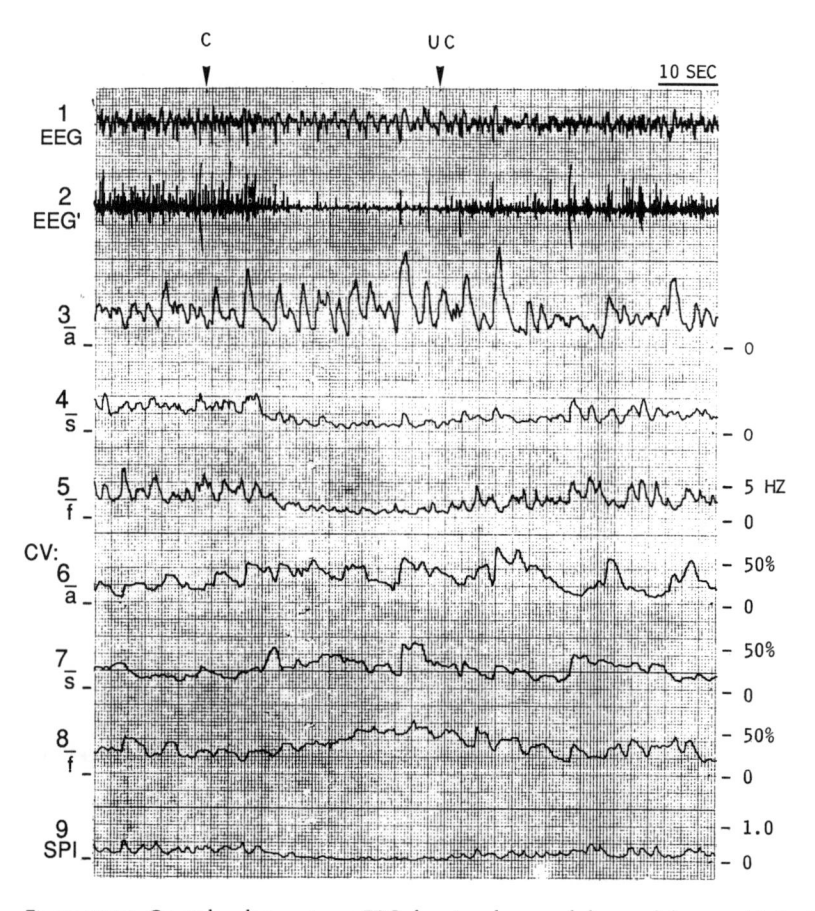

Figure 17.12 Carotid endarterectomy EEG showing decreased slow and decreased fast activity.

frequency can be taken as an approximate indication of the relative content in the EEG of the two.

With the fifth type of response (no change of slow or of fast activity; see figure 17.14) used as a reference, it is evident that in each of the remaining four types a decrease in the running mean frequency follows a latent period after the clamping, irrespective of the behavior of the slow activity and the fast activity (i.e., the running mean amplitude and the running mean slope, respectively) considered individually. (An additional measure was also explored, namely the quotient of the running mean amplitude and the running mean frequency (cf. Riehl 1963); the quotient is not actually an independent determination, since running mean frequency is partly determined by running mean amplitude. In any case, this measure was not found to be as reliable an indication of EEG changes of the various types in this series as the running mean frequency.)

In figure 17.11, it is evident that the running mean slope (Trace 4) in the second type of response is suggestive of relatively constant slope in the period after clamping, in contrast to the marked increase in the running mean amplitude (Trace 3). Such a constant-slope behavior is also evident in the EEG

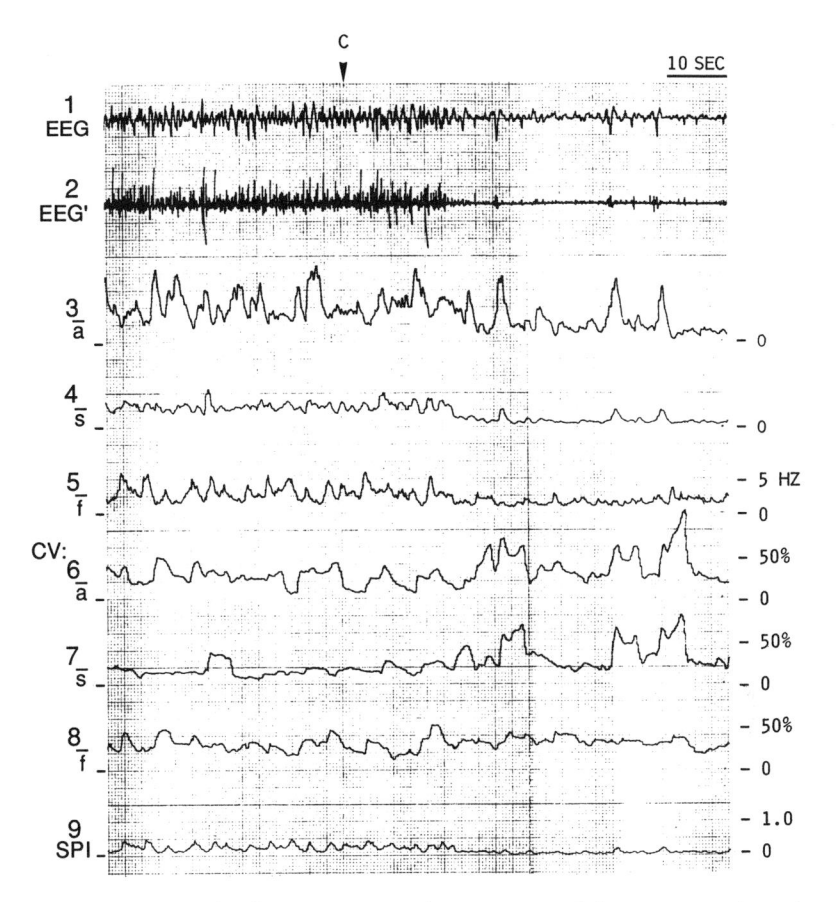

Figure 17.13 Carotid endarterectomy EEG showing increased slow activity with no change in fast activity.

shown in figures 17.15 and 17.16, but only on the side opposite the clamping (figure 17.16). For the side ipsilateral to the clamping, the running mean slope decreases after clamping (figure 17.15). Comparison of the results for the two sides suggests that for this EEG the effects of clamping were also reflected on the opposite side, but to a less pronounced degree—i.e., that a constant-slope effect indicates a more moderate degree of impairment of cerebral circulation than does a decreasing running mean slope, after clamping. (Blume and Sharbrough (1987) discuss moderate vs. major or severe EEG changes during clamping in relation to the reversibility of the changes resulting from decreased cerebral perfusion.)

Overall, these results for EEG monitoring during carotid endarterectomy indicate that the running mean amplitude and the running mean slope represent considerable improvements over the earlier measures of "fast activity" (4–30 Hz) and "slow activity" (0.8–1.0 Hz) that were derived by analog filtering (Barlow 1984). Moreover, the quotient of the running mean slope and the running mean amplitude, i.e., the running mean frequency, would appear to offer the basis of determining and signaling a significant change in the EEG,

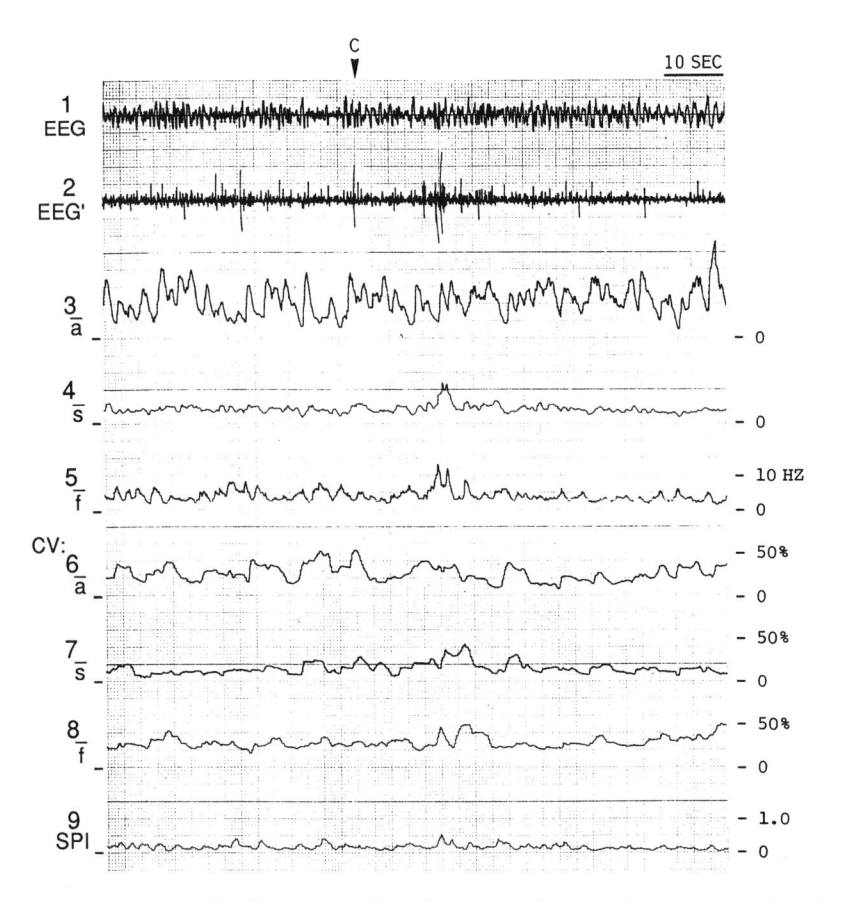

Figure 17.14 Carotid endarterectomy EEG showing no change in slow activity and no change in fast activity.

if a reference value were taken immediately before or immediately after clamping and if subsequent values were expressed as (e.g.) a percentage of the pre-clamping reference (i.e., trend monitoring). In contrast to the earlier method of adaptive segmentation, which was necessarily an off-line (after-the-fact) method of analysis, the present method is an on-line one and could be employed in the operating room. (For multi-channel EEG monitoring recordings, one possible display would consist of a topographic map of the scalp employing a color scale for the running mean frequency, progressing from blue for the beta range through green for the alpha range, orange for the theta range, and red for the delta range of activity; such a display would not, however, indicate differences of amplitude between the two sides.) Artifact is, of course, always a possibility in EEG monitoring.

In brief: These limited results suggest that the relatively simple on-line technique of multi-channel determination of running mean frequency may merit further exploration and comparative evaluation in relation to other techniques, including other methods of determining average frequency (e.g., Hjorth's normalized slope descriptors—see chapter 25) for EEG monitoring (Binnie 1986; Pronk 1986; Blume and Sharbrough 1987; Daube et al. 1990).

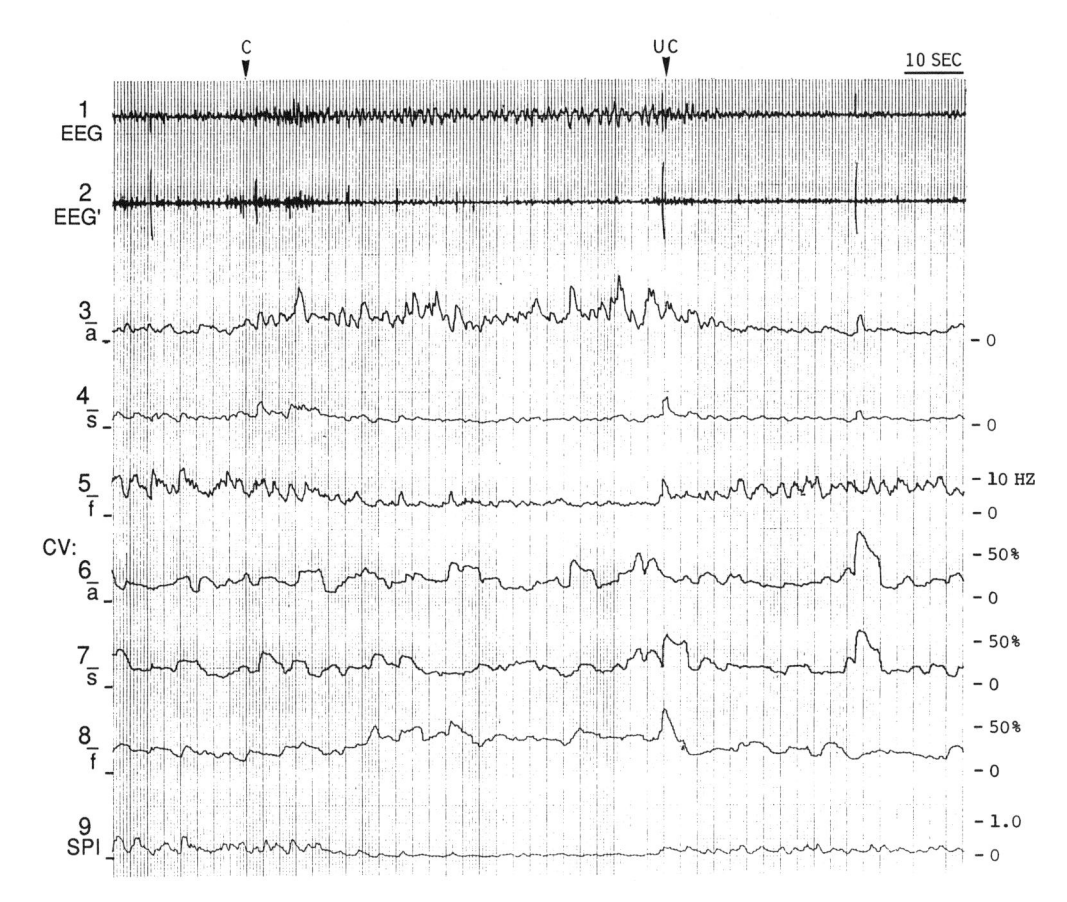

Figure 17.15 Analysis of a bilateral EEG recording before, during, and after carotid clamping: EEG from the same side as the clamping. Identification of traces as in figure 17.10. Note that the running mean slope tends to decrease during the clamping.

Continuous write-outs of running means of amplitude and frequency do not have the disadvantage that may be encountered in compressed spectral arrays when a flat spectrum indicating a sudden decrease in EEG voltage may be hidden for a time behind the immediately preceding spectra. (The latter can be diminished by the use of an isometric display, as shown in figure A.3 of appendix A, or eliminated by using a density spectral array.)

Running Means of Amplitude and Frequency as Preprocessed Measures for Adaptive Segmentation

It was pointed out above in the section on quasi-linear methods that adaptive segmentation entails a rather complex and time-consuming procedure of determining running mean amplitude and running mean frequency from autocorrelation functions.

The question arose at the very beginning of the present work of whether the running mean amplitude and the running mean frequency would suffice as preprocessed data for segmentation. (Indeed, as was pointed out in the intro-

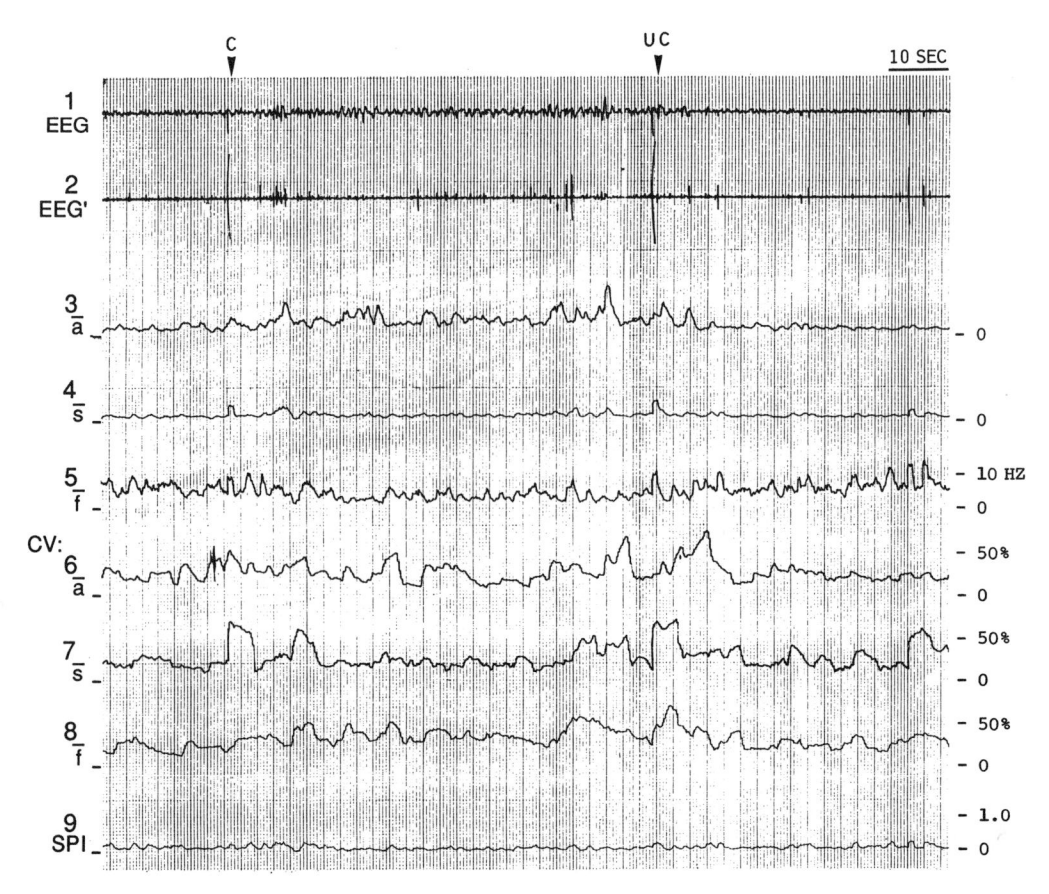

Figure 17.16 Analysis of a bilateral EEG recording before, during, and after carotid clamping: EEG from the side opposite to clamping (same recording as for figure 17.15). Note that the running mean slope remains relatively unchanged during the clamping.

duction, it was with this question that the present approach originated.) The question can be considered in relation to figure 17.17, in which the same EEG section as in figure 17.7 was analyzed. During the three high-voltage paroxysmal bursts, the running mean amplitude (trace 3) increases, there is a small increase in the running mean slope (trace 4), and there is evidently a decrease in the running mean frequency (trace 5) . There are also changes in the Coefficients of Variation for amplitude (trace 6) and for frequency (trace 8), and to a lesser extent for the SPI (trace 9). Although these measures indicate the occurrence of the paroxysmal events, they do not very well indicate the onset and the termination of the two paroxysms. In any event, determining the latter would be a task for the computer program (algorithm) for segmentation, which should be adaptable to such preprocessed data on mean amplitude and mean frequency. (The onset of the paroxysms could be relatively well marked by some combination of the beginning of the rise of the Coefficient of Variation for the runing mean amplitude and for the running mean slope (traces 6 and 8, respectively). The Coefficients of Variation are, of course, normalized, and are therefore independent of the original EEG amplitude

262   Chapter 17

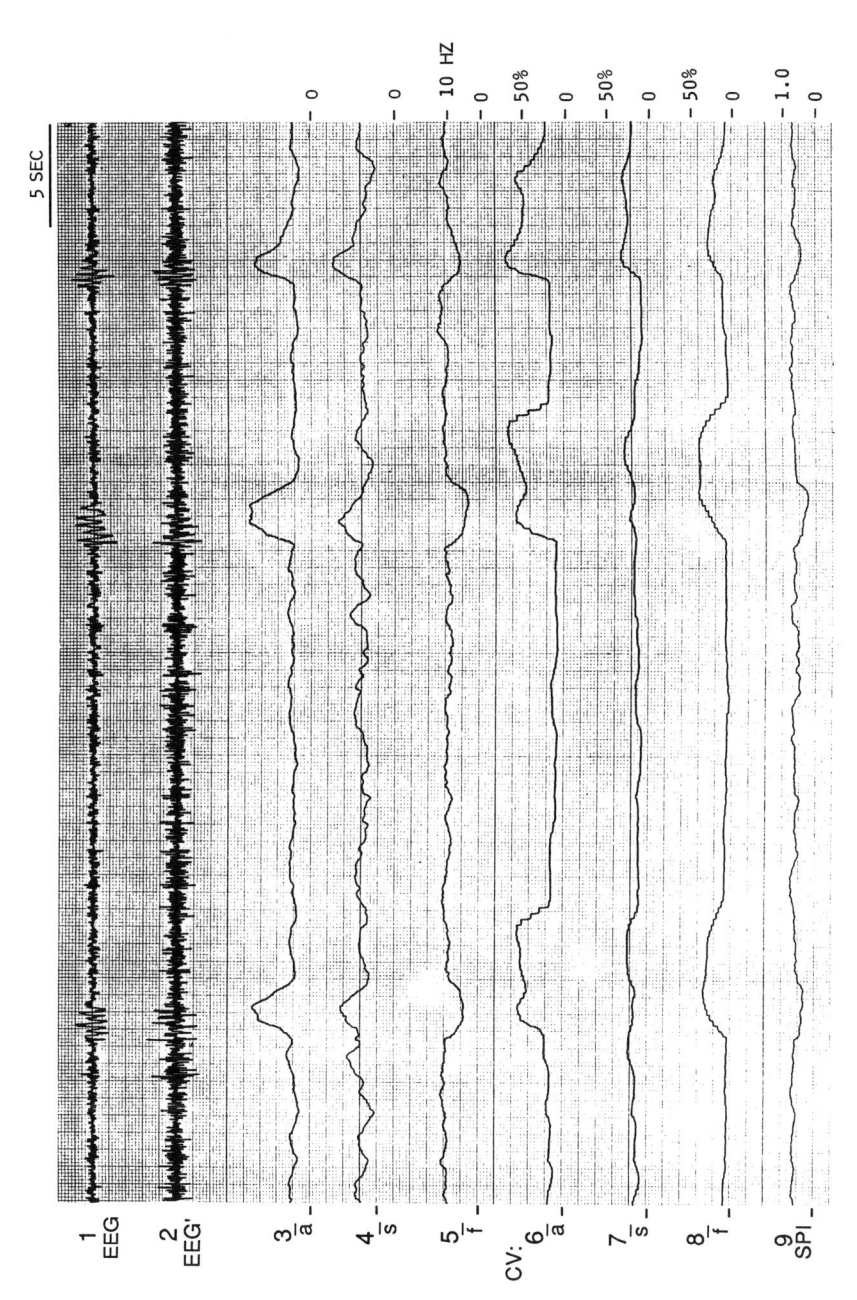

Figure 17.17 Analysis of the same EEG (007) as in figure 17.7, showing changes during three paroxysms (bursts). Trace identification as in figure 17.10. (Trace 4 is the running mean slope displayed at twice the scale factor as in figures 17.10–17.16.)

(trace 1). It is clear that repositioning of the leading edge of the averaging windows for the running means so as to coincide with the segment boundary would be necessary for marking a segment boundary at the end of the paroxysms (figure 17.7). (The decrease in the Spectral Purity Index (trace 9) during the paroxysms can be attributed to the greater spread of frequency components at those times.)

In brief: It appears that the running mean amplitude and the running mean frequency could serve as preprocessing techniques for the adaptive segmentation of EEGs. On the other hand, it is perhaps questionable that segmentation according to amplitude and slope would be more efficacious than segmentation according to amplitude and frequency, if the basic difficulty in the combined techiques of adaptive segmentation and clustering of the resultant segments lies in the clustering process, as mentioned above, rather than in the segmentation process. In any event, this question has been set aside with the emergence of the extrema-slopes hypothesis.

Relationships among Multi-Channel EEG Recordings

Although the question of the extension of the extrema-slopes hypothesis to multiple EEG channels is not dealt with in this book, it is clear that the Coefficient of Determination, used in the present studies as a quantitative measure of the degree of similarity between the running means and the instantaneous envelopes of the EEG and of its first derivative, could be a convenient index of the degree of similarity between the envelope of the EEG signals from two recording sites, e.g., comparable (homotopic) points on the two sides of the scalp. One such application could be that of comparing bursts of activity of the two hemispheres in premature infants, the degree of synchrony of which is useful in estimating levels of maturation (Lombroso 1987; Niedermeyer 1987b; Hrachovy et al. 1990).

In relation to topographic displays of multi-channel EEG data, which have become increasingly widely used (see, e.g, Dubinsky and Barlow 1980 and Duffy 1986), running mean frequencies, displayed on a map of the scalp on a gray or color scale, may be attractive as a parameter for display, since running mean frequency is easier to compute as the quotient of mean slope to mean amplitude (using, e.g., a 0.5-sec averaging window) than it is via the formal spectrum derived from the fast Fourier transform.

Detection of Interictal Epileptiform Events

Perhaps the most potentially useful application of the present set of techniques for analyzing the EEG would be that of the detection and identification of epileptiform events by combined simultaneous analysis of both the spike (or sharp-wave) and the slow-wave components in the interictal spike-and-slow-wave complex of focal epilepsy (chapter 8). In considering this possibility, however, it should be noted that the slow-wave component of a spike-and-slow-wave complex may be distributed more widely than the spike component, and attenuated less than the spike component, in scalp recordings (Abraham and Ajmone-Marsan 1958; Klass 1975). Nonetheless, since the slow-wave component is often present in the interictal scalp discharge, its inclusion in computerized methods of detecting and identifying epileptiform transients seems reasonable in any case.

Such a combined evaluation of spike and of slow-wave component is well established for detection of repetitive (and also irregular) patterns, such as 3-Hz spike-wave events (see below). However, in the case of spike-and-slow-wave complexes or sharp-and-slow-wave complexes, it is often the case that detection and identification of only the spike component is attempted (see, e.g., Gotman 1986). An exception is the approach of Ma et al. (1976), who implemented an automated pattern-recognition technique and found that 75 percent of spikes were followed by slow waves lasting from 130 to 500 msec.

It has been customary to define the spike (sharp wave) itself in terms of certain parameters, such as amplitude and slope, evaluated at certain times (e.g., rising or falling phase, inflection points, half-waves) (Frost 1985; Gotman 1980; Ktonas 1987). Additionally, such running measures as instantaneous amplitude (not to be confused with the instantaneous envelope of the EEG), instantaneous slope, and instantaneous curvature have been used (an earlier review appears in Barlow 1979). (A simplified arithmetic detector for EEG sharp transients (Qian et al. 1988), which employed a slope-duration detector, can be considered as a simplified method of using the instantaneous envelope of the first derivative of the EEG as one of the criteria for detecting sharp transients.)

But such arbitrarily selected features of interictal spike-and-slow-wave epileptiform events tend to vary, since the original EEG waveforms of such events vary even at the same recording site on the scalp (see figure 17.18,

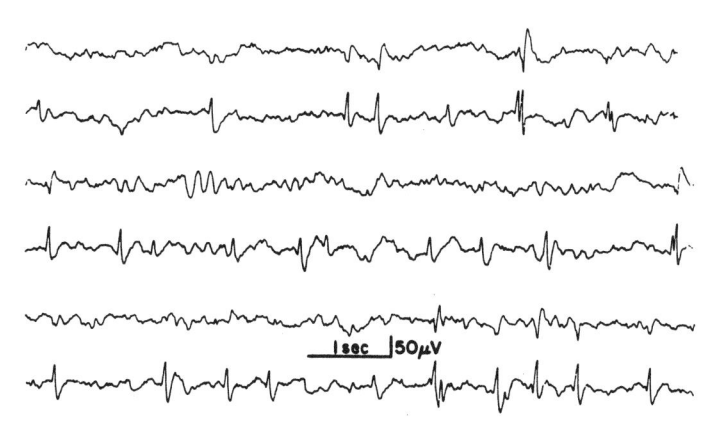

Figure 17.18 Variability of spike morphology at the same recording site in a 6-year-old patient. Three paired left-sided (bipolar) traces are shown, the upper trace of each pair is the midtemporal to posterior-temporal (T3–T5) derivation, the lower trace being the posterior-temporal to occipital derivation (T5–O1). Note that the spike (negative at the active electrode, T5) is inconstantly present in the upper trace, and that an associated slow-wave is often present. (From Niedermeyer 1987c.)

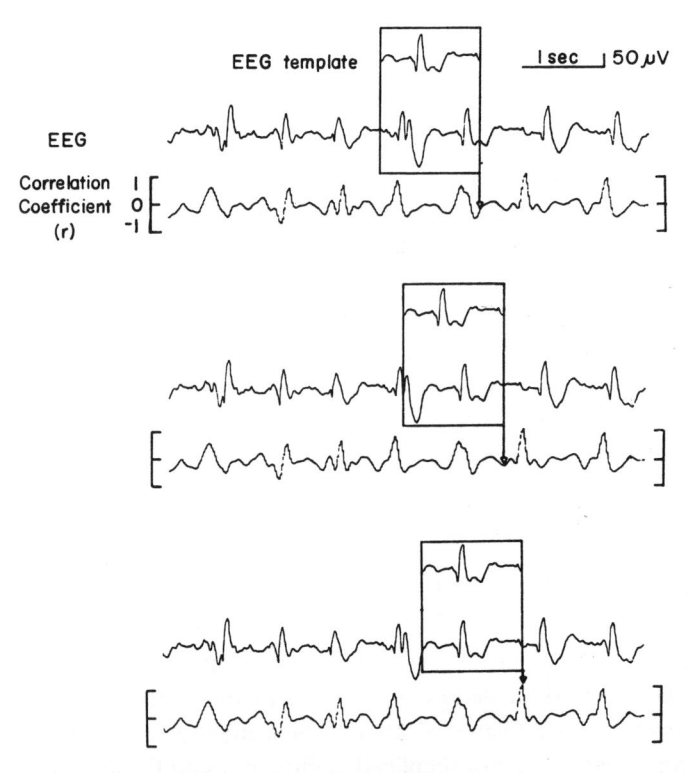

Figure 17.19 Template matching of an epileptiform pattern with an EEG. The same portion of the computer write-out is reproduced three times; in each instance, the rectangle indicates the time window for comparison of template and EEG. In the first two panels there is no match, but in the third the template and the EEG match exactly (since the template was taken from this section of the EEG) and hence the correlation coefficient reaches a peak of 1.0. However, because of the variability of the preceding and following epileptiform events, the peak value of the correlation coefficient is also quite variable; for all other events, it is less than 1.0. (From Barlow and Dubinsky 1976.)

or figures 3 and 5 in Frost 1985), rendering reliable detection of such events (e.g., by template matching—see figure 17.19) more difficult. A part of this variability may result from superimposed background EEG activity, but at least some of the variability may be inherent in the epileptiform-transient generating mechanism. Indeed, *epileptiform discharges* is used as a general term for spikes (less than 80 msec) and sharp waves (80–200 msec) (Daly 1990). In computerized studies, the distinction is usually ignored. But even this clinical usage omits mention of the slow-wave component.

If the extrema-slopes hypothesis is indeed an appropriate one for epileptiform patterns, then appreciable variability of spike or slow-wave patterns (or, more generally, of spike-and-slow-wave complexes) would not be surprising, since the exact waveform of a given event would then be at least partially dependent on its immediately preceding history, even for identical modulations, according to the hypothesis. It is conceivable, however that the variability of the immediately prior EEG history would introduce less variability into the instantaneous envelope of spike-and-slow-wave complexes than into the instantaneous EEG itself during an epileptiform transient.

It thus seems possible that the use of the information provided by the instantaneous envelopes of the EEG and of its first derivative (chapter 8), or in combined form as their quotient, the instantaneous frequency (chapter 29), could provide a basis for more reliable detection of interictal spike-and-slow-wave epileptiform events. The possibility could be tested by determining whether the variability of the waveshape (morphology) of the instantaneous envelope of the EEG and of its first derivative, or in their combined form, the instantaneous frequency, was smaller than the variability in the instantaneous amplitudes, slopes, and curvatures of the original spike-and-slow-wave complexes themselves. (The instantaneous frequency takes all of the latter three measures into account, although in practice the evaluation of the instantaneous frequency can be seriously impeded by "noise" in the EEG.)

A further possibility would be to employ the instantaneous measures themselves in template-matching schemes. At least, the present approach formally takes the slow-wave component of the complex into account. (The incorporation of the slow-wave component of the spike-and-slow-wave complex into a method of detecting and identifying the complex as a whole should be distinguished from the use of ongoing delta activity as an aid in localization of epileptic foci, e.g., during electrocorticography (Panet-Raymond and Gotman 1990).)

Further, the incorporation of the complete spike-and-slow-wave complex (rather than the spike component alone) into methods for improving the efficacy of computerized detection of epileptiform events, such as context-dependent and state-dependent detection (i.e., of altering spike-detection thresholds according to the type of background EEG activity; see Glover et al. 1989, Gotman 1990a, and Gotman and Wang 1991) could perhaps improve the detection efficiency still more, at least for certain types of epileptiform patterns.

As was mentioned in chapter 8, there is some suggestion of an exponential decrease in the instantaneous envelope of the first derivative of the EEG for spike-and-slow-wave complexes. If this is indeed the case, then it may be possible to characterize a spike-and-slow-wave event by a single number, namely the slope of a logarithmic plot of the instantaneous envelope of the first derivative of the EEG. (A possible alternative is a logarithmic plot of the instantaneous frequency of the EEG.) The detection of a spike-and-slow-wave complex would then consist of identifying such a "decay constant" over a duration of time commensurate with (or perhaps somewhat less than) the usual duration of such events (e.g., 0.5 sec). In view of "noise" arising from the background EEG in such a determination, some smoothing (e.g., with a transversal filter; see chapter 23) may be necessary; such "windowing" would have the added advantage of diminishing muscle artifact, not infrequently a problem in the detection of epileptiform activity (Barlow 1986).

Characterizing interictal epileptiform transients in this way may also aid in formulating more precise definitions of such events, at least for computerized detection, since the definitions for clinical EEG practice (Chatrian et al. 1974) are not very satisfactory for formulating computerized detection regimes (Ktonas et al. 1981; Ktonas 1987).

Detection of 3-Hz Spike-Wave Activity

The detection of 3-Hz spike-wave patterns is, in general, a simpler problem than the detection of spike-and-slow-wave complexes, because the 3-Hz spike-wave pattern is often repetitive (although often less so in sleep), because it is much more widely distributed, and because interference from unrelated background EEG activity is less likely. The results presented in chapter 8 suggest that a relatively simple detection routine for the 3-Hz spike-wave pattern could be template matching of the logarithm of the instantaneous frequency; the expected waveform for the latter is a repetitive sawtooth. Alternatively, a detection scheme could, in principle, be based on the expectation that the first derivative of the logarithm of the instantaneous frequency would be relatively constant, save for a transient at the transition point between the end of a slow wave and the next spike; the associated noise level, however, may be prohibitive.

Asymmetry of Spike Waveforms

A much-discussed question in relation to the interictal epileptiform spike is that of whether the leading or the trailing portion (i.e., the first or the second half-wave) of a spike or sharp wave has the greater slope. From visual inspection of scalp-recorded EEGs, Gloor (1977) concluded that the first half-wave was steeper. Ktonas et al. (1981) found that, for the EEGs from two patients, the slope of the trailing edge was greater than that of the leading edge for spikes, but not for sharp waves.

Gotman (1980), who studied a larger series of monophasic spikes and sharp waves, also found that, when there was such a difference, which was the case in 30 percent of instances, the slope of the second half-wave was greater than that of the first. Gotman contrasted this finding in humans with findings from the topical penicillin model of focal epilepsy, in which the first half-wave of spikes was markedly steeper than that of the second.

In preliminary results from studies on epileptic spike morphology of recordings from intracerebral electrodes, which were mentioned in the same report, Gotman (1980) found that both types of slope asymmetries were frequently encountered. Lemieux and Blume (1983) found that about half of the epileptiform events they studied in electrocorticograms had unequal slopes, the first half-wave being the steeper. These authors did not include the early spike component of the spike-wave pattern, in view of the fact that it appeared only inconsistently; attention had been drawn to such an early spike component in the classical 3-Hz spike-wave pattern by Weir (1965).

For scalp-recorded spikes in spike-and-slow-wave complexes, Blume and Lemieux (1988) found that the difference between slopes of the first and second half-waves depended on the technique by which slopes were determined. Thus, the slope for the entire first half-wave was usually equal to or greater than that for the second half-wave, whereas if the slopes of only the upper half of the spike were measured the slope before the peak was usually less than that after the crest of the peak. Blume and Lemieux (1988) pointed out that Gotman's (1980) use of the latter method accounted for the apparent discrepancy between his results and those of Gloor (1977).

In determinations of the slopes of spikes, the possibility of distortion resulting from inadequate low-frequency response should be kept in mind. This effect is such that, for a spike approximated by one cycle of a monophasic triangular wave, the slopes will be equal if there is an adequate high-frequency response. On the other hand, if an inadequate high-frequency response results in slight prolongation of the rise time and also of the fall time of the spike, then determining the slope on the basis of the entire half-waves will result in equal values, whereas if the determination is based only on the upper halves of each half-wave the second half-wave (i.e., the trailing edge) of the spike will have the greater slope. This effect is at least partially consistent with the above-mentioned distinction made by Blume and Lemieux (1980); it is also consistent with the present findings that the instantaneous envelope of the slope was greatest at the onset of the spike component, progressively decreasing thereafter, apparently in the manner of an exponential decay (chapter 8).

In any event, it is evident that the technique of evaluating the instantaneous envelope of the first derivative of the EEG throughout the course of a spike or a sharp wave could provide a definitive answer to the question of the relative slopes of their several portions. The results presented in chapter 8 suggest that it is the earliest component of the spike that has the greatest slope.

Evaluation of Spike Parameters in Relation to Clinical Seizure Control

An easier problem to attack than the above-mentioned question of possible subtle manifestations of epileptiform activity is that of tracking possible changes in epileptiform patterns as a result of medication. Frost and Kellaway (1981) found that bringing focal motor epilepsy under clinical control was accompanied by a change in spike parameters, i.e., a decrease in amplitude and duration and an increase in the normalized sharpness (defined as the ratio of the second derivative at the major peak to the amplitude of the latter). These results could be considered to be consistent with a smaller active area of the epileptic focus.

Subsequently, Frost et al. (1986) reported that control of seizures in focal epilepsy was associated with a decrease in interictal spike amplitude and duration, an increase in normalized sharpness (as defined above), and a decrease in the composite spike parameter (CSP). The CSP was defined as

$$\text{CSP} = \frac{k(\overline{A} \cdot \overline{D})}{\overline{S/A}},$$

where, for each sample of spikes, $\overline{A}$ is the mean amplitude, $\overline{D}$ is the mean duration, $\overline{S/A}$ is the mean normalized second-derivative value at the peak (i.e., the sharpness), and k is a constant scaling factor. Frost et al. point out that the CSP, which is decreased by a decrease in spike amplitude or duration or by an increase in the normalized sharpness, provides a single characterizing parameter for a given spike sample.

Since the present parameters of the instantaneous envelope of slope and the instantaneous frequency are based on the EEG and on its first and second derivatives, some parallel may be expected between their behavior and the CSP of Frost et al. (1986). An important difference is that the present measures are computed for the entire interictal spike-and-slow-wave complex, including the slow-wave component, not only for the spike component. If anti-epileptic medication results in changes in the slow-wave component as well as in the spike component, then the slope of a logarithmic plot of the instantaneous envelope of the first derivative of the EEG (or possibly of the instantaneous frequency) for the duration of a spike-and-slow-wave complex might be comparatively evaluated with the composite spike parameter as a possible index of the efficacy of medication for epilepsy.

Detection of Possible Subtle (Non-Ictal, Non-Interictal) EEG Manifestations of Epilepsy

If epilepsy is taken to be a reflection of an abnormal preponderance of cortical excitatory over inhibitory activity, then it might be supposed that some more subtle indication of such an imbalance might be present continuously (Symonds 1962), not just during an interictal epileptiform event or an ictal manifestation. The verification of the presence of the latter manifestions may require long-term monitoring for some days (Gotman 1982; Gotman et al. 1985; Kaplan and Lesser 1990). Detecting such subtle manifestations (if, indeed, any are present) is a formidable problem. This question has not been examined in relation to the extrema-slopes hypothesis; however, the Coefficient of Variation of the instantaneous frequency, or of the instantaneous envelope of the first derivative of the EEG, might be examined. It should be kept in mind, in this conection, that the ictal EEG manifestations can be different from even the overt interictal manifestations. As an example, the spike-and-slow-wave complex appearing in the temporal regions of the scalp as an interictal manifestation, in contrast to quasi-rhythmic theta (e.g., 6–7 Hz) activity as an initial ictal manifestation in complex partial seizures (temporal-lobe seizures), could be cited.

As was mentioned in chapter 7, the beginning of a change from a constant-slope pattern to a constant-frequency pattern that was encountered in a limited number of slow-wave EEGs may be such a subtle EEG manifestation, in this case, of the 3-Hz spike-wave epileptiform pattern.

A possible difficulty in such a proposed test for epileptogenicity is that the EEG pattern of intermittent rhythmic delta slowing (see chapter 13) can also occur in metabolic disorders, among other diseases. This possibility has not been examined.

As relatively simple on-line, real-time, running means of amplitude, slope, and frequency, their Coefficients of Variation and the Spectral Purity Index may be useful measures in the evaluation of changes in EEG activity before, during, and after electrical seizure activity (Simon et al. 1976).

18 Limitations of the Scope of the Present Work

Although the basic hypothesis and its associated model are relatively comprehensive in scope, there have necessarily been limitations in the compass of the work itself. Thus, only a limited number of types of normal and abnormal EEG patterns, as well as a limited number of examples of each type, and only a single channel of each, have been examined in relation to the hypothesis. In contrast, the standard clinical EEG usually includes at least 18 channels recorded simultaneously from combinations of electrodes distributed over the scalp. But if a sufficient diversity of single-channel EEG patterns are examined, then the lack of study of simultaneously recorded multi-channel EEGs becomes somewhat less important.

Further, the technique of reconstitution of EEGs—which is specifically based on the extrema-slopes hypothesis in determining the instantaneous envelopes of the EEG and of its first derivative and in reconstituting the latter pair of signals by means of the oscillator model—gives every indication of being able to handle any type of EEG pattern, irrespective of the degree of complexity.

The EEGs studied have been entirely limited to scalp recordings; no recordings from the surface of the brain (electrocorticograms) or from electrodes in the substance of the brain have been studied. Nonetheless, the hypothesis may be relevant to EEG recordings made from the exposed cortex (more exactly, the neocortex), or from other parts of the brain (e.g., the hippocampus). (Recordings of the former type could be of particular interest in view of the unusual and unanticipated, but predictable, relationship between the spectra of Type 3 and Type 4 waves described in chapter 5 (figures 5.9–5.11.)

The question of multi-channel EEGs in relation to the extrema-slopes hypothesis raises the question of interactions between two or more oscillator models, a matter that has not been specifically examined. On the other hand, tests that have been carried out indicate that, in the case of rhythmic oscillations (e.g., simulated alpha), the oscillator model is clearly capable of mutual entrainment with another oscillator model, as would be expected. Mutual entrainability of two oscillators, or of an ensemble, requires that they be nonlinear—a requirement met by the present oscillator model. It may be pointed out, in this connection, that some of the methods of analysis that have been employed for testing the extrema-slopes model for a single EEG channel are also applicable to pairs of channels in multi-channel EEG recordings, e.g., the Pearson Product-Moment Correlation Coefficient and its square, the Coefficient of Determination. These measures can be employed to determine the similarity of the envelopes of two simultaneously recorded EEG signals. Examples include the question of synchrony and asynchrony of the envelopes of bilateral alpha activity, as contrasted with the synchrony and asynchrony of individual waves of bilateral alpha activity themselves (Garoutte and Aird 1958; Hoovey et al. 1972), and the maturational aspects of synchrony and asynchrony of envelopes of bursts in the premature infant (mentioned in chapter 17 above). (Lopes da Silva et al. (1989) have pointed out, however, that the most reliable techniques for exploring relationships among activities from different scalp area may be rather cumbersome, entailing nonlinear methods.)

The number of epileptiform patterns examined has been limited. Thus, although the 3-Hz spike-wave pattern, the slow (2–2.5 Hz) spike-wave pattern of the Lennox-Gastaut syndrome, and the spike-and-slow-wave complex pattern of focal epilepsy have been considered (chapters 4 and 8), EEG patterns during other types of seizures (such as those associated with generalized tonic-clonic convulsions) have not been explored. (In the latter, the onset is often marked by the relatively sudden onset of a "desynchronized" pattern, proceeding rapidly to rhythmic, about 10 Hz activity of rapidly increasing voltage, followed by theta and delta slowing with polyspike-and-wave complexes (Niedermeyer 1987e).)

Maturational aspects of the EEG, beginning from the *tracé discontinu* (periods of activity alternating with periods of much lower voltage or no activity) of the early premature infant, are not explictly discussed. Among other questions is that of the transition from relatively irregular to more nearly regular or rhythmic activity in early childhood (in terms of the oscillator model, a shift from preponderantly Type 4 (irregular) waves to a mixture of Type 3 (rhythmic) and Type 4 (irregular) waves, and the gradual increase in frequency of the posterior rhythm eventually to become the alpha rhythm in those individuals whose EEGs exhibit the latter. From the perspective of the extrema-slopes hypothesis, such a progressive increase in frequency could readily be accounted for by a progressive increase in the average level of the EEG slope, but an alternative possibility is a progressive increase in the frequency of the intrinsic oscillations of the oscillator model. (Actually, the two alternatives are ultimately equivalent.)

In the consideration of the EEG in non-REM sleep, sleep spindles (as a form of rhythmic activity, at about 14 Hz in the adult) have not been explicitly discussed, nor have vertex sharp transients, except to note that that the quasi-frequency of the latter approximates that of the irregular background EEG (i.e., about 5 Hz; see chapter 6) for Stage 2 sleep.

The phenomenon of postictal slowing after generalized seizures (which contrasts with the lack of such slowing after the "absence seizures" that are often associated with the 3-Hz spike-wave pattern) is not dealt with, save that, in the generalized formulation (chapter 16) based on the extrema-slopes hypothesis, the slowing implies a predominance of inhibition over excitation (chapter 16) during the postictal period. (In connection with extreme postictal slowing, it is of interest that an unusual configuration of the oscillator model results in output waves that can be very slow indeed (1 Hz or less); the configuration is similar to that for Type 3 (rhythmic or constant-frequency) waves, except that the otherwise identical input modulations for extrema and slopes are of opposite, rather than the same, polarity.)

The sometimes clinically difficult problem of distinguishing between the normal variant pattern of "small sharp spikes" ("benign epileptiform transients" or "benign sporadic sleep spikes") and true interictal spike-and-slow-wave complexes (Westmoreland 1990) has not been explored.

The question of event-related potentials, including stimulus-evoked potentials (in particular, for flash stimuli), and their interrelationships with the ongoing EEG activity (Barlow 1960, 1962a; Barlow and Trabka 1961; Barlow and Estrin 1971; Lansing and Barlow 1972), has not been explicitly considered. One of the effects of flash stimuli appears to be that of resetting the phase of a subpopulation of alpha-activity generators so as to be time-locked to the stimuli (i.e., the "rhythmic sensory afterdischarge")—an effect which, like the mutual entrainment cited above, requires a nonlinear physiological mechanism. Tests with the oscillator model indicate such a capability of being reset in phase by an externally applied pulse, analogous to a flash stimulus as would be expected with a nonlinear oscillator (Barlow 1962c). (On the other hand, there is evidence that the phase of most alpha-generating units appears not to change after the alpha-blocking period associated with event-related potentials (Goldstein 1970).)

Some particular topographic features of the EEG have not been discussed. For example, in children, is the *posterior* predominance of (normal) high-voltage hyperventilation-induced slowing, in contrast to the (abnormal) *anterior* predominance of 3-Hz spike-wave activity, a matter of intrinsic organization of the cerebral cortex, or is this difference a matter of the nature of the particular corticothalamic interrelationships? (In contrast, the normal background EEG voltage is usually lower anteriorly (the "desynchronized" pattern) than posteriorly (e.g., for alpha activity.)

Attention has been drawn several times to the fact that, in the reconstitution of EEGs on the basis of the instantaneous envelopes of the originals and of their first derivatives (chapter 9), the polarity of the original EEG is not in general retained (although with some special additions to the relevant electronic circuit (chapter 29) the ambiguity can be diminished somewhat). This limitation, which is most noticeable for asymmetrical patterns such as the mu rhythm (figure 4.11) and for epileptiform events (figure 9.9), is an inherent characteristic of the reconstitution of EEGs on the basis of the respective instantaneous envelopes. At the least, it is apparent that the generally negative polarity of epileptiform spikes and sharp waves is determined by some factor other than the instantaneous envelope of the slope of the spike, since the latter is lacking in information about the sign of the instantaneous slope. On the other hand, the problem is encountered only in the reconstitution of asymmetrical EEG problems, not in their characterization (e.g., traces 2 and 3 in figure 8.6, and traces 7 and 8 in figure 9.9).

In the discussion of the relationship of the present findings to underlying physiological mechanisms, the perspective is one in which the EEG is taken as a reflection primarily of synaptic events. The possibility of any additional contributions to the EEG resulting from electrical transmission (as opposed to chemical transmission), or that of intracellular rhythmic processes, is not taken into account.

Additional questions that may be asked of the extrema-slopes hypothesis (or, for that matter, of any model of the EEG) could include the following:

• Is the very high voltage (300 mV or more, as compared with, e.g., 50 mV for alpha activity) that can be seen in the 3-Hz spike-wave pattern fully explained by widespread synchronization anteriorly in the cortex?

• Why does hyperventilation-induced or sleep-induced slowing promote the 3-Hz spike-wave pattern?

• What is the basis of the clinically sometimes appreciable similarity between the low-voltage irregular posterior pattern in drowsiness (Stage 1 non-REM) and the low-voltage irregular pattern of the "desynchronized EEG" of the alert (eyes open) state?

19 A Methodological Note on the Wiener Clock Hypothesis for the Alpha Rhythm

In a series of publications, Norbert Wiener (1955, 1956, 1957) advanced the concept that the alpha rhythm might be a reflection of a relatively stable clocking mechanism of the brain, to serve a gating function. Wiener ascribed the hypothesized stable clocking mechanism to mutual entrainment of an ensemble of nonlinear alpha-rhythm generators such that the frequencies of the individual members of the ensemble would have a tendency to be pulled toward a central frequency, in a manner analogous to that in which large numbers of some species of fireflies flash synchronously. A mathematical model for the hypothesis was added later (Wiener 1958, 1961); the model was considered in chapter 14 above. In the power spectrum of the ensemble of alpha generators (i.e., in the alpha rhythm as recorded from a pair of electrodes on the scalp), Wiener pointed out, the "brain clock" hypothesis implied that a spectral dip should be found on either side of the spectral peak (the latter ideally a very narrow band—see figure 19.1), representing the effect of such an attraction to the central frequency (the center of gravity of the frequencies, so to speak). To test the hypothesis, spectra (obtained by Fourier transformations of autocorrelation functions of EEGs) were examined for the predicted spectral shape (Wiener 1961; see also Barlow 1985a).

In chapter 17 above, it was pointed out that variations in the amplitude of a pure sine wave due to modulation by another sine wave of lower frequency results in spectral broadening—i.e., in more than one spectral peak (figure

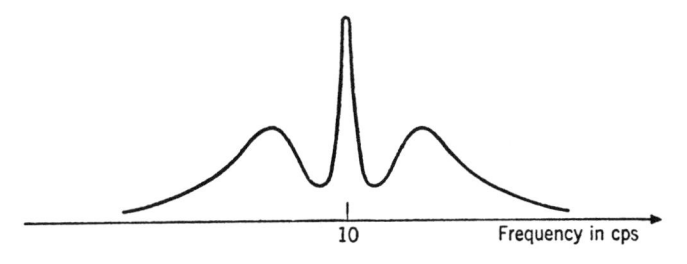

Figure 19.1 Idealized spectrum according to Wiener for an ensemble of alpha-wave generators that are mutually entrained. The dips in the spectrum on either side of the peak indicate a relative dearth of oscillators having these frequencies that results from the mutual pull of frequencies toward the center frequency of 10Hz. (From Wiener 1958.)

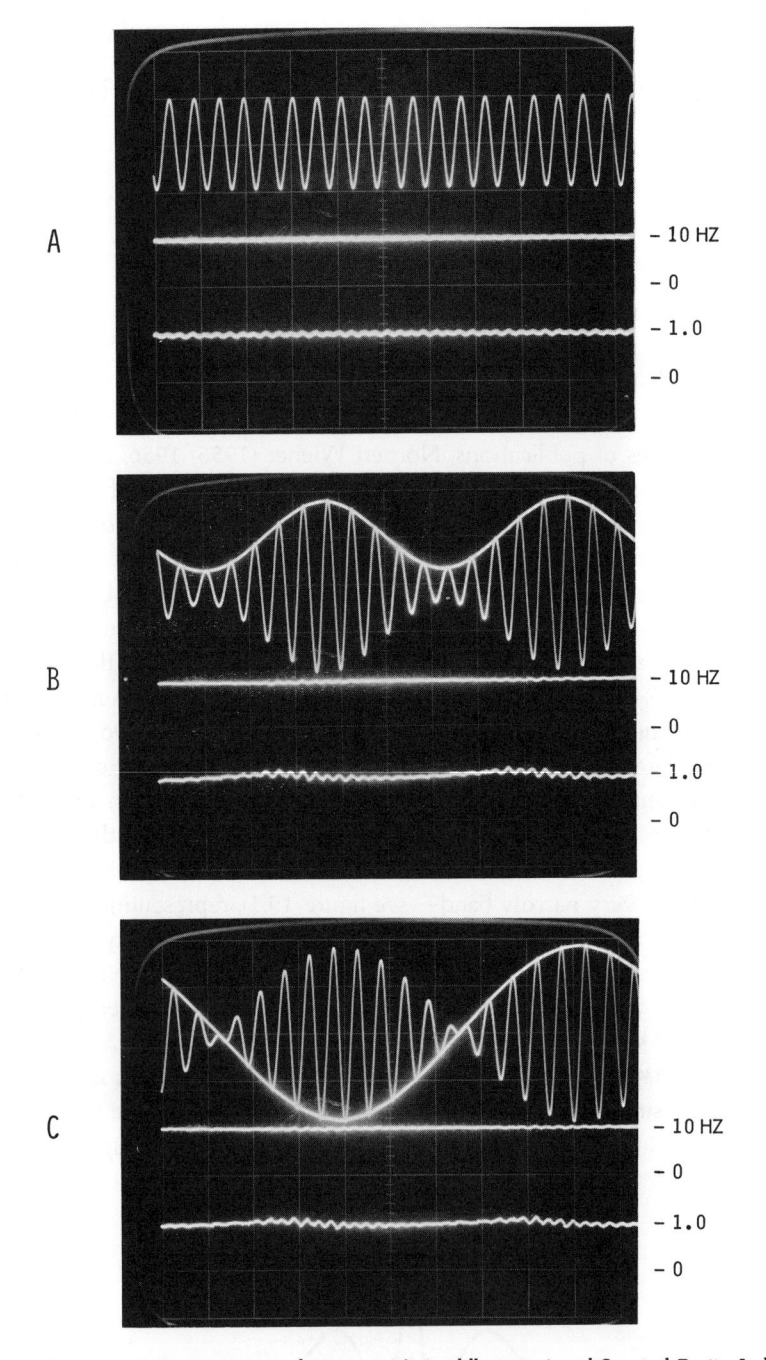

Figure 19.2 Running mean frequency (f) (middle traces) and Spectral Purity Index (SPI) (bottom traces) for a 10-Hz sine wave that is unmodulated (A), multiplied by a 1-Hz sine wave having a DC offset (B), and multiplied by a 0.5-Hz sine wave without a DC offset (C). (The low-frequency sine waves in part B and in part C are superimposed on the 10-Hz sine wave so as to indicate the envelope of the latter; in both B and C the amplitude of the 10-Hz sine wave waxes and wanes at a rate of 1 Hz, but the two resultant waveforms differ in detail.) Note that

278   Chapter 19

17.2). (If the modulation is irregular, a fairly smooth broadening of the peak can be expected.) Such multiple peaks arise from the fact that Fourier analysis carries out the operation of determining which combination or superposition of constant-amplitude sine and/or cosine waves fits the original pattern in question. Thus, even an alpha rhythm that is very stable in frequency at 10 Hz but which waxes and wanes at about 1 Hz (thus producing the familiar alpha "spindles") could, upon spectral analysis, be represented by a broadened peak around, rather than a relatively narrow band at, 10Hz. In carrying out the spectral analysis, it is intrinsically assumed that a linear process characterizes the generator of the pattern. However, if the generator actually entails a nonlinear process (as Wiener assumed)—for example modulation or multiplication—the answer given by Fourier analysis may be inappropriate (even if the result is a mathematical equivalent of the original), and the resulting "artificially" broadened spectrum may be misleading.

The evidence amassed in this book concerning the extrema-slopes hypothesis, which is inherently and intrinsically a nonlinear model of the EEG, suggests that alpha-generating mechanisms of the brain are themselves nonlinear, and that therefore the appropriateness of spectral analysis (a linear technique) as a method of testing Wiener's "brain clock" hypothesis may be questioned. In the present oscillator model, the frequency of rhythmic (i.e., Type 3) waves can be quite stable indeed, despite their waxing and waning amplitude.

Goldstein (1970) found that waves of alpha activity appearing after alpha blocking (induced by intermittent lighting of a viewing area) appeared to be phase-locked to the pre-blocking waves; these results were considered by Goldstein to be consistent with the idea of a basic pacemaking system unaffected by periods of alpha blocking. It could, therefore, be informative to re-explore the question of the degree of phase coherence between waves of spontaneous alpha activity in successive spindles by means of techniques such as the one employed by Goldstein. (Walter (1959), using the multi-channel helical scan toposcope, perhaps a particularly appropriate method for this question, found a relatively high degree of such phase coherence, and hence frequency stability, for resting alpha activity.) The implementation of such techniques might be facilitated by conversion of the EEG (preferably of continuous or almost continuous alpha activity) to a uniform amplitude, a transformation that could in principle be accomplished by dividing the original EEG by its instantaneous envelope.

---

the running mean frequency (10 Hz) and the Spectral Purity Index (1.0) are the same in the three cases (except for minimal computational fluctuations evident for the SPI in B and in C). In contrast, the spectra for the waves in B and C differ from one another (as well as from the spectrum for the 10-Hz unmodulated wave (A) that consists of a single line at 10 Hz), as can be appreciated from figures 17.2 and 17.3. (Smoothing window for the running mean frequency and the SPI: 0.5 sec.)

As a more direct approach of determining the frequency stability of the alpha rhythm in subjects, the instantaneous frequency, in combination with its variability (evaluated e.g., by means of the Coefficient of Variation) and the Spectral Purity Index, could be examined in EEGs that have been bandpass filtered so that only alpha activity remained. These measures are not affected by waxing and waning of alpha activity (figure 19.2), in contrast to the results of Fourier methods (chapter 17).

The above discussion is not intended to be a commentary on the validity of Wiener's brain clock hypothesis of the alpha rhythm (commentaries can be found in Walter 1962, Storm van Leeuwen 1978, and Barlow 1985a). Rather it is intended as a commentary on the methodology to evaluate the frequency stability of the alpha rhythm as an element in the "brain clock" hypothesis, and to suggest that spectral analysis, a basically linear tool, may underestimate the frequency stability of the alpha rhythm.

20 Résumé

THE BASIC HYPOTHESIS AND THE ASSOCIATED MODEL

The basic hypothesis that is advanced and tested in this book is that an EEG signal can be considered as reflecting a self-oscillatory system, the extrema (positive and negative peaks) and slopes of the output waves of which are modulated independently. (Modulation of extrema, in which the positive and negative extremes (or reversal points) are varied, is to be distinguished from modulation of amplitude, which is a scaling or multiplicative operation.) The hypothesis had a fortuituous origin in the course of testing a new, simple method of obtaining the running (moment-to-moment) frequency of an EEG signal, as an alternative to the determination of running frequency via computing the autocorrelation function, for use in adaptive segmentation of the EEG (a method of detecting significant changes in the EEG pattern).

The method of determining the running frequency was found to be satisfactory, but it gave an indication of a hitherto apparently undescribed feature of certain EEG patterns: that the slopes of the waves varied somewhat less than other parameters, such as amplitude and frequency. Originally observed in the EEG during drowsiness but subsequently found not to be constantly present in that state, the feature of constant slope (more exactly, relatively constant slope) was found to be characteristic of deeper stages of non-REM sleep.

In probing the features of such constant-slope waves, an electronic analog model was built to simulate the constant-slope waves. This model (apparently not described before) could readily be modified to generate waves of constant frequency and variable amplitude (thus simulating waxing-and-waning alpha waves). Further simple modifications of the electronic model (which is termed the *oscillator model*) permitted simulation of epileptiform patterns and of irregular EEG patterns (e.g., the "desynchronized EEG").

The oscillator model, which evolved progressively, was capable, in its final form, of simulating a wide variety of normal and abnormal EEG patterns from subjects of different ages and in various states. In essence, the simulation of such a variety of EEG patterns was accomplished by separately modulating the extrema and the slopes of the basic oscillations of the oscillator model. Waves having such combined modulation of extrema and slopes have different features from the waves of combined amplitude and frequency modulation.

METHODS OF TESTING THE HYPOTHESIS

Three approaches to the testing of the hypothesis were taken:

• Simulation of actual EEG patterns by means of the oscillator model, as described above. This method was limited to visual comparisons of simulated and actual EEG patterns and to comparisons of their summary features, such as the means of various parameters (e.g., frequency).

• Testing of predictions concerning actual EEGs, based on the hypothesis and on the behavior of its associated oscillator model. For this purpose, methods of evaluating a number of measures were developed especially for testing the predictions. These measures included running means of amplitude, slope, frequency, and curvature (sharpness); the Spectral Purity Index (a new measure of the degree of rhythmicity having a value of 1.0 for a sine wave of arbitrary frequency even if varying in amplitude); the running Coefficient of Variation; the running Pearson Product-Moment Correlation Coefficient; and the square of the latter, the running Coefficient of Determination. Finally, to supplement the aforementioned running means (evaluated over 0.5-sec and 2.0-sec windows), the instantaneous envelopes of the EEG and of its first derivative as well as the instantaneous frequency were evaluated by new methods especially developed for the purpose. (Details of these methods of analysis and their implementation, together with a detailed description of the oscillator model itself and other relevant developments, are described in part IV of the book.)

• Direct testing of the extrema-slopes hypothesis by reconstituting actual EEG signals on the basis of their instantaneous envelopes and the instantaneous envelopes of their first derivatives. The on-line real-time reconstitution is accomplished by using the latter pair of signals as modulating signals for the extrema and slopes inputs, respectively, of the oscillator model, the output of which can then be compared with the original EEG (save for an ambiguity of polarity that is intrinsic to the method).

RESULTS OF THE TESTS

Simulation of EEG Patterns by Means of the Oscillator Model

It was found possible to simulate a relatively wide variety of EEG patterns, which can be grouped under four principal types of waves from the oscillator model.

Waves of relatively constant slope but variable amplitude (Type 1 waves): EEG patterns in Stages 3 and 4 of non-REM sleep, normal hyperventilation-induced slowing, abnormal random (polymorphic) delta slowing.

Waves of relatively constant amplitude but variable slope (Type 2 waves): the 3-Hz spike-wave pattern.

Waves of relatively constant frequency but variable amplitude and slope (Type 3 waves): rhythmic activity—in particular, alpha activity, with its characteristic waxing-and-waning envelope.

Waves of variable amplitude, slope, and frequency, i.e., irregular waves (Type 4 waves): the "desynchronized" or irregular low-voltage EEG pattern of the waking, alerted, eyes-open state, and the spike-and-slow-wave-complex pattern.

In addition, particular features of certain EEG patterns could be simulated by means of the oscillator model—e.g, the DC shift during the 3-Hz spike-wave pattern, and other asymmetrical patterns such as the picket-fence shape of the mu rhyhm.

Testing of Predictions Concerning Features of Various EEG Patterns

Using the measures described above (running means, etc.), it was found that the prediction of a smaller variability of the running mean slope (i.e., constant slope) than of the running mean amplitude for the EEG during sleep was confirmed for the EEG in Stages 3 and 4 of non-REM sleep, but not for Stage 1 (for which constant-slope waves were infrequent) or Stage 2 sleep. On the other hand, suggestively identifying characteristics of Stage 2 sleep (i.e., a running mean frequency of about half the alpha frequency, little changed by vertex sharp waves), and a relatively well marked transition between Stage 2 and Stage 3 sleep emerged (i.e., the onset of the constant-slope feature). No clear distinction between the EEGs of Stage 1 and REM sleep was found.

The prediction of a relatively variable instantaneous envelope for the slope in the 3-Hz spike-wave pattern was confirmed, with the added unexpected finding that the transition from spike to slow-wave is progressive or smooth, rather than abrupt, the instantaneous envelope of the slope decaying exponentially from the beginning of the spike at least to a point well into the slow wave.

In view of the familiar waxing and waning of alpha waves, the frequency of which varies relatively little, it was not surprising that the expectation of a smaller variability of frequency than of amplitude or slope for EEG alpha activity was confirmed. Not anticipated was the finding, from the tests of the oscillator model (which was confirmed by analyses of actual EEG recordings), that the frequencies of individual "alpha waves" could vary according to their particular positions in an alpha spindle (figures 5.4. and 5.5). Thus, the frequency of the highest-amplitude alpha waves in a spindle (i.e., at the peak of the spindle) could be slightly greater than, or equal to, or slightly less than that for the waves of lowest amplitude, at the valley of a spindle. In the oscillator model, these effects were obtained by imposing small (amplitude) differences in the input modulations for the extrema and the slopes; there was no such variation of frequency with amplitude if the two modulations were identical.

The prediction of completely independent amplitude and slope features of "desynchronized" EEG activity was not confirmed in the evaluation of the degree of relationship between the two (as evaluated by the Coefficient of Detemination); instead, the two were invariably found to be partially related. This finding may be anticipated in part on the basis of the central limit theorem of statistics and in part on a neurophysiological basis. On the other hand, there were some unanticipated findings. First, an inherent characteristic of the Type 4 waves was found to be that their spectra should show a decrease for frequencies above that of the corresponding Type 3 waves. Confirmation for such a behavior emerged from analyses of alpha-type and "desynchronized" EEGs from the same individual, a finding that may place the apparent attenuation by the scalp of at least some types of higher-frequency activity (above 15 Hz—see chapter 12) in a different perspective. Further, the prediction that the epileptiform pattern of spike-and-slow-wave complexes could be characterized by parallel but non-identical behavior of their instantaneous envelopes and those of their first derivatives was confirmed, the latter suggesting an exponential decline (although not as well delineated as in the case of the 3-Hz spike-wave pattern, perhaps because of "noise" from the background EEG for the former).

Reconstitution of EEGs on the Basis of Their Instantaneous Envelopes

The resemblances between original EEGs and their reconstituted versions (the latter obtained by using the instantaneous envelopes of the originals and of their first derivatives as input modulating signals for the oscillator model) were quite satisfactory, for a variety of normal and abnormal EEG patterns, in this test in which the EEGs were reconstituted without reference to the four basic types of output waves of the oscillator model mentioned above.

SIGNIFICANCE OF THE RESULTS—EVALUATION OF THE HYPOTHESIS

The results summarized above offer corroborative evidence in favor of the extrema-slopes hypothesis. Even those instances in which specific predictions are not borne out (e.g., the prediction of complete independence of the envelopes of extrema and of slopes in the "desynchronized" EEG) do not undermine the basic hypothesis; rather, they represent a "prediction error" on the part of the author.

The summary of results thus far has concerned the extrema-slopes hypothesis from a merely phenomenological standpoint, i.e., as though the EEG originated from a "black box." Of interest beyond this limited perspective is the question of whether the hypothesis can be related to the presumptive generating mechanisms of the EEG. For this purpose, selected aspects of the anatomy, the physiology, and the pathophysiology of EEG-generating mechanisms are reviewed as a preliminary to a more comprehensive evaluation of the hypothesis. The basic extrema-slopes model is a nonlinear, multiplicative one, since it entails dual modulation; both anatomical and physiological evidence for such operations by the cortex are cited.

Taking into account these additional perspectives, a formulation for EEG activity is advanced, based in part on evidence indicating that neocortical inhibitory activity in a given small region (e.g., a cortical column) is predominantly or perhaps entirely locally generated and that, by the same token, distant (primarily thalamocortical and corticocortical) input to a given small cortical region (excluding the relatively diffusely distributed input from certain brain-stem nuclei) is predominantly or perhaps exclusively excitatory. In this formulation, disease primarily of the cortex gives rise to focal epileptic EEG manifestations as a result of a deficiency of intracortical inhibitory mechanisms (as previously suggested by others). (An important exception of primarily cortical disease having epileptic manifestations is Alzheimer's disease, in which mainly the larger pyramidal cells—presumably the "powerhouses" of epilepsy—are affected.)

On the other hand, disease primarily affecting subcortical white matter, resulting in an interference with excitatory input to the cortex, results in abnormal (theta and delta) slowing in the EEG. Further, primarily cortical mechanisms are envisaged to underlie the basic oscillatory mechanism of the EEG (as previously suggested by others), the oscillations of which are viewed as intrinsic oscillations the extrema and slopes of which are modulated. The formulation further proposes that the general level of inhibitory cortical activity and its variability are determined, at least in part, by the general level of excitatory cortical input and its variability.

In turn, in the formulation, except for focal epileptic activity, the instantaneous envelope of the EEG is proposed to be inversely related to the overall level of excitatory input to the area of the cortex reflected at the overlying EEG recording electrode. In the case of epileptiform activity, the envelope of the EEG is suggested to be primarily dependent on the intracortical cortical excitatory drive.

The instantaneous envelope of the first derivative of the EEG, on the other hand, is proposed to be inversely related to the overall level of intracortically generated inhibitory activity in the region of the cortex represented at the overlying recording electrode.

The physiological details of the above-described formulation are necessarily left unspecified, in view of their undoubtedly enormous complexity; indeed, much smaller ensembles of cells, not to mention intrinsically oscillatory single cells (e.g., in invertebrates), can give rise to oscillations.

In any case, at an operational level, the ratio of these two variables (i.e., the two instantaneous envelopes) is proposed as a measure of the relative preponderance of excitation and inhibition, and their quotient, after appropriate normalization, is just the instantaneous frequency. It thus follows that, for rhythmic activity such as alpha activity, localized excitation and inhibition are in balance; for instantaneous frequencies higher than the alpha activity excitation predominates over inhibition, and for instantaneous frequencies lower than the alpha frequency inhibition predominates over excitation. In this scheme, epileptiform activity results when there is an initial disproportionate predominance of excitation (of abrupt onset), which may then give way progressively to a predominance of inhibition, with a corresponding swing of the instantaneous frequency from above the alpha frequency range to below the latter, repetitively (in the case of the 3-Hz pattern) or singly (in the case of the interictal pattern of the spike-and-slow-wave complex of focal epilepsy). Conversely, a preponderance of inhibition over excitation (and consequent lower instantaneous frequencies) would correspond either to abnormal slowing in the EEG or to Stages 3 and 4 of non-REM sleep. (Non-REM Stages 1 and 2 and Stage REM are not so well characterized, although each has its individual features, in the formulation.)

It is also suggested that the variability of the instantaneous frequency, as a measure of the instantaneous variations of the relative preponderance of areal excitation and inhibition, as delineated above, may provide a general indication of the level or intensity of information processing by part of the neocortex underlying the electrode (or, in some combination, of the pair of electrodes, in the case of a bipolar EEG recording).

In view of the enormous complexities of the cortex, the possibility of specifying the details of the generating mechanisms for the respective modulating signals for extrema and slopes, envisaged in the extrema-slopes hypothesis, appears remote. Indeed, these "signals" may appear only intrinsically (as "hidden variables"), in some diffusely distributed manner, rather than explicitly. The generating mechanisms of the modulating signals thus remain even more ill-defined than the physiological basis of the oscillator mechanisms themselves, as presumably representing the activity of very large ensembles of cortical columns and their interactions. (A possible model for the latter is offered in appendix B in the form of an adaptive signal processor, originally built for a quite different purpose, which has some remarkable properties.) Indeed, perhaps oscillator mechanisms and modulating mechanisms are so inextricably intertwined in the cortex as not to be separable.

It is emphasized, however, that the basic extrema-slopes hypothesis, which in essence characterizes a great diversity of EEG patterns by merely two parameters, was originally evolved as a unifying approach to account for such a wide variety of EEG patterns, and in this respect "stands on its own feet," irrespective of the speculative inferences that have been attempted concerning possible physiological implications of the hypothesis in relation to basic EEG-generating mechanisms.

IMPLICATIONS FOR AND APPLICATIONS TO COMPUTERIZED EEG ANALYSIS

Some conventional methods of EEG analysis and the relationship to them of the methods specifically developed for testing the extrema-slopes hypothesis are considered, with particular reference to spectral (Fourier) and related techniques and their inherent limitations as basically linear techniques. (Spectral analysis in relation to Norbert Wiener's concept of the alpha rhythm as a brain clock is considered as a particular instance of the latter limitation.) The present methods of running means of amplitude and frequency, and also the Spectral Purity Index, are compared with the related but not identical approach of Hjorth's normalized slope parameters.

Possible applications of the present methods in characterizing EEG signals, detecting changes in the EEG pattern (e.g., alpha-blocking, paroxysmal slowing), sleep staging, detecting epileptiform EEG activity (including possible subtle manifestations), intra- and perioperative monitoring, EEG maturation in the premature infant, and interchannel comparisons of multi-channel EEG recordings are considered.

IV Technological Chapters

21 Introduction to Technological Chapters

A number of techniques not previously applied to electroencephalography have been specially developed for the testing of the extrema-slopes hypothesis. All the devices used are of the author's own design and construction, and are analog rather than digital (excluding the digital counting and addressing circuits), reflecting the author's extensive experience with analog techniques.

The specific devices were constructed (sometimes in more than one implementation) as the needs arose. Descriptions of the various units (none of which have been published before) are gathered here for convenience. For the most part, functional block diagrams or schemas, rather than detailed circuits, are provided, since any duplication of the processes is likely to be carried out with digital computers rather than with analog components. In any event, the implementation of all of the units should be within the capabilities of a competent electronics engineer.

The descriptions are presented in a logical sequence. The basic element, the oscillator model, is considered in chapter 22. This is followed, in chapter 23, by descriptions of certain essential building blocks, i.e., a precision rectifier, a transversal or rectangular filter, and a tapped delay line, which are employed repeatedly in the overall computing facility. The units for deriving the basic measures of running means of amplitude, slope, and curvature are considered in chapter 24, together with two essentially equivalent methods of obtaining derivatives: by means of an operational amplifier and by means of successive differences in a sampled-data approach.

The methods for obtaining the derived measures, which include the running mean frequency, the Spectral Purity Index (a measure of rhythmicity), the Coefficient of Variation, the Pearson Product-Moment Correlation Coefficient and its square, the Coefficient of Determination (which is related to the coherence), as well as the interrelationships among these measures, are discussed in chapter 25.

The next several chapters are concerned with units for acquiring or modifying EEG data and with the simulation of modulating signals for the oscillator model. The specially instrumented photo-optical scanner required for retrieval of EEGs from closely adjacent or even interleaving adjacent ink traces is described in chapter 26, together with a highly portable two-channel FM cassette tape recorder used for temporary storage of the output of the photo-optical scanner. A general-purpose "time machine" for temporary storage is discussed in chapter 27; this device has independent read-in and read-out rates, e.g., for analysis of individual epileptiform transients. Noise generators (e.g., for generating modulating signals for the oscillator model) having different characteristics (Gaussian and rectangular probability density distributions, $1/f$ Gaussian noise) are considered in chapter 28.

Several techniques for obtaining the instantaneous envelope (in the form of the magnitude of the analytic signal, to use the commmunications engineering term) of an EEG and of its first derivative (the pair being essential for reconstituting EEGs by means of the oscillator model) are considered in chapter 29, along with a method (developed in connection with this work) which has the special feature of applicability to relatively wideband signals instead of to merely narrowband (rhythmic) ones (e.g., alpha activity). Interfacing of the units for instantaneous envelopes with the oscillator model, for the reconstitution of EEGs, is also discussed in chapter 29.

ELECTRONIC COMPONENTS

For reference the electronic components (chips) are listed below (exclusive of standard digital components, such as binary counters):

Quad operational amplifier: TC084C (FET input)

Quad comparator: 2901

Multiplier (1%): Analog Devices 534 series

Arithmetic Computing Unit (ACU) for high-precision arithmetic operations: Analog Devices 538 series

Multiplexer, 16-channel: Analog Devices 7506 and 506A series

D/A Converter, 12-bit: Analog Devices 562 series

22 The Oscillator Model

A block diagram of the oscillator model (so termed because its output waveforms constitute models for EEG patterns) is shown in figure 22.1. The oscillator model consists of two parts: a generator of triangular waves, the extrema and slopes of which can be modulated independently, and a shaping or smoothing unit, in which the triangular waves are converted to quasi-sinusoidal form. An alternative would have been to incorporate the special features of the smoothing unit (i.e., parabolic or combined parabolic-quartic smoothing) into the basic oscillator itself, so that the smoothed waves would be generated directly. The final output waves would have been the same in either case, although the latter design would possibly be considered to be the more appropriate as a model for a biological phenomenon, since triangular waves do not appear explicitly.

THE TRIANGULAR-WAVE GENERATOR

The oscillator model can be considered to be basically a voltage-controlled oscillator (VCO) having a triangular-wave output, but modified so that not only the slopes but also the extrema of the triangular waves can be modulated. (It is essential to distinguish between modulation of extrema and modulation of amplitude; the former results in changes both in amplitude and in frequency, whereas in the latter only the amplitude changes—compare figure 1.1C with figure 1.1A.)

   As shown in figure 22.1, the triangular-wave oscillator consists of an integrator and a comparator arranged in such a way that when the integrator's output voltage reaches a level specified by the reference voltage into a comparator (the other input being the integrator's output voltage itself) the charging current to the integrator is reversed in polarity, as is the polarity of the reference voltage into the comparator. The two independent modulating inputs make possible four major modes of the oscillator model, with four corresponding types of output waves:

Mode 1: modulation of extrema only (Type 1 waves—constant slope)

Mode 2: modulation of slopes only (Type 2 waves—constant amplitude)

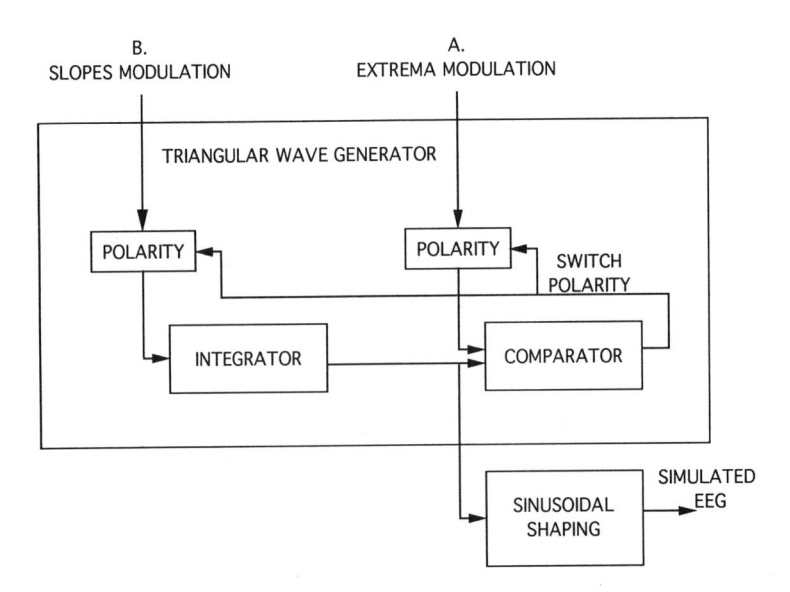

Figure 22.1 Block diagram of the oscillator model, consisting of the basic triangular-wave generator and a quasi-sinusoidal shaping unit. The triangular-wave generator is essentially a voltage-controlled oscillator but is modified so that both extrema and slopes can be modulated. Such a dual-modulation oscillator (not to be confused with combined amplitude-frequency modulation) may not have been described previously.

Mode 3: congruent modulation of both extrema and slopes (Type 3 waves—constant frequency)

Mode 4: independent modulation of extrema and slopes (Type 4 waves—irregular).

The characteristic of constant slope for Type 1 waves is evident in the second trace of figure 22.2A, in contrast to Types 2 and 3 waves, for which slope is not constant (second traces of figures 22.2B and 22.2C, respectively). (The process of obtaining the smoothed versions of the waveforms, shown in the bottom traces of figures 22.2 and 22.3, is considered below). Type 1 waves, modulated only in their extremes and having constant (absolute) slope (figure 22.2A) may not have been previously described.

An example of very irregular Type 4 waves resulting from Mode 4 operation of the oscillator model with independent random inputs is shown in figure 22.3B; (figure 22.3A is the control); of course, slopes are also not constant (not shown in figure 22.3) for Type 4 waves.

CONVERSION OF TRIANGULAR WAVES TO A PARABOLIC APPROXIMATION OF SINUSOIDAL FORM

It might be supposed that the conversion of the basic triangular-wave output of the oscillator model could be accomplished in a straightforward manner by conventional filtering. This is not, however, the case, since the frequency of the output waves generally depends in a complex manner on the input

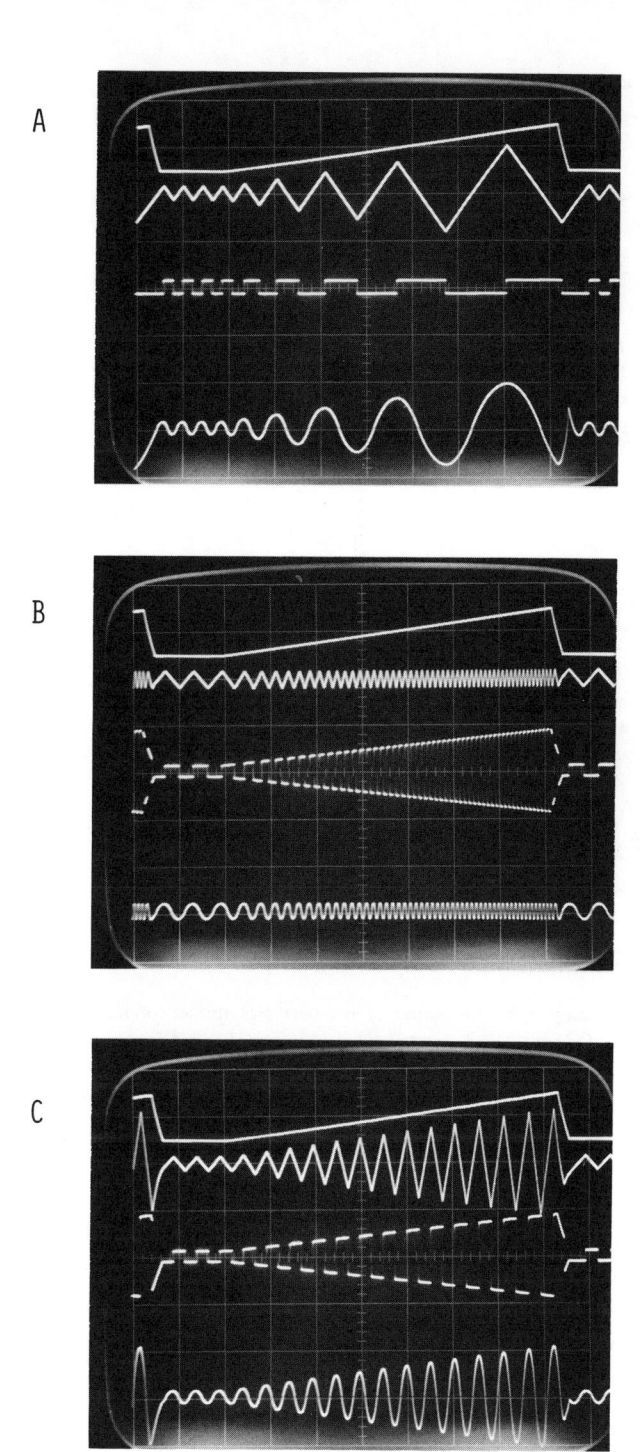

Figure 22.2 Characteristic features of extrema and slopes for (A) Type 1 (constant-slope) waves, (B) Type 2 (constant-amplitude) waves, and (C) Type 3 (constant-frequency) waves. In each instance, trace 1 is a modulating waveform (a ramp), trace 2 is a triangular wave output of oscillator model, trace 3 is the first derivative of trace 2, and trace 4 is a smoothed version of the triangular wave. Note that the derivative (trace 3) of the triangular wave (trace 2) is constant only in part A (i.e., for constant-slope waves).

The Oscillator Model

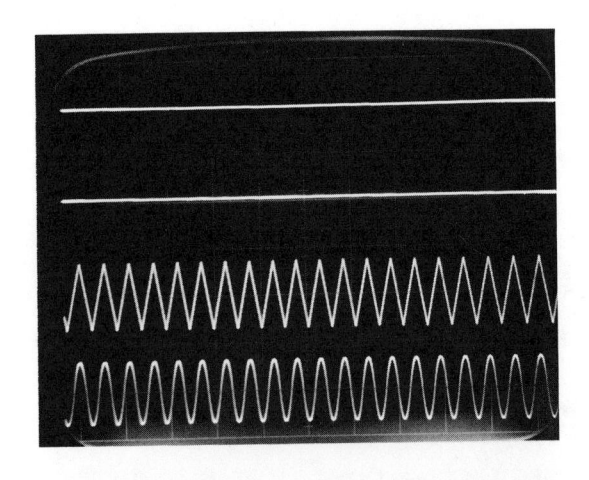

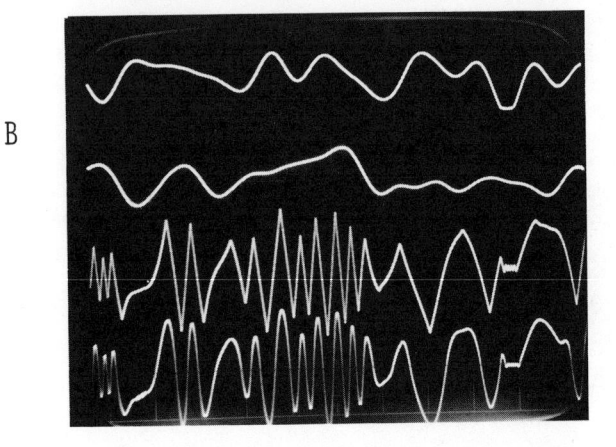

Figure 22.3 Examples of the output of the oscillator model for independent modulation of extrema and of slopes, i.e., Type 4 (irregular) waves (B), and for no modulation (i.e., for DC inputs). (A) Trace 1: extrema modulation. Trace 2: slopes modulation. Trace 3: triangular-wave output. Trace 4: smoothed output. Note that the envelope of the extrema of traces 3 and 4 is the same as trace 1, and that the slopes of the waves in traces 3 and 4 parallel the slopes modulation (trace 2).

modulating signals. Therefore, a completely new general-purpose waveshaping circuit was designed for the purpose. The inputs to the shaping unit from the basic oscillator include the triangular waves themselves and the extremes-modulation signal for the oscillator.

The shaping equation is based on the trigonometric expansion

$$\cos x = 1 - \frac{x^2}{2!} + \frac{x^4}{4!} - \frac{x^6}{6!} + \frac{x^8}{8!} \cdots. \tag{1}$$

Initially, only the first two terms, $1 - x^2/2!$ (i.e., a parabolic correction) were employed, but subsequently the first three terms were used, thus including the quartic term ($x^4/4!$). (It is probable that in practice the parabolic correction would have sufficed, but the derivation of the instantaneous envelope of the

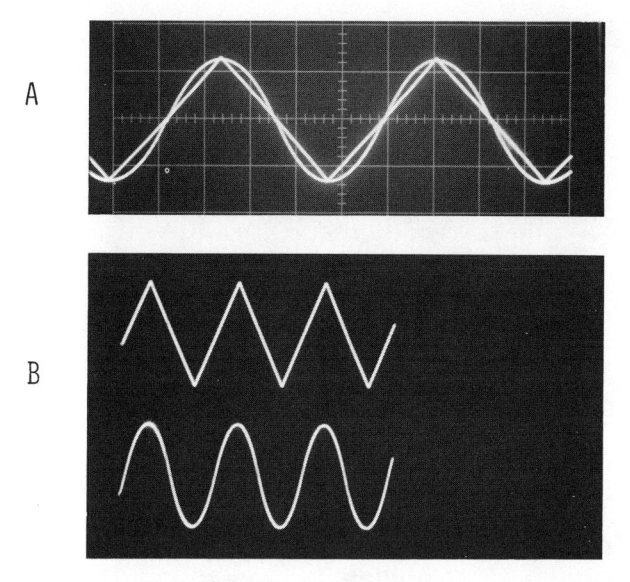

Figure 22.4 (Same as lower left of figure 2.4.) (A) Triangular wave and superimposed parabolic approximation to a sine wave; the two waves coincide at the baseline and at their positive and negative peaks. (B) Same, except that the two traces are separated and are displayed on a slower time base.

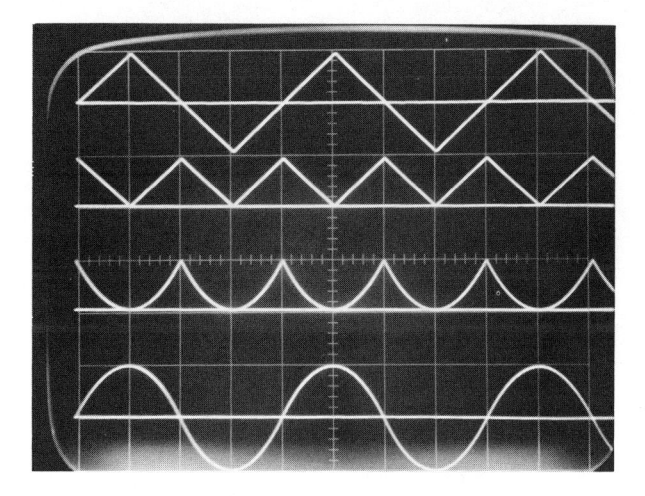

Figure 22.5 Abbreviated version of the parabolic smoothing procedure, illustrated for constant-amplitude triangular waves. Trace 1: original triangular wave. Trace 2: after full-wave rectification. Trace 3: after squaring and normalization. Trace 4: after reversing the polarities of alternate parabolas. Baselines are included with each trace. (No DC offset is shown in trace 4.) Note that the waveform in trace 4 is virtually indistinguishable from a sine wave.

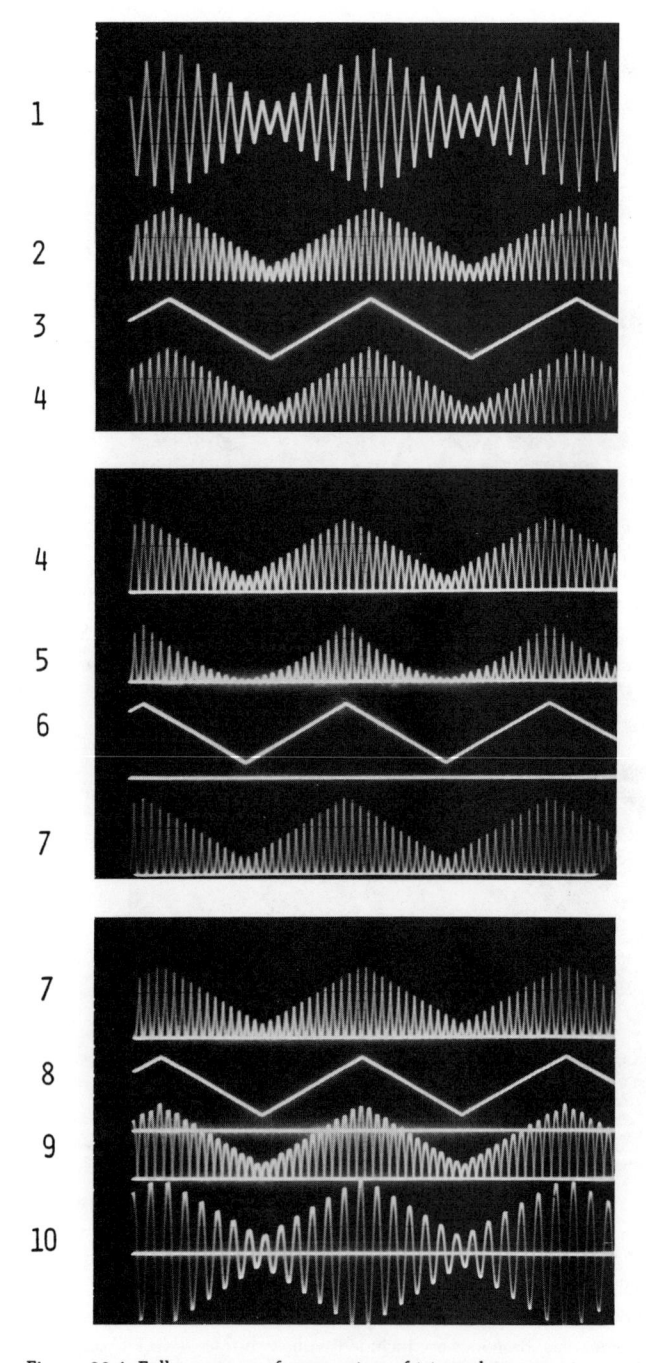

Figure 22.6 Full sequence of conversion of triangular waves to quasi-sinusoidal form by parabolic approximation. Note that the three sets of traces are not in temporal alignment. Baselines are included for the repeats of traces 4–10. Trace 1: original triangular waves from oscillator model. Trace 2: after full-wave rectification. Trace 3: original extrema-modulating signal. Trace 4 (shown twice): after subtracting trace 2 from trace 3. Trace 5: after squaring trace 4 (note the parabolic form of the individual waves as well as of their envelope). Trace 6: repeat of trace 3. Trace 7 (shown twice): restoration of linearity of the envelope of the parabolas after dividing trace 5 by trace 6 (note that the individual waves retain their parabolic form, but the envelope of the waves is now triangular instead of parabolic). Trace 8: repeat of trace 3 (baseline partly overlaps trace 9). Trace 9: after subtraction of trace 7 from trace 8. Trace 10: after inversion of alternate parabolas in trace 9 (note that the amplitude of the resulting quasi-sinusoidal wave is the same as that of the triangular wave in trace 1).

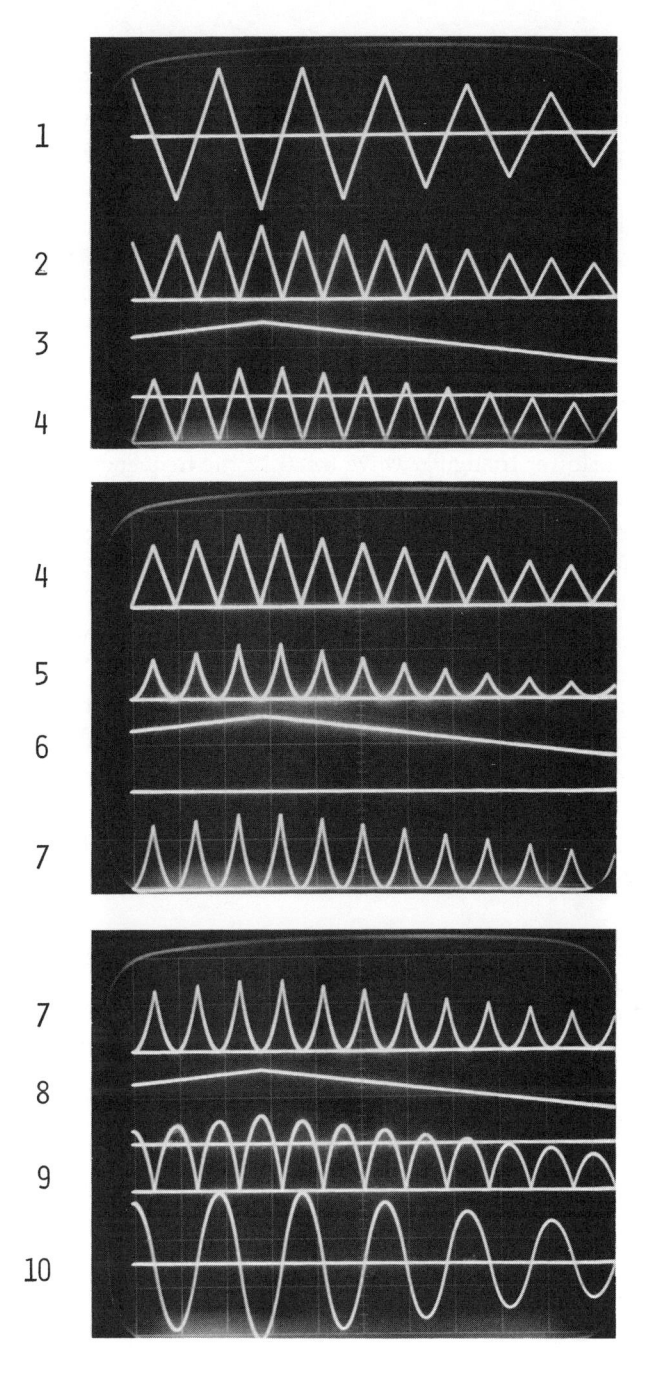

Figure 22.7 Same sequence as in figure 22.6, but on faster time base and with baselines added to all traces. (The baseline for trace 3 partially overlaps trace 4, and the baseline for trace 8 partially overlaps trace 9.)

first derivative of a signal (chapter 29) entails the second derivative of the signal, which, for EEG patterns simulated by the oscillator model, would have been triangular rather than quasi-sinusoidal in form if only the parabolic correction had been used. The quartic correction was therefore included. The parabolic and the combined parabolic-quartic approximations are virtually indistinguishable by eye.)

The transformation of the triangular waves to the parabolic approximation of the quasi-sinusoidal form (i.e., through the second term on the right in equation 1) is illustrated in figure 22.4. An abbreviated depiction of the process, to illustrate the basic principle, is shown in figure 22.5 for triangular waves of constant amplitude. The full sequence is shown in figure 22.6, and on a faster time base in figure 22.7, for a triangular wave congruently modulated by a slower triangular wave (of 1/12 the frequency) in extrema and in slopes so that the frequency of the output waves of the oscillator model remains constant (Mode 3 of the oscillator model). The bottom trace (trace 10) in both figures shows the resulting parabolic approximation, which is essentially indistinguishable by eye from sinusoidal form.

Figure 22.8 shows that this sequence of transformations functions equally well for triangular waves the extrema and slopes of which have been independently modulated by two random signals. (Additional examples of the smoothing procedure for a wide range of waveforms of the basic triangular-wave generator appear in chapter 4.)

MORE EXACT (PARABOLIC + QUARTIC) APPROXIMATION TO A SINE WAVE

As already mentioned, only the parabolic approximation to sinusoidal form was initially employed. Subsequently, for reasons that will now be considered, the closer approximation to sinusoidality afforded by additional inclusion of the quartic term ($x^4/4!$) was implemented in the smoothing unit.

In chapter 3 it was pointed out that the third major test of the extrema-slopes hypothesis, for which EEGs are reconstituted (by means of the oscillator model) on the basis of their instantaneous envelopes and the instantaneous envelope of the first derivative of the EEGs, used as paired input modulating signals for the oscillator model. However, as detailed in chapter 29, determining the instantaneous envelope of the first derivative of a signal (i.e., an EEG) entails obtaining the second derivative of the signal as well as its first derivative. But the derivative of a parabolic approximation to a sine wave is a triangular wave, as can be appreciated from the expression

$$\frac{d(x^2)}{dt} = 2x.$$

This process can be viewed as the reverse of that depicted in figure 22.4, i.e., as a transformation from a parabolic wave to triangular wave (except for the

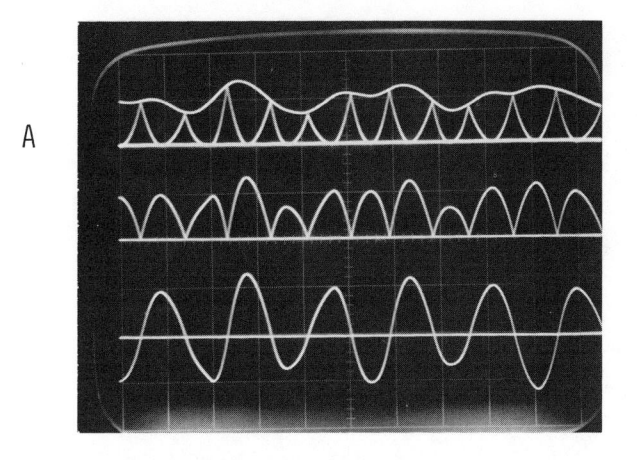

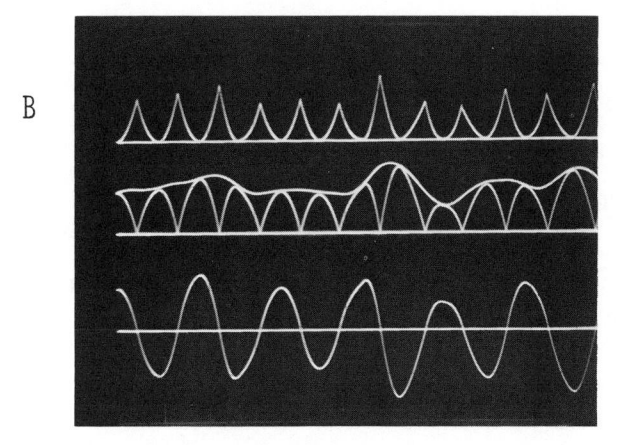

Figure 22.8 Sinusoidal conversion process for triangular waves (not shown) having their extrema and slopes independently modulated by two random signals (only that for the extrema modulation is shown). Baselines are included for each trace. (A) Top trace: original modulating signal. Trace 2: triangular waves after squaring and division by the modulating signal. Trace 3: after subtraction of trace 2 from trace 1. Trace 4: after inversion of alternate half cycles; note the resulting irregular waveform. (B) Same as A, except that the extrema-modulating signal is shown superimposed on the series of parabolas before inversion. Note that the modulating signal is the envelope for the apexes of the parabolas in trace 2 of part A and also for the parabolas after subtraction from the modulating signal in trace 3 of part B.

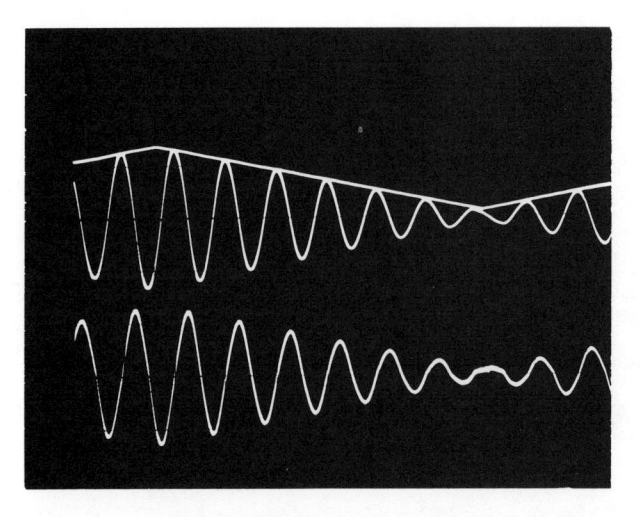

Figure 22.9 Combined parabolic and quartic approximation to a sine wave (trace 2, comparable to trace 10 of figure 22.6 or 22.7), and its first derivative (trace 3), which appears to be sinusoidal but is actually parabolic. Without the additional quartic correction, trace 3 would once again be a triangular wave, comparable to trace 1 in figure 22.6 or 22.7. (For the combined quartic and parabolic correction, the steps indicated by traces 4–7 of parts A and B of figure 22.6 are carried out separately for the quartic component. The result of the latter is then added to the parabolic correction to yield the combined correction.)

absence of the 90° phase lead that is introduced by differentiation). On the other hand, the derivative of a true sine wave is a cosine wave (a sine wave shifted in phase by 90°), rather than a triangular wave. It was because of this poor approximation resulting from inclusion of only the first two terms of equation 1 that the quartic correction was subsequently added. The efficacy of the additional quartic correction is apparent in the lowest trace in figure 22.9, which is the derivative of the modulated, quartically approximated wave shown as the middle trace. Had the middle trace incorporated only the parabolic approximation, the bottom trace would have been triangular rather than sinusoidal.

SPECTRA OF THE FOUR BASIC TYPES OF WAVES FROM THE OSCILLATOR MODEL

As discussed in chapter 2, the two independent modulating inputs (for extrema and for slopes, respectively) of the oscillator model permit four types of output waves, corresponding to four principal modes of the oscillator model (not including mixed modes): waves of constant slope (Type 1), waves of constant amplitude (Type 2), waves of constant frequency (Type 3), and irregular waves (Type 4). For further understanding of these four types of waves in relation to conventional analyses, figure 22.10 shows their respective spectra, using a pair of independent low-frequency triangular waves as input modulating waveforms for the oscillator model. (Triangular waves have a

Figure 22.10 Power spectra (on an arbitrary scale linear for power) for the four types of waves from the oscillator model, with a pair of low-frequency triangular waves of different frequencies used as input modulating waveforms. (Frequency in this figure and in figures 22.11 and 22.12 are in Hz.) In comparison with the narrow spectrum for Type 3 (constant-frequency) waves having a peak at 9 Hz, the spectrum for Type 1 (constant-slope) waves is skewed toward the lower frequencies, the spectrum for Type 2 (constant-amplitude) waves tends to be flat and symmetrical about 9 Hz, and the spectrum for Type 4 (irregular) waves is relatively flat up to 9 Hz and decreases for frequencies higher than 9 Hz.

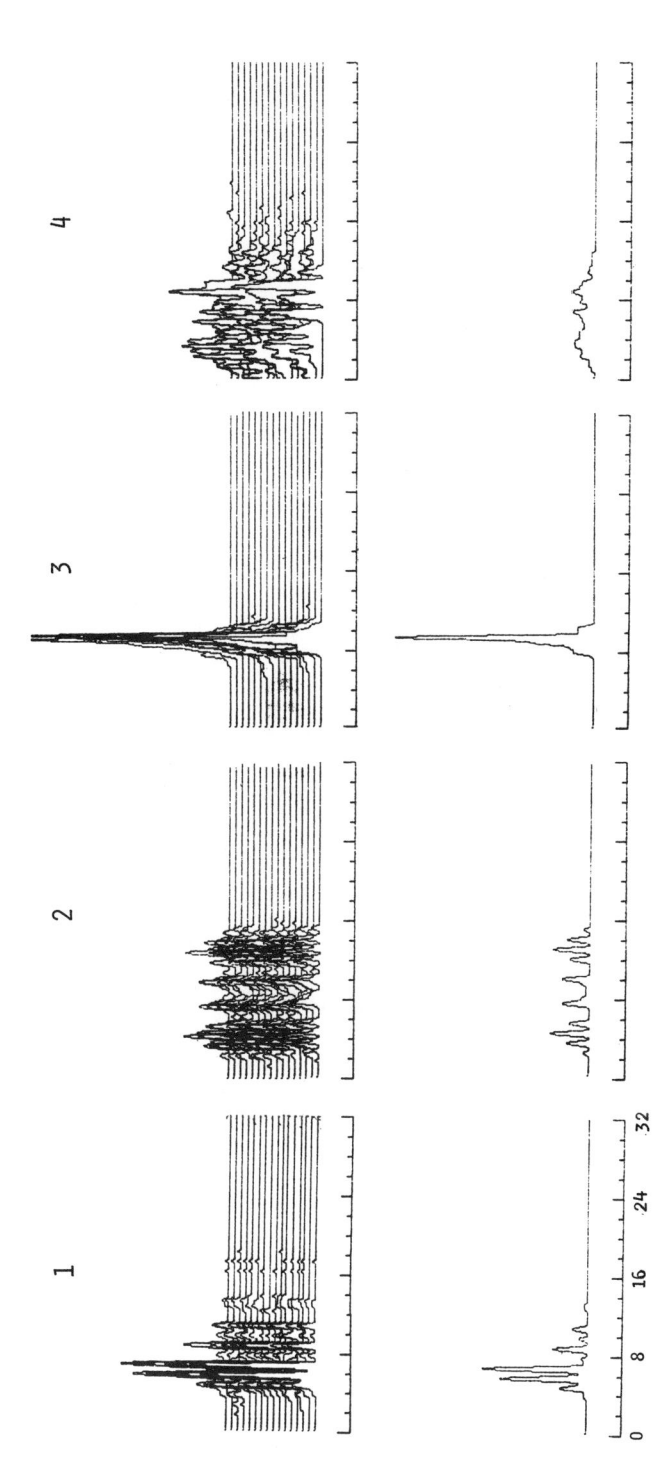

303   The Oscillator Model

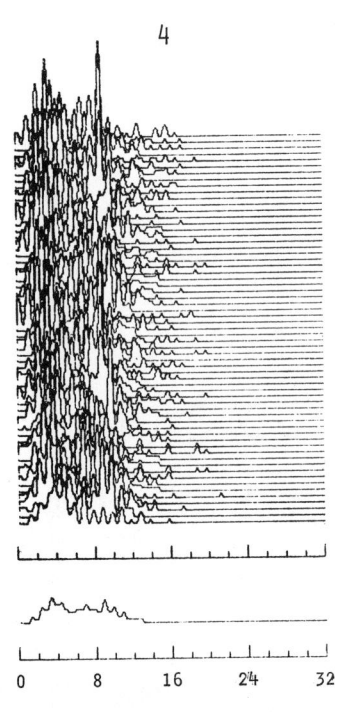

Figure 22.11 Repeat computation of figure 22.9 for Type 4 waves, but for 64 instead of 16 samples. As in figure 22.9, the spectrum is relatively flat below about 9 Hz but decreases for frequencies above 9 Hz.

rectangular amplitude distribution (probability density) function; i.e., every amplitude is equally probable.)

Figure 22.10 suggests that, in comparison with the narrow spectrum for Type 3 (constant-frequency) waves having a peak at 9 Hz, the spectrum for Type 1 (constant-slope) waves is skewed toward the lower frequencies, the spectrum for Type 2 (constant-amplitude) waves tends to be flat and symmetrical about 9 Hz, and the spectrum for Type 4 (irregular) waves is relatively flat up to 9 Hz and decreases for still higher frequencies. The spectrum for Type 4 waves is repeated in figure 22.11 for 64 instead of 16 samples, and the same behavior as in figure 22.10 is apparent.

For further characterization of the spectra of the four types of waves, a pair of independent random (rather than the periodic triangular wave) low-frequency noise signals having a rectangular amplitude distribution (probability density) function (details in chapter 28) were used for modulating the oscillator model. The results for using such random modulations are shown in figure 22.12, and it is evident that the forms of the spectra are much the same as the corresponding ones in figure 22.10. (Ordinary random noise having a Gaussian (chapter 29) rather than a rectangular amplitude distribution function would not be satisfactory for this purpose, since modulation of slopes (which is equivalent to frequency modulation) by a random signal having a Gaussian distribution would result in a spectrum having a Gaussian shape rather than the flat shape that results for the Type 4 waves in figure 22.12.)

Figure 22.12 Same as figure 22.10, but with two independent random noise signals each having a rectangular amplitude distribution (probability density) function as input modulating waveforms for the oscillator model. The distinctive features of the spectrum for each type of wave are much the same as in figure 22.10.

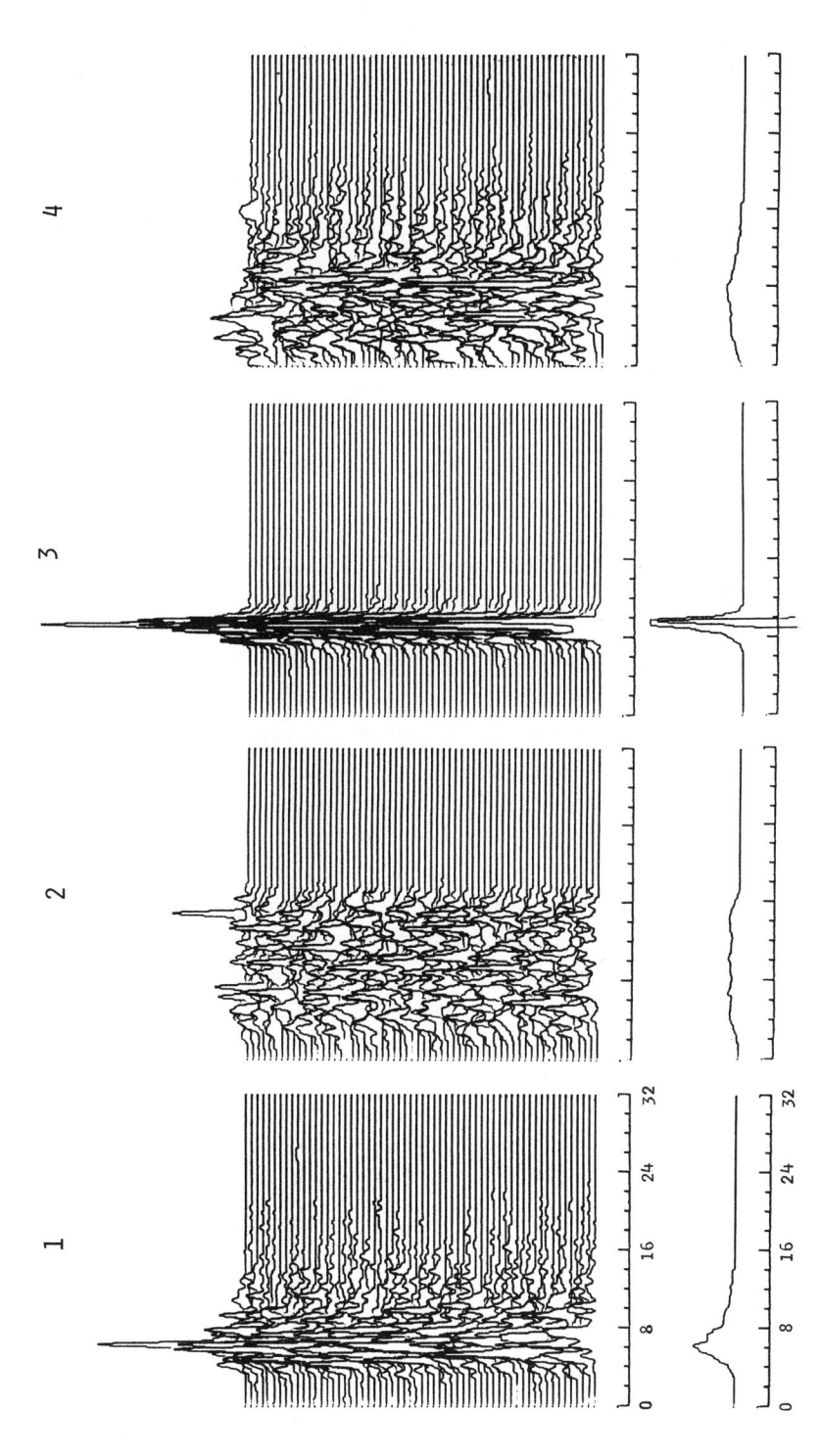

To recapitulate: The power spectrum of Type 1 waves (modulation of extrema only) has a peak at the lower-frequency end (figures 22.10, and 22.12), as expected, since for such waves amplitude and frequency are inversely related, and hence the waves of largest amplitude are at the low-frequency end. (On a log power vs. log frequency plot, a straight line would have resulted, in accordance with the relation $a = k/f$, where a is amplitude (log power), f is frequency, and k is a constant.

The power spectrum of Type 2 waves (modulation of slopes only) yields a flat spectrum centered at 9 Hz, the intrinsic frequency of the oscillator model.

For Type 3 waves, the spectrum has the expected peak at the intrinsic oscillating frequency (9 Hz, for congruent modulation of extrema and slopes), the width of the spectrum reflecting the variations in amplitude of the waves (an inherent feature of Fourier analysis that is discussed in chapter 17).

Type 4 waves have a very interesting spectrum; it is flat for frequencies below the intrinsic oscillating frequency of 9 Hz (the frequency of the corresponding Type 3 waves), but it progressively decreases for frequencies higher than the latter frequency, approximately. *This is an inherent and striking, if unanticipated, characteristic of Type 4 waves of the oscillator model.* The spectrum clearly shows a decreases for frequencies higher than 9 Hz. (Comparable EEG results are shown in figure 5.9.)

In summary: When one is modulating with signals having rectangular amplitude distributions (probability density functions) (in contrast to Gaussian probability density distributions—see above) for Type 1 (constant-slope) waves, the spectrum is skewed toward the low-frequency end; for Type 2 (constant-extrema) waves, the spectrum is flat and centered at the intrinsic oscillating frequency (e.g., 9 Hz); for Type 3 (constant-frequency) waves, the spectrum is narrow and centered at the intrinsic oscillating frequency; for Type 4 (irregular) waves, the spectrum has a cutoff (i.e., a progressive attenuation at higher frequencies) at the intrinsic oscillating frequency and is flat for lower frequencies.

23 Precision Full-Wave Rectifier; Transversal Filter; Tapped Delay Line

PRECISION FULL-WAVE RECTIFIER

In a number of applications in this work (e.g., in evaluating running means and the Spectral Purity Index), the need arose for a full-wave rectifier having an extremely wide dynamic range of 10,000 to 1, corresponding to a range from 10 to 0.001 V. For a signal that ranges in value from 0.1 V at 1 Hz to 10 V at 10 Hz, the range of amplitude for the signal itself is 100 to 1 (10 to 0.1 V), but the corresponding range of the first derivative is 1,000 to 1 (10 to 0.01 V), and that of the second derivative is 10,000 to 1 (10 to 0.001 V). Such a dynamic range is necessary in the computation of the instantaneous envelope of a signal (chapter 29), since the latter is based on the original signal, its first derivative, and its second derivative. Such a characteristic was found to be beyond the capability of conventional full-wave rectifier circuits made up of combinations of diodes and operational amplifiers, because the cutoff characteristics of the diodes were not sharp enough for the present purposes. A precision full-wave rectifier circuit was thus designed and implemented.

A block diagram of the precision full-wave rectifier is shown in figure 23.1. After buffering to provide low source impedance, the signal is fed to a comparator, the output of which indicates the polarity of the signal with respect to ground (the reference input for the comparator). The signal is also inverted, and the inverted and uninverted forms of the signal are fed to a pair of FET switches which are operated by switching voltages in opposite phase from the output of the comparator. The polarity of the output can be reversed by interchanging either the signal voltages to the two FETs or their switching voltages. The extremely sharp cutoff characteristic was achieved in this way, and the circuit was found to meet the above-stated requirements satisfactorily.

A TRANSVERSAL (RECTANGULAR, BOXCAR) FILTER

A circuit that has been used very extensively in this work is that of the transversal, rectangular, or boxcar filter. Ordinarily understood to be a digital filter of the finite impulse response (FIR) type, as indicated in figure 23.2, the transversal filter has been implemented in sampled analog form in the present application, as shown in figure 23.3. In this form, it consists simply of one or

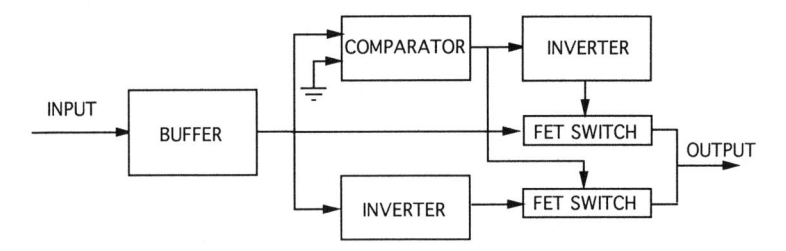

Figure 23.1 Block diagram of precision full-wave rectifier. The use of a pair of FETs operated by switching (polarity) voltages derived from the comparator results in a very sharp cutoff characteristic and a wide dynamic range.

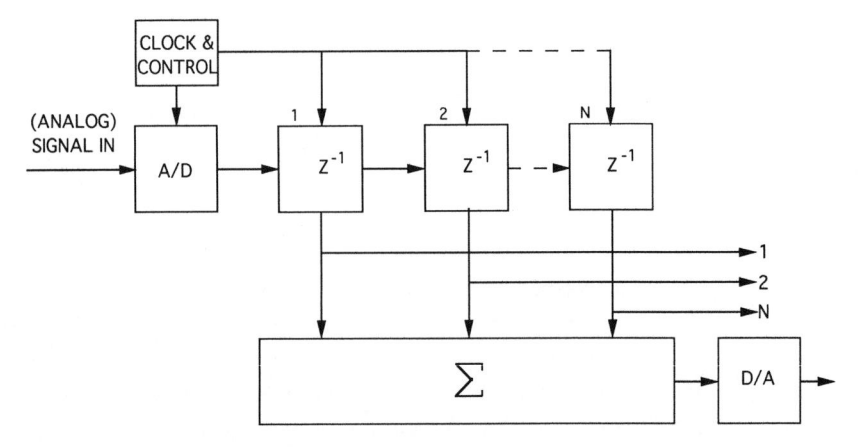

Figure 23.2 A digital implementation of a transversal filter, constituted of shift registers, an A/D and a D/A converter, and a sequential summating (accumulator) unit. The notation z^{-1} indicates a time delay of one unit, equal to the reciprocal of the rates of operation of the A/D and the D/A converters.

more 16-channel analog multiplexers, the 16 outputs of which are temporarily stored in condenser-based hold circuits; the outputs of the latter are then continuously summated, in self-normalized form, by means of the precision resistors. The output of the transversal filter for a square-wave input is shown in figure 23.4.

From figures 23.2–23.4 it is evident that the transversal filter is equivalent to a running integral over a time window of duration equal to the time for one full cycle of the multiplexer; such a transversal filter is thus a form of low-pass filter. As in any sampled data system, care must be taken to avoid the possibility of aliasing, i.e., that signal frequencies higher than the Nyquist frequency (twice the sampling frequency) have been removed by appropriate filtering.

An important distinction between such a low-pass transversal filter and a (single-stage) low-pass RC filter is that, by definition and by design, the transversal filter weighs all samples equally, whereas the RC filter assigns the more recent samples progressively greater weights according to a decaying exponential curve. Figure 23.5 shows the output of a transversal filter (having 64 rather than 16 points) and of a single-stage RC low-pass filter, for a

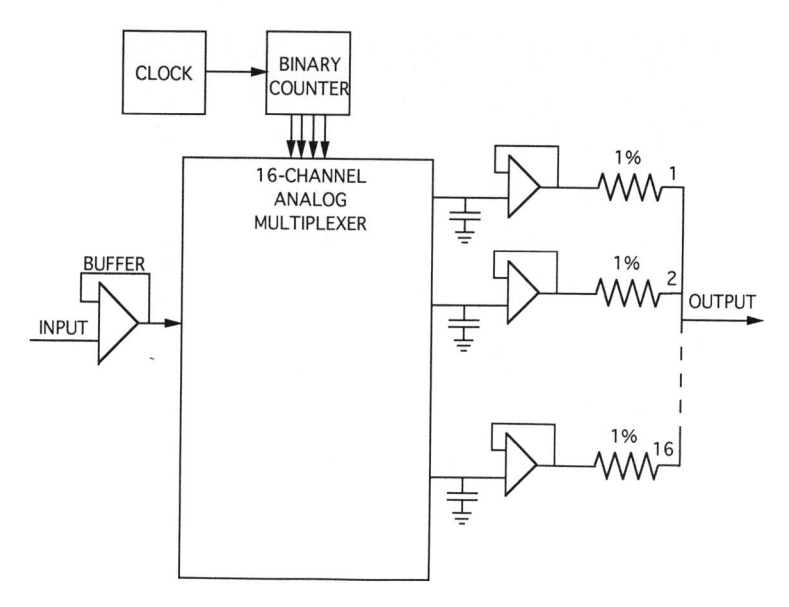

Figure 23.3 Sampled analog implementation of a 16-point transversal filter using a 16-channel analog multiplexer and an array of hold circuits with equally weighted outputs. The number of points can readily be extended simply by incorporating more multiplexers, hold circuits, and summating (1%) resistors.

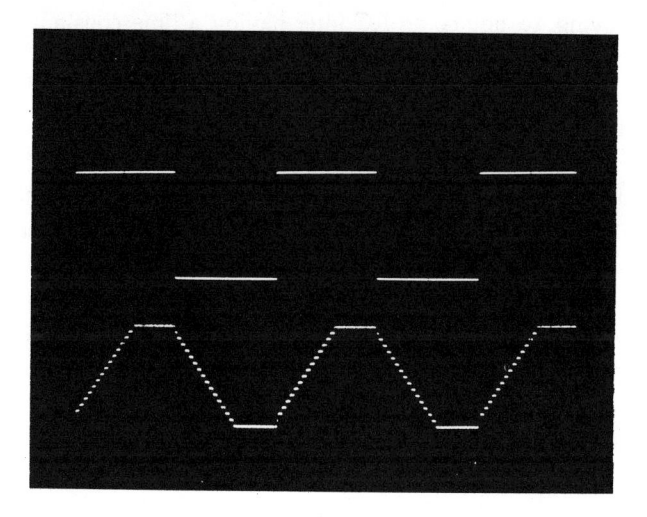

Figure 23.4 Output of a 16-point transversal filter for a square-wave input. The averaging window duration is $\frac{1}{4}$ the period of the square wave.

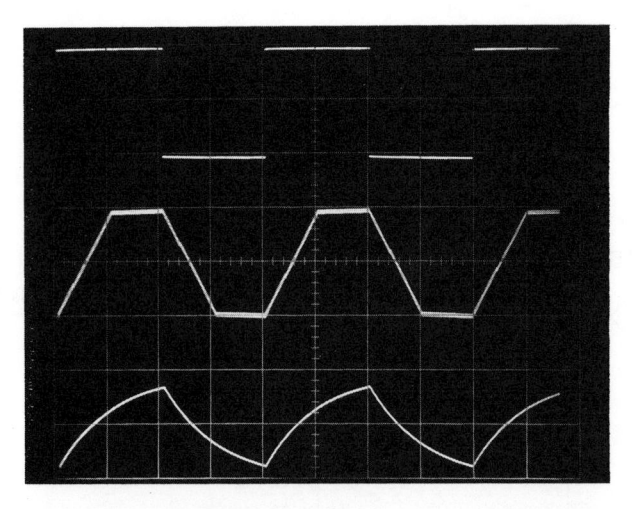

Figure 23.5 Smoothing of a square wave by transversal filtering or rectilinear averaging (top trace—width of the 64-point averaging window is ¼ the period of the square wave) and by simple RC low-pass filtering (bottom trace—"width" of window is specified by RC time constant).

square-wave input. In actual computation of running means, the transversal filter is preceded by one stage of RC filtering; in the case of a 0.5-sec transversal filter having 16 points, an RC filter having a time constant of 0.1 sec is used.

Interpolation by Means of a Transversal Filter

Another application of the transversal filter (or perhaps a different view of the operation) is that of interpolation between sample values. In this application, the duration of the transversal filter is matched to the interval between sample points. Figure 23.6 illustrates the use of the transversal filter for interpolation. For a step-function input, one transversal filter results in linear interpolation. If its output is then passed through an identical, synchronously operated transversal filter, quadratic interpolation results; this can be quite smooth, as is evident from the bottom trace in figure 23.6. The capability of a transverse filter for interpolating was employed in simulating epileptiform waveforms, as follows.

In the simulation of epileptiform transients in the form of spike-and-slow-wave complexes (figure 4.20), it was necessary to have a pair of waveforms for modulating the extrema and the slopes of the oscillator model. A waveform having an abrupt rise followed by an exponential decay sufficed for the modulation of the slopes, but a more complex waveform, having a gradual rise and a more gradual fall, was found to be necessary for modulating the extrema. A simple low-pass RC filter followed by a high-pass RC filter was not found to be entirely suitable.

A satisfactory solution (figure 4.20) was found in multiplexing and then smoothing the DC output of a series of 16 potentiometers connected to the

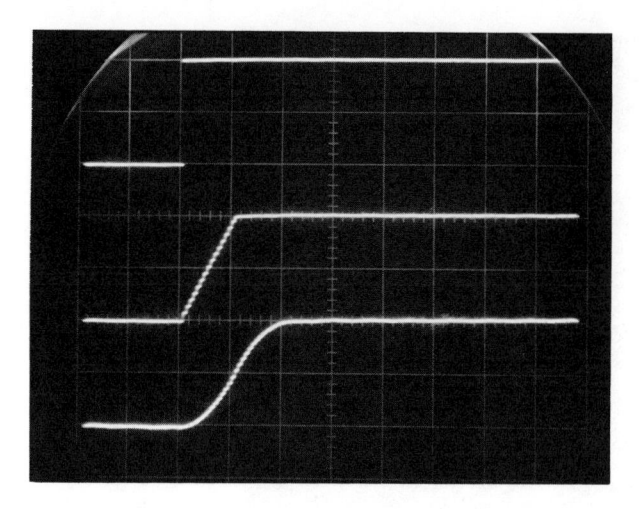

Figure 23.6 Use of the transversal filter as an interpolator. Top trace: step function. Middle trace: output of first transversal filter, with resultant linear interpolation. Bottom trace: output of second transversal filter, with resultant quadratic interpolation.

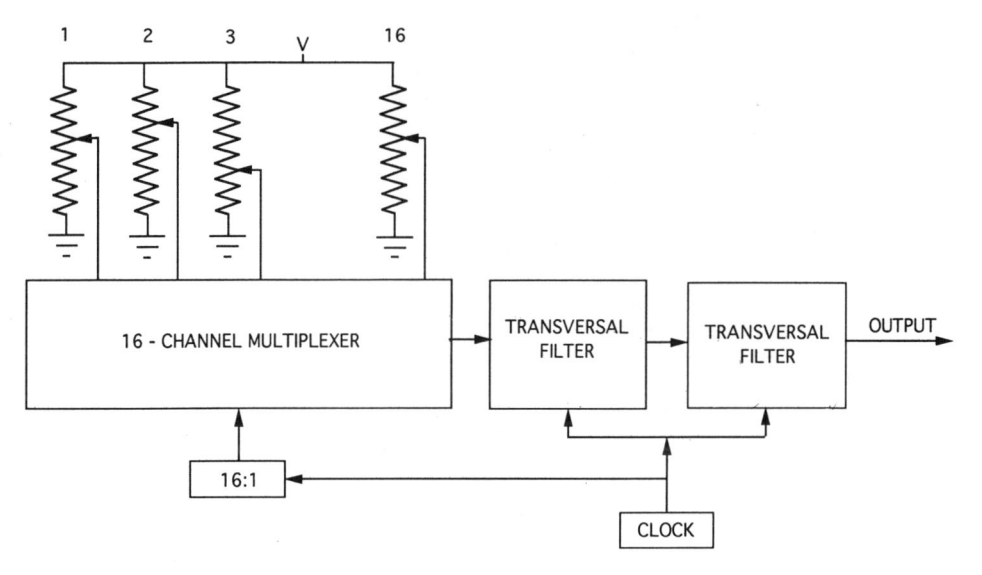

Figure 23.7 Schema for generating an arbitrary waveform of 256 points by multiplexing and interpolation (smoothing) of the output of an array of 16 manually adjusted potentiometers.

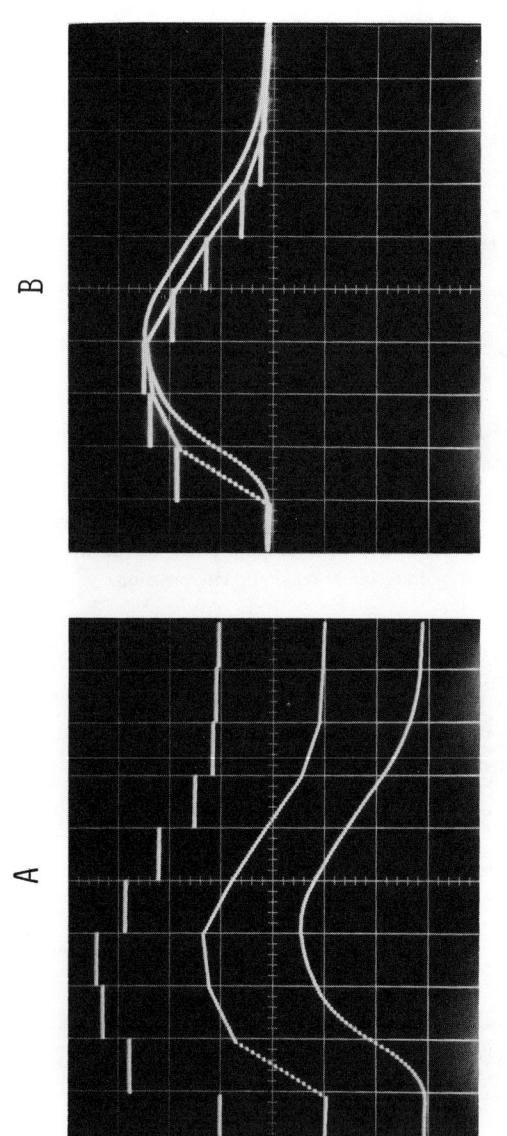

Figure 23.8 (A) Generation of a transient having an arbitrary waveform. Top trace: multiplexer output for the 16 DC input voltages. Middle trace: linear interpolation by means of a transversal filter. Bottom trace: quadratic interpolation by means of a second transversal filter. (The transversal filters operate at a clock rate of 16 times the input multiplexer.) Note the time delay introduced by each of the transversal filters; it is shown more clearly in part B.

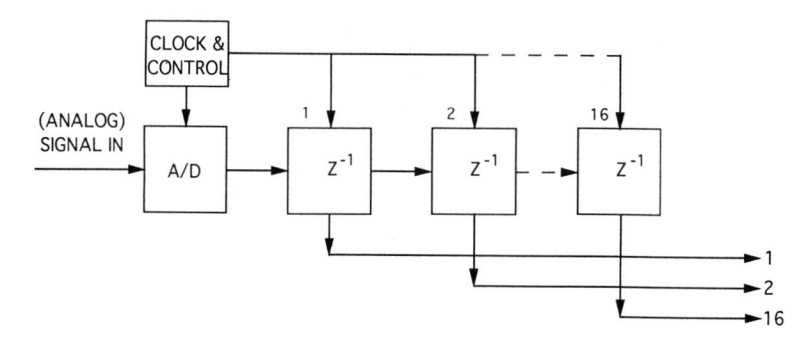

Figure 23.9 Block diagram of a 16-tap digital delay line. The symbol z^{-1} indicates one unit of delay. Note the components in common with those of figure 23.2.

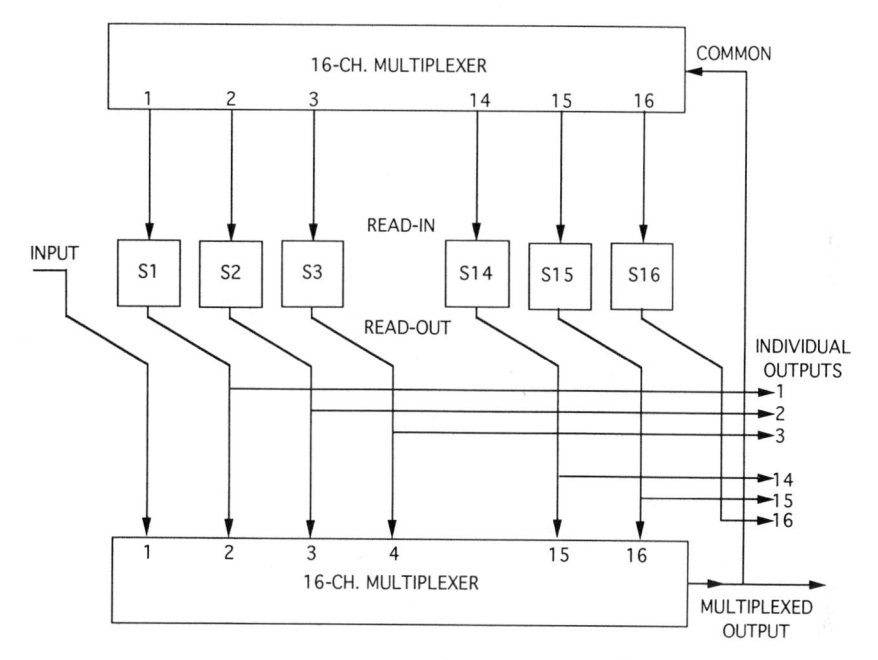

Figure 23.10 Schema of a 16-tap analog delay line made up of two synchronously driven 16-channel analog multiplexers. The outputs are available in either individual or multiplexed form.

same supply voltage, as shown in figure 23.7. The coarse steps are linearly interpolated with the first transversal filter, and quadratically interpolated with a second transversal filter, as shown in figure 23.8.

TAPPED ANALOG DELAY LINE

In several applications in the EEG data processing in this work, a tapped delay line is used: for obtaining time derivatives by the method of successive differences (chapter 24); in time-scaling (chapter 27); in computing and displaying event-related potentials, spectra, and autocorrelation functions (appendix A); and in the adaptive signal processor (appendix B). Like the transversal filter

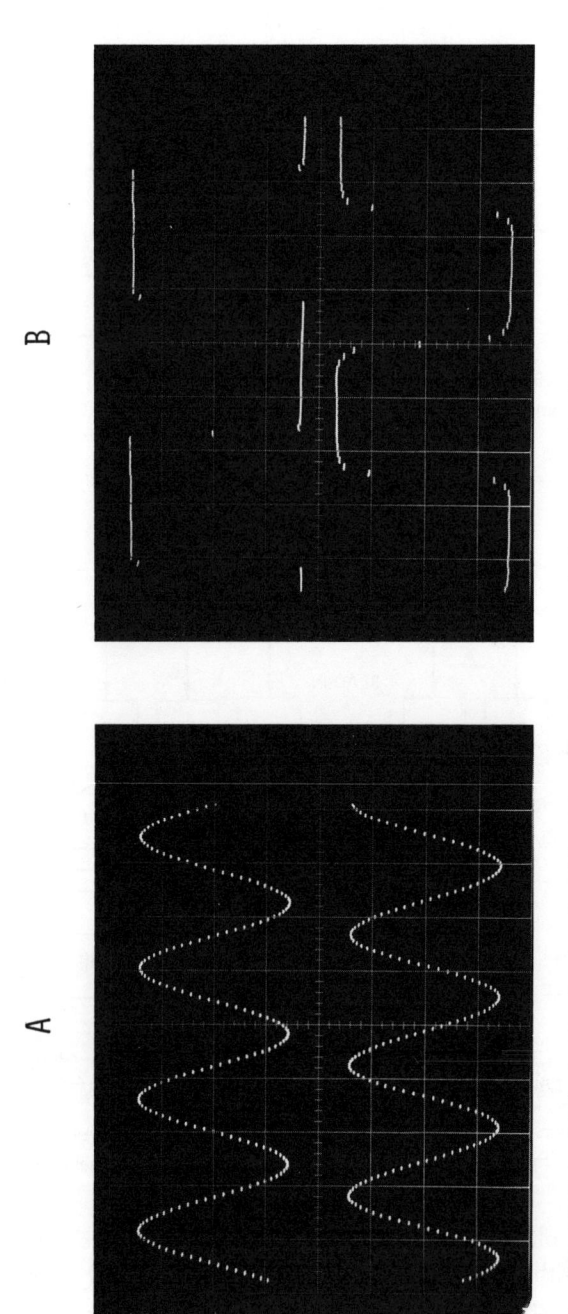

Figure 23.11 Output at the first tap (top trace) and the sixteenth tap (bottom trace) of a 16-tap analog delay line for an input 10-Hz sine wave (A) and for a 10-Hz square wave (B). The relative delay between the two taps is 0.25 sec, or $\frac{1}{4}$ the wavelength of the 10-Hz waves. Some loss of high-frequency response at the sixteenth tap is apparent for the square wave.

described above, a tapped delay line is normally implemented digitally (e.g., by means of shift registers), with separate readouts provided for each delay (as indicated in figure 23.9 for a 16-tap unit). An analog implementation of a 16-tap delay line is shown in figure 23.10.

As indicated in figure 23.10, the analog tapped delay line (which has a DC response) consists of two synchronously driven 16-channel multiplexers, which serially transfer, via their interconnected common terminals, the stored voltages between adjacent condenser-based storage units. The outputs are available both in individual and in multiplexed form, the latter from the interconnected common terminals of the multiplexers (figure 23.10). In essence, the unit operates as a "bucket brigade" (cf. Pratt et al. 1982), as does a charge-transfer device; however, in the present unit voltage rather than charge is transferred. Figure 23.11 shows the output of taps 1 and 16 of the delay line for 10-Hz sine-wave and 10-Hz square-wave inputs.

24 Basic Measures

The running means of amplitude and slope (or their moving averages) are computed in connection with the second type of tests of the extrema-slopes hypothesis (chapter 3). In the form of their quotient, the running mean slope and the running mean amplitude are also employed for computing the running mean frequency (chapter 25), and in combination with the running mean curvature (sharpness), to evaluate the Spectral Purity Index. As will be explained in chapter 25, the Spectral Purity Index is a new measure that indicates the degree of rhythmicity of a signal; it has a maximum value of 1.0 for a pure sine wave.

The same procedure is used for computing the running mean amplitude, slope, and curvature of a signal (figure 24.1). The signal for which the running mean is to be computed (i.e., the original signal, its first derivative, or its second derivative) is passed through a precision full-wave rectifier (chapter 23) so that all values are made positive, thus yielding absolute values of the signal. The full-wave rectified signal is then smoothed with a short time-constant (0.1 sec) RC filter, and then is passed through a 16-point transversal filter (chapter 23) having a nominal window duration of 0.5 sec (clock rate: 32 Hz), corresponding to a flat frequency response down to 1 Hz.

For obtaining the first and second (time) derivatives of a signal, two alternative approaches were explored and were found to give equivalent results. The first was that of conventional operational-amplifier based differentiation (figure 24.2A); the second was the method of successive differences (figure 24.2B). The first method was actually used, because of its relative simplicity.

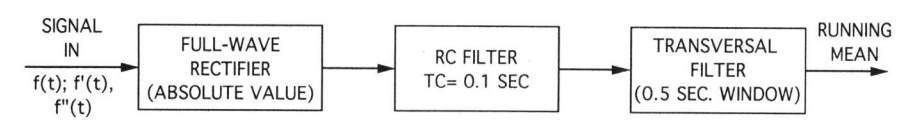

Figure 24.1 Schema of derivation of running (absolute) mean by full-wave rectification, short-time-constant RC filtering, and transversal filtering. Three units identical to the one shown are used to obtain the running means of a signal, its first derivative, and its second derivative.

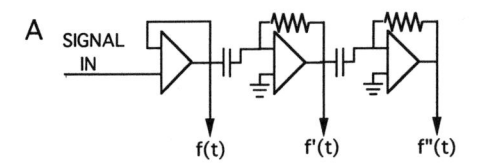

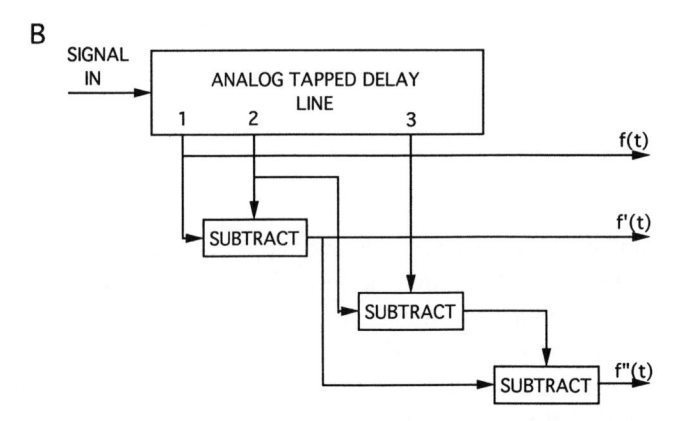

Figure 24.2 Schema of successive differentiation by conventional operational amplifiers (A) and by the method of successive differences (B). The latter unit consists of a tapped analog delay line (chapter 23) made up of a pair of eight-channel analog multiplexers with interconnected common terminals.

25 Derived Measures

RUNNING MEAN FREQUENCY

That the running mean frequency of a signal could be evaluated as the quotient of the running mean slope and the running mean amplitude was suggested by the fact that, for a sine wave of constant amplitude, the output of an operational-amplifier-based differentiation is linearly proportional to the input frequency. Normalization with respect to the input amplitude would then yield the frequency of the input irrespective of the amplitude, within a constant of proportionality. The latter is very simply evaluated by calibrating the system with a single precise frequency (e.g., 10.00 Hz). A preliminary description of this approach, but using a digital computer (in an application to the study of spontaneous alpha blocking), has been published (Goncharova and Barlow 1990).

A block diagram of the unit for determining running mean frequency is shown in figure 25.1. The units for evaluating the running means of amplitude and slope are identical (chapter 24), their inputs being, respectively, the original signal and its first derivative. Figure 25.2 shows the linearity of the system for a sine-wave input over the range 1–40 Hz.

Figure 25.3 shows the output of the system for a 10-Hz (center frequency) sine wave that was frequency-modulated by a square wave, so that the modulated frequency alternated between 5 and 15 Hz. The transition time is determined by the width of the averaging windows—in this case, 1.0 sec. (The clock frequency for the transversal filters was 16 Hz.) Figure 25.4. illustrates the operation of the system for noise signals of various characteristics; the mean frequency is indicated in each case, and the values are very close to the expected ones. (For wideband noise of 1.0–20 Hz, the mean frequency obtained by this method was approximately 12.5 Hz.)

Some limitations of this method of determining running mean frequency, and a comparison with Hjorth's normalized slope descriptors, are considered in chapter 17.

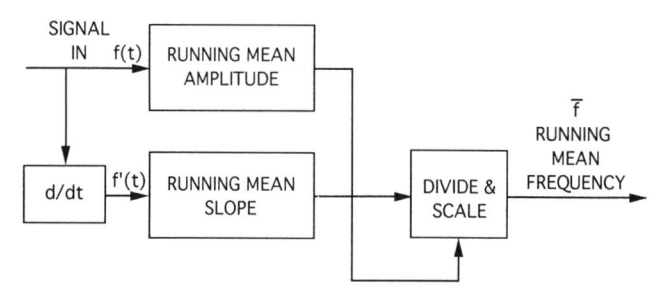

Figure 25.1 Block diagram of unit for evaluating running mean frequency ($\bar{f}$). The units for evaluating running mean amplitude and running mean slope are the same as the standard unit shown in figure 24.1. When the running mean frequency unit is used in conjunction with the photo-optical scanner for retrieving EEGs from ink recordings (chapter 26), the paper speed for the latter may be the same as or different from the original EEG paper speed; the scale factor is selected accordingly.

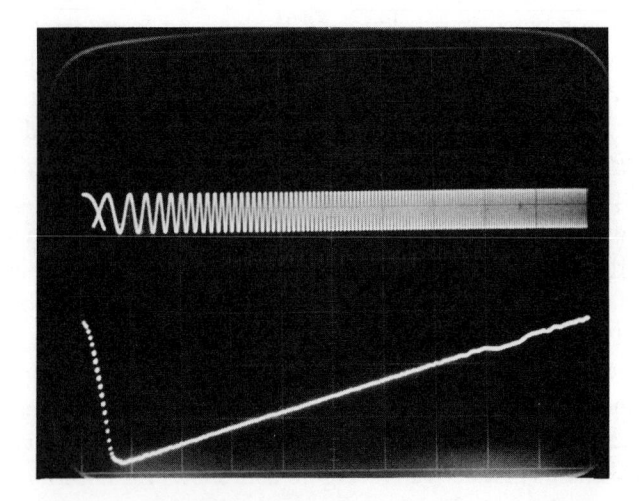

Figure 25.2 Derivation of running mean frequency (bottom trace) for a swept sine wave: 1–40 Hz (trace 1), indicating linearity of the system. (Photographed from a repetitive sweep.)

SPECTRAL PURITY INDEX (SPI)

In the course of a study of spontaneous alpha blocking (Goncharova and Barlow 1990), in which the just-described method of obtaining the running mean frequency was employed extensively, a need developed for an indication of frequency spread around the mean frequency (corresponding to width of a peak in a spectral plot). Initial results from the above-cited study indicated that, in some instances, the mean frequency of an EEG changed only minimally during periods of lower amplitude when the EEG appeared upon visual inspection to be rather irregular (i.e., during spontaneous alpha blocking). Such a finding suggested that the range of frequencies around the mean increased. It was to provide a quantitative measure of this effect that the Spectral Purity Index (SPI) was formulated.

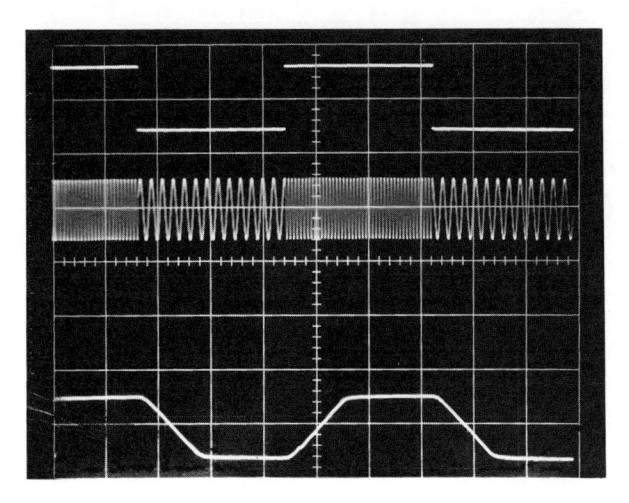

Figure 25.3 Running mean frequency (bottom trace) for a 10-Hz sine-wave frequency modulated by a square wave (top trace) resulting in an alternation between 5 and 15 Hz (middle trace). The transition time for the mean frequency (bottom trace) is the same as the duration of the averaging window of the transversal filter (in this case, 1.0 sec).

Since the running mean frequency is a single number (rather than an ensemble of numbers), it was desirable that a measure of the bandwidth of an EEG signal also be a single number. Further, it was desirable that such a number be dimensionless, i.e., completely normalized, so that its value would not be dependent on either amplitude or frequency. Finally, it was desirable that the measure have the value 1.0 for a sine wave, irrespective of the amplitude and frequency of the latter.

Inasmuch as the running mean frequency of a signal was based on determinations of running mean amplitude and running mean frequency, it appeared logical that a measure of bandwidth of a signal could be derived from some combination of the running means of its amplitude, slope, and curvature (sharpness), reflecting features of the original signal, its first derivative and its second derivative, respectively. Initially, an expression was worked out by dimensional analysis (so as to be dimensionless); then the expression was confirmed theoretically. The measure was termed the Spectral Purity Index, since it has a maximum value of 1.0 for a sine wave of (in principle) any amplitude and any frequency.

The expression for the (running) Spectral Purity Index is:

$$\text{SPI} = \frac{\bar{s}^2}{\bar{a}\bar{c}}, \tag{1}$$

or, alternatively,

$$\text{SPI} = \frac{\bar{f}\bar{s}}{\bar{c}}, \tag{2}$$

where $\bar{a}$, $\bar{s}$, $\bar{c}$, and $\bar{f}$ are the running means of amplitude, slope, curvature, and frequency, respectively.

Derived Measures

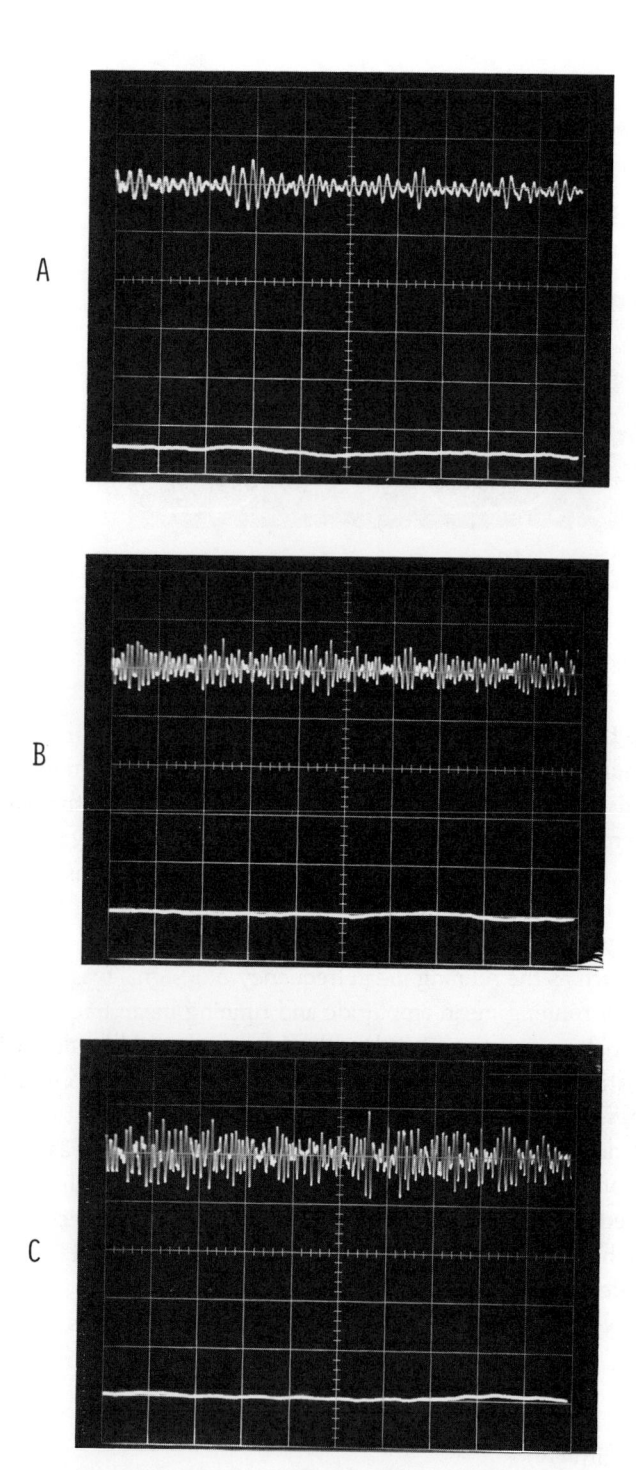

Figure 25.4 Running mean frequency (bottom traces) of several noise signals (top traces). (A) Noise centered at 5 Hz (24-dB rolloff outside passband). (B) Same as in part A, but centered at 10 Hz. (C) 5–15-Hz band-limited noise. The corresponding running mean frequencies (bottom traces) are approximately 5 Hz, 10 Hz, and 10 Hz, respectively.

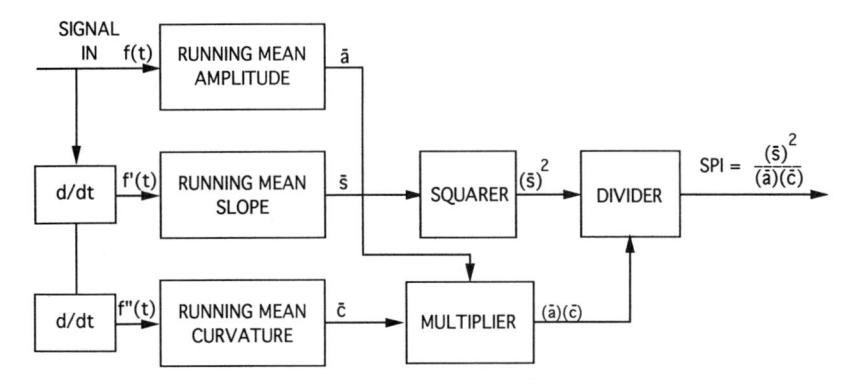

Figure 25.5 Block diagram of unit for computation of the Spectral Purity Index. The running-mean units are identical, and are the same as in figure 25.1. The differentiations are accomplished with operational amplifiers. The resultant means for amplitude, slope, and curvature are denoted as indicated. Note that each is a mean of absolute (positive or zero) values.

The implementation of equation 1, for which high-precision analog arithmetic computing units (chips) are used, is indicated in the block diagram of figure 25.5.

The manner in which the Spectral Purity Index provides an amplitude- and frequency-independent measure of the width of the frequency band of a signal (and thus an indication of the width of its spectrum) can be understood by reference to the sequence of curves in figures 25.6 and 25.7 and the following considerations. For a sine wave of fixed amplitude but variable frequency (figure 25.6A, top curve), the running mean (absolute) value of its slope (i.e., its first derivative) varies as the first power of its frequency (second curve), and the running mean (absolute) value of its curvature (i.e., its second derivative) varies as the square of its frequency (fourth curve). Further, the square of the running mean absolute value of its slope, which is the numerator in the expression for the SPI, also varies with the square of its frequency (third curve), which has the same shape as the product of the running mean curvature and the running mean amplitude (fifth curve), since the latter is constant (first curve). The fifth curve is the denominator of the expression for the SPI (expression 1), and hence the SPI itself, normalized to have a value of 1.0 (extreme right curve in figure 25.6A) is independent of frequency for a sine wave of fixed amplitude.

The comparable sequence of curves for the counterpart of the above, i.e., a sine wave of variable amplitude but fixed frequency (top curve in figure 25.6B), is as follows. The running mean (absolute) value of its slope varies as the first power of its amplitude (figure 25.6B, second curve), and the running mean value of its curvature varies as the square of is amplitude (fourth curve). The square of the running mean absolute value of its slope (third curve) varies as the square of the amplitude. The latter curve, which is the numerator in the expression for the SPI (expression 1), has the same shape as the product of the running mean curvature and the running mean amplitude (fifth curve), which

Derived Measures

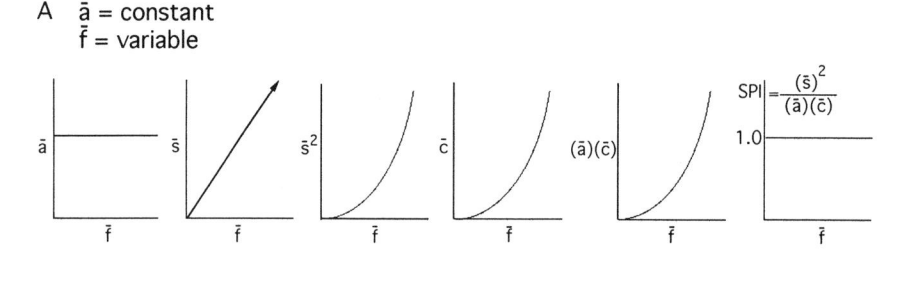

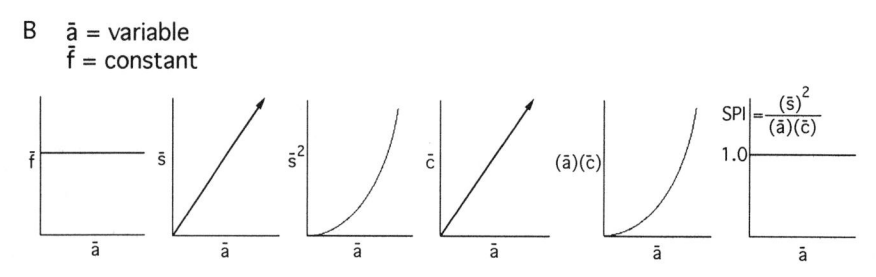

Figure 25.6 Characteristics of mean slope ($\bar{s}$), square of mean slope ($\bar{s}^2$), mean curvature ($\bar{c}$), and Spectral Purity Index (SPI) for (A) sine waves of constant amplitude but variable frequency and (B) sine waves of constant frequency but variable amplitude. Note that the Spectral Purity Index (extreme right) is 1.0 in both cases.

is the denominator of the SPI expression; hence, the SPI, normalized to have a value of 1.0, is independent of amplitude for a sine wave of fixed frequency (extreme right curve in figure 25.6B).

However, if a range or a band of frequencies is present (figure 25.7), rather than a single frequency, the Spectral Purity Index will have a value less than 1.0, because frequency components higher than the mean frequency will be represented in the running mean absolute curvature to a disproportionately greater extent than components of frequencies lower than the mean frequency. This effect increases linearly with the bandwidth; hence the Spectral Purity Index decreases with increasing bandwidth as

$$(f_0 - \Delta f)/f_0, \tag{3}$$

or

$$(1 - \Delta f/f_0), \tag{4}$$

in which f_0 is the mean frequency and Δf is the half-width of the frequency band around it, assuming the frequency spectrum is flat betweeen $(f_0 + \Delta f)$ and $(f_0 - \Delta f)$. Thus, an SPI of 1.0 implies a line spectrum (i.e., a pure sine wave), and an SPI of 0.9 indicates a bandwidth of $0.11(f_0)$ (i.e., for $f_0 = 10$ Hz, a range of frequencies from 8.9 to 11 Hz). See table 25.1.

SPI values of less than 0.5 (i.e., $\Delta f_0/f_0$ greater than 1.0) necessarily imply a bandwidth of frequencies asymmetrical about f_0—i.e., a greater expanse (but lower amplitudes) of higher frequencies than of lower ones, relative to the mean frequency, f_0.

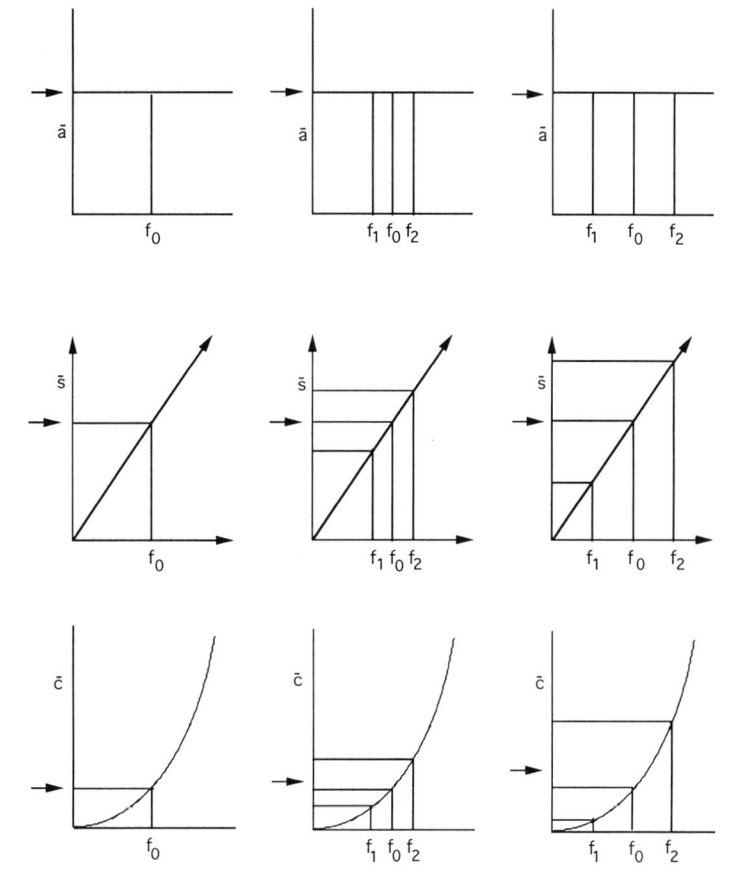

Figure 25.7 Characteristics of running means of amplitude, slope, and curvature as the range of frequencies in a signal (i.e., its bandwidth) progressively increases (first, second, and third columns). Note that in the expression SPI = $(\bar{s})^2/(\bar{a})(\bar{c})$, as the frequency band (f_1-f_2) increases from left to right, $(\bar{a})$ (first row) and $(\bar{s})$ (second row)—and therefore $(\bar{s}^2)$—remain constant (denoted by arrows), but $(\bar{c})$ (third row) increases progressively (note progressive upward shift of the arrows), because of the greater weighting of the frequency components that are above the mean frequency as compared with the weighting of frequency components below the mean frequency (note arrow at left). Therefore, $(\bar{a})(\bar{c})$ becomes larger than $(\bar{s})^2$, and hence the Spectral Purity Index becomes less than 1.0.

Table 25.1

SPI	$\Delta f/f_0$
1.0	0
0.9	0.11
0.8	0.25
0.7	0.42
0.6	0.66
0.5	1.00
0.4	1.5
0.3	2.3
0.2	4.0
0.1	9.0

The measures of running mean frequency and the Spectral Purity Index are compared with Hjorth's normalized slope parameters in chapter 17.

A Digital Implementation of the Spectral Purity Index

As is the case with all the measures described in this book, implementation on a general-purpose digital computer should be relatively straightforward.

An example of the result of determination of the Spectral Purity Index during spontaneous alpha blocking is shown as the bottom trace of figure 25.8. The running mean amplitude, slope, and frequency are shown in the upper traces. From this figure it is apparent that, during the alpha blocking in this instance, there was a decrease in the Spectral Purity Index (i.e., a widening of the band of frequencies), although there was no change in the mean frequency.

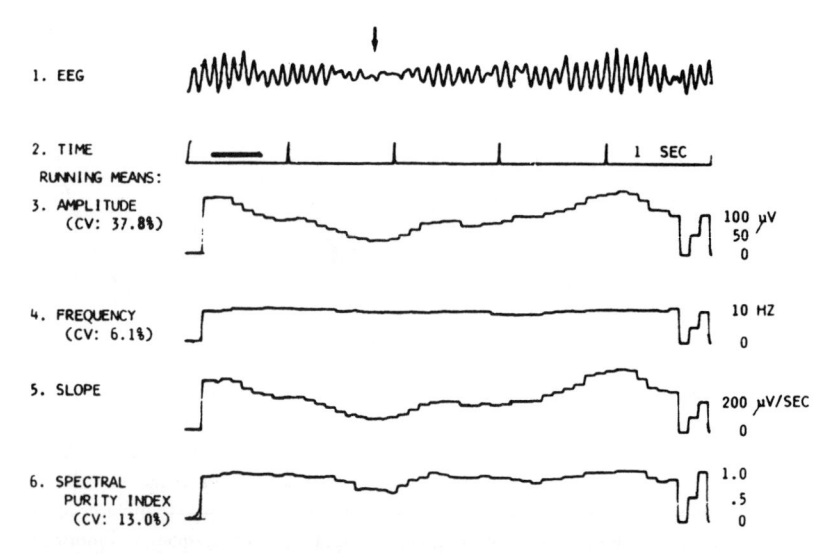

Figure 25.8 Example of digital implementation, by Irina I. Goncharova (now of the Brain Institute, Moscow), of the Spectral Purity Index (bottom trace) together with the running means of amplitude (trace 3), frequency (trace 4), and slope (trace 5), in a case of spontaneous alpha blocking. Note the decrease in the Spectral Purity Index during the brief period of alpha blocking although the running mean frequency remains essentially unchanged. (From Goncharova and Barlow 1990.)

COEFFICIENT OF VARIATION (CV)

The Coefficient of Variation (CV) is defined (Sokal and Rohlf 1973; Goncharova and Barlow 1990) in terms of a percentage as the quotient of the standard deviation (SD) to the mean (M):

$$CV(\%) = (SD/M) \cdot 100. \tag{5}$$

This quotient can be viewed as the standard deviation normalized for the mean.

In the present work, the Coefficient of Variation is evaluated on a running basis, i.e., for a moving window of generally four times the duration of the averaging window for the basic running means (i.e., those of amplitude, slope, and curvature).

In equation 5, the numerator can be replaced by its definition as the square root of the difference between the mean of the squares and the square of the mean, divided by the mean:

$$CV = \frac{\sqrt{(\sum Y_i^2)/n - Y_m^2}}{Y_m}. \tag{6}$$

Here Y_i represents the individual sample values and Y_m the mean of the samples. Since the Coefficient of Variation is a normalized measure (note the denominator in equation 6), it is insensitive to a change in scale of the original signal (EEG).

The steps in the evaluation of the Coefficient of Variation are shown in figure 25.9. The system is calibrated by using a signal that has the maximum possible Coefficient of Variation, i.e., 100%. For this purpose a square wave is used that has a positive DC offset that is half the peak-to-peak amplitude; i.e., the "negative" phase of the square wave is at 0 DC. The output CV is then adjusted for full-scale value, i.e., 100% or 1.0.

For the present work, the length of the averaging window indicated in equation 3, i.e., the length of the transverse filter, was usually four times that of the transversal filter used for obtaining the basic running means (amplitude, etc.).

RELATIVE VARIABILITY

In some instances, it was desirable to have an index of the relative variability of the running mean slope and the running mean amplitude. From the definition of the standard deviation (the numerator in equation 3), it is evident that, if two processes have the same mean but the standard deviation of the second is twice as great as that of the first, then the second process can be said to have twice as much variability as the first. Therefore, measures having different variabilities can be compared by taking the quotient of their Coefficients of Variation, since the latter are normalized with respect to the respective means. Thus, if the second of two measures is twice as variable as the first, the ratio of their CVs is 2:1; and for the reverse, 1:2, the corresponding quotients

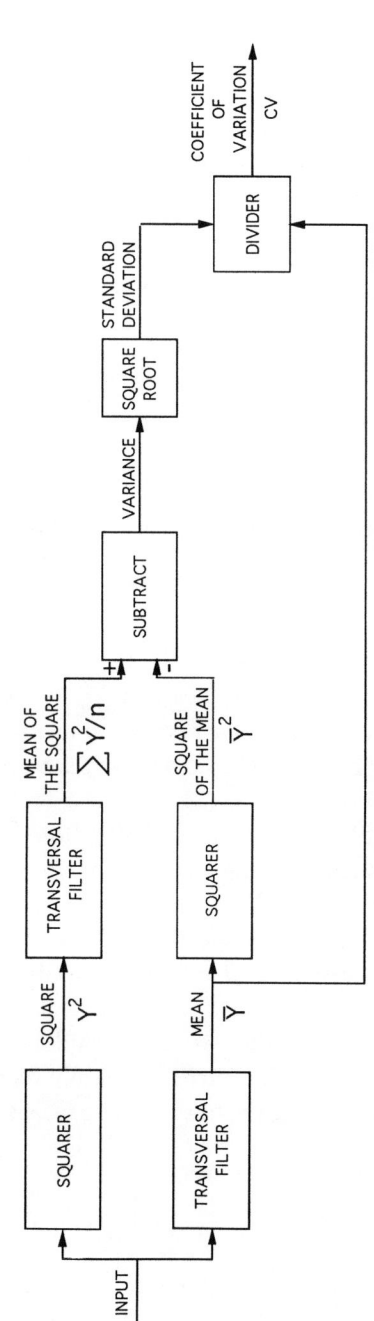

Figure 25.9 Block diagram of unit for computing the running Coefficient of Variation (CV) as the standard deviation divided by the mean.

being 2.0 and 0.5. The quotient of the two is itself not convenient, however, because its scale is not a linear one. A linear scale is, however, conveniently obtained by taking the logarithm of the quotient of the respective Coefficients of Variation—in the present case, of slope (s) and amplitude (a):

$$\log(\text{Relative variability } (\bar{s}, \bar{a})) = \log\left(\frac{\text{CV}(\bar{s})}{\text{CV}(\bar{a})}\right). \tag{7}$$

A value of zero indicates that the slope and the amplitude are equally variable; a negative value indicates that the slope is less variable than the amplitude; a positive value indicates that the slope is more variable than the amplitude. Appropriate scaling can be chosen so that, e.g., a value of -0.5 could indicate that amplitude is twice as variable as slope, and $+0.5$ the converse. Since each of the Coefficients of Variation in equation 4 is insensitive to a change in scale of the original measure (i.e., running means of amplitude, slope), the quotient of the two Coefficients of Variation or the relative variability is also independent of any change in scale (e.g., a change of the sensitivity setting of the original EEG recording).

THE PEARSON PRODUCT-MOMENT CORRELATION COEFFICIENT

The Pearson Product-Moment Correlation Coefficient (PPMCC), r, is a quantitative measure of the degree of similarity between two non-zero-mean processes or time series (e.g., the running mean amplitude and the running mean slope, in the present application), defined as follows:

$$r_{12} = \frac{\sum y_1 y_2}{\sqrt{(\sum y_1^2)(\sum y_2^2)}}, \tag{8}$$

where y_1 and y_2 denote the sample values of the two time series after the removal of the respective mean values from each (Sokal and Rohlf 1973). The PPMCC, which is the same as the normalized cross-correlation computed only at zero lag, has a value of 1.0 for two identical time series (after removal of the respective mean or DC component from each), and a value of -1.0 if one series is the negative of the other. The value fluctuates around 0 for two unrelated time series, the amplitude of the fluctuation being determined by the averaging time in relation to the frequency content of the two time series (Barlow and Dubinsky 1976, figure 2).

The block diagram of the unit for evaluating the Pearson Product-Moment Correlation Coefficient, including the elimination of the means of the two time series, is shown in figure 25.10. The first two components for each input channel (i.e., a transversal filter and a multiplexer) serve to compute the running mean of the most recent 16 points, which is subtracted from each of the 16 sample values in multiplexed form. The remainder of the computation represents a straightforward implementation of equation 8, including squaring, summating (in transversal filters), multiplication, taking the square root, and division. The unit is so adjusted that, if the input signals are too low in

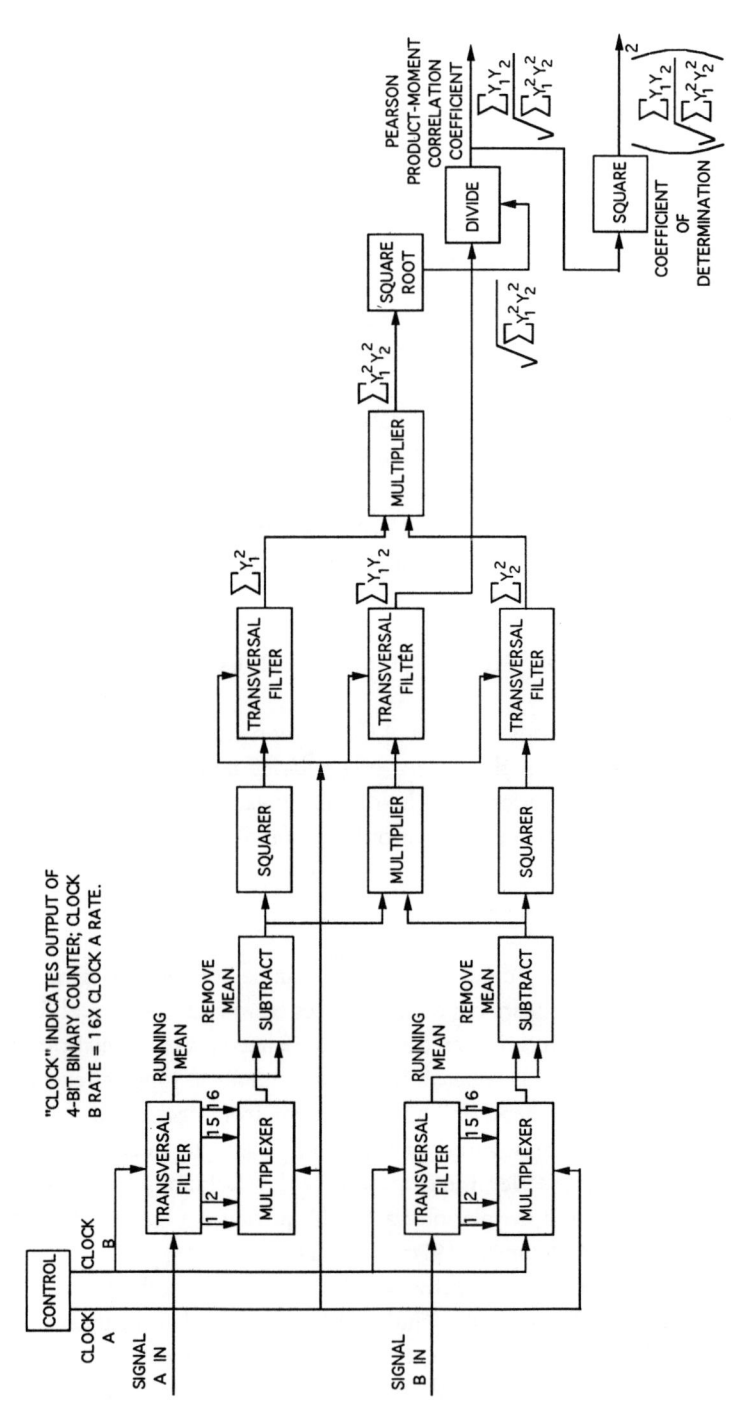

Figure 25.10 Block diagram of unit for computing the running Pearson Product-Moment Correlation Coefficient. The clock (A) for the transversal filters operates at $\frac{1}{16}$ the rate of the clock (B) for the other units, so that the computation of a point on the output curve (based on the most recent 16 data points stored in the transversal filter) is completed at the sampling rate for the input to the transversal filter. The last squarer (lower right) is included for computing the Coefficient of Determination, the square of the PPMCC.

amplitude for accurate determination of the PPMCC, the output value of the latter is greater than 1.0. (Squaring, the last operation in figure 25.10, is used for obtaining the Coefficient of Determination, as described below.) The time interval over which the PPMCC is computed can be extended by adding a transversal filter to the output.

THE COEFFICIENT OF DETERMINATION

The Pearson Product-Moment Correlation Coefficient can range in value from +1.0 (for two identical signals of the same polarity) to −1.0 (for two identical signals of opposite polarity). If the indication of relative polarity is not desirable or necessary, the square of the PPMCC—which is termed the Coefficient of Determination (CD) (Sokal and Rohlf 1973)—may be preferred. The Coefficient of Determination, a measure of the degree of relatedness of two signals irrespective of their polarity, ranges in value from 1.0 (for two identical signals, irrespective of their relative polarity) to 0 (for two unrelated signals). The CD is more sensitive than the PPMCC to differences between two time series; for example, for a PPMCC value of 0.8, the CD is 0.64. Figure 25.11 illustrates the evaluation of the Coefficient of Determination for three pairs of Gaussian noise signals that are identical, partially related, and completely independent, respectively.

As employed in the present work, the CD is determined not from the original two signals but rather from derived measures, such as running means of their amplitudes and slopes, in which direct information concerning individual frequency components and their phases is not retained. The PPMCC and the CD, as normalized measures, are both insensitive in principle to a change in scale factor of one or both the two time series; nonetheless, requirements of computational accuracy in the several steps entailed necessitates adequate signal levels. A condition of inadequate signal levels is indicated in the PPMCC unit by an output greater than 1.0.)

THE COEFFICIENT OF DETERMINATION VS. THE COHERENCE FUNCTION

The CD, a normalized quantity (its maximum value is 1.0), should be distinguished from the Coherence Function (Walter et al. 1966; Lopes da Silva 1987b). The Coherence Function is a measure of relatedness between two signals or time series frequency by frequency, irrespective of the relative phases of a given frequency component in the two signals. The Coherence Function is normalized; i.e., its maximum value at any given frequency is 1.0. The Coherence Function is accompanied by a Phase Spectrum, indicating the phase relationship between the same frequency components in the two signals.

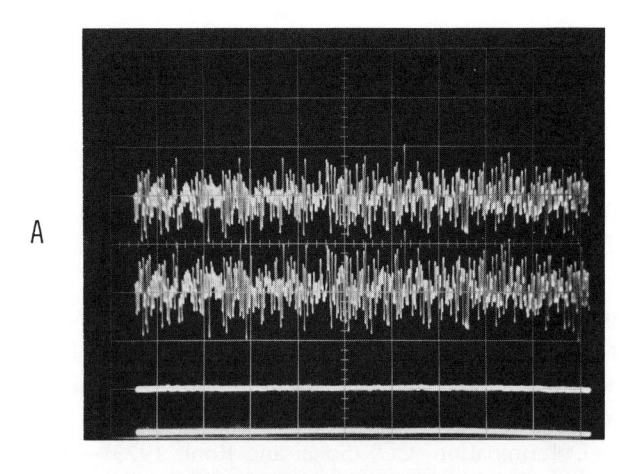

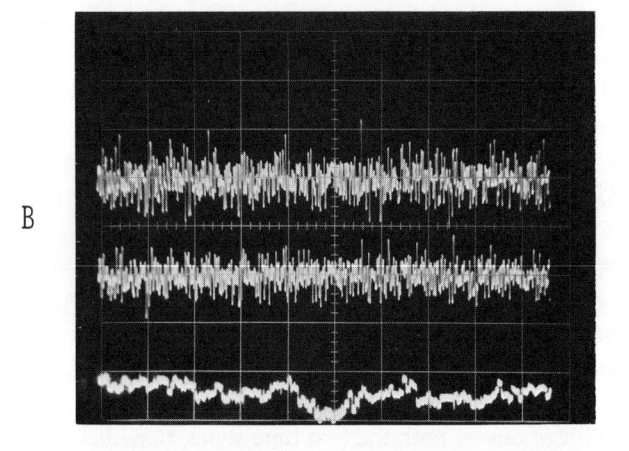

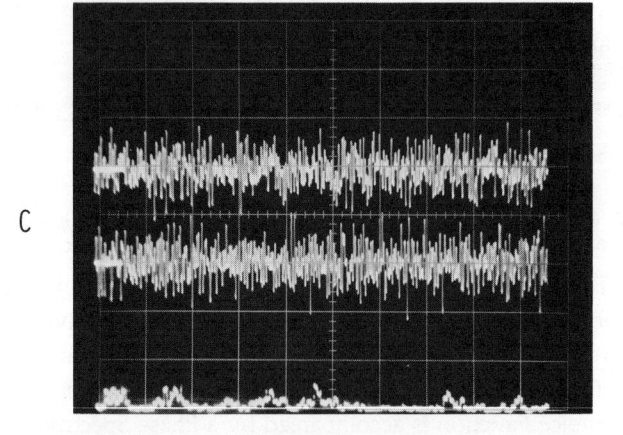

Figure 25.11 Write-out of Coefficients of Determination of two Gaussian noise signals that are identical (A), partially related (B), and completely independent (C). The respective values of the CDs are approximately 1.0 (note baseline at the bottom in Part A), 0.5, and 0.1. Note the random (statistical) fluctuations in parts B and C, associated with the relatively short averaging window used.

RELATIONSHIPS AMONG THE SPECTRAL PURITY INDEX, THE RELATIVE VARIABILITY, THE PEARSON PRODUCT-MOMENT CORRELATION COEFFICIENT, AND THE COEFFICIENT OF DETERMINATION; RECAPITULATION

As was indicated in chapter 3, the running mean frequency and the running Spectral Purity Index provide information concerning the mean frequency and the frequency spread of an EEG. (The Spectral Purity Index gives information that can be compared with the spectral width of a Fourier spectrum.) The Coefficient of Variation provides a quantitative index of the relative variability of a given measure; a linear indication of the relative variability of two measures is conveniently given by the logarithm of the quotients of their respective Coefficients of Variation. The Pearson Product-Moment Correlation Coefficient and its square, the Coefficient of Determination, provide a measure of the degree of similarity between, e.g., the running mean amplitude and the running mean slope.

In the case of a sine wave, the Spectral Purity Index is 1.0, the Coefficients of Variation of the running means of slope and amplitude are both 0 (and hence the logarithm of their ratio is undefined), and the Pearson Product-Moment Correlation Coefficient for the running means of amplitude and slope is 1.0, as is the Coefficient of Determination.

For moderately rhythmic alpha activity, the running means of amplitude and slope will be very similar in waveform. The running mean frequency will be that of the alpha frequency. The Spectral Purity Index will be close to 1.0 (even for alpha activity that varies appreciably in amplitude). The Coefficients of Variation of the running mean slope and amplitude will be approximately the same, their values depending on the duration of the alpha spindles (the higher, the shorter the spindles). The quotient of the two coefficients of variation (i.e., the Relative Variability) will be about 1.0, and hence its logarithm will be 0 (signifying equal variability of the two running means). The Pearson Product-Moment Correlation Coefficient and the Coefficient of Determination for the running mean amplitude and running mean slope will be approximately 1.0, since the latter two waveforms are very similar.

For rather irregular EEG activity, the running means of amplitude and slope will differ in their waveform. The running mean frequency will correspond to the middle of the frequency band of the EEG. The Spectral Purity Index will be less than 1.0. The Coefficients of Variation for the running mean slope and amplitude may be similar or different, according to the predominant type of EEG waves (chapter 2). The logarithm of the quotient of the two Coefficients of Variation may be 0 (e.g., for rhythmic activity), less than 0 (for constant-slope waves), or greater than 0. The Pearson Product-Moment Correlation Coefficient and the Coefficient of Determination will be less than 1.0, according to the degree of irregularity of the EEG.

26 Photo-Optical Scanner for Data Retrieval from EEG Ink Recordings

The device that permits the reconversion of EEG ink recordings to electrical form, and therefore permits access to a wide variety of existing ink-recorded EEGs, was described in its original form in a series of publications some years ago (Barlow 1967a, 1968, 1971; Barlow and DiPerna 1967, 1968). It uses the principle of phase-modulated analog sampling (Barlow 1967a), illustrated in figure 26.1. A block diagram of the original scanner is shown in figure 26.2. A specially constructed photo-optical scanning pen (which resembles a standard EEG writing pen for a Grass electroencephalograph) is operated at 60 Hz, with the same signal (save for a small phase shift) used as the input to a pair of sample-and-hold circuits triggered by the leading and trailing edges of the photopulses, respectively, for upward or downward motion of the scanning pen. The summed output of the two sample-and-hold circuits (thus correcting for trace width of the EEG) constitutes the final output.

Since the original publications, a number of improvements and simplifications have been made in the circuitry. One of the most important was the introduction of a "floating threshold" for the photopulse, which automatically corrects for variations in its amplitude due to variations in ink density, width of trace, reflectivity of paper (etc.) of the original ink-recorded EEG, and for variations in sensitivity of the photocell in different scanning pens.

COMPENSATION FOR SELF-OVERLAPPING OF AN EEG INKED TRACE

Two additional major problems, partly interrelated, arose in connection with the present work. The first resulted from the overlap or confluence of upgoing and downgoing portions of relatively high-amplitude EEGs written out on a relatively slow time base—a situation that occurs during all-night sleep recordings written out on a time base of 10 or 15 mm/sec, as compared with the paper speed of 30 mm/sec usually used for waking EEG recordings. (Correction for non-confluent traces is afforded by using the pair of sample-and-hold circuits, one triggered by the leading edge and the other triggered by the trailing edge of the photopulse, and summating the two (Barlow and DiPerna 1968).)

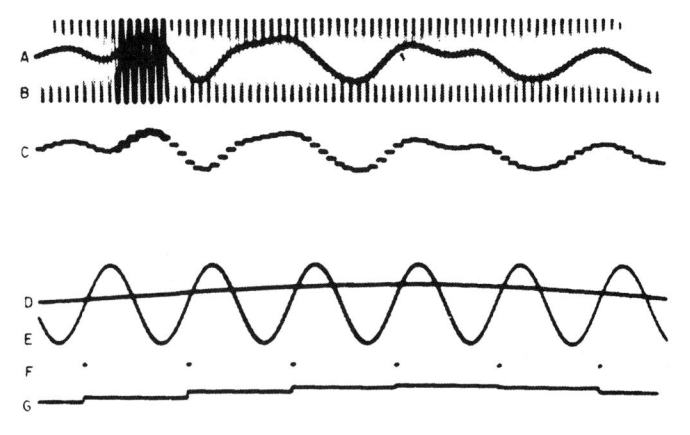

Figure 26.1 The principle of phase-modulated analog sampling. Trace A: curve to be transcribed (scanned waveform). Trace B: scanning waveform. Trace C: output of sample-and-hold circuit. Traces D, E, and G: intensified portions of traces A, B, and C, respectively, but on a faster time base. Trace F: pulses indicating coincidence of scanned (trace D) and scanning (trace E) waveforms. (From Barlow 1967a.)

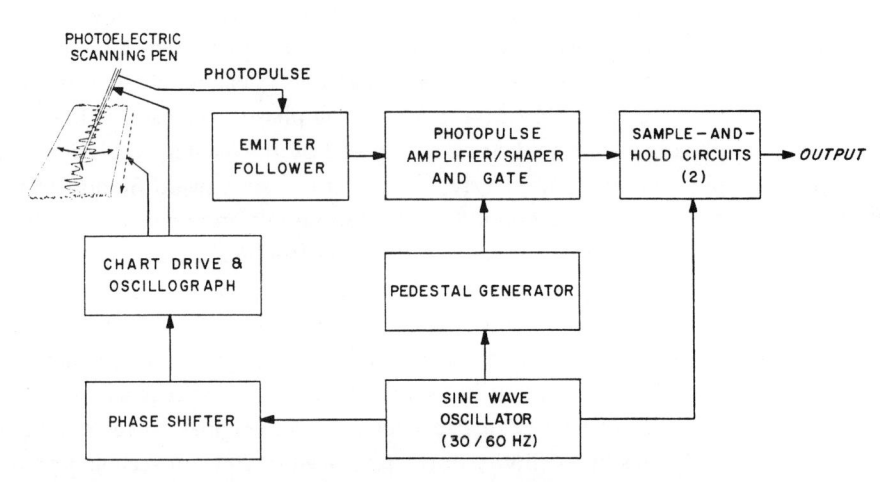

Figure 26.2 Block diagram of original photo-optical scanner. The chart drive and the oscillograph are those of a standard (Grass) electroencephalograph with the standard writing pen replaced by a photoelectric scanning pen. (From Barlow and DiPerna 1968.)

If, however, the upgoing and downgoing portions of the trace overlap to an appreciable degree, as depicted in figure 26.3, equal summation of the output of the two sample-and-hold circuits will result in an attenuation of the output. However, the problem can be diminished by summating a variable proportion, rather than an equal mixture, of the outputs of the two sample-and-hold circuits. Such a variable proportion, or ratio, was obtained from the running quotient of the derivatives of the leading and the trailing edges of the photopulse, such that the output of the two sample-and-hold circuits corresponding to the higher derivative is given the greater weight. The result is that the output of the weighted and summated sample-and-hold units tends to follow the *outside* of an inked trace that partially overlaps itself, thus minimiz-

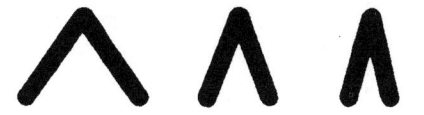

Figure 26.3 Depiction of a self-confluent trace resulting from its finite width. Note the progressive partially overlapping upward and downward portions of the trace with increasing steepness (slope) of the trace.

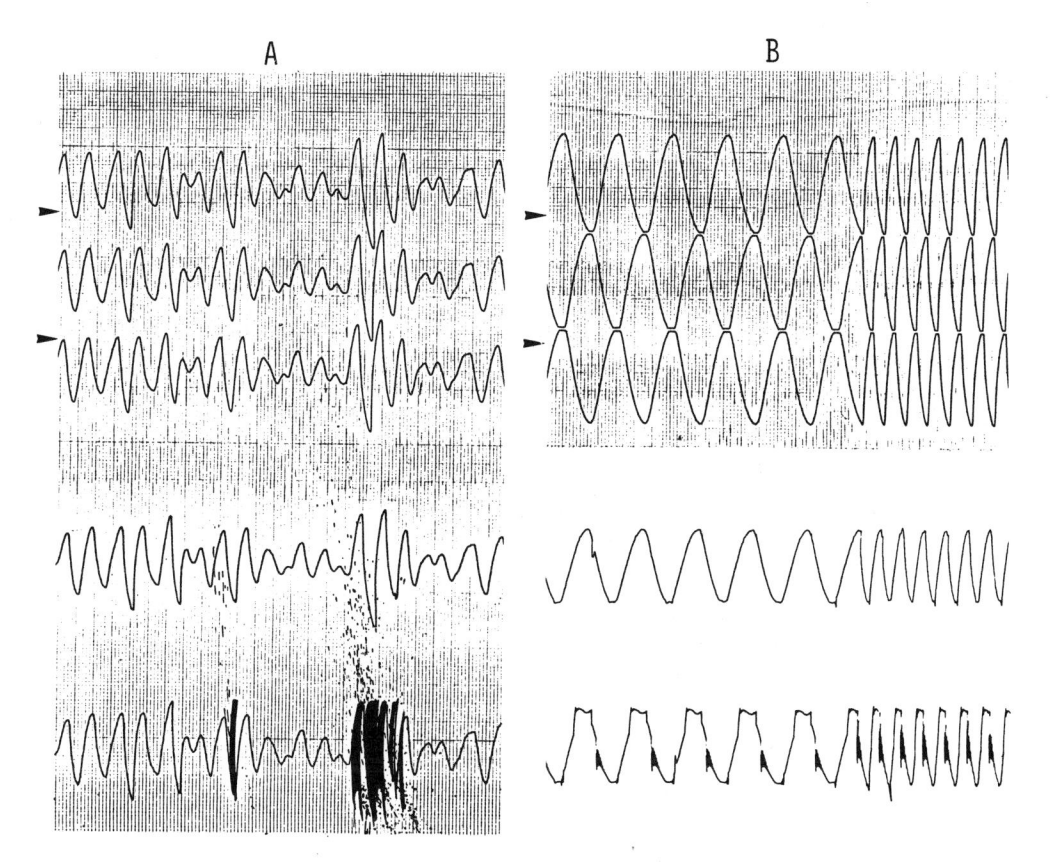

Figure 26.4 The two types (A and B) of adjacent-trace overlap that result in interference in the photo-optical scanning process and require different methods for their elimination. Of the top three traces in each, the second trace is scanned in each instance (the arrows mark the limits of excursion of the tip of the scanning pen); the fourth trace shows the write-out with the interference removed, and the fifth trace shows the write-out without the elimination of the interference. In part A, the traces interleave (in-phase interference); however, one can eliminate the interference by rendering the scanning pen "blind" except to a very narrow horizontal band centered on the trace being scanned at a given instant. In part B, the adjacent traces are opposed (anti-phase interference) and hence a trace-counting procedure is necessary.

ing loss of amplitude in the final output. (The relative portions of the sample-and-hold circuits were obtained by a pair of multipliers functioning effectively as a ganged pair of potentiometers operating in a fade-in/fade-out manner.)

ELIMINATION OF ADJACENT-TRACE INTERFERENCE

Certain EEG recordings, such as those from deeper stages of non-REM sleep and 3-Hz spike-wave patterns, may be of sufficiently high amplitude on the write-out to extend into the region of one or both of the adjacent channels, therefore interfering with the photo-optical scanning of the adjacent trace. There are two types of adjacent-channel interference, as indicated in figure 26.4. The first, resulting from interleaving of traces, is more likely to be encountered in referential EEG recordings; the second, resulting from closely adjacent extrema, in bipolar recordings.

The first form of interference (figure 26.4A) can be eliminated by making the scanning pen "blind" except to a narrow vertical band centered at the inked trace—an effect that is accomplished by deriving a pedestal from the combined output of the two sample-and-hold circuits, which is used for enabling (gating) the photopulse. (The photopulse is activated only during upward motion of the photo-optical scanning pen.)

The second form of interference (figure 26.4B) cannot be eliminated by the procedure just described. Instead, the solution lies in automatically counting up the number of interfering traces (generally, but not invariably, only one) between the correct inked-trace intersection (after which the sample-and-hold trigger pulses are inactivated) and the peak of the excursion of the scanning pen, and then counting down, reactivating the aforementioned trigger pulses when the downward-motion count matches the upward-motion count. The counting procedure is repeated anew after each baseline crossing of the tip of the scanning pen.

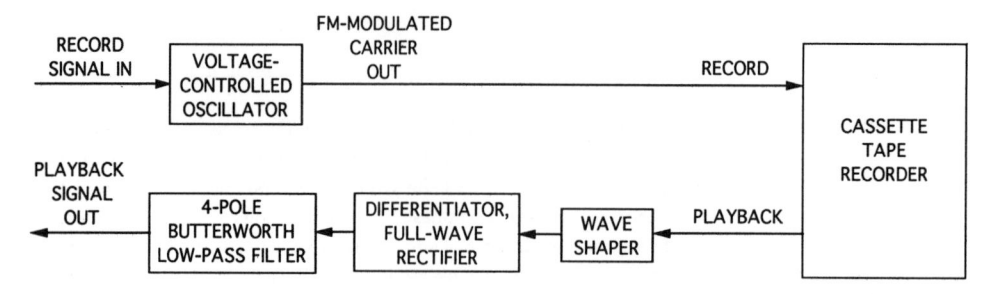

Figure 26.5 Block diagram of two-channel FM cassette tape recorder system for storage of the output of the photo-optical scanner. The FM modulator is a conventional comparator-based voltage-controlled oscillator circuit (center frequency: 5 kHz). The playback signal from the cassette recorder is reconverted to a square wave by means of a comparator, is differentiated and full-wave rectified, and is then passed through a four-pole Butterworth filter having a cutoff frequency of 500 Hz, provision being made for adjusting the level and DC offset of the final output. (Only one channel is shown.)

TEMPORARY MAGNETIC-TAPE STORAGE OF OUTPUT OF PHOTO-OPTICAL SCANNER

In some instances, it was desirable to store the output of the photo-optical scanner temporarily after retrieval of ink-recorded EEG data (e.g., for optimizing various parameters of analysis). Figure 26.5 shows a block diagram of a simple two-channel FM system, operated in conjunction with a Walkman-type portable cassette recorder, that was used for this purpose.

27 Time-Scale Converter ("Time Machine")

In the study of the amplitude and slope characteristics of certain epileptiform transients (e.g., the 3-Hz spike-wave pattern and the spike-and-slow-wave complex), it became necessary to have a means of "capturing" such transients as they were photo-optically scanned from clinical EEG ink recordings played back at a lower speed than the original write-out-paper speed, and then reading them out repetitively with a speedup factor (of, e.g., 3–6), for computation and display (figures 8.6 and 8.7). A time-scale converter or "time machine" was built for this purpose.

A block diagram of the converter is shown in figure 27.1. At an initiating signal (e.g., a button-press just before the epileptiform event reaches the tip of the photo-optical scanning pen), 64 samples of the input EEG waveform are read into a 64-cell storage unit (utilizing condensers and FET-input operational amplifiers) by means of a 64-channel (4×16) multiplexer. The readout signal, derived from the 64 storage units via a second 64-channel multiplexer, is then passed through two cascaded stages of transversal filtering (chapter 23), the clock rate for the synchronously driven transverse filters being 16 times the clock rate for the second 64-channel multiplexer. The first transversal filter functions as a linear interpolator; the second, operating on the output of the first, produces a parabolic interpolation. With the interpolation, the original 64 sample points are smoothed to a total of $64 \times 16 = 1024$ points (figure 27.2).

The readout clock is independent of the read-in clock rate of 60 Hz (which is derived from the photo-optical scanner); hence, the readout can be at a slower or at a faster rate than the read-in, so that a change of time scale can be made. Further, the readout can be made in reverse as well as forward time, since up/down counters are used in the readout. Finally, the readout can be either repetitive or as a single sweep (e.g., on an x-y plotter). An optional time base of 1024 points is generated for the readout by means of a D/A converter. The latter timebase was used for the example shown in figure 27.2.

In other applications of the device that do not involve the photo-optical scanner or curve reader, the read-in component has its own clock, which can be completely independent of the readout clock. In other applications, two units, operated conjointly, are used, e.g., in autocorrelation (appendix A).

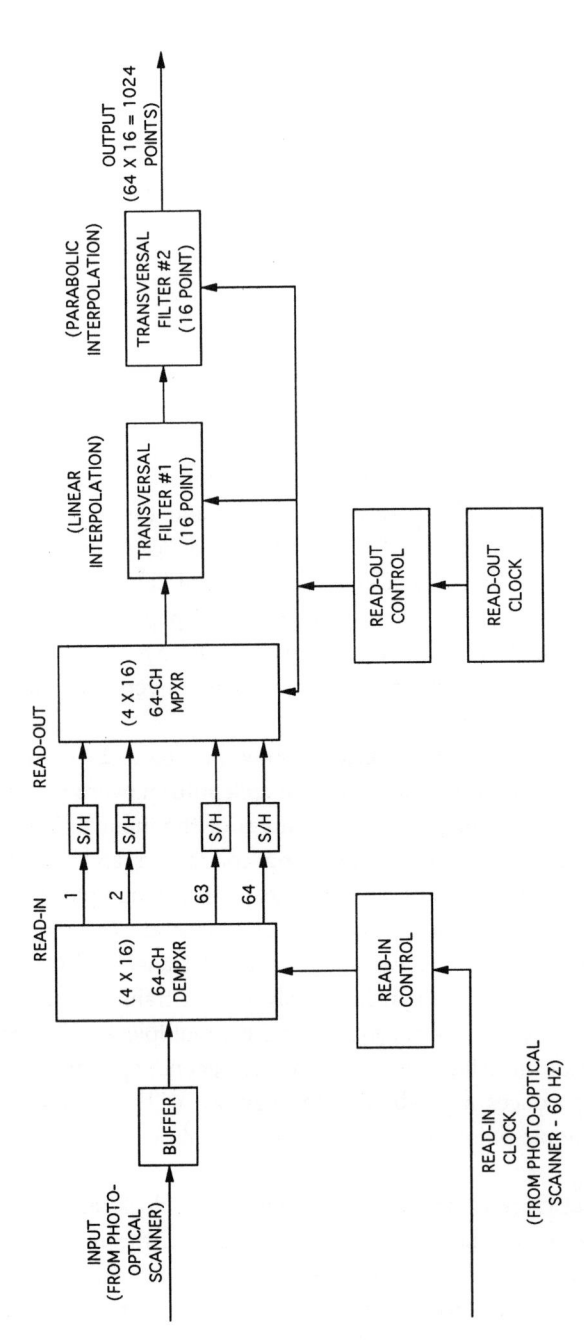

Figure 27.1 Block diagram of the epileptiform transient-capture device ("time machine"). The read-in clock rate from the photo-optical scanner (chapter 26) is 60 Hz. Note the independent readout clock and the two transversal filters, which provide parabolic interpolation to 1024 points from the original 64 sample points.

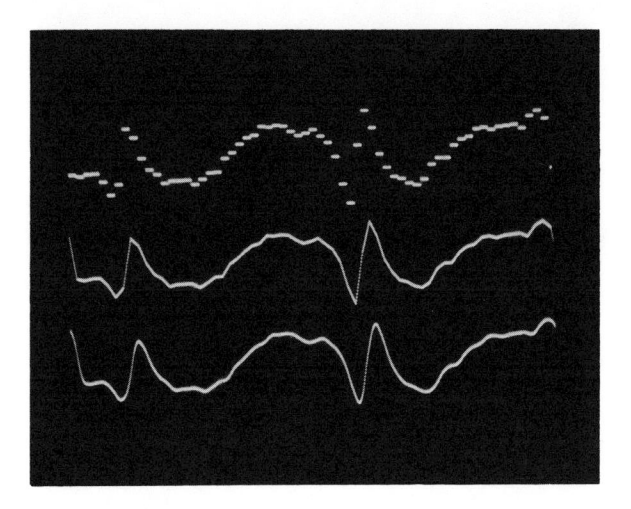

Figure 27.2 Example of operation of the "time machine." Top trace: 64-point readout of two epileptiform events. Middle trace: after 16-point linear interpolation of top trace by means of a transversal filter. Bottom trace: after a second (cascaded) 16-point interpolation with a second transversal filter, resulting in parabolic smoothing. (The two transversal filters are operated synchronously.) Note the slight delay introduced by each of the interpolations. (The sweep was repetitive, so that the transient at the extreme left represents the smoothing between the last sample point at the right and the first sample point at the left.) Speedup factor: 10 × (sweep duration: 50 msec). Original read-in time for 64 points: 500 msec.

It is in view of its flexibility that the unit is called a "time machine." (See appendix A for additional applications.) It can be compared with a digital (storage) oscilloscope except for having the additional capability of a readout on the same or a different time base. The readout can be simultaneous with the read-in, and its sampling rate can be faster, slower, or the same as that of the read-in.

28 Random-Noise Generators

Of the three types of random noise signals considered in this chapter, the first two have Gaussian (normal) and rectangular amplitude distribution (or probability density) functions, respectively. The third type of noise signal is one for which amplitude varies inversely with frequency, i.e., noise having a constant-slope characteristic. All are assumed to have a zero mean (i.e., no DC component).

In the following discussion, two curves will be referred to: the probability density function and its integral. The latter is termed the *cumulative distribution function*, and is sometimes referred to as simply the *distribution function*. In the case of a Gaussian or normal process (e.g., Gaussian electronic noise), the probability density function (which corresponds to the probability of the instantaneous occurrence of a given amplitude) has the familiar bell-shaped curve, and its integral is the familiar sigmoid curve of the cumulative distribution function (figure 28.5A). For Gaussian noise, the most probable amplitude is 0 (the highest point on the probability density curve), the probability of occurrence of a given amplitude diminishing with increasing amplitude, positive or negative. Gaussian noise is therefore said to have a Gaussian (bell-shaped) amplitude distribution.

In the case of a rectangular probability density function, in which every amplitude between the positive and negative limits is equally probable, the curve has the shape of a rectangle, the limits corresponding to the left and right sides (negative and positive limits) of the rectangle (figure 28.5B). The corresponding cumulative distribution function is 0 to the left of the left side of the rectangle, rises linearly to a value of 1.0 at the right side of the rectangle, and remains constant beyond that value.

In the simulation of certain types of EEG patterns (i.e., Type 4 waves; see chapters 2 and 4), it was necessary to have independent modulating signals for the extrema and for the slopes of the waves generated by the oscillator model (chapter 22). At first sight, it would seem that two independent random noise signals, i.e., signals having a Gaussian (normal) probability density function, could be used as the two modulations. However, the joint probability density function for two such signals, plotted in three dimensions, is not a flat surface; instead, it peaks in the vicinity of 0, as indicated in figure 28.1. (Such a joint probability density function can be imagined as the result of rotating the

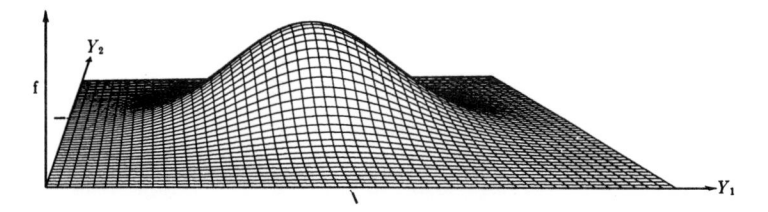

Figure 28.1 Idealized joint probability density function, in the form of a bell-shaped mound, for two independent Gaussian noise signals. The zero points on the Y1–Y2 coordinates are marked, and correspond to the point of highest joint probability (*f*). (From Sokal and Rohlf 1973.)

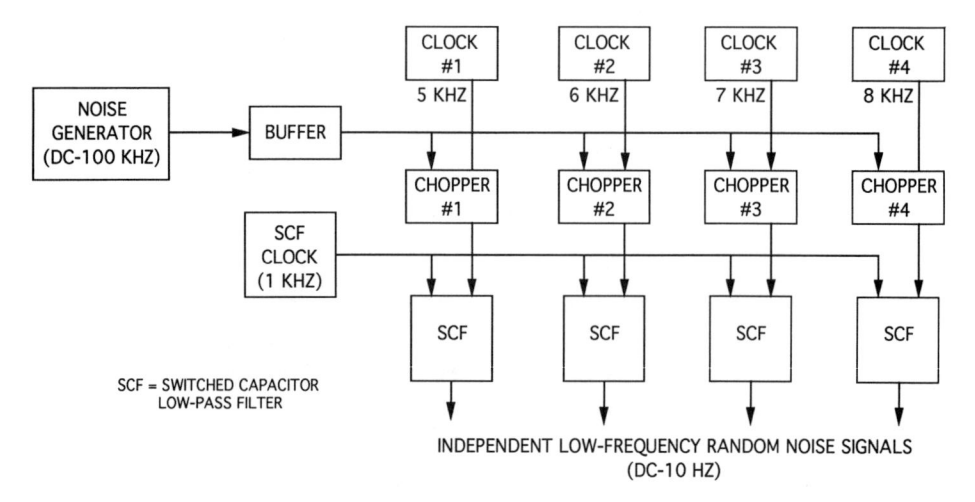

Figure 28.2 Block diagram of a four-channel low-frequency noise source. The choppers (polarity reversers) are FET switches. The clock-frequency input to the low-pass switched-capacitor filters (SCF) determines their cutoff.

previously mentioned bell-shaped curve through 360° about the vertical axis.) Therefore, two random signals having rectangular, rather than Gaussian, amplitude distribution functions were used as the modulating signals for extrema and for slopes.

Such a platform-like rectangular joint probability density can be obtained by using two independent random signals, each having a rectangular or uniform probability density (Lee 1960, pp. 190–195; Bendat and Piersol 1966, p. 660) instead of a Gaussian probability density. The generation of such a pair of signals is considered below.

FOUR-CHANNEL RANDOM NOISE HAVING A GAUSSIAN PROBABILITY DENSITY (GAUSSIAN NOISE)

A block diagram for four channels of a Gaussian-noise generator (any two of which can be used as random input modulations for the oscillator model) is shown in figure 28.2. Four basically independent DC–10 Hz noise signals

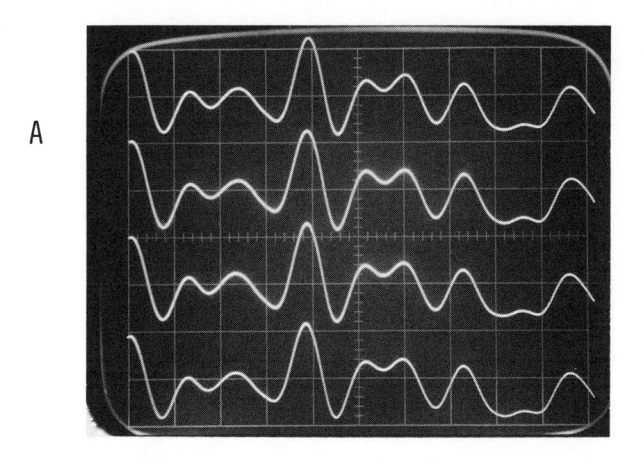

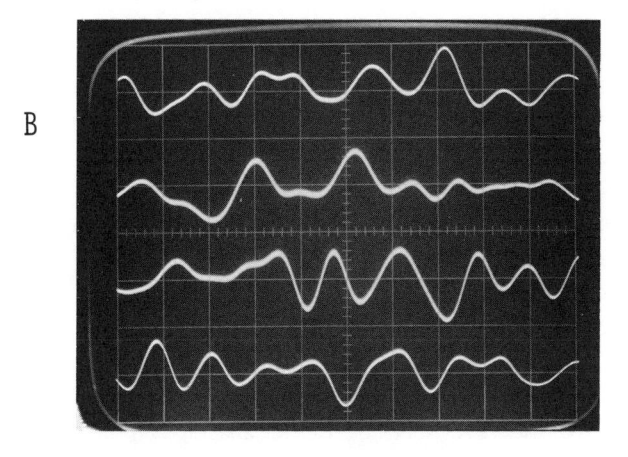

Figure 28.3 Sample of the four Gaussian noise signals, each of bandwidth DC–10 Hz, for identical (A) and non-identical (B) clock frequencies for the four switched-capacitor filters in figure 28.2.

(figure 28.3B)) are generated from a single wide-band commercial noise generator (DC–100 kHz) by heterodyning with four separate frequencies, followed by low-pass filtering with switched-capacitor filters having a cutoff of 10 Hz.

CONSTANT-AMPLITUDE VARIABLE-BANDWIDTH QUASI-GAUSSIAN NOISE GENERATOR

In the circumstance that a single channel of random (Gaussian) noise suffices, a minor revision of the block diagram of figure 28.2 results in an interesting and useful feature. The revision is that the same clock frequency be used for the heterodyning as for operating the switched-capacitor filter (the upper cutoff frequency of which is 1/100 the input clock frequency). The result is that the output amplitude of the low-frequency noise is independent of the upper frequency limit selected. This characteristic results from aliasing of the input wideband noise, and it is in marked contrast with the dependence of

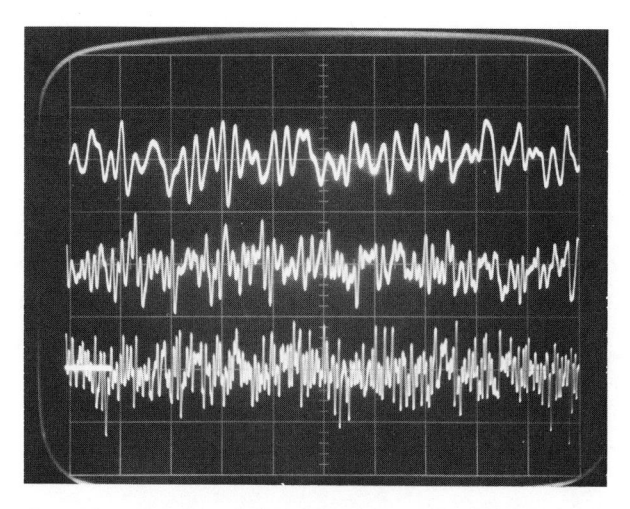

Figure 28.4 Sequence of Gaussian noise signals of different bandwidths, showing the independence of amplitude and bandwidth. For these results, the same clock frequencies (0.5, 1.0, and 2.0 kHz for traces 1, 2, and 3, respectively) were used for the choppers and for the switched-capacitor filters (figure 28.3), yielding quasi-Gaussian noise output signals of DC to 5, 10, and 20 Hz.

output noise amplitude on bandwidth that characterizes the output of a (relatively) wide-band noise generator used in conjunction with a variable electronic low-pass filter. For the latter combination, the higher the low-pass filter cutoff point, the greater the amplitude of the noise—an inconvenience when random signals of different bandwidths but equal amplitudes are needed as test signals. The constant-amplitude, variable-bandwidth noise may not be truly Gaussian, however, because of the aliasing. Figure 28.4 illustrates the relative independence of output level from the unit for different upper cutoff frequencies.

TWO-CHANNEL RANDOM-NOISE GENERATOR HAVING A RECTANGULAR (UNIFORM) PROBABILITY DENSITY

In order to obtain a random signal having a rectangular (uniform) density function, i.e., in which all amplitudes are equally probable, within the specified positive and negative limits, the principle of transformation of probability densities can be used, by which a normal or Gaussian density can be converted to a rectangular one (Lee 1960). The two densities are shown in figure 28.5.

Basically, in the present approach, the transformation is accomplished by on-line multiplication of the sample values of a Gaussian noise signal by the corresponding sample points on the Gaussian density curve. A block diagram of the unit for carrying out the transformation is shown in figure 28.6, and selected corresponding waveforms are shown in figure 28.7. A 50-Hz triangular wave, in conjunction with 10-kHz high-pass noise, a comparator, a 600-Hz low-pass filter, and a differentiator, is used to generate a Gaussian probability

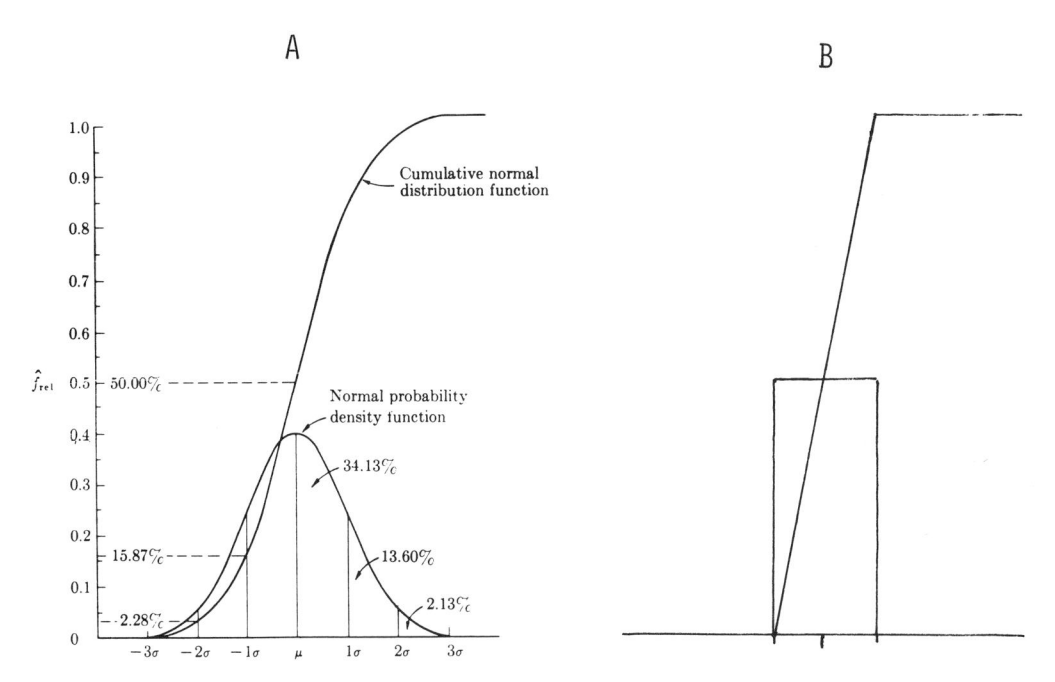

Figure 28.5 Gaussian (normal) probability density function and cumulative normal distribution function (A), and rectangular (equally probable) probability density function and cumulative rectangular density function (B). (Curves at left from Sokal and Rohlf 1973.)

density curve repetitively at 100 Hz (one curve for each half cycle of the triangular wave). The same 50-Hz triangular wave and a DC–10 Hz Gaussian noise signal are combined to generate sampling pulses which simultaneously sample the low-frequency (DC–10 Hz) noise and sample the Gaussian density curve at the corresponding point. Finally, multiplying the individual low-frequency noise samples by the corresponding sampled values from the (repetitive) Gaussian probability density converts the DC–10 Hz random signal from a Gaussian probability density to a rectangular probability density.

The actual form of the transfer function for this transformation can be derived as shown in figure 28.8. The middle trace shows a 0.5-Hz triangular wave (note the slow time base) which, for the purpose of displaying the transfer function, replaces the DC 10-Hz noise signal indicated at the left in figure 28.6. The top trace in figure 28.8 shows the Gaussian probability density curve sampled at 100 Hz, i.e., the output of the sample-and-hold circuit at the lower right in figure 28.6. The third trace in figure 28.8 is the running product of the first two traces and depicts the transfer function as a complete curve between successive positive and negative peaks of the 0.5-Hz triangular wave, the successive curves being reversed end-for-end.

From inspection of the latter curves, it is evident that the points on the triangular wave having the greatest positive and the greatest negative values are attenuated whereas intermediate points are magnified, the maximum of magnification occurring at points slightly outside the ones corresponding to one standard deviation from the peak of the Gaussian density curves (top

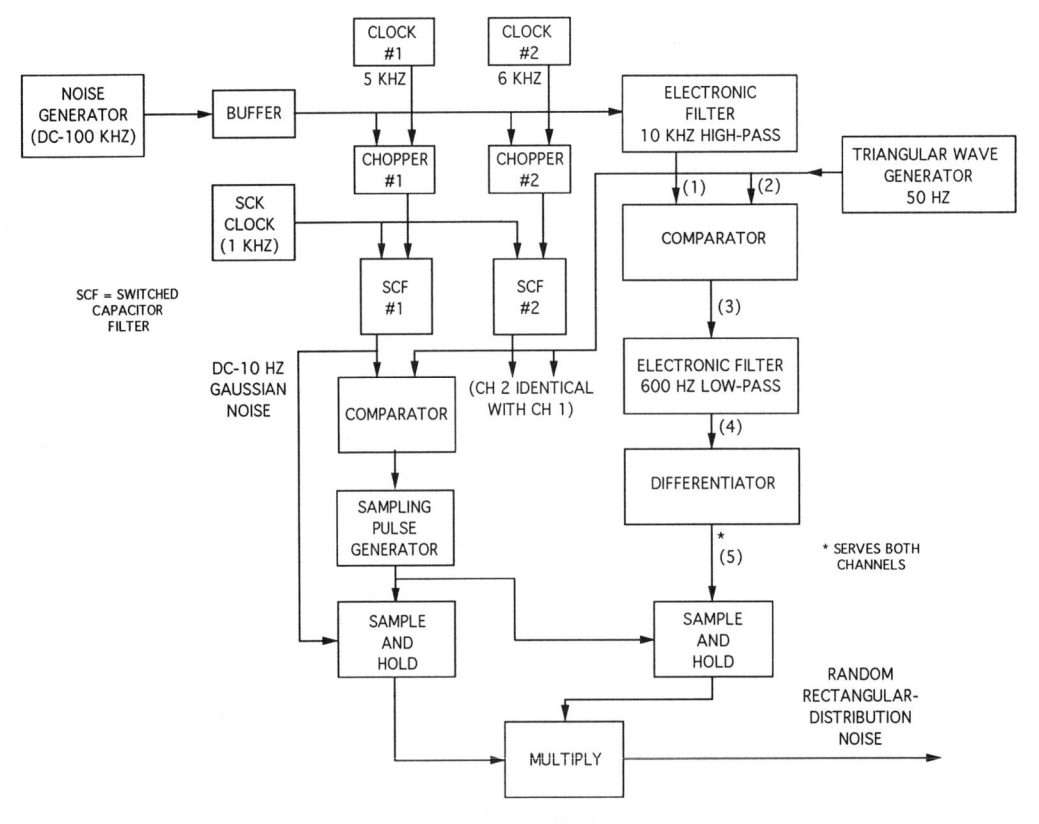

Figure 28.6 Block diagram of two-channel unit for conversion of the density of a random signal from a Gaussian probability density to a rectangular probability density. The numbers in parentheses correspond to the traces in figure 28.7. The components on the right side generate a Gaussian probability density repetitively at a rate of 50 Hz, by means of the 10-kHz high-pass Gaussian noise, a 50-Hz triangular wave, a comparator, an electronic 600-Hz low-pass filter (24 dB/octave), and a differentiator. The same 50-Hz triangular wave is intersected, in a comparator, with a low-frequency (DC–10 Hz) Gaussian signal (figure 28.3B) to generate a sampling pulse. The latter is used to sample the low-frequency Gaussian noise signal, and simultaneously to sample the Gaussian density curve at the point that corresponds to the sampled value of the low-frequency noise. These two sampled voltages are then multiplied, yielding the desired random noise signal having a rectangular density.

trace). It is this variable scaling that transforms the Gaussian distribution of the DC–10 Hz signal at the left in figure 28.6 to the rectangular distribution at the output.

Figure 28.9 shows the distribution or cumulative probability curves (i.e., the integrated probability density curves) for the random low-frequency Gaussian noise signal (top trace) and for the random low-frequency rectangular probability density noise signal derived from the former (bottom trace). The essentially linear form of the curve for the rectangular distribution, between the two limits of the latter, contrasts with the sigmoid shape of the curve for the Gaussian distribution.

An example of the actual transformation of a random low-frequency signal having a Gaussian probability density function into a random low-frequency

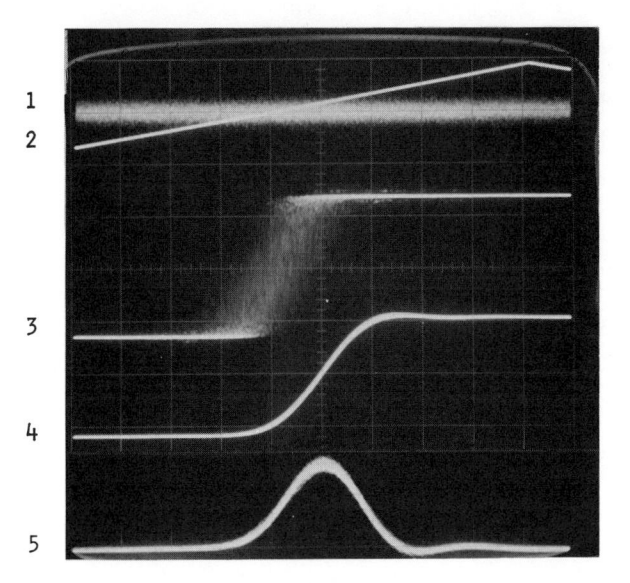

Figure 28.7 Waveforms indicating the operation of the Gaussian to rectangular density transform unit. Top trace: 50-Hz triangular wave. Trace 2: 10-kHz high-pass Gaussian noise. Trace 3: output of comparator having the signals of trace 1 and trace 2 as input. Trace 4: low-pass (600-Hz cutoff) of the signal of trace 3 to yield the Gaussian cumulative probability curve. Trace 5: differentiation of trace 4 to yield the Gaussian probability density curve. The slight overshoot in traces 3 and 5 arises from the four-pole low-pass filtering of trace 3.

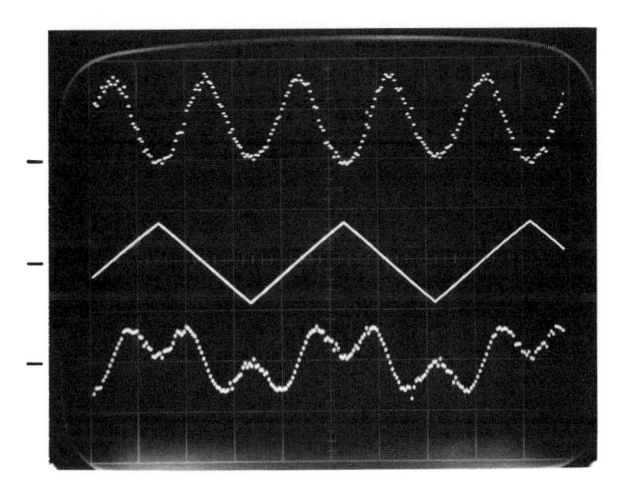

Figure 28.8 Repetitive generation of the transfer function (trace 3) for forming a rectangular probability density function, by multiplication of a sampled Gaussian probability density function (trace 1) by a 0.5-Hz triangular wave (trace 2). Baselines as indicated.

Random-Noise Generators

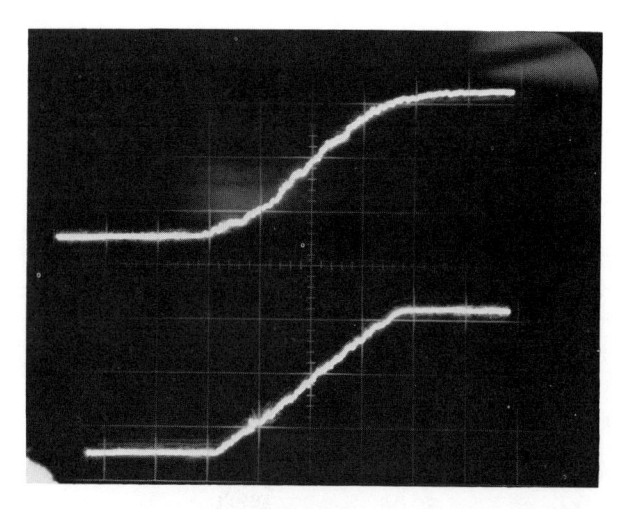

Figure 28.9 Cumulative distributions for random signals having a Gaussian density (top trace) and a rectangular density (bottom trace). Note the sigmoid and linear forms, which are comparable to the two curves in figure 28.5.

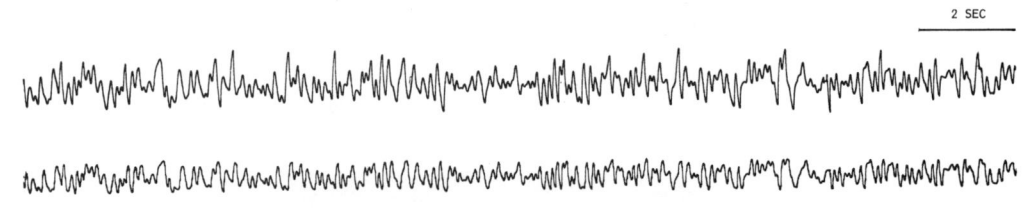

Figure 28.10 Conversion of a random signal having a Gaussian probability (amplitude) density function into a random signal having a rectangular (equally probable) density function. Frequency range of the input random Gaussian noise: 0.1–10 Hz. Note the positive and negative limits of the excursions of the output signal, corresponding to the sides of the rectangles in figure 28.5B.

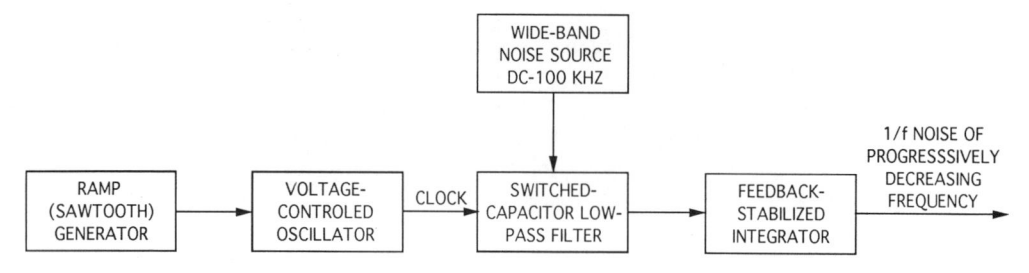

Figure 28.11 Block diagram of unit for generating random Gaussian noise having a $1/f$ amplitude characteristic (i.e., a constant mean absolute slope). A sample write-out is shown in figure 6.2.

signal having a rectangular probability density function is shown in figure 28.10. The transformation is such that the smaller values are amplified and the larger values are progressively compressed, so that the limits of the rectangular density are apparent as the upper and lower limits on the write-out. In the lower trace, all values of the instantaneous amplitude within the above limits are equally probable. In the upper trace, the most probable amplitude value is 0, the remaining values of the instantaneous amplitudes being progressively less probable with increasing amplitude according to the Gaussian (normal) distribution.

RANDOM (GAUSSIAN) NOISE HAVING CONSTANT MEAN ABSOLUTE SLOPE (1/f-AMPLITUDE NOISE)

Figure 28.11 illustrates the generation of random noise having a Gaussian probability density function and an amplitude characteristic that is inversely proportional to frequency (which can be used to simulate EEG patterns having a relatively constant running absolute mean slope; see chapter 6). The ramp generator imposes progressively lower low-pass filtering, by means of the switched-capacitor filter, of the wide-band noise. The resulting low-pass white noise is then passed through a feedback-stabilized integrator, the output of which is 1/f noise having constant mean slope. A write-out of the resulting signal as the cutoff frequency of the low-pass filter progressively diminishes (figure 6.2) resembles the behavior of the EEG during progressively deeper non-REM sleep.

29 Instantaneous Envelope of the EEG and of Its First Derivative; Interfacing with the Oscillator Model

In view of the importance of the instantaneous envelope of the EEG and of its first derivative (most especially for the fast transients of epileptiform activity —see figures 8.6, 8.7, and 9.9) as the basis of the third approach to the testing of the extrema-slopes hypothesis (chapter 3), the importance of the latter method itself as the most comprehensive one (functioning as it does for any type of EEG pattern), and the fact that a new approach to deriving the instantaneous envelope has been developed specifically for the present work, the background of, and methods for, the derivation of the instantaneous envelope of a signal are considered in some depth in this chapter.

BACKGROUND—THE ALPHA ENVELOPE AND FREQUENCY

In the second group of tests (chapter 2) of the extrema-slopes hypothesis of the EEG, running means of the EEG and of its first derivative were obtained by means of full-wave rectification and RC filtering (time constant 0.1 sec), followed by averaging over a 0.5-sec window with a 16-point transversal (rectangular) filter. The latter window duration was selected so as to permit analysis of EEG frequency components down to 1 Hz (half-period 0.5 sec). In the third group of tests of the hypothesis, the EEG is reconstituted by means of the oscillator model using, as the two modulating inputs, the instantaneous envelope of the EEG and of its first derivative.

For rhythmic EEG activity (e.g., alpha activity or drug-induced beta activity), the envelope is comparatively easy to obtain. The relatively simple method of rectification followed by smoothing has been described by several workers. Pasquali (1969) described a six-phase (i.e., three phases, each full-wave rectified) circuit for alpha activity in the range 9–12 Hz. Lansing and Barlow (1972) used a 7–14-Hz bandpass filter to select alpha activity, which was then full-wave rectified and low-pass filtered (two cascaded RC filters), to obtain the alpha envelope. Tatsuno et al. (1980; see also Tatsuno 1981) used squaring instead of rectification, followed by smoothing in the form of a moving average (running mean). These workers obtained the instantaneous frequency from the durations of the successive half-waves. A method of obtaining the envelope by means of a sample-and-hold circuit activated by

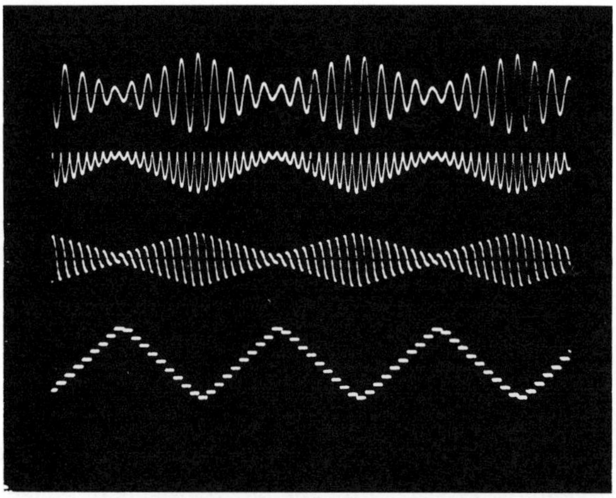

Figure 29.1 Envelope detector employing a peak detector in combination with a sample-and-hold circuit. Trace 1: original narrow-band signal (a 10-Hz sine wave modulated by a 1-Hz triangular wave). Trace 2: after full-wave rectification (shown inverted). Trace 3: after differentiation of trace 2 (the discontinuities in the latter correspond to the sharp peaks in the former). Trace 4: output (× 2) of the sample-and-hold circuit. (Trigger pulses for the latter were generated upon baseline crossings of the signal of trace 3.)

successive positive and negative peaks of a sine wave modulated by a triangular wave is shown in figure 29.1.

In all of the above-described methods for obtaining the alpha envelope, an averaging (smoothing) window of greater or lesser duration is employed, and hence from none can the instantaneous envelope of the EEG be obtained. The latter signal, together with the instantaneous envelope of the first derivative of the EEG, is necessary for faithful reconstitution of an EEG pattern, especially for epileptiform activity as already mentioned, as required for the third type of tests of the extrema-slopes hypothesis. For this purpose, the temporal resolution afforded by simple methods such as that depicted in figure 29.1 is not adequate.

In their review of methods of deriving the envelope of the EEG, Ktonas and Papp (1980) included the peak amplitude and zero-crossing method, already considered (figure 29.1), and the determination of frequency by phase-locked demodulation. The latter is basically a frequency-demodulation technique, with an inherent frequency smoothing (in order to maintain the stability of the phase-locked loop). It does not provide the envelope; however, in principle, the latter could be obtained by means of a coherent rejection technique (see figures 3 and 5 of Barlow 1986), although the limitations imposed by loop stability would exist.

DETERMINATION OF INSTANTANEOUS EEG ENVELOPE AND INSTANTANEOUS FREQUENCY

In their review, Ktonas and Papp (1980) also included three methods of obtaining the instantaneous envelope and the instantaneous frequency using

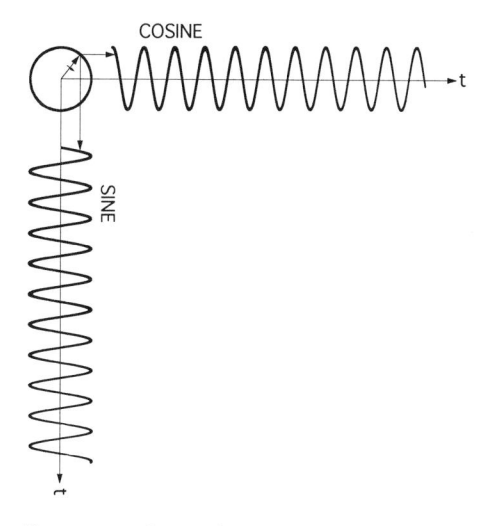

Figure 29.2 Sine and cosine components of a point undergoing uniform circular (simple harmonic) motion about the origin. The sine and cosine waves are of fixed amplitude and fixed frequency. (The curves in this figure and in figures 29.3–29.5 are from oscilloscope photographs.)

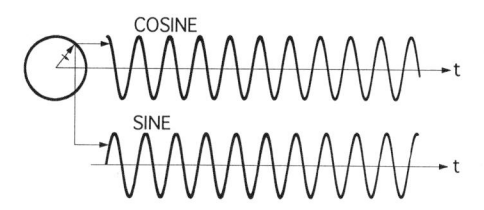

Figure 29.3 Same as figure 29.2 except that the sine and cosine components are shown in vertical alignment; note the 90° phase difference.

mathematical approaches. These methods—in-phase and in-quadrature filtering, complex demodulation, and Hilbert transformation—can be considered together, as they all entail the concept of the analytic signal, a vector that rotates about and advances along the time axis in a three-dimensional space having x, y, and t axes, such that the length of the vector (i.e., its magnitude) is the magnitude of the instantaneous envelope and the rate of rotation of the vector (i.e., the rate of increase of the phase angle) corresponds to the instantaneous (angular) frequency. Thus, in this scheme, the signal is depicted as a point that spirals around the time axis, the distance from the axis being the instantaneous envelope of the signal.

The concept of the analytic signal can be understood by reference to figure 29.2. Figure 29.2A (upper left) shows a point undergoing uniform circular motion (simple harmonic motion) about the origin, the projection of the motion of which onto axes at right angles to one another yields the pair of sine and cosine waves, respectively, as shown. The sine and cosine waves are depicted adjacent to one another in figure 29.3. If the x, y, and t axes are combined, and the sine and cosine waves are included (figure 29.4), and their

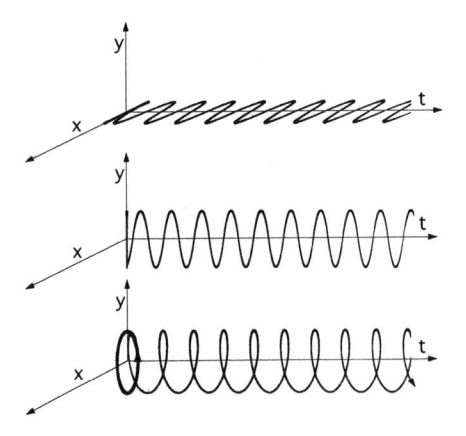

Figure 29.4 Same as figures 29.2 and 29.3 except that the sine and cosine components are shown in three-dimensional space (x, y, t) as the two top traces. If the sine and cosine waves are combined in the three-dimensional space, the spiral shown in the third trace results. The spiral traces out the motion of the tip of a vector originating on the time axis; the vector is termed the *analytic signal*, and its magnitude is given by the distance from its tip to the time axis, t. It is the latter that is the instantaneous envelope; in this case it is constant.

instantaneous values are projected into the three-dimensional space, then the motion of the resultant point traces out the tip of a vector originating on the time axis. The vector is termed the *analytic signal* (Middleton 1960; Bracewell 1986), and its length is the magnitude of the analytic signal. Variations in instantaneous envelope result in a spiral of greater or lesser diameter, and variations in instantaneous frequency result in a spiral of tighter or more distantly spaced turns about the time axis, t. The length of the vector from the t-axis is termed the *magnitude* or *modulus* of the analytic signal, or, in the present discussion, the *instantaneous envelope* of the original signal.

For obtaining the instantaneous magnitude (length) of the analytic signal in figure 29.2C, the trigonometric equivalent of the Pythagorean theorem,

$$x^2 + y^2 = r^2, \text{ or } r^2 = \sqrt{x^2 + y^2},$$

can be used; it is

$$\sin^2 x + \cos^2 x = 1$$

for a circle of radius 1 (e.g., the circle in figure 29.2), where x is now redefined as the angle (in radians) of the vector in figure 29.4 that rotates about the t-axis.

The squares of the sine and cosine waves in figure 29.3 are shown in figure 29.5 as the third and fourth traces, together with their sum (the fifth trace). These results are in accord with the trigonometric identities

$$\sin^2 x = (1 - \cos 2x)/2$$

and

$$\cos^2 x = (1 + \cos 2x)/2,$$

so that

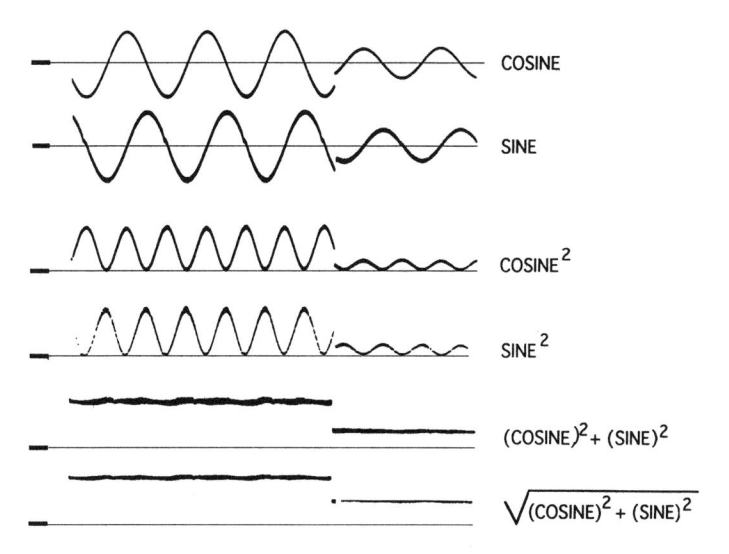

Figure 29.5 Schema to indicate that the square of a sine wave is a cosine wave of twice the frequency with a DC component of half the amplitude, and that the square of a cosine wave is the same, except 180° out of phase, so that the sum of the two results in a steady or fixed value, which is the square of the magnitude of the analytic signal corresponding to the sine-cosine pair. Note the effect of a decrease (on the right) of amplitude (to $\frac{1}{2}$) of the cosine and sine waves. Baselines as indicated.

$\sin^2 x + \cos^2 x = (\frac{1}{2} - \cos 2x/2) + (\frac{1}{2} + \cos 2x/2) = 1.$

The sum of the squares is therefore constant as long as the amplitude of the simple harmonic motion is constant (figure 29.5, trace 5). The square root of this quantity (figure 29.5, trace 6) is, then, the magnitude of the analytic signal, i.e., the desired instantaneous envelope. It changes instantly if the original sine and cosine (figures 29.2, 29.3) change their amplitude, as shown on the right side of the traces in figure 29.5.

Thus, in contrast to the techniques of obtaining the envelope of the EEG considered above, all of which entail some smoothing or averaging, there is, at least in principle, no smoothing or time lag in the determination of the instantaneous envelope; hence the name.

From figures 29.2–29.5, it is clear that obtaining the analytic signal, and in turn the instantaneous envelope, entails the use of sine-cosine pairs, or, more generally, of in-phase and in-quadrature signals (the latter implying a phase shift of 90° or one-fourth of the period), for all frequency components with respect to the in-phase or original signal.

METHODS OF OBTAINING THE IN-PHASE AND IN-QUADRATURE SIGNALS

The three methods listed by Ktonas and Papp (1980) of obtaining the analytic signal, and thus the instantaneous envelope function, are as follows (mathematical details can be found in Ktonas and Papp (1980), to supplement the descriptive summary below).

In the method of in-phase and in-quadrature filtering, a pair of digital filters are used, of which the characteristics of the in-quadrature filter are those of the Hilbert transform (defined below) of the in-phase filter. The outputs of the two filters thus constitute an in-phase and in-quadrature pair, from which the instantaneous envelope is obtained as the square root of the sums of the squares of the in-phase and the in-quadrature signals.

In the method of complex demodulation (see also Bingham et al. 1967, Childers and Pao 1972, and Levine et al. 1972), a sine-and-cosine pair having the same frequency as the signal to be analyzed are each multiplied by the latter. The resultant products are low-pass filtered (to eliminate higher-frequency components in the cross-products), and the instantaneous envelope is obtained as the square root of the sum of the squares of the output signals from the low-pass filters.

In the method of the Hilbert transform, the in-quadrature signal is created from the original in-phase signal, as explained below, and the instantaneous envelope is obtained as the square root of the sums of the squares of the two signals.

In all three methods, the instantaneous frequency is obtained as the time rate of rotation of the analytic signal, or, equivalently, as the time rate of change of the angle whose tangent is given by the quotient of the in-quadrature component to the in-phase component.

THE HILBERT TRANSFORM

Among these three methods, the method of the Hilbert transform is particularly attractive for the present purposes, because it does not require prior information concerning the unmodulated or center frequency of the signal. The latter is necessary in the method of complex demodulation for setting the frequency of the "local oscillator," and also in the method of in-phase and in-quadrature filtering, for specifying the characteristics of the filters. (The band-width limitations of all three methods are discussed below.)

The Hilbert transform (Middleton 1960; Bracewell 1986; Siebert 1986) creates an in-quadrature version of the original in-phase signal by shifting each and every frequency component by 90°. Thus the Hilbert transform of a sine wave is a cosine wave, and the Hilbert transform of a cosine wave is a negative (inverted) sine wave. For waves of a single frequency, taking the Hilbert transform is equivalent to differentiating (except for a scale factor), which also shifts the phase by 90°; however, for a range of frequencies, differentiation results in an increase of amplitude proportional to the frequency, whereas no such amplitude change with frequency occurs with the Hilbert transform.

The Hilbert transform can be carried out in either the frequency domain or the time domain. For transforming in the frequency domain, a section (or successive sections) of the in-phase signal is Fourier transformed (e.g., via the Fast Fourier Transform) into its sine and cosine components at each frequency. The sine and cosine components are interchanged (i.e., multiplying the sine

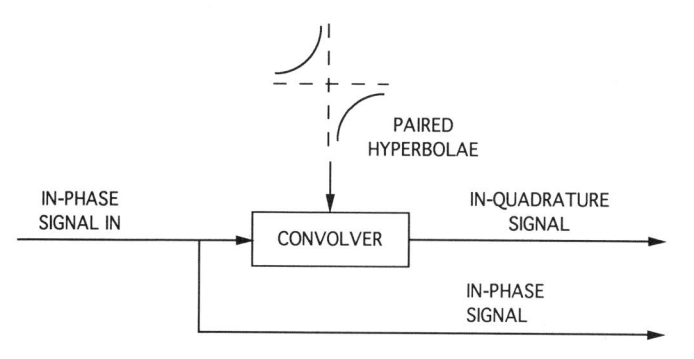

Figure 29.6 Schema to indicate the manner in which convolution of a sine wave with a pair of hyperbolas results in a cosine wave, i.e., a shift of 90°.

and cosine coefficients by $-j$, the square root of -1), and inverse Fourier transformation then yields the section of the signal in in-quadrature form. This approach results in piecemeal (section-by-section) derivation of the Hilbert transform, and, in turn, the instantaneous envelope.

For obtaining the Hilbert transform in the time domain, the in-phase signal is convolved (figure 29.6) with (i.e., multiplied by) a pair of back-to-back hyperbolas (termed the *kernel*), each hyperbola being symmetrical about the $-45°$ axis. The resultant cross-products are summated continuously in a process that will be considered in more detail below.

The manner by which a convolution of a sine wave with a pair of hyperbolas can shift a sine wave by 90° to form a cosine wave (a result that at first sight may seem very odd indeed) can be understood from figure 29.7. Since this process is a linear one (i.e., doubling the amplitude of the sine wave doubles the output cosine wave), the input signal can, in principle, have any arbitrary spectrum; i.e., the signal can be arbitrarily complex (e.g., white noise).

A limitation of all of the three of the above-described techniques for obtaining the instantaneous envelopes is that they are ordinarily restricted to use on relatively narrow-band signals (i.e., in the case of the EEG, largely to rhythmic patterns such as alpha activity and sleep spindles). A method of circumventing this limitation is discussed below.

APPLICATIONS TO EEG

Complex demodulation has been applied to the study of alpha activity or event-related rhythmic EEG activity by Walter (1968), Dick and Vaughan (1970), Childers and Pao (1972), Childers (1973), Nogawa et al. (1976), Étévenon (1977), Naitoh and Lewis (1981), and Ktonas and Papp (1980). The latter authors applied complex demodulation to simulated alpha activity and to sleep spindles, for determination of instantaneous envelope and instantaneous frequency. Tatsuno (1981) has described a method of complex demodulation in the frequency domain.

Dick and Vaughan (1970) pointed out that the reference or demodulation frequency in the method of complex demodulation is never exactly the same

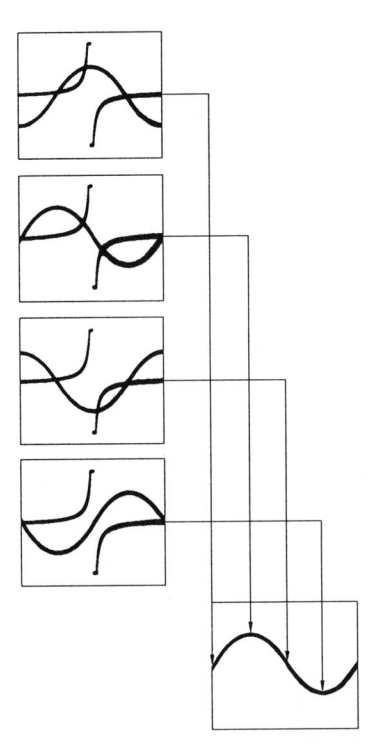

Figure 29.7 Sample waveforms for the schema shown in figure 29.6. When the transition between the two hyperbolas coincides with the baseline crossing of the sine wave, the products of the two curves are positive on both sides of the transition, and hence the products will summate to a nonzero number. On the other hand, if the transition between the two hyperbolas coincides with a positive or with a negative peak of the sine wave, then the products of the curves will be positive on one side of the transition and negative on the other side (since the hyperbolas have opposite signs on the two sides of the transition), and hence the products will summate or integrate to 0.

as the center frequency of the signal being analyzed (e.g., an alpha rhythm), and they suggested incorporating a phase-locked loop from which the reference frequency would be obtained. Hileman and Dick (1971) described such a system, constituting a system for complex demodulation with a phase-locked loop and yielding the center frequency of alpha activity as well as the instantaneous phase fluctuations about the center frequency.

Adey and Walter (1963) used the in-phase and in-quadrature filtering method formulated by Goodman (1960) for continuous measurement of the phase and amplitude characteristics of hippocampal wave trains during delayed response training in cats.

Devyatkov et al. (1973) used the method of the Hilbert transform to examine sections of unfiltered EEGs for nonstationarities—the latter being indicated by changes in the slope of the curve of increasing phase angle with time, i.e., the accumulated number of waves beginning from a given time (Goodman 1960). The derivative of the latter curve yielded the instantaneous frequency. Accordingly, these authors termed their method *phase-frequency* analysis.

The analytic signal can be viewed as being obtained from the original signal by suppressing negative frequencies and doubling the result (Bracewell 1986, p. 270), a process that can be compared with that entailed in single-sideband radio transmission (Hartley 1928; Siebert 1986).

In investigating rhythmic activity in the EEG, Étévenon (1977) used the frequency-domain version of the Hilbert transform to obtain the in-quadrature version of short (0.5-sec) EEG sections. The envelope (or modulation, in Étévenon's terminology) of the rhythmic activity was then obtained as the running square root of the sums of the squares of the original EEG section and its Hilbert transform.

Witte et al. (1990, 1991) used the Fourier-based Hilbert-transform approach to obtain spatio-temporal maps of the instantaneous amplitude of the EEG, including EEGs with epileptiform spikes.

TWO COMPUTING TECHNIQUES FOR OBTAINING THE HILBERT TRANSFORM AND THE INSTANTANEOUS ENVELOPE OF THE EEG

The Conventional Hilbert Transform

Figure 29.8 shows a block diagram of a sampled-data system for deriving the envelope of a signal as the magnitude of the analytic signal obtained from the paired in-phase and in-quadrature signals, the latter obtained by the time-domain Hilbert transform method. The signal, after any desired or necessary filtering (including anti-alias filtering), is fed to an analog tapped delay line (chapter 23) having 16 taps and a DC response. (The output of the ninth tap is taken as the in-phase signal, since this point in the delay line corresponds to the midpoint of the kernel, i.e., the paired hyperbolas, used in the convolution operation.) The 16 most recent sampled data points are available in multiplexed form from the delay line. The pair of hyperbolas, in sampled form, is generated repetitively by means of an analog divider having as its input a 16-step ramp (figure 29.9, lower trace), from which the value of 0 is purposely excluded (to avoid division by 0). The ramp is obtained from a D/A converter fed by a 4-bit (count-of-16) binary counter (figure 29.8).

The 16 sequential points of the hyperbolas are multiplied by the corresponding 16 most recent sample points. The resultant products are demultiplexed into 16 sample-and-hold circuits, whose outputs are summated in a 16-point transversal filter to yield a single point on the curve of the Hilbert transform (i.e., the in-quadrature signal). The data samples in the delay line are then shifted one cell, the oldest data point is discarded, and a new data point added. The entire computational process repeats, and so on.

The instantaneous envelope of the original signal is then obtained, as indicated in figure 29.10, as the running square root of the sum of the squares of the in-phase signal and the in-quadrature signal.

Figure 29.11A shows, for the above-described unit, the in-phase and in-quadrature pair for a sine wave; Figure 29.11B displays the pair for a narrow-band noise signal. Figure 29.12 shows the in-phase and in-quadrature signals

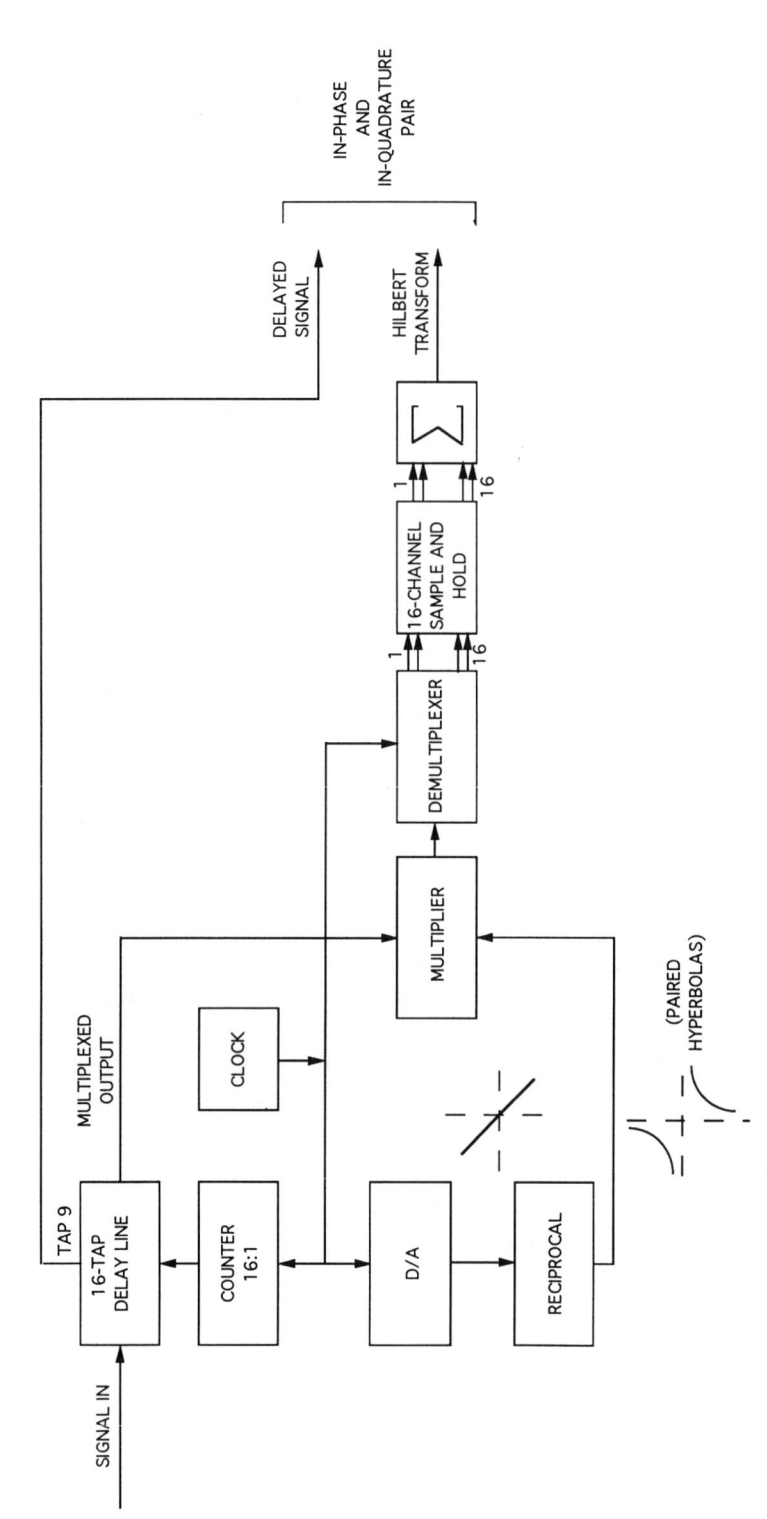

Figure 29.8 Block diagram of a sampled-data system for obtaining the Hilbert transform of a signal. The 16-point paired hyperbolas (formed by means of an analog electronic divider fed by a ramp generated from a D/A converter driven by a four-bit counter (i.e., count of 16—see figure 29.9) are multiplied in rapid succession by the most recent 16 samples of the input signal (available in multiplexed form from the 16-tap analog delay line). The 16 products are summed in a transversal filter to yield one point on the output curve, the latter being the Hilbert transform. The entire computation is repeated for the next most recent 16 points, i.e., after the oldest data sample is discarded and a new one taken into the tapped delay line (sampling rate 50 Hz; multiplication rate 50 × 16 = 800 Hz).

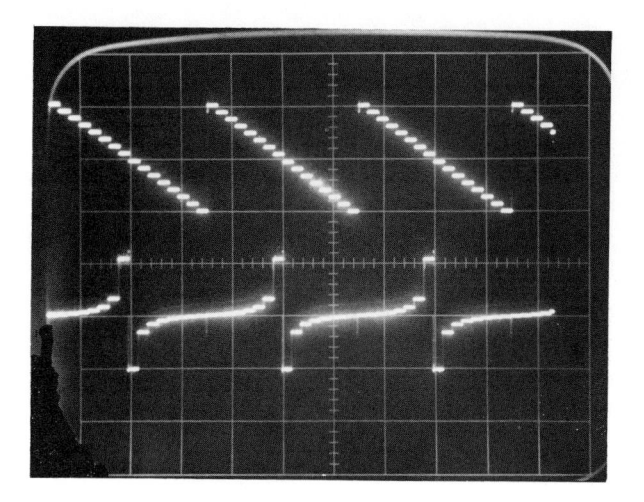

Figure 29.9 Generation of a pair of hyperbolas (lower trace) from a 16-step ramp (upper trace) by means of an analog multiplier chip arranged as a divider. (The ramp is generated from a D/A converter fed by a count-of-16 (four-bit) counter.) There are thus 16 points on each pair of hyperbolas, the value of 0 being purposely excluded so as to avoid the problem of the reciprocal of 0.

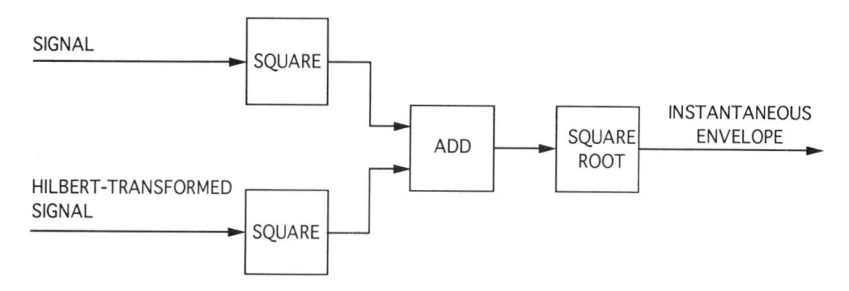

Figure 29.10 Derivation of the instantaneous envelope from an original signal (the in-phase signal) and its Hilbert transform (the in-quadrature signal).

for a narrow-band noise signal with the instantaneous envelope (magnitude of the analytic signal) superimposed on the in-quadrature signal. (Although not shown explicitly in the figure, the instantaneous envelope would equally well superimpose on the in-phase signal.)

This system, as well as the alternative system described below, computes the instantaneous envelope continuously (at the sample rate—nominally 50 Hz), on line and in real time.

From inspection of the instantaneous envelope shown in figure 29.12, it is evident that the time-domain implementation depicted in figure 29.8 for the derivation of the instantaneous envelope by means of the Hilbert transform would be quite satisfactory for obtaining the envelope of even a moderately irregular train of alpha waves. However, for the reconstitution of EEGs as a part of the third type of test of the extrema-slopes hypothesis, the instantaneous envelope of the first derivative of the EEG as well as the instantaneous

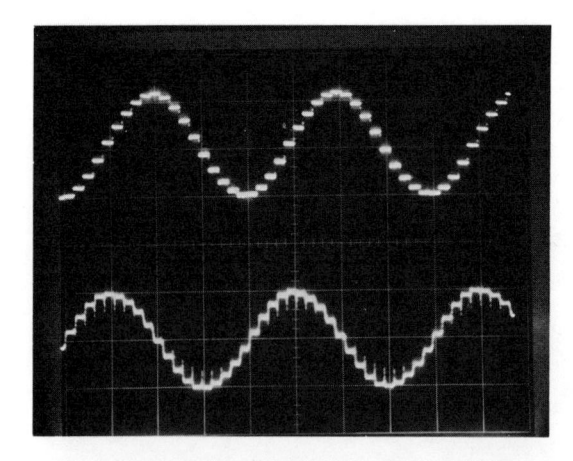

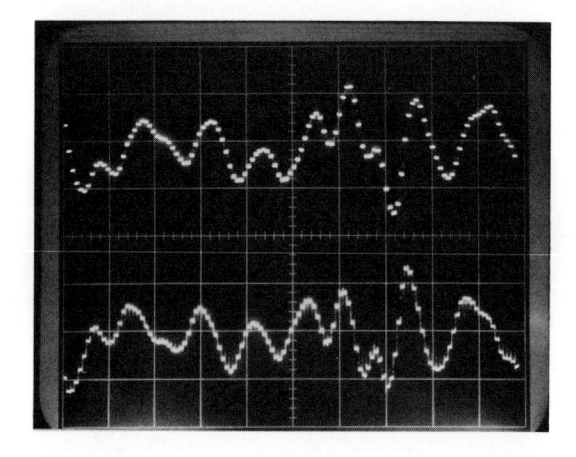

Figure 29.11 Original (in-phase) and Hilbert-transform (in-quadrature) signals for (A) a 10-Hz sine wave and (B) band-limited noise (1–20 Hz), obtained by the system of figures 29.8 and 29.10. In the Hilbert-transformed signal, each and every frequency component is shifted (advanced) in phase by 90° for that frequency.

envelope of the EEG itself is needed. For obtaining both envelopes simultaneously, two complete systems of the type just described would be necessary. Moreover, a sampling rate of 50 Hz is not really adequate for epileptiform patterns. Fortunately, the implementation of a quite different system, which had suggested itself in the course of work with the one just described, greatly simplified these problems.

Instantaneous Envelope by Paired Integration and Differentiation— Bypassing the Hilbert Transform

The approach to be described had its origin in the consideration that, for a sine-wave signal, a differentiator (e.g., an operational-amplifier differentiator) introduces a phase lead of 90°, and an integrator (e.g., an operational ampli-

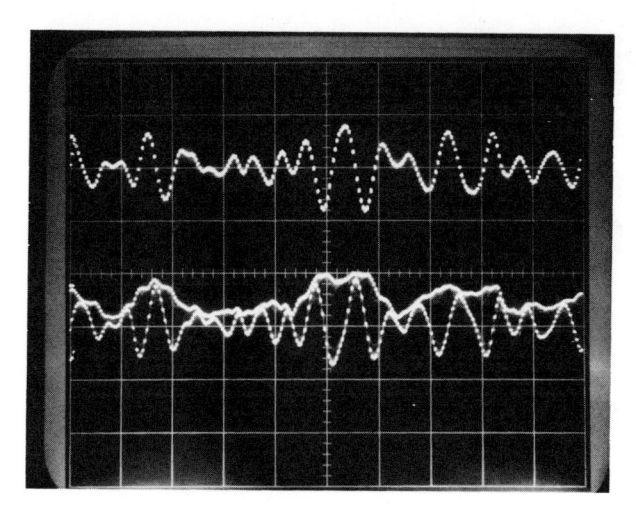

Figure 29.12 In-phase and in-quadrature (Hilbert-transform) signals for 10-Hz narrow-band noise, together with the instantaneous envelope, computed by the sampled-data system (figures 29.8 and 29.10). Note that the envelope "fits" both the in-phase and the in-quadrature signals.

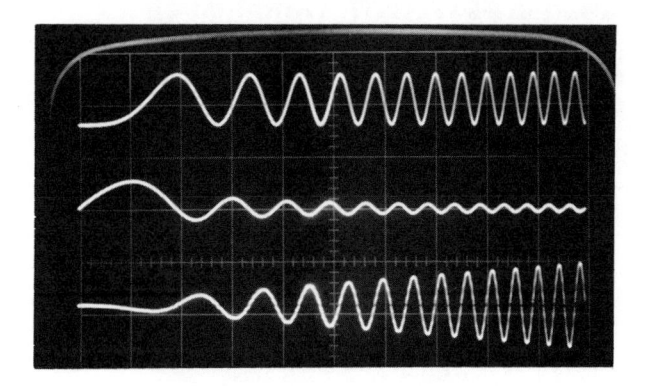

Figure 29.13 Output of an electronic (operational-amplifier) feedback-stabilized integrator (trace 2) and an electronic differentiator (trace 3) for a sine wave swept in frequency from 1 to 40 Hz (trace 1). As the frequency increases, the output amplitude decreases for the integrator but increases for the differentiator.

fier) introduces a phase lag of 90°, irrespective of the frequency of the sine wave. Since differentiation and integration are linear operations (i.e., superposition holds), the same 90° shifts occur for a signal of any combination of frequencies.

For the sine-wave signal, the resulting phase-shifted signals are 180° out of phase with one another; but inverting the one or the other puts the integrated and differentiated signals in phase with one another, and puts both in quadrature (i.e., at 90°) with respect to the original signal. However, the amplitude of both signals is frequency-dependent, as is evident from traces 2 and 3 of figure 29.13; the amplitude of the differentiated signal is directly proportional to the frequency, whereas the amplitude of the integrated signal is inversely

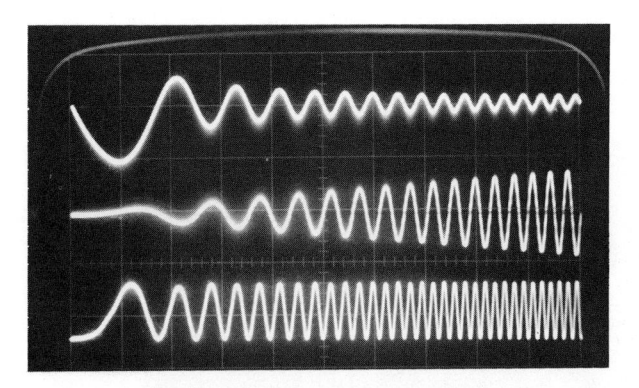

Figure 29.14 Product (trace 3) of an integrated (trace 1, shown in uninverted form) and a differentiated (trace 2) frequency-swept sine wave (1–40 Hz). (The latter is shown as the top trace in figure 29.13.) Note that the product (trace 3) is of constant amplitude, has a minimum of 0 (figure 29.15, trace 1), and has a frequency that is twice that of traces 1 and 2.

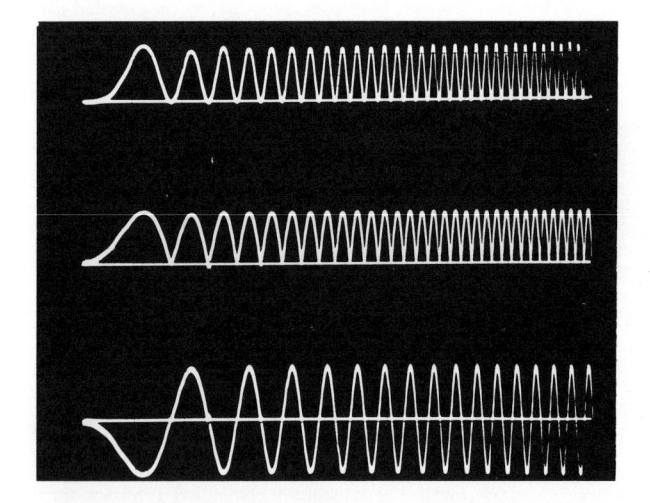

Figure 29.15 In-quadrature (Hilbert-transform) signal (trace 3) obtained as a result of alternating the polarity of successive half-cycles of the square root (trace 2) of the product (trace I) of the integrated and differentiated sine wave shown in figure 29.14. The baseline is shown for each trace.

proportional to the frequency. The question then became one of whether this pair of signals could be combined in some way to form a frequency-independent in-quadrature signal, as does the formal Hilbert transform.

Experiments confirm what theory would have predicted: Simply adding the two was not satisfactory; the amplitude of the resulting product was not frequency-independent. However, multiplication of the two signals yielded a frequency-independent product of double the original frequency, as shown in trace 3 of figure 29.14. The in-quadrature signal is then obtained by taking the square root (figure 29.15, trace 2) of the product signal (trace 1) and inverting alternate half-cycles (trace 3). That the signal thus obtained is indeed the in-quadrature signal can be verified by comparison of the top and bottom

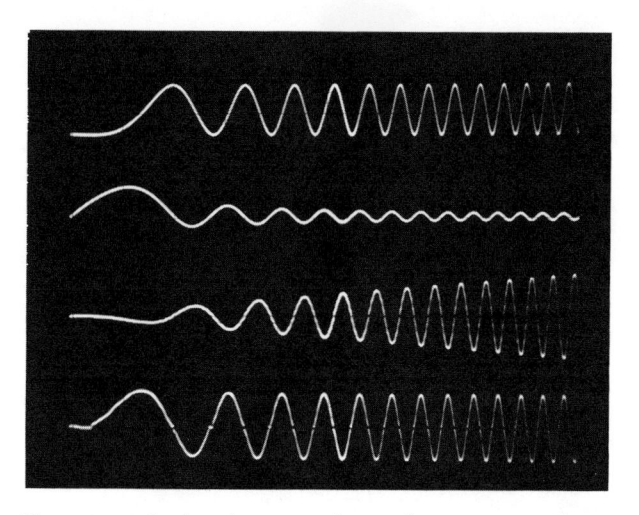

Figure 29.16 In-phase (trace 1) and in-quadrature (trace 4) signals, the latter obtained from the integrated (trace 2) and the differentiated (trace 3) in-phase signal by the method shown in figure 29.15. Note that both the integrated and the differentiated signals are 90° out of phase with the in-phase signal, as is, of course, the in-quadrature signal (trace 4).

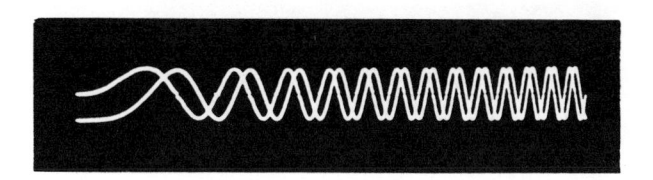

Figure 29.17 Superimposition of in-phase and in-quadrature signals (traces 1 and 4 in figure 29.16, respectively) to show more clearly the 90° phase shift, irrespective of the frequency.

traces of figure 29.16; these two traces are shown superimposed in figure 29.17. A block diagram of this method of obtaining the in-quadrature (Hilbert transform) signal is shown in figure 29.18.

Now, the instantaneous envelope of a signal is given by the square root of the sums of the squares of its in-phase and in-quadrature versions, as was indicated in figure 29.10. But it is now evident that the product of the integrated signal and the differentiated signal is just the square of the in-quadrature signal (figure 29.14, traces 1, 2, and 3; figure 29.15, traces 1 and 3), and hence the step of obtaining the in-quadrature signal can be bypassed. In brief, the combined integration-differentiation approach yields the square of the in-quadrature signal directly. This "short-cut" has additional important consequences, which will be considered below.

This process of obtaining the instantaneous envelope by adding the square of the in-phase signal to the square of the in-quadrature signal (i.e, the Hilbert transform of the in-phase signal) and taking the square root of the sum (figure 29.10) is illustrated in figure 29.19A for a sine wave modulated by a lower-frequency sine wave, and in figure 29.19B by a lower-frequency triangular wave. In each case, the recovered instantaneous envelope is superimposed on

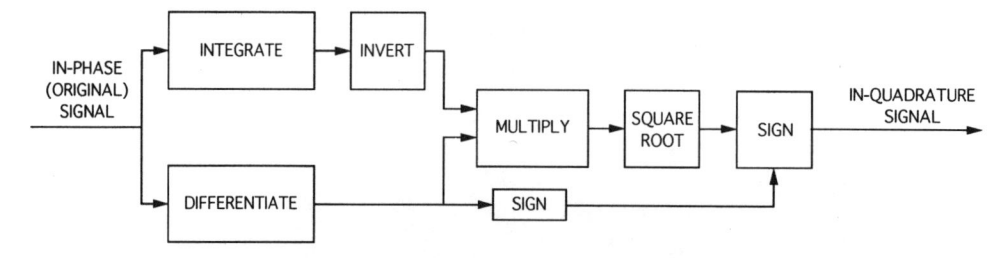

Figure 29.18 Block diagram of derivation of the in-quadrature (Hilbert-transform) signal by paired integration and differentiation of the in-phase signal.

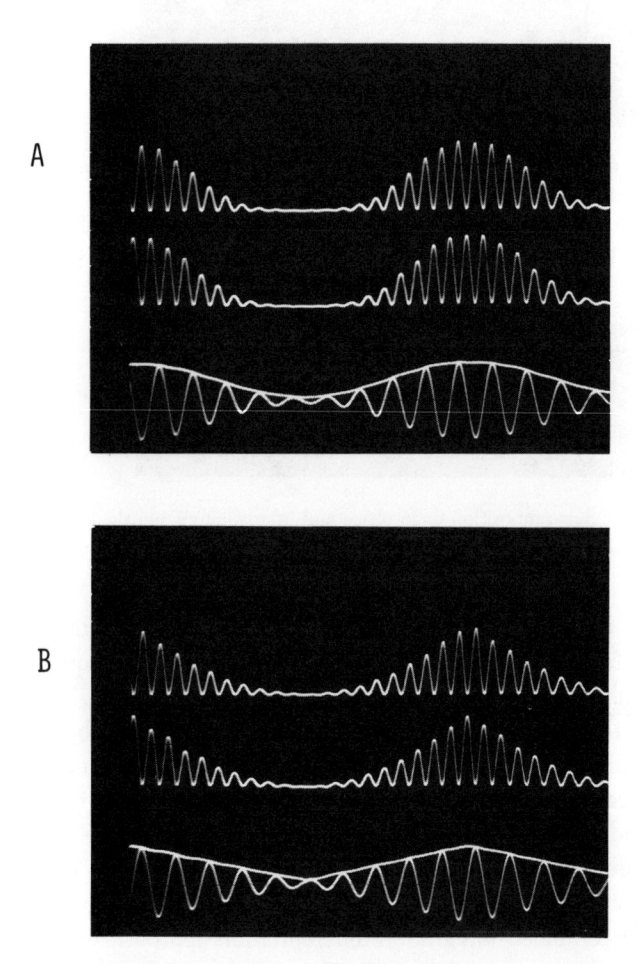

Figure 29.19 Instantaneous envelopes of a 10-Hz sine wave modulated by a 1-Hz sine wave (A) and by a 1-Hz triangular wave (B), obtained as the square root of the sum of the square of the in-phase signal (trace 1, in parts A and B) and the square of the in-quadrature signal (trace 2, in parts A and B), the latter obtained as the product of the integrated and the differentiated in-phase signals, respectively. The original in-phase signal before squaring is shown in the bottom trace in parts A and B, with the respective instantaneous envelope superimposed. (In this method, the in-quadrature signal does not appear explicitly.) Note that the instantaneous envelope is a continuous curve, in contrast to the sampled results shown in figures 29.11 and 29.12.

370   Chapter 29

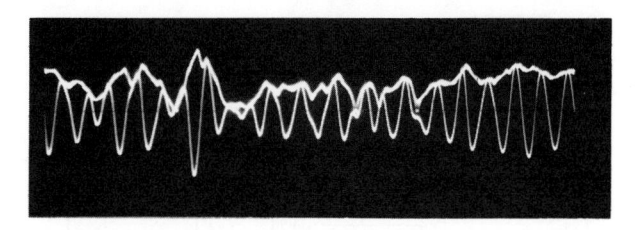

Figure 29.20 Instantaneous envelope of 10-Hz narrow-band noise by the method of paired integration and differentiation.

the original (in-phase) signal. Figure 29.20 shows narrow-band noise with its instantaneous envelope superimposed.

INSTANTANEOUS ENVELOPE OF A SIGNAL AND OF ITS FIRST (TIME) DERIVATIVE

For the reconstitution of a signal on the basis of its instantaneous envelope and the instantaneous envelope of its first derivative, the latter must of course be computed simultaneously with the former. This procedure is accomplished as indicated in figure 29.21. In general, the same principles as depicted in figure 29.18 are implemented for obtaining the instantaneous envelope of the first derivative of the signal. Thus, the instantaneous envelope of the original signal is obtained from the original signal itself, its integral, and its first derivative, whereas the instantaneous envelope of the first derivative of the signal is obtained from the signal itself, its first derivative, and its second derivative.

The instantaneous envelope of a sine wave that is swept in frequency and is simultaneously modulated by a triangular wave is shown in figure 29.22. The same set of waveforms is shown in figure 29.23 for an asymmetrical EEG.

THE INSTANTANEOUS FREQUENCY

By analogy with the determination of the running mean frequency as the ratio of the running mean slope and the running mean amplitude, the instantaneous frequency can be determined as the ratio of the instantaneous envelope of the first derivative of a signal to the instantaneous envelope of the signal itself. This method of obtaining the instantaneous frequency can be considered as the equivalent of computing the latter as the time rate of change of the phase of the analytic signal. (For the latter, see Middleton 1960, p. 100, and Bracewell 1986, p. 271.)

RAPIDITY OF RESPONSE

As was previously mentioned, the reconstitution (from the paired instantaneous envelopes of an EEG and its first derivative) of EEGs having epileptiform patterns, as well as of other EEG activity entailing fast transients,

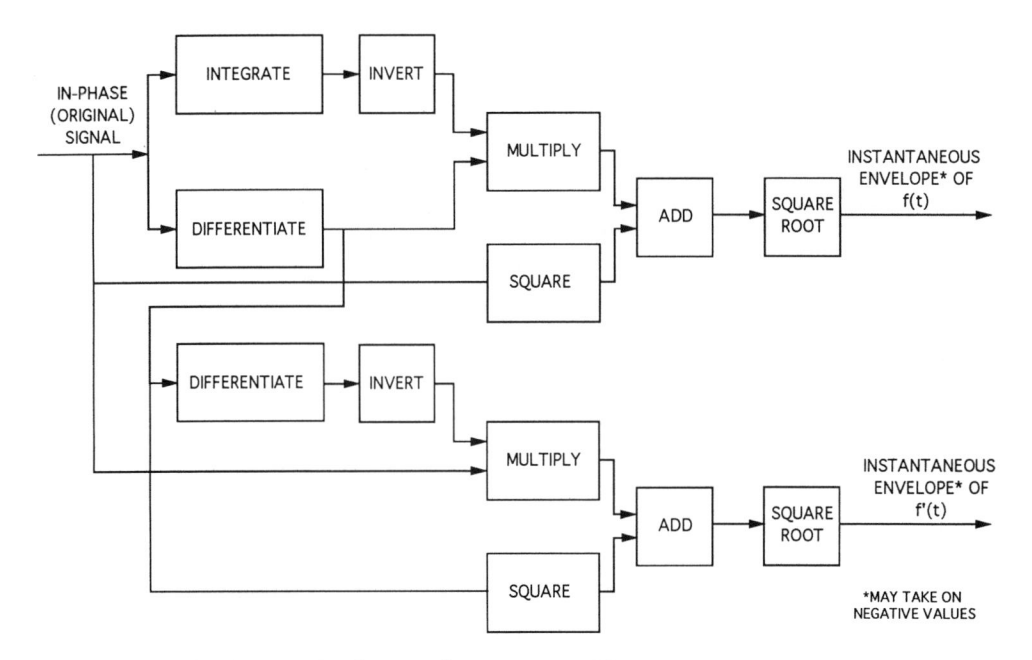

Figure 29.21 Simultaneous determinations of the instantaneous envelope of a signal and of its first derivative by the method of paired integration and differentiation. The instantaneous envelope of the original signal is computed in the same way as depicted in figure 29.18, by combined integration and differentiation of the original signal. The instantaneous envelope of the first derivative of the original signal is, correspondingly, computed from its integral (which is just the original signal again, since the successive operations of integration and differentiation counteract one another—see figure 9.2), and its derivative, i.e., the second derivative of the original signal. (See also figure 29.25B.)

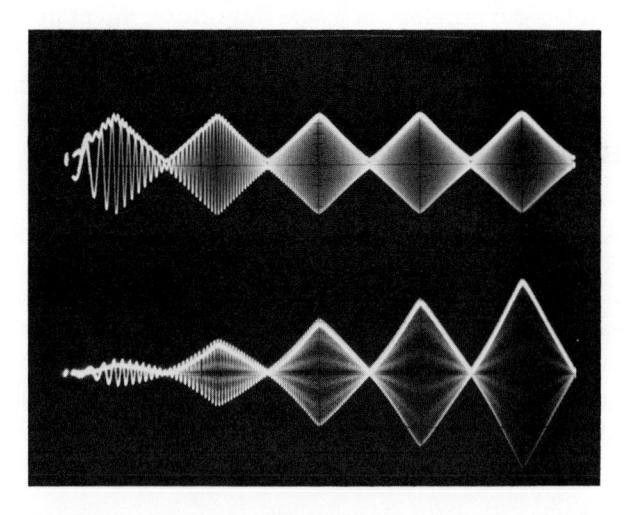

Figure 29.22 Simultaneous determinations of the instantaneous envelope of a swept sine wave (1–40 Hz) that is modulated by a 0.4-Hz triangular wave (upper traces), and of its first derivative (lower traces). The envelopes are superimposed on the tops of the respective original traces. Note the linear increase in the amplitude of the peaks of the instantaneous envelope of the first derivative (lower traces) as the sine wave increases in frequency.

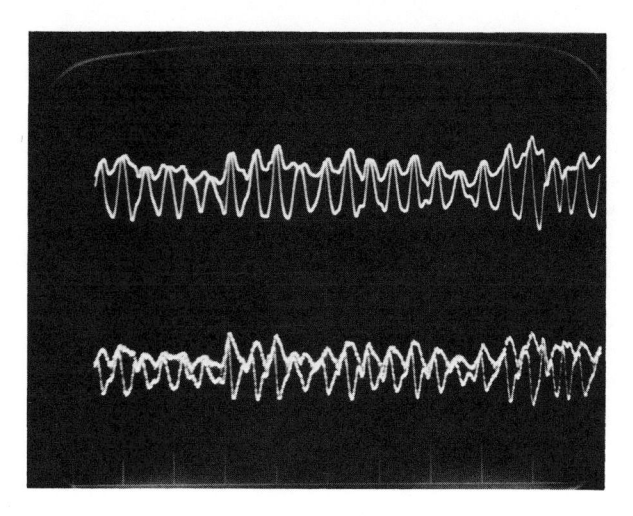

Figure 29.23 Instantaneous envelopes of an asymmetrical EEG and of its first derivative. Note the rapid and continuous changes of both envelopes, corresponding to the positive and negative phases of the original EEG.

necessitates a rapid response time in the derivation of the respective instantaneous envelopes. The rapidity of response of the determination of the instantaneous envelopes of a signal and of its first derivative is illustrated in figures 29.24A and 29.24B for stepwise changes in amplitude and frequency, respectively. In each case, the original sine wave is shown in trace 1, its instantaneous envelope in trace 2, the instantaneous envelope of the first derivative in trace 3, and the instantaneous frequency in trace 4. Quite rapid responses to the instantaneous changes are evident.

INSTANTANEOUS ENVELOPE OF RELATIVELY WIDE-BAND SIGNALS

It is the usual practice that determination of the instantaneous envelope is carried out only for relatively narrow-band signals, such as a modulated carrier frequency, or (in the case of the EEG) only for rhythmic activity such as alpha activity or sleep spindles. Indeed, the analytic signal, and therefore the instantaneous envelope, is generally considered to have meaning only for relatively narrow-band signals (Devyatkov et al. 1973).

One method of dealing with relatively wide-band signals is to break them up into several narrower bands, and to determine the instantaneous envelope for each band separately. This procedure was followed by Bullock (1988a, figure 6), who separated the EEG of the turtle (1–40 Hz) into four bands (1–5, 5–10, 10–20, and 20–40 Hz) by means of bandpass filters and then obtained the instantaneous envelopes via the conventional Hilbert-transform method. Additional studies using this approach are described in Bullock and Başar 1988 and, for the human electrocorticogram, in Bullock et al. 1990.

Since the present purpose of determining the instantaneous envelopes was to reconstitute EEGs on the basis of their instantaneous envelopes and the

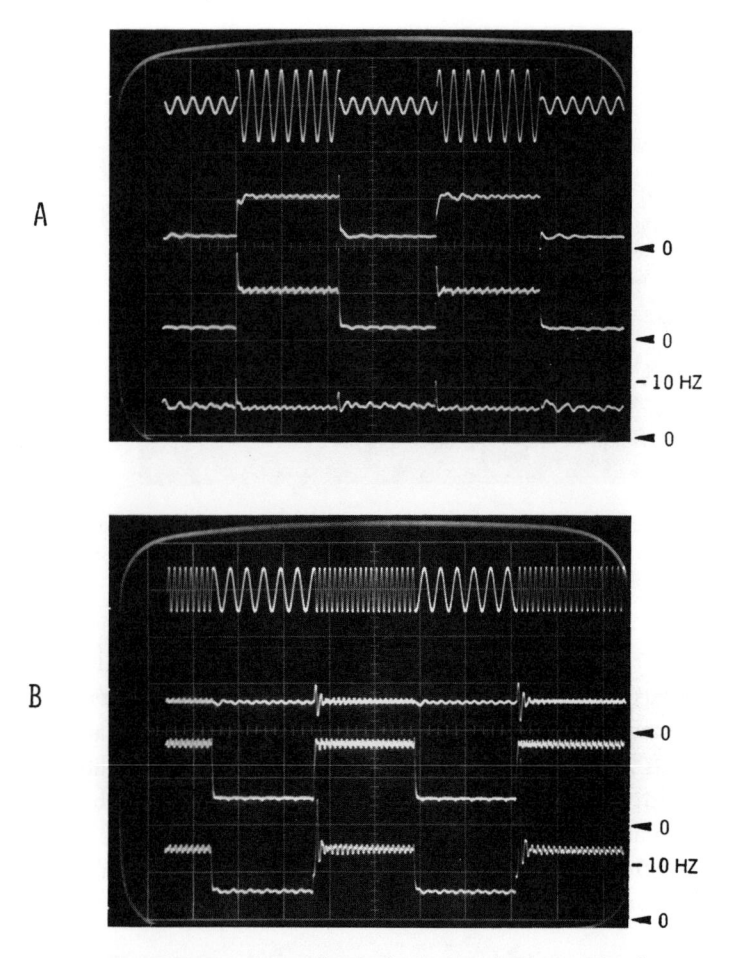

Figure 29.24 Instantaneous envelopes of (A) an amplitude-modulated 7-Hz sine wave and (B) a frequency-modulated 10-Hz sine wave, and of their respective first derivatives (the latter are not shown). The original signals are shown in the top traces (modulating signal in each case: 0.5 Hz square wave). Second traces: instantaneous envelope of the original signals. Third traces: instantaneous envelopes of the first derivative of the original signals. Bottom traces: instantaneous frequency (note the calibration). The baselines for traces 2–4 are indicated by the arrows at right. Note the rapidity of the responses to the step-like changes in the original signal. Note also that the instantaneous frequency for amplitude modulation (trace 4 in part A) remains essentially constant, whereas for frequency modulation the instantaneous amplitude (trace 2 in part B) remains essentially constant.

instantaneous envelope of their first derivative, the above-mentioned "parcellation" approach would not have been satisfactory. However, a special feature of the combined integration-differentiation method of obtaining the instantaneous envelope permits this method to be used even with relatively wide-band signals. This unanticipated feature of the combined integration-differentiation method of obtaining the instantaneous envelope, in contrast to the above-mentioned limitation of the conventional Hilbert-transform method, can be understood from the following comparison of the two methods, and concerns the manner in which the square of the in-quadrature signal is derived.

In the Hilbert-transform method (figure 29.25A), as previously noted, the instantaneous envelope (i.e., the magnitude of the analytic signal) is obtained as the square root of the sums of the squares of the in-phase and the in-quadrature signals. Since the squares, and therefore the sums of the squares, are invariably positive or zero, the square of the instantaneous envelope (and therefore the instantaneous envelope itself) is invariably positive or zero. In the combined integration-differentiation method (figure 29.25B), however, the square of the in-phase signal (which is always positive or zero) is added, not to another positive or zero quantity, but to a quantity that can be positive, zero, or negative—namely, the product of the integrated in-phase signal and the differentiated in-phase signal. A positive value of the latter product will occur whenever the inverted integrated signal and the differentiated signal are of the same polarity, as is the case for a sine wave (figure 29.11, trace 3; the integrated signal—trace 2—is shown before inversion) or for a narrow-band signal. On the other hand, a negative value of the product will occur when the inverted integrated signal and the differentiated signal are of opposite polarity, as can occur for a relatively wide-band signal. In such a case, if the magnitude of this product exceeds the magnitude of the square of the in-phase signal, the sum of the two (i.e., the square of the instantaneous envelope) will be negative.

Under these conditions, the instantaneous envelope itself would be imaginary, as the square root of a negative number. In the actual computation, however, the sign can temporarily be reversed, the square root obtained, and the negative sign then restored.

It is this information about negative values of the instantaneous envelope that cannot be conveyed by the Hilbert-transform method. (The limitation is not in the Hilbert transform itself, but rather in the subsequent step of squaring.) Negative values of the instantaneous envelope of the first derivative of a signal occur during periods when the polarity of the second derivative of the original signal is the same (rather than opposite, as is the case for a sine wave), as that of the original signal—e.g., for the "notched" waveform in trace 1 of figure 29.26.

For narrow-band signals, the instantaneous envelopes obtained by the standard Hilbert-transform method and the paired integration-differentiation method will be identical, since, as previously mentioned, the product of the integrated signal and the differentiated signal is always positive for such

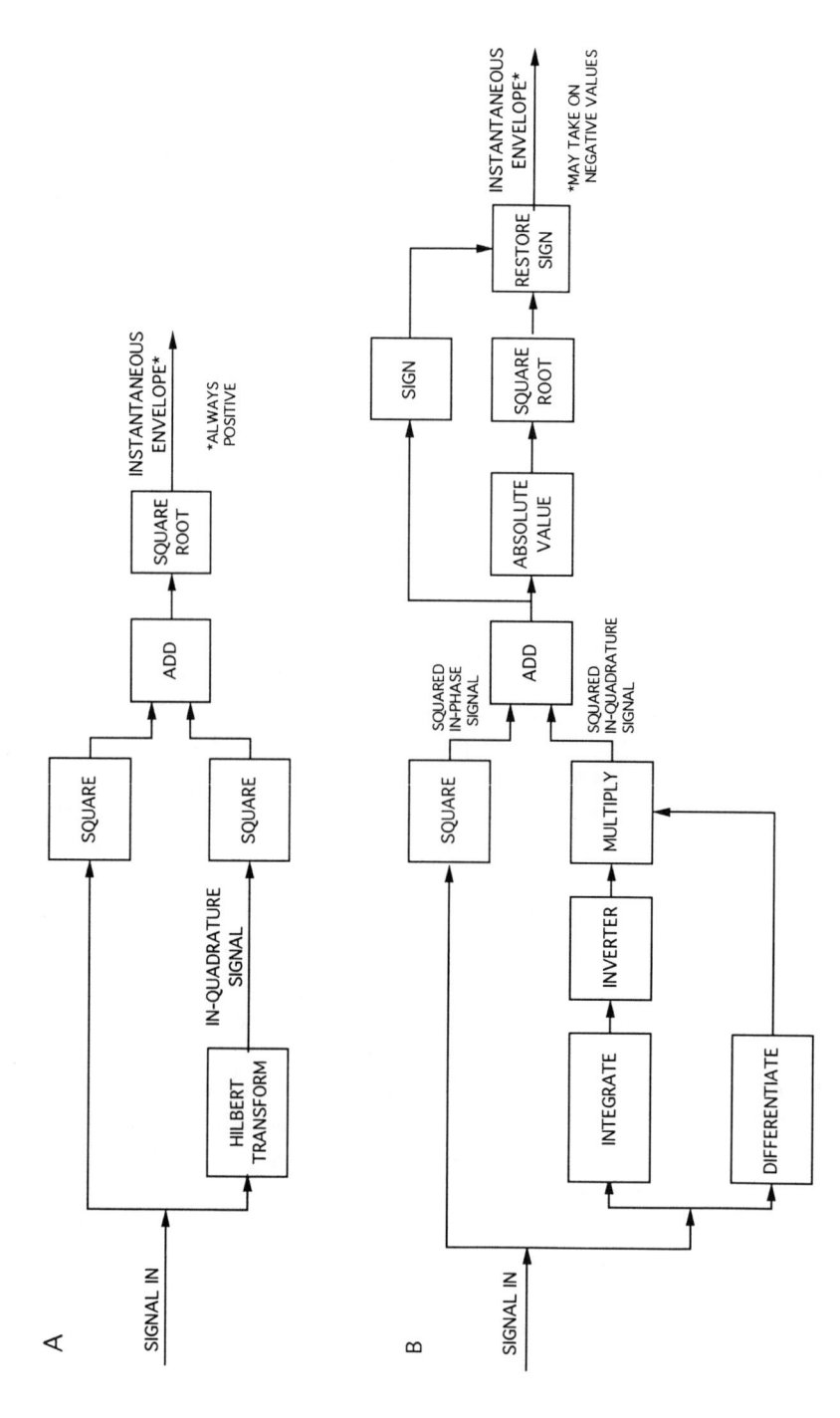

Figure 29.25 Comparison of derivation of instantaneous envelope by (A) the conventional Hilbert-transform method and (B) the paired integration-differentiation method. Note that the square of the in-quadrature signal appears in the second method, but the in-quadrature signal itself does not appear explicitly. Note also that in the combined integration-differentiation method, negative values of the square of the magnitude of the analytic signal (i.e., the square of the instantaneous envelope) can occur; these are rendered as negative values of the instantaneous envelope, whereas only positive values can occur in the conventional Hilbert-transform method (A).

376   Chapter 29

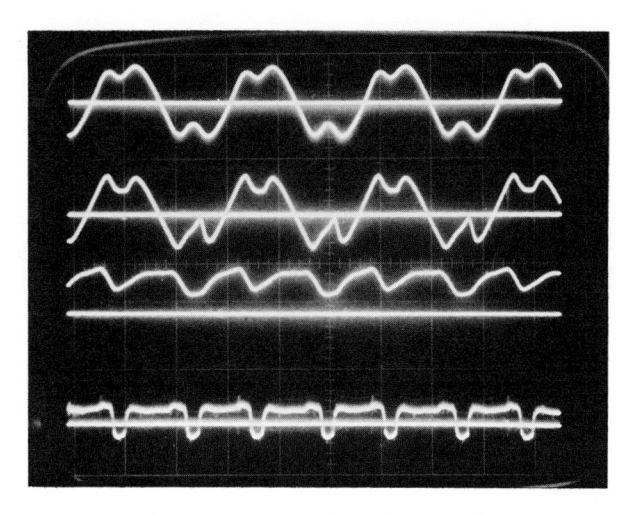

Figure 29.26 Instantaneous envelopes of a signal having negative excursions of the instantaneous envelope of its first derivative. Trace 1: original signal. Trace 2: reconstituted signal. Trace 3: instantaneous envelope of original signal. Trace 4: instantaneous envelope of the first derivative of the original signal. Note that the negative swings of the latter correspond to the reversals of curvature (notches) of the original signal, and of the reconstituted version (trace 2). Baselines are shown for each trace.

signals. The instantaneous envelopes obtained by the two methods will also be identical for relatively wide-band signals if the absolute value of the product of the integrated signal and the differentiated signal is always taken, so that no negative values occur. (Taking the product of the integrated signal and the differentiated signal can, in some respects, be compared with taking the product of a complex function with its complex conjugate, instead of squaring the complex function.)

From the preceding discussion, it is clear that the wider the bandwidth of a signal, the more probable are negative values of the magnitude of its instantaneous envelope. Accordingly, for narrow-band signals such as alpha activity in the EEG, the Hilbert-transform method of deriving the instantaneous envelope is quite satisfactory. However, for the case of relatively complex EEG signals (e.g., the "desynchronized" EEG), the Hilbert-transform method would not be satisfactory.

In the example of a signal having a notched waveform shown in figure 29.26, the instantaneous envelope of the first derivative becomes negative (trace 4)—an effect that is in turn reflected in the corresponding portions of the reconstituted version (trace 2).

RECONSTITUTING EEGS: INTERFACING THE INSTANTANEOUS ENVELOPES UNIT WITH THE OSCILLATOR MODEL

For the reconstitution of EEGs on the basis of their instantaneous envelopes and those of their first derivatives, the unit for deriving the pair of instantaneous envelopes is interfaced with the oscillator model (chapter 22). The

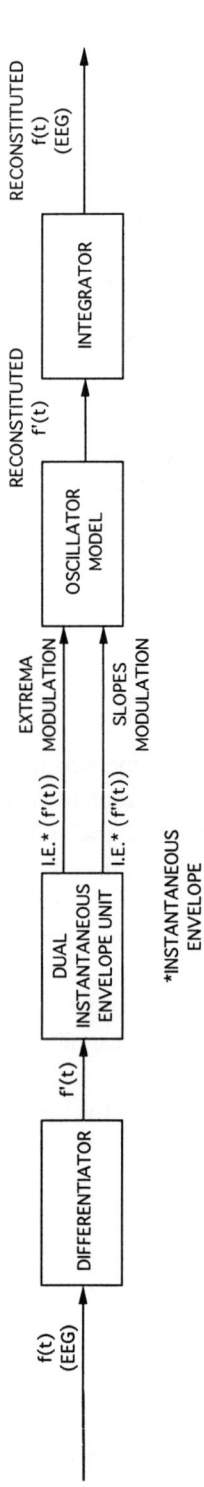

Figure 29.27 Block diagram of interfacing of the instantaneous-envelopes unit with the oscillator model. With this form of interfacing, the polarity of the reconstituted EEG is arbitrary with respect to that of the input EEG. The insertion of the differentiator in the input to the instantaneous-envelopes unit and the integrator in the output of the oscillator model increases the overall bandwidth of the combined system.

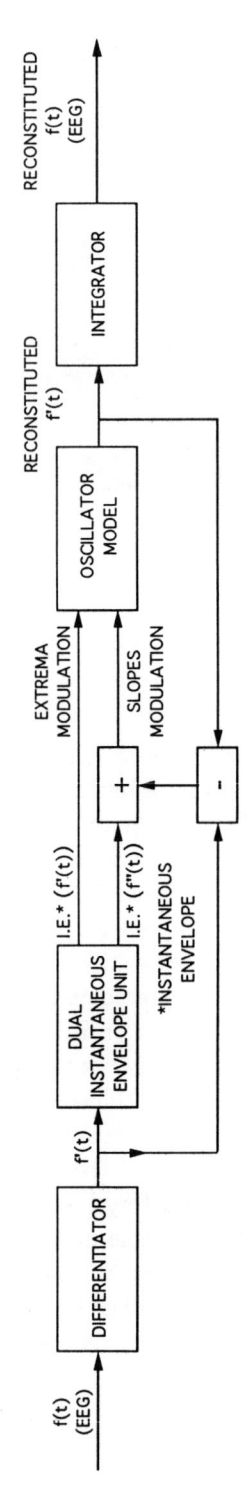

Figure 29.28 Arrangement for diminution of polarity error between the reconstituted and the original EEG by employing a feedback loop for the slopes-modulation signal. The error signal is obtained by comparing the first derivative of the original with that of the reconstituted signal (which is actually the output of the oscillator model, before integration of the latter signal, in the configuration shown).

interfacing is straightforward in that the instantaneous envelope of an EEG is fed to the extrema-modulation input of the oscillator model, and the instantaneous envelope of the first derivative of the EEG is fed to the slopes modulation of the oscillator model. Although unnecessary for narrow-band EEGs (e.g, for alpha activity), overall improved performance of the reconstitution process is achieved by inserting a differentiator before the input to the instantaneous-envelopes unit and a feedback-stabilized integrator after the output of the oscillator model, as illustrated in figure 29.27. Especially for constant-slope EEGs (and for other EEGs of increased slow-wave content), the insertion of the differentiator-integrator pair increases the overall bandwidth of the system, since the original $1/f$ spectral characteristics of such EEGs is transformed into a flat spectral characteristic. This procedure can be viewed as "pre-whitening" (i.e., converting the spectrum to a relatively flat one) of such EEGs for processing.

As previously mentioned, the polarity (phase) of the individual waves of the reconstituted signal is necessarily arbitrary with respect to the original, since phase information is not retained in the process of reconstitution. Thus, EEG spikes are as likely to be reconstituted with a polarity opposite to that of the originals as with the same polarity. In contrast, actual EEG spikes of true epileptic origin are characteristically negative at the active electrode.

The ambiguity of polarity of the reconstituted signal can be diminished, although not eliminated entirely, by incorporating a feedback loop to minimize the error in the first derivative of the reconstituted signal as compared with that of the original EEG, as indicated in figure 29.28.

Even with the incorporation of the paired differentiator-integrator and the phase-correcting feedback loop, however, the reconstituted trace is not a perfect replica of the original, as is evident from figure 9.9. The difference between the two actually arises, not from the derivation of the respective instantaneous envelopes of the original signal and of its first derivative (which are instrinsically "blind" to polarity), but in the reconstitution process that utilizes the oscillator model.

Despite these limitations, the extension of the basic technique of computing the instantaneous envelopes (in effect providing for the handling of complex or imaginary numbers) appreciably extends the bandwidth of signals that can be studied in this way.

Appendixes

A Some Traditional Methods of EEG Analysis: On-Line Real-Time Analog Implementation

As was mentioned in chapter 21, the pursuit of the extrema-slopes hypothesis of the EEG has entailed extensive development of new electronic circuitry, described in detail in chapters 22–29. In turn, experience with the resulting circuits has suggested new approaches, employing analog techniques, to some traditional data-processing techniques in electroencephalography and related fields. These "spinoffs" or dividends from the basic work are described here and in appendix B.

SPECTRAL ANALYSIS: COMPRESSED SPECTRAL ARRAYS

Spectral (frequency or Fourier) analysis of EEGs has been carried out in several ways. (For a short account of the early history of analysis of physiological oscillations, see Walter 1987.) The approaches have included a harmonic analyzer (Grass and Gibbs 1938), special-purpose frequency analyzers (Walter 1943a, 1943b), Fourier transformation of autocorrelation functions (Barlow et al. 1959), use of the discrete Fourier transform (Walter et al. 1966), and, finally, an expedited form of the latter: the fast Fourier transform, which has been the standard method for some years (Dumermuth and Molinari 1987).

In the present implementation, the Fourier transform or spectrum is computed in a manner that is similar to the one used in the discrete Fourier transform, except that the computation is carried out by analog means, in real time, and recursively (i.e., on a running basis). With this approach, spectra can be computed so as to supplement the more succinct measures of running mean frequency and the Spectral Purity Index (chapter 25).

The block diagram of the spectral analyzer unit shown in figure A.1 consists of the time-scale converter and the spectral analyzer itself. The output of the time-scale converter is a repetitive version of its input (more specifically, of the portion of the input signal stored at any given instant), which thus appears at the output on a contracted time scale. The basic spectral analyzer includes an optional Hanning or cosine window (generated from a triangular wave as a parabolic approximation to a cosine wave, as in figure 2.3, lower left) for tapering the EEG data so as to avoid "leakage" of spectral components into adjacent spectral regions (Dumermuth 1977), and a system for generating paired sine and cosine waves the frequency of which can be swept over the

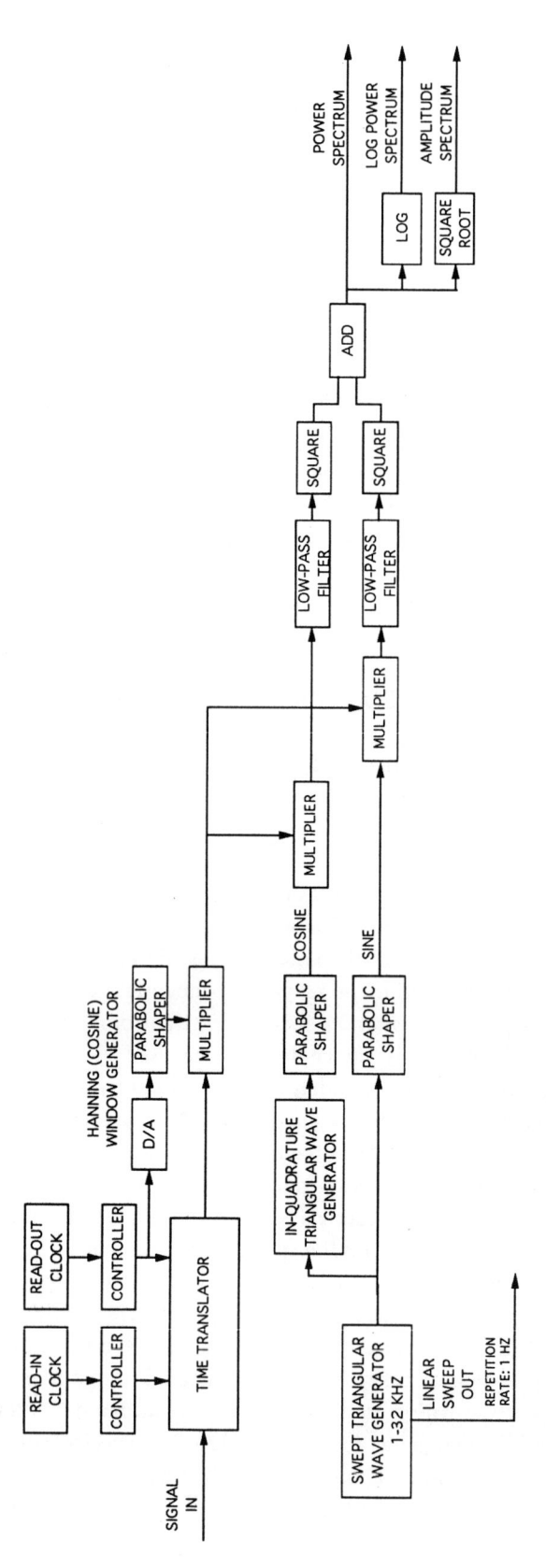

Figure A.1 Block diagram of the Analog Spectrum Analyzer.

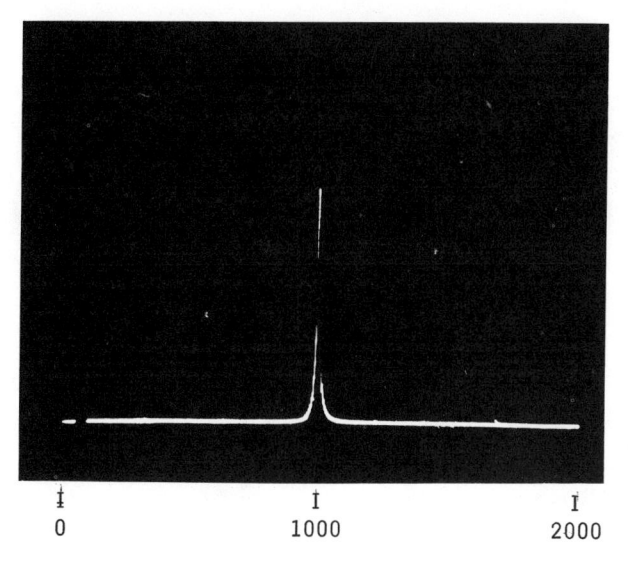

Figure A.2 Power spectrum for a 1,000-Hz sine wave. Analysis (sweep) time: 13 sec. (The shorter the sweep time, the wider the spectrum.)

desired frequency range. (The sine-cosine pair are also generated by parabolic approximation from a pair of triangular waves 90° out of phase with one another.)

As the frequency of the triangular wave is swept over the desired range, the input signal is heterodyned separately against the sine and cosine waves by means of the pair of multipliers, and the resulting outputs are low-pass filtered and squared to recover the sine and cosine components of the original signal at the current frequency of the frequency sweep. The output is available in three forms: as the power spectrum, as the amplitude spectrum (i.e., the square root of the power spectrum), or as the log power spectrum. An example of the output of the spectral analyzer alone for a 1000-Hz sine-wave input is shown in figure A.2.

For spectral analysis of EEGs, the time-scale converter is interposed between the output of the photo-optical scanner (chapter 26) and the spectral analyzer. A 60-Hz read-in rate (synchronized with the sampling frequency of the photo-optical scanner, i.e., the frequency of the photo-optical scanning pen), in combination with a 6-kHz readout rate, yields a speedup factor of 100. For a sweep time of the sine-cosine pair of 1 sec (e.g., a sweep from 100 to 3200 Hz), spectra of successive non-overlapping 1-sec EEG epochs are calculated on line in real time. With some additional electronic circuitry, the spectra can be displayed on an oscilloscope screen as compressed spectral arrays with hidden line suppression in isometric view, as illustrated in figure A.3. Further, with the averaging unit described below, blocks of successive spectra could be averaged. With some further circuitry, the spectra can be recorded (with a 1-sec delay) continuously for an unlimited time on an incremental or digital plotter.

A B

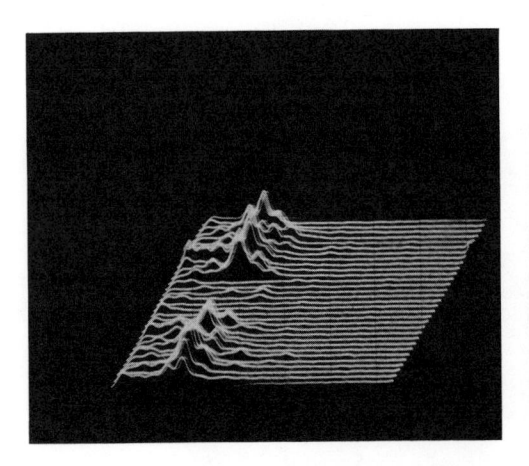

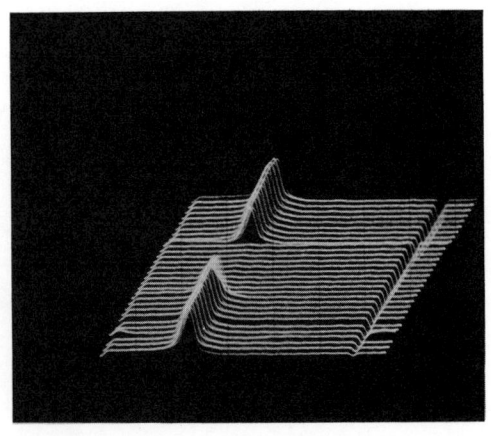

Figure A.3 (A) On-line real-time calculation of a compressed spectral array (1–32 Hz) with hidden line suppression and in isometric view for successive non-overlapping 1-sec epochs of a 30-sec photo-optically scanned parieto-occipital EEG recording, showing alpha blocking during the middle 10-sec period when the eyes were open. (B) Similar analysis, but for a 10-Hz sine wave, attenuated 1:10 in amplitude during the middle 10 sec. In both instances, the amplitude spectrum (square root of the power spectrum) is displayed. (Hanning window not used in these examples.)

AVERAGING OF WAVEFORMS: EVENT-RELATED POTENTIALS, SPECTRA

It is not infrequently convenient to have available a very simple on-line real-time averaging device for averaging (or summation, if there is no normalization) of waveforms such as those of event-related potentials, or those of spectra.

For such computations, a special adding circuit is incorporated into the functioning of the second (readout) unit of the time-scale converter, as indicated in figure A.4B. In brief, the current input point (voltage) is summed with the voltage on the current storage condenser (1 out of 64), and restored in the same storage condenser. These steps are carried out during the first and the second phase, respectively, of each clock cycle. An example of a summated waveform is shown in figure A.5. (True averaging, as opposed to summation, can readily be accomplished by dividing the summed waveform by the number of waveforms averaged; such a voltage can be obtained as the output of a D/A converter driven by the necessary number of decade counters to accommodate the number of summated waveforms.)

AUTOCORRELATION AND CROSS-CORRELATION

Autocorrelation and cross-correlation are sometimes used in the analysis of EEGs (e.g., figure 17.7; see Gevins 1987 for a review). In the case of data

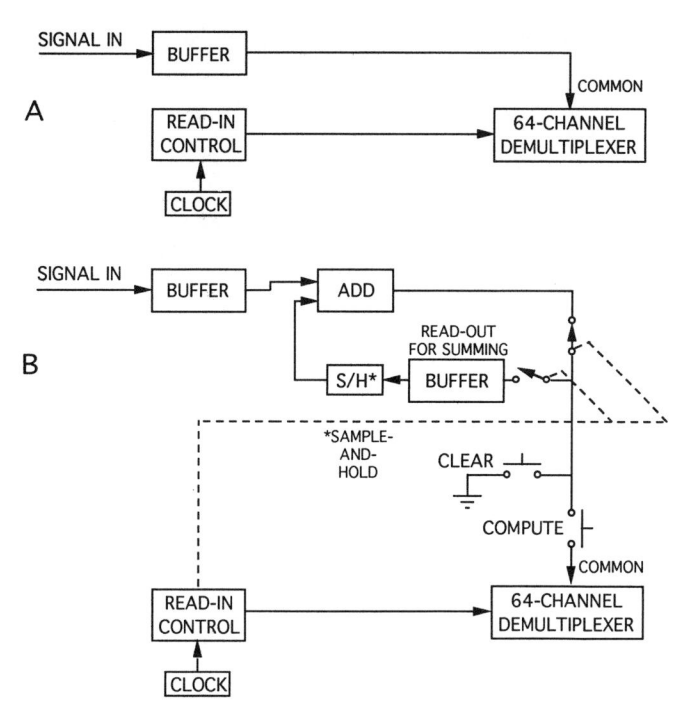

Figure A.4 Block diagram of the basic read-in portion of the "time machine" before (A) and after (B) the incorporation of the subunit for summation.

sampled at regular (periodic) intervals, they are defined by the relation

$$R_{xy}[k] = \frac{1}{N} \sum_{n=0}^{N-1} \{x[n]y[n+k]\},$$

where $x[n]$ and $y[n]$ are the values (voltages) of a pair of time series, x and y, at time n; k is the time shift or relative lag of $y[n]$ with respect to $x[n]$; and N is the number of samples over which the correlation function is computed. If the two time series are the same ($x = y$), R_{xx} is the autocorrelation function of the single time series; if they are different, R_{xy} is the cross-correlation function for the two time series (Gevins 1987).

Evaluation of the autocorrelation function can be carried out by means of two "time machines," with a multiplier unit interposed between the two, as indicated in figure A.6. Since autocorrelation requires the summation of a series of cross-products of two signals at a series of lags, provision must be made for a series of delays. This is accomplished by the multiplexed tapped delay line in the form of the first "time machine," the second multiplexer of which is operated at 64 times the rate of the first, its starting address being incremented with each new sample of the input signals(s). The cross-products of the fixed delay (32 delay units) and the variable delay ($k = 1$ through 64 delay units) are computed serially by the multiplier. In the first half of a fast clock cycle, the resultant cross-products are summated with the previously computed and summated cross-products as the latter are read from the

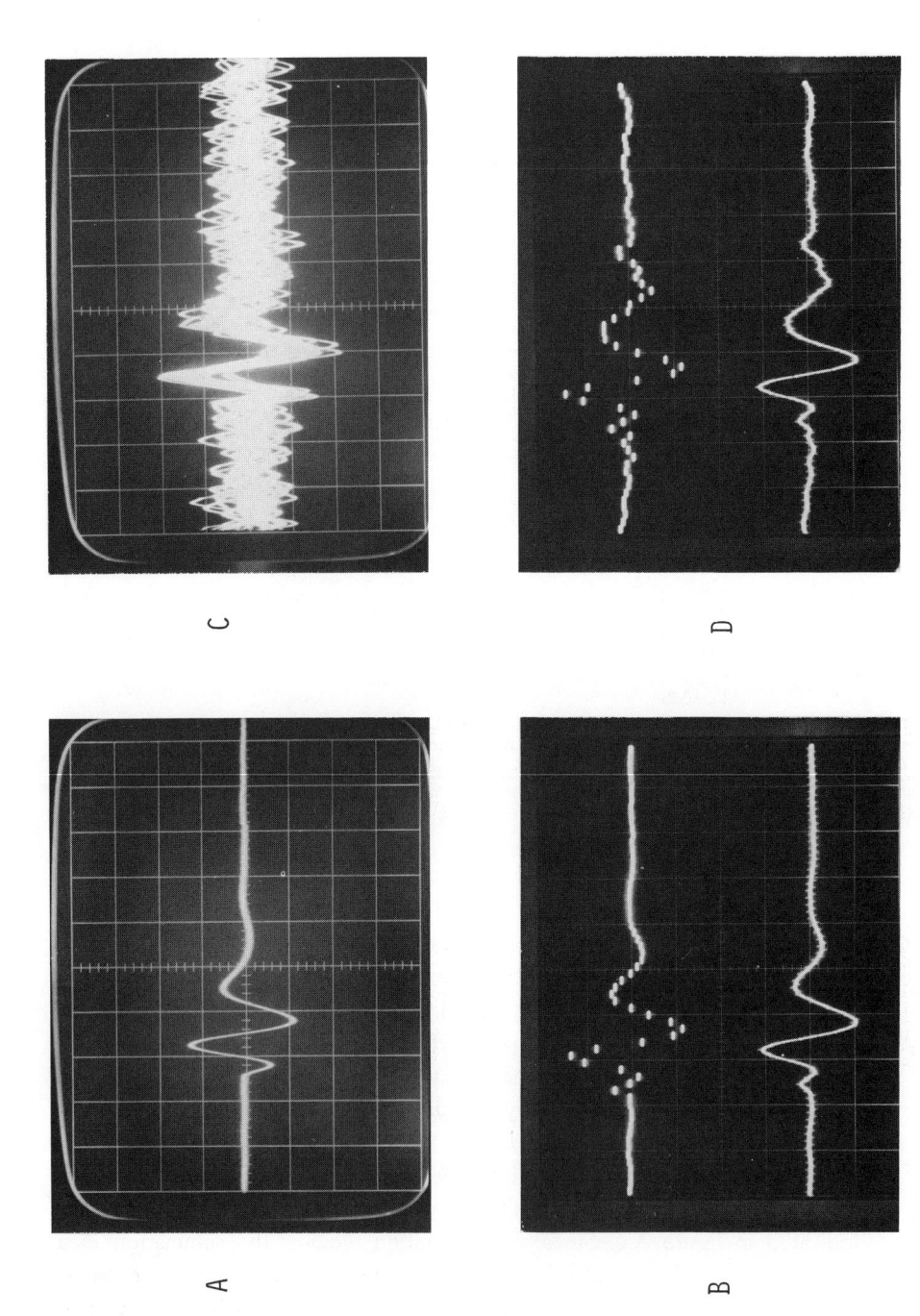

Figure A.5 Examples of averaging of waveforms. In part A a single trace of a simulated event-related potential is shown, and in part C ongoing "background" activity in the same frequency range has been added. The corresponding 64-point averages are shown in the upper traces in parts B and D, respectively, and the lower traces show the results after parabolic interpolation (figure 27.2).

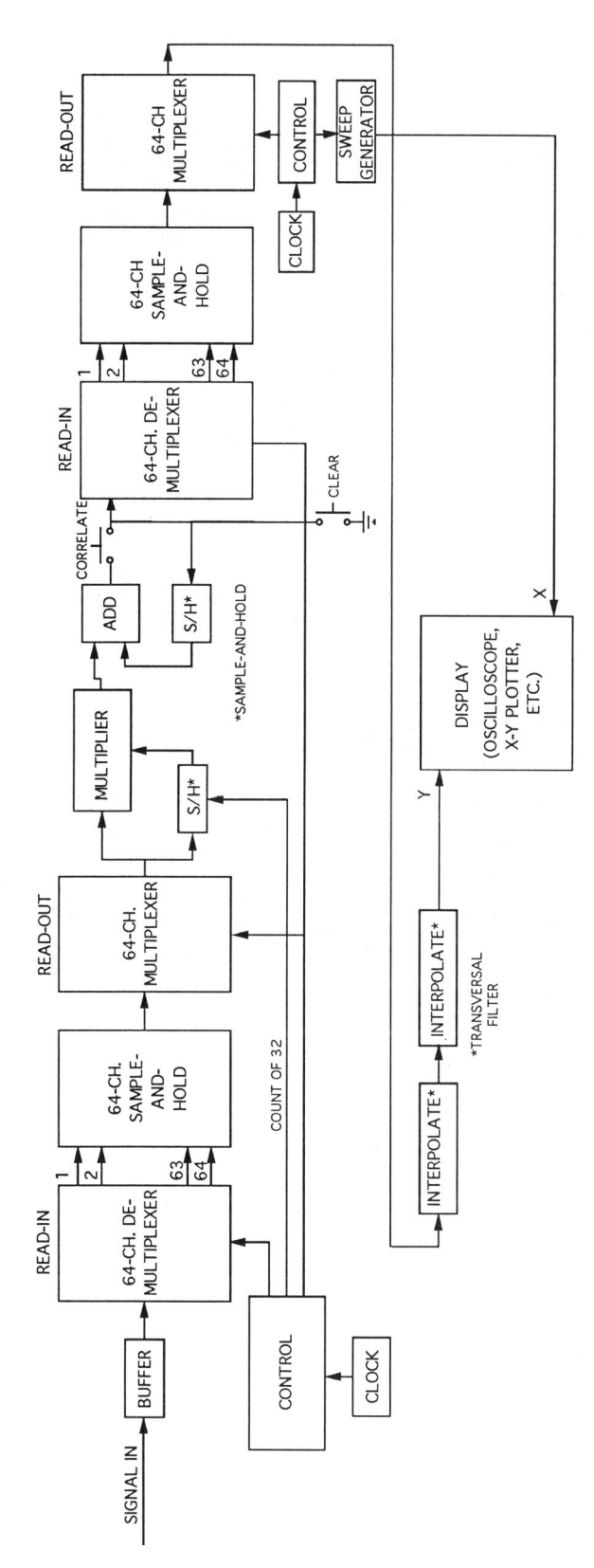

Figure A.6 Block diagram of the unit for autocorrelation. (An additional "time machine" is required for the second signal, in computing crosscorrelation functions.)

Traditional Methods of EEG Analysis

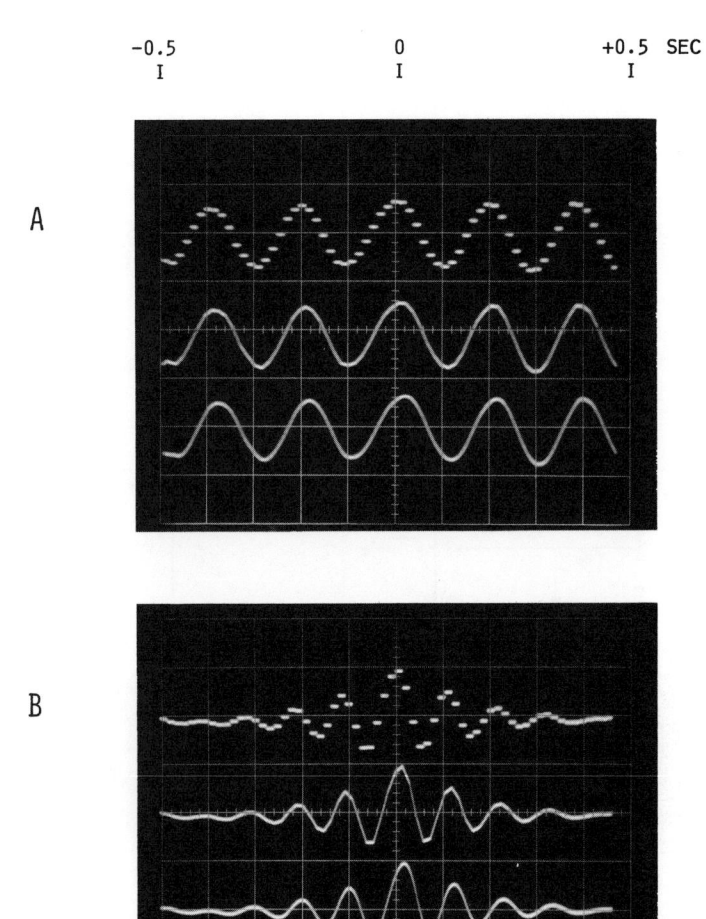

Figure A.7 Autocorrelation functions (autocorrelograms) for (A) a 5-Hz sine wave and (B) 10-Hz band-limited noise (24-dB rolloff on either side of the center frequency). Top traces: autocorrelation functions of 64 points. Middle traces: after one stage of linear interpolation. Bottom traces: after two stages of linear interpolation (i.e., after parabolic interpolation). Note that the successive interpolation procedures result in successive slight shifts of the peak to the right (compare trace 2 and 3 with trace 1 in each instance). Time shift (lead/lag) in sec.

sample-and-hold circuits of the second "time machine." In the second half of a fast clock cycle, the new summations are stored in the respective sample-and-hold units of the second "time machine" in a manner quite similar to that used in the averager described above (figure A.4). (Cross-correlation requires a separate "time machine," to delay the second signal input by 32 delay units.) The correlogram is read out by the second multiplexer of the second "time machine" at the desired rate for repetitive display on an x-y oscilloscope, or, at a lower speed, on an x-y plotter. The x-axis signal for the latter devices is derived from the D/A converter (figure A.6).

Examples of an autocorrelogram of a 5-Hz sine wave (which should be a cosine wave of the same period) and of 10-Hz band-limited noise (which is expected to have the form of a symmetrically damped 10-Hz cosine wave) are shown in figure A.7.

B Eliminating or Minimizing Artifact by Paired Sampling and by Coherent Rejection; Analog Adaptive Signal Processing

In this appendix, several methods of signal processing (or, perhaps more exactly, signal nulling) of progressively increasing sophistication will be considered. These methods are based in part on the electronic-circuit developments carried out in connection with the work on the extrema-slopes hypothesis. The first technique is that of eliminating 60-Hz interference by paired in-phase sampling and subtraction. The second technique, that of frequency-independent coherent rejection of interference or artifact, can be viewed as an extension and a generalization of the principles of the first technique. The third technique, that of adaptive signal processing, represents a further extension of the principles of the first two techniques together with an analog tapped delay line (chapter 23), since it entails the nulling of an arbitrary signal on the basis of the signal's own immediate past. Brief accounts of the first two techniques appeared in Barlow 1986. Despite some limitations, the powerful technique of adaptive signal analysis is relevant not only to the characterization of physiological processes but perhaps to their modeling as well.

ELIMINATION OF 60-HZ ARTIFACT BY PAIRED ANALOG SAMPLING

Although 50-Hz or 60-Hz filters are routinely provided on electroencephalographs and polygraphs, the phase-shift characteristics of these may be undesirable in some applications. One alternative is to utilize a computer-based 60-Hz filter having a linear phase-shift characteristic (i.e., it delays all frequencies by the same amount of time) (Gotman 1982). An alternative is to subtract from the EEG a version of itself that has been delayed by half the wavelength of a 60-Hz wave (i.e., 8.33 msec), which eliminates the 60-Hz interference; that procedure was originally implemented with a magnetic delay drum (Barlow 1967b; see also Barlow 1986). A much simpler implementation that yields the same results can be obtained by utilizing the principle of paired sampling and summation (figure B.1). Such a device can be considered as a two-point transversal filter (chapter 23).

As figure B.1 shows, 60-Hz in-phase and out-of-phase sampling pulses are used to sample the EEG contaminated by 60 Hz. In the summation of the two

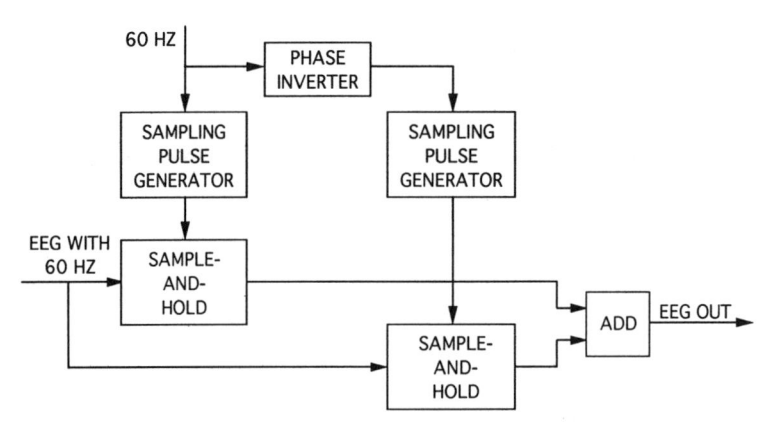

Figure B.1 Block diagram of the paired sampling (two-point) and summation technique of eliminating 60-Hz interference.

sampled waves, the 60-Hz signal is eliminated (figure B.2), leaving a 120-Hz sampled version of the original EEG. (The output signal could be smoothed by means of transverse filters (chapter 23), if desired.) Since the Nyquist frequency for a 120-Hz effective sample rate is 60 Hz, the original signal should be filtered to eliminate any frequency components above 60 Hz, so as to eliminate the possibility of aliasing of such frequency components. (If necessary, the 60-Hz signal used to trigger the sampling circuits can be derived from the contaminated EEG itself.) In figure B.3, the frequency response of the filter is compared with that of Gotman's 60-Hz filter and with the response of a commercial 60-Hz notch filter on an EEG instrument; its use in a clinical EEG recording is illustrated in figure B.4.

The paired sampling filter can also be used to minimize or eliminate moderately rhythmic EEG activity, such as sleep spindles (figure B.5), pharmacologically induced rhythmic fast (beta) activity, or even alpha activity. (In such applications, anti-aliasing filtering may be necessary.)

ARTIFACT MINIMIZATION BY COHERENT REJECTION (AUTOMATIC NULLING)

(This section will also serve as a preliminary to the next section, on adaptive signal processing.)

In the previous section it was apparent (figure B.2) that, although the filter has a linear phase-shift characteristic (all frequencies are delayed by a fixed amount), the attenuation characteristics of this type of filter are not very sharp; i.e., there is attenuation of frequencies below 60 Hz as well as at 60 Hz. In contrast, in the method of coherent rejection, the attenuation characteristic is very sharp, so that frequencies even very close to 60 Hz are not affected either in amplitude or in phase. In this approach it is desirable, although not essential, that the artifact or interference be available separately from the EEG, but with the same waveform (although not necessarily of the same amplitude) with

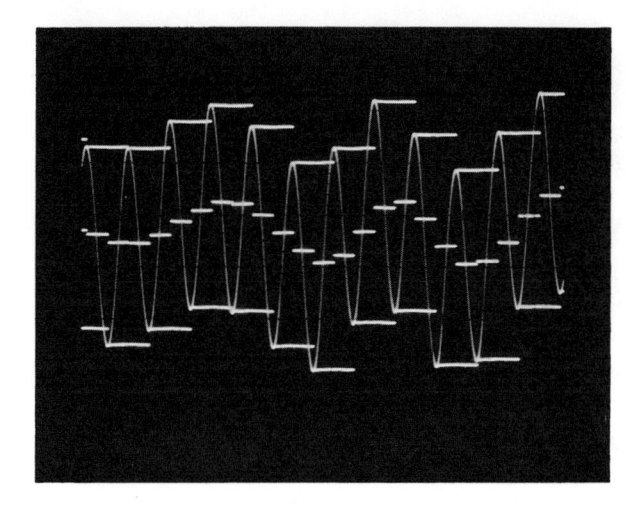

Figure B.2 Waveforms for the unit, showing the original EEG with superimposed 60-Hz contamination, the paired samples (at the positive and negative extrema of the superimposed 60 Hz), and their sum, a 120-Hz sampled version of the EEG with 60-Hz interference removed (middle trace). The phasing of the paired samples with respect to the 60-Hz interference is immaterial.

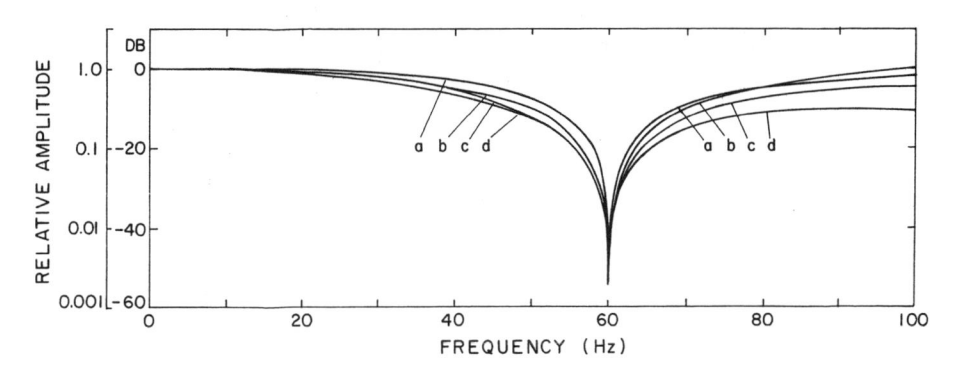

Figure B.3 Frequency response of (a) a commercial 60-Hz notched filter for EEG (Grass Instruments Co. Model 8 Electroencephalograph), (b) the paired-sampling filter, (c) Gotman's three-point digital filter, and (d) a quadruple sampling filter (same as b, except four sample points per cycle instead of two). Filters b, c, and d have a linear phase-shift characteristic with frequency (i.e., the filters introduce a fixed time delay for all frequency components within the passband; see Gotman 1982 and Barlow 1986). The paired-sampling filter (c) and the quadruple-sampling filter (d) should be supplemented with anti-aliasing filtering above 60 Hz if needed.

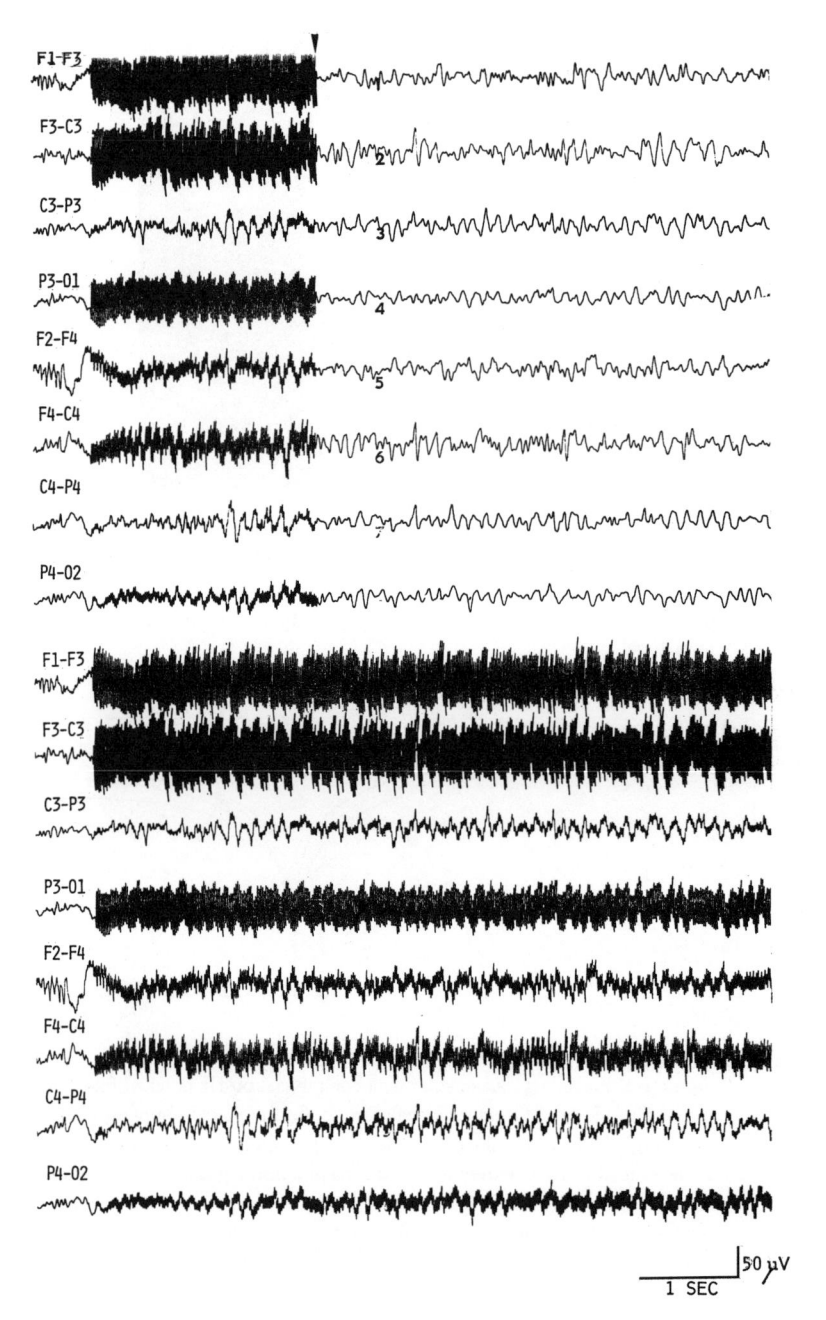

Figure B.4 Use of the paired sampling 60-Hz filter in multi-channel form for a clinical EEG recording in which 60-Hz interference had been purposely exaggerated. The top eight and the bottom eight channels are identical except that the 60-Hz paired-sampling filter had been inserted into each of the top eight channels, and all of the filters were turned on at the arrow.

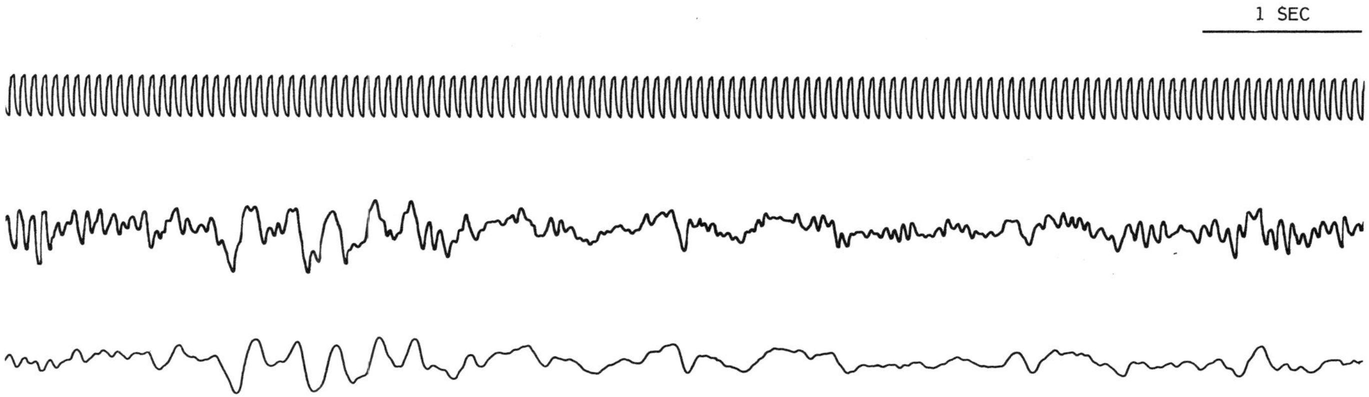

Figure B.5 Elimination of sleep spindles (trace 3) by paired sampling and summation of an original EEG (trace 2). The sampling pulses were generated by a sine wave (trace 1) set to the same frequency (15 Hz) as that of the sleep spindles. Note especially the elimination of sleep spindles from among the train of vertex sharp waves.

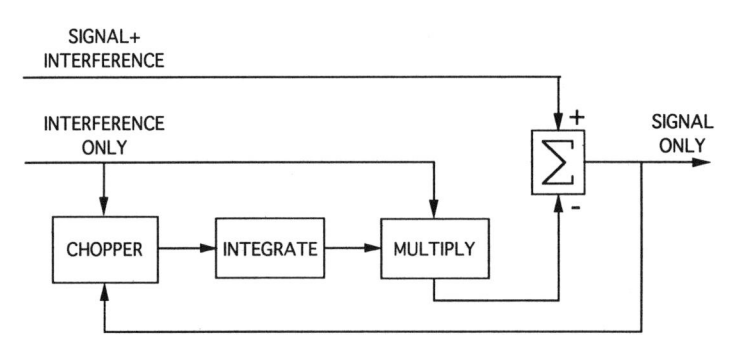

Figure B.6 Block diagram of the unit for automatic nulling or coherent rejection.

which it appears (as an artifact or as interference) in the EEG. However, both the waveform itself and its recurrence rate can be arbitrary; indeed, the recurrence can be aperiodic.

Basically, the unit functions by automatic nulling, via a feedback loop, of the interference or artifact in the EEG. Its principle of operation is essentially similar to that of a phase-locked loop in frequency tracking, except in the automatic nulling unit it is the amplitude (which is ordinarily stable) of the interference that is tracked.

Figure B.6 is a block diagram of the unit. The EEG with the interference signal and the interference signal alone are fed to a coherent or phase-sensitive detector in which the interference signal drives a chopper that synchronously alternates the polarity of the contaminated signal. (The chopper or synchronous detector consists of a comparator, an inverter, and a pair of FET switching transistors.) The output of the coherent detector, the DC component of which is the error signal, drives the integrator in a direction such that the amplitude of the interference signal emerging from the multiplier is of the same amplitude and polarity as that of the interference component of the EEG, so that the interference is eliminated in the subtraction unit. (The polarity of the interference signal alone is immaterial, since the polarity of the output of the integrator is driven in the correct direction in any case.) The operation of the phase-sensitive detector can be understood in the case in which only the interference signal is present in the "EEG." In such a case, the synchronous detector in effect carries out a full-wave rectification of the interference signal, the DC component of which drives the integrator, and in turn the multiplier, to the point at which the inputs of the two interference signals into the subtractor are exactly equal; at that point, there is no output from the subtraction, and hence no error signal.

Examples of the elimination of 60-Hz interference are shown in figure B.7 for two conditions: (A) when an independent source of the 60-Hz interference is available and (B) when no independent source of the 60-Hz source is available. In the latter case, the contaminating signal is extracted from the contaminated EEG itself (e.g., during playback from magnetic tape).

Physiological artifacts such as blinks and EKG potentials can also be removed by coherent rejection (Barlow 1986). The elimination of EKG artifact

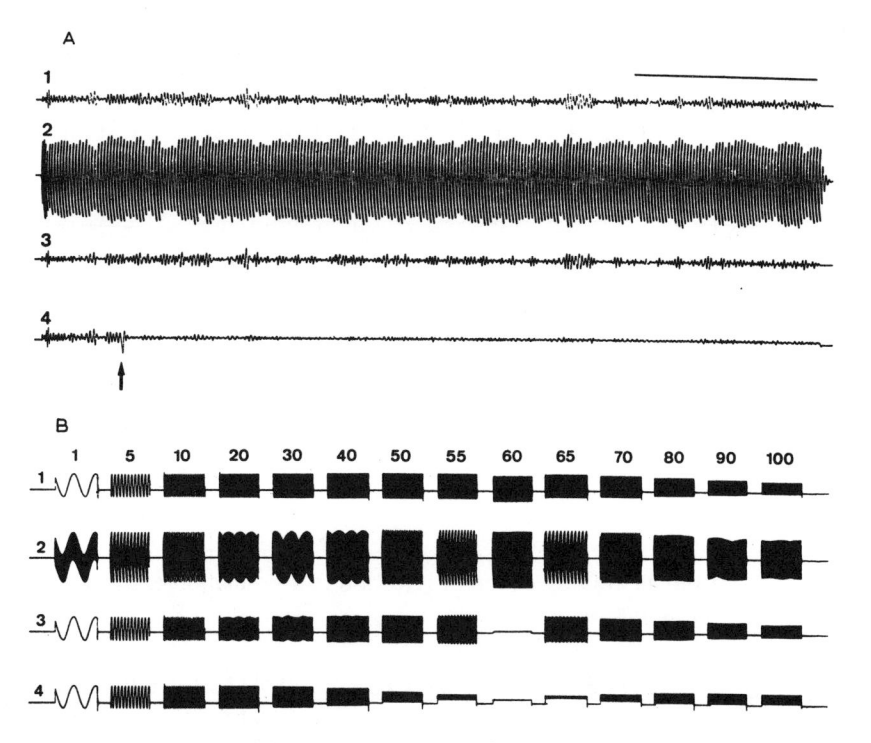

Figure B.7 Precision, no-phase-shift 60-Hz notch filter, having two modes of operation. (A) Mode 1: an independent source of the 60 Hz is available (e.g., from the power line) at the time of the original recording for the nulling of the interference. Trace 1: bandpass electronic noise centered at 60 Hz (24 dB/octave attenuation above and below the center frequency). Trace 2: same signal, after mixing with 60-Hz sine wave; the amplitude variation results from beating of frequencies in the two signals. Trace 3: output of the filter; the trace is indistinguishable from the original (trace 1), which indicates the extreme narrowness of the filter and the high rejection at 60 Hz (approximately 40 dB or 100:1). Trace 4: output of conventional EEG 60-Hz notch filter (switched in at the arrow); the original signal is no longer recognizable because of attenuation and phase distortion of the frequencies near 60 Hz. (B) Mode 2: no independent source of the 60-Hz interference is available, and hence the latter is extracted from the contaminated EEG itself (e.g., during playback from a magnetic tape recording), by means of a phase-locked loop. Trace 1: series of sine waves of various frequencies. Trace 2: same, after mixing with the 60-Hz interference. Trace 3: output of the filter. Trace 4: output of conventional EEG 60-Hz notch filter. The rejection at 60 Hz in this mode of operation is approximately 40 dB; the notch is not as narrow as for mode 1, but is nonetheless quite narrow; note lack of attenuation of sine waves at 55 and 65 Hz. (From Barlow 1986.)

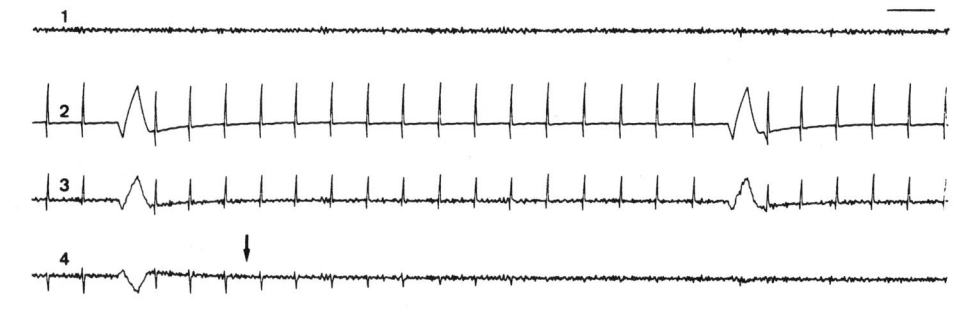

Figure B.8 Simulated automatic nulling of EKG artifact in an EEG. Trace 1: simulated EEG (irregular low-voltage). Trace 2: simulated EKG, including two QRS complexes having an altered waveform. Trace 3: EEG (same as trace l) contaminated by EKG. Trace 4: progressive automatic nulling of the EKG artifact, beginning at the arrow, including the QRS complex of altered waveform (initial amplitude and polarity of the artifact is arbitrary). Time marker: 1 sec. (From Barlow 1986.)

from an EEG by coherent rejection in a simulation experiment is illustrated in figure B.8.

ADAPTIVE SIGNAL PROCESSING (KALMAN OR ADAPTIVE FILTERING, AUTOREGRESSIVE MODELING, LINEAR PREDICTION WITH TIME-VARYING PREDICTOR COEFFICIENTS)

The next logical step in the sequence after the above-described automatic nulling or coherent rejection is to combine several such nulling circuits and a tapped delay line. The result is an *adaptive signal processor* (Goodwin and Sin 1984; Widrow and Stearns 1985), also known as a *Kalman filter* and as a *linear predictor with time-varying (predictor) coefficients*. In contrast to nulling by coherent rejection, which requires that the contaminating component be available separately in "pure form," adaptive signal processing permits a signal (even one having time-varying characteristics) to be self-nulling, in effect, by forming a model of itself.

The following discussion places the consideration of this unit in perspective relative to other topics in this book.

As was described in chapter 17, one of the methods of modeling the EEG is *autoregressive modeling*, in which a model is made of an EEG by regressing the EEG on itself in a manner akin to the manner in which a regression equation can be derived for two variables. This process is also termed *linear prediction*, since the next sample point on the curve is predicted on the basis of a linear combination of the immediate past of the signal. In essence, the prediction of the next sample point is made from the sum of some small number (e.g., 5) of the immediately preceding sample points, each weighted according to the corresponding prediction (or autoregressive) coefficient. The difference between the predicted value and the actual value constitutes the error signal, ordinarily random in character, which is in turn used to "tune" or adjust the prediction coefficients themselves. The prediction coefficients are

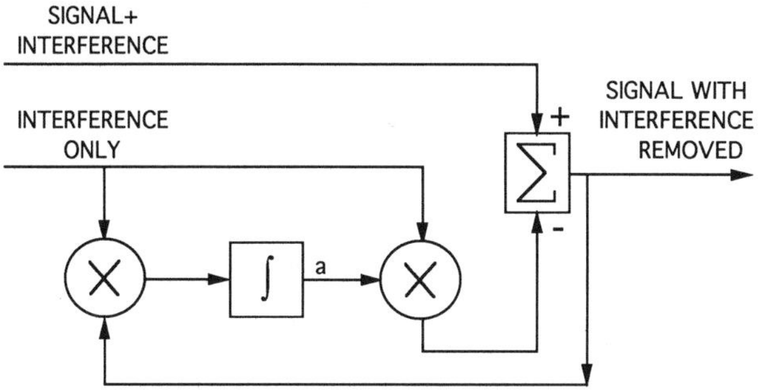

Figure B.9 Block diagram of the coherent rejection filter of figure B.6 except that a multiplier is used for the phase-sensitive detector instead of a chopper. The output of the integrator is the multiplier coefficient *a*.

considered as parameters of the model of the EEG, and hence the approach can be considered a parametric method of EEG analysis. From them, the spectra of the EEG can be derived—a procedure that has some advantages, as well as some disadvantages, in comparison with the more familiar Fast Fourier Transform (FFT) method (Lopes da Silva and Mars 1987).

For application of linear prediction or autoregressive analysis with fixed coefficients, the signal being analyzed must be "stationary" (i.e., must have relatively unchanging statistical characteristics, such as mean amplitude and mean frequency). However, nonstationary signals can also be analyzed if the predictor coefficients track or follow the changes in the signal. This is the case for Kalman filtering or linear prediction with time-varying coefficients (Barlow 1985c, Lopes da Silva and Mars 1987). Using the autoregressive or predictor coefficients for a given signal in combination with a random (Gaussian) noise signal, it is possible to generate a signal that is statistically indistinguishable from the original signal.

Mathematically, an adaptive signal processor can be characterized by the relation

$$y_k - a_1 y_{k-1} + a_2 y_{k-2} \cdots a_n y_{k-n} = e, \tag{1}$$

in which y_k is the actual value of the next sample point; the $a_i y_{k-i}$ terms indicate the prior samples of the signal (available from the taps of a tapped delay line), multiplied by the corresponding predictor coefficients; and e is the difference between the first and the remaining terms on the left (i.e., the error, the sequence of values of which constitutes the error signal). If the signal is predicted perfectly (e.g., for a sine wave), the error signal will be 0 after the predictor coefficients have become adapted to the signal. The autoregressive coefficients $a_1, \ldots, a_n$ constitute the autoregressive model of the original signal.

The analog adaptive signal processor, as mentioned above, is based on an ensemble of coherent rejection units and a tapped delay line. The block diagram of the coherent rejection unit shown in figure B.9 is the same as the one in figure B.6 except that the phase-sensitive detector is now a multiplier

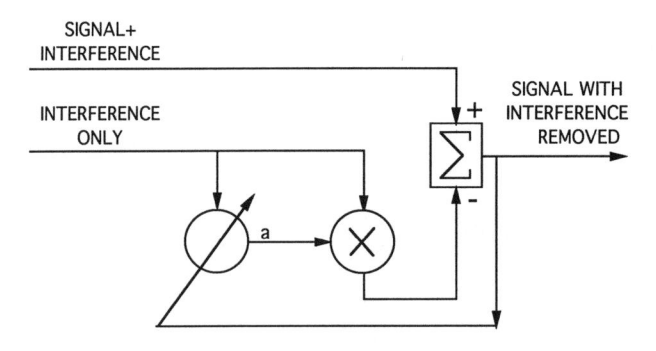

Figure B.10 Block diagram of the coherent rejection filter of figure B.9 in simplified form.

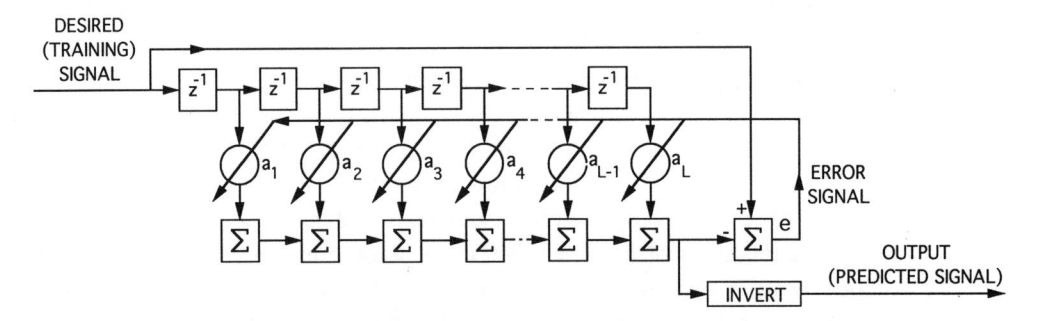

Figure B.11 Block diagram of the adaptive signal processor.

instead of a chopper; the two are equivalent in function. This version of the coherent rejection unit thus consists in essence of two multipliers, an integrator, a summator, and a feedback loop, and is shown in simplified form in figure B.10. A block diagram of the Adaptive Signal Processor itself is shown in figure B.11, and the basic resemblance to figure B.10 is evident.

For the coherent rejection filter (figures B.9, B.10), the interfering signal is, as previously mentioned, available as a separate input, for which the amplitude and the polarity required for nulling the interference component of the contaminated signal are determined by the error (feedback) signal to the multiplier serving as a phase-sensitive detector, in conjunction with the integrator and the second multiplier.

In the case of the adaptive signal processor (figure B.11), several such feedback loops are employed in conjunction with the tapped delay line. The several delayed and weighted versions of the original signal constitute the elements for subtraction. The amplitude and the polarity in each instance are determined by the predictor or autoregressive coefficients, $a_1, a_2, \ldots, a_n$ (see equation 1 above), the latter coefficients being evaluated automatically and simultaneously by the circuit.

To recapitulate: The coherent rejection filter in effect nulls the interference from the contaminated signal by subtracting the necessary amount (amplitude and polarity) of the former from the latter. The adaptive signal processor, on the other hand, nulls the signal itself (leaving only the small random error

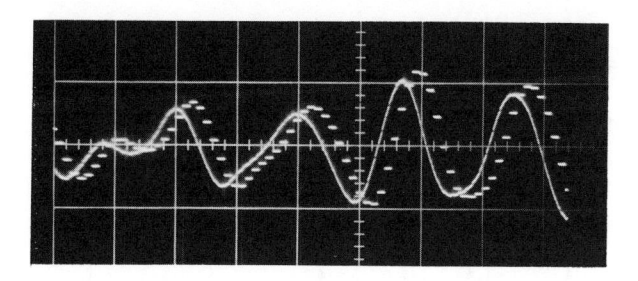

Figure B.12 Example of the operation of the Analog Adaptive Signal Processor as a linear predictor. The continuous curve is the predicted output, which is one sampling interval ahead of the most recently sampled version of the input (which, being slightly displaced to the right on the oscilloscope display on which time moves from left to right, trails slightly in time). (Signal: 25-Hz band-limited noise. Sampling rate: 420 Hz.)

signal) by subtracting from it a predicted version based on the immediate past of the signal.

In the present implementation of the adaptive signal processor, as many as eight predictor coefficients can be evaluated; to avoid using 16 multipliers (two for each coefficient), only two are used, the respective multiplications being carried out sequentially, by multiplexing, followed by demultiplexing into the respective sample-and-hold circuits. Since the coefficients themselves are multiplexed, they can be viewed in rapid sequence on an oscilloscope, or, if desired, written out sequentially on a slow time base on an x-y plotter. Further, the coefficients can be zeroed, or, alternatively, they can be kept fixed or "frozen." A change of the frequency characteristics of the input signal results in automatic adaptation of the predictor coefficients, the adaptation time being determined by the time constant of the resistor-capacitor combination used in the integrators.

As has been mentioned, the adaptive signal processor has the capability of up to eight (the number is readily selectable) predictor coefficients (i.e., the order of the autoregressive filter). A discussion of the order or number of predictor coefficients appears in Lopes da Silva and Mars 1987; frequently employed values for EEG signals are 5 and 6. An example of the operation of the adaptive signal processor functioning as a linear predictor is shown in figure B.12.

One of the applications of linear predictors or autoregressive models is that of determination of power (density) spectra (see Lopes da Silva and Mars 1987 for details), as an alternative to the FFT method (Barlow 1985c). Although the spectra so obtain are already smoothed (raw FFT spectra, in the form of periodograms, are not), the linear-predictor method has the disadvantage that the resolution is poorer at the lower-frequency end than at the high-frequency end. (This feature was confirmed when spectra were derived from the predictor or autoregressive coefficients obtained with the present adaptive signal processor.) This difficulty can be overcome by using longer samples for analysis of lower frequencies; the use of varying sample lengths

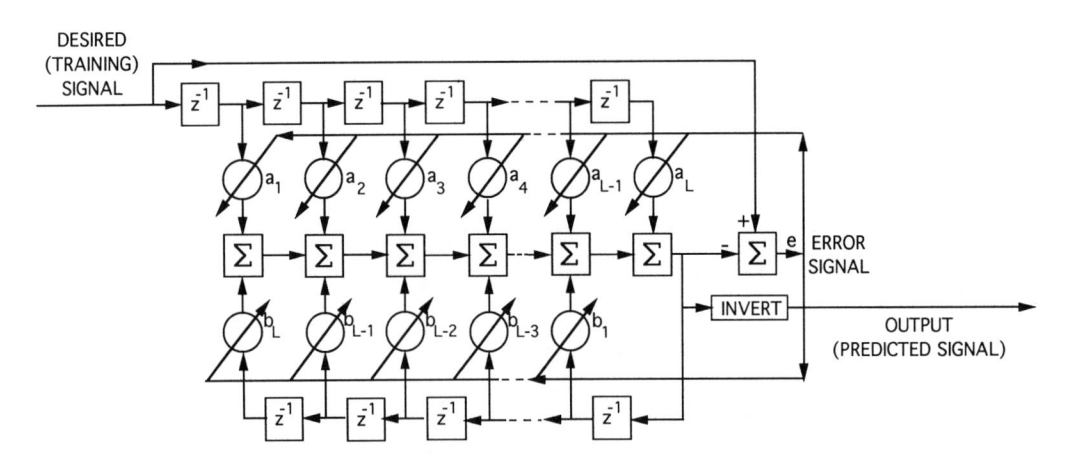

Figure B.13 Block diagram of an adaptive signal processor having an infinite impulse response (IIR), in which the predicted signal as well as the error signal is fed back, each having its own set of coefficients.

for different parts of the spectrum, however, can itself be an inconvenience in practice.

The adaptive signal processor described to this point is the so-called *finite impulse response* (FIR) type (Widrow and Stearns 1985, p. 420), in which the predictor coefficients are evaluated on the basis of the error signal. In the *infinite impulse response* (IIR) type of adaptive signal processor, the output or predicted signal is also fed back, as shown in figure B.13; this entails the evaluation of a separate set of coefficients, the "b" or recurrent coefficients. (Technically, the IIR type of adaptive signal processor is termed a *pole-zero* system, in contrast to the zeros-only FIR type (Widrow and Stearns 1985, p. 420).) If all the "b" coefficients are set to, and kept at, zero, the IIR configuration reduces to the FIR configuration, since the recurrent loop is effectively eliminated. Although in principle the IIR type of adaptive signal processor has the advantage of providing a closer fit, it has the major disadvantage of tending toward instability during the adaptive process when there is a momentary gain of greater than unity in the second ("b") feedback loop (Goodwin and Sin 1984, section 11.3.1; Widrow and Stearns 1985, p. 154). As a result, the coefficients may become very large (so that they do not "converge"), and consequently the predicted signal may saturate. (This disadvantage was confirmed with the present adaptive signal processor when it was operated in the IIR configuration.) Accordingly, the IIR type of adaptive signal processor has in the past had limited application (Widrow and Stearns 1985, p. 154).

Adaptive Modeling and System Characterization

One of the applications of adaptive signal processing is that of mimicking the characteristics of an unknown system or a system having unknown characteristics (Widrow and Stearns 1985). A block diagram for this application is

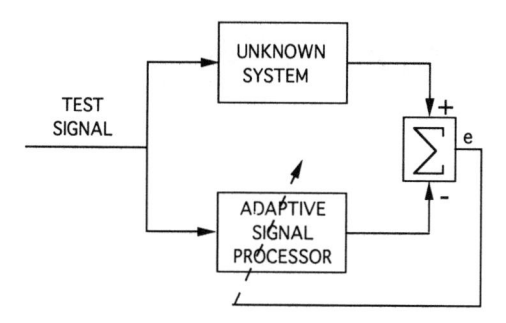

Figure B.14 Block diagram of arrangement for duplicating the characteristics of an unknown system (in this case, an analog electronic filter). (Based on figure 9.1a of Widrow and Stearns 1985.)

shown in figure B.14. The adaptive signal processor adjusts itself so that its output matches that of the unknown system. Examples of such an application are shown in figures B.15 and B.16 for both the FIR (A) and the IIR (B) configuration. The "unknown system" in this case was a variable analog electronic filter. In the case illustrated in figure B.15, the adaptive signal processor was automatically "trained" (adapted) to match the response (trace 2) of the electronic filter set as a band-reject filter to a repetitive swept sine wave (trace 1). The result, i.e., the output of the adaptive signal processor to the swept sine wave, after the adaptation, is shown in trace 3. Comparison of this trace in figure B.15A with the third trace in figure B.15B indicates that the IIR configuration gives a closer approximation to the training signal (note the clearer null at the center of the band-reject region), and therefore models the analog filter more closely, than the FIR configuration.

The same comparison is shown in figure B.16 for the same swept sine wave but for the analog filter set for narrow band-pass filtering at 10 Hz. Again the superior performance of the IIR configuration is evident (note the narrower band-pass region for the latter). (Difficulties with instability during adaptation in obtaining the results shown in figures B.15 and B.16 were minimized by using relatively low levels of the test signal, i.e., the swept sine wave.)

Applications and Implications of Adaptive Signal Processing

Pronk (1986) has remarked that, although autoregressive modeling of the EEG has given promising results in several research studies, it has not been applied to continuous perioperative monitoring because of the high demand for computer-processing capability. The present approach of analog implementation of an adaptive signal processor for autoregressive modeling may offer a more attractive possibility in this connection than the usual digitally implemented approach.

The process of readaptation to an abrupt change in the input signal is remarkable. When viewed on an oscilloscope screen, the error signal abruptly increases in amplitude, and then decreases progressively as the predictor co-

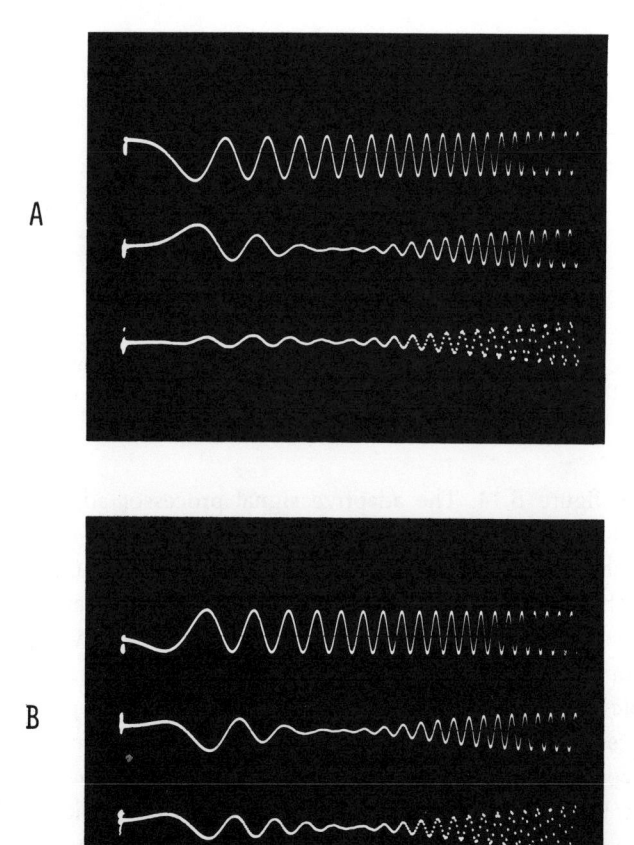

Figure B.15 Modeling of the characteristics of an analog band-reject filter (5-Hz low-pass paralleled with 19-Hz high-pass, 24 dB/octave attenuation) with the Adaptive Signal Processor in (A) FIR (finite impulse response) and (B) IIR (infinite impulse response) configurations. Trace 2 in each instance is "training signal," i.e., the output of the analog filter to a swept sine wave (trace 1). Trace 3 in each case is the output of the Adaptive Signal Processor. Comparison of the third traces in Parts A and B indicates that the latter, corresponding to the IIR configuration, provides the closer approximation to the output signal from the analog filter (second traces), thus modeling the latter more closely.

efficients (also displayed on the oscilloscope) individually and simultaneously readjust themselves. Moreover, adaptation to a second signal (e.g., a sine wave of a different frequency) can occur in such a way that adaptation to the first signal remains largely intact.

Such a process of self-adaptation suggests itself as a possible model for the processes of habituation (note the term *adaptive* signal processing) and dishabituation. Indeed, the term *learning curve* has been used in reference to adaptive signal processors (Widrow and Stearns 1985, p. 61). As specific biological counterparts, habituation of the arousal reaction (Sharpless and Jasper 1956) could be suggested. The EEG counterpart of the arousal reaction is the "activation" pattern of irregular low-voltage fast activity that supplants

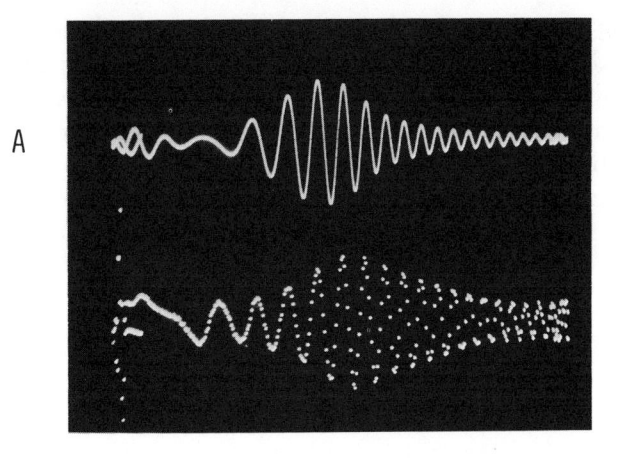

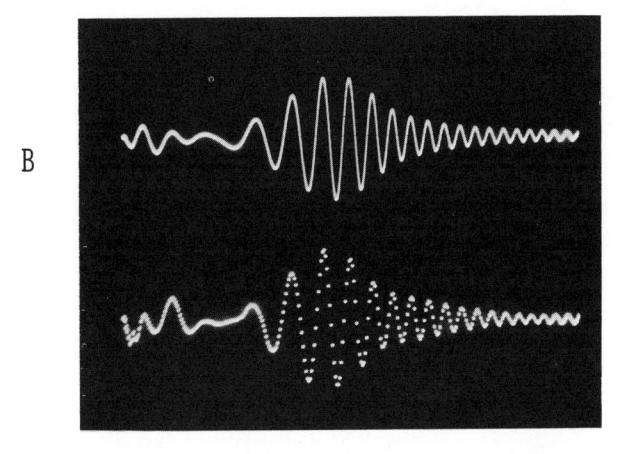

Figure B.16 Same as figure B.15, except for a narrow-band analog filter (10 Hz, 24 dB/octave attenuation on either side of the center frequency). (The swept sine wave, the same as in figure B.11, is not shown.) (A) IIR configuration. (B) FIR configuration. As in figure B.15, the IIR configuration provides the closer approximation to the "training" signal.

the large-amplitude low-frequency components of sleep. As habituation (or adaptation) to a repeated, initially unfamiliar stimulus occurs, both the behavioral arousal and the EEG activation diminish in degree. (The converse effect, dishabituation, occurs when a new or altered stimulus occurs.) Further, the "freezing" (and possible storage) of the predictor coefficients can be viewed as a kind of memory process. Leakage (e.g., exponentially) of the predictor coefficients (stored as a voltage) could, in turn, be compared with the fading of memory. Finally, the characteristics of the adaptive signal processor can be altered by imposing an external (or previously stored) set of predictor or weighting coefficients, thus providing the possibility of a basis for recognition of a particular signal, corresponding to the particular set of coefficients, for which the error signal would be minimized.

At a more basic level, the question may be raised of whether there may be physiological counterparts of adaptive signal processing in the cerebellum (including its nuclei) and in the cerebral cortex (e.g., at the level of the cortical column (chapter 11)) in conjunction with subcortical nuclei. In the latter connection, the possibility of instability of the infinite-impulse-response form of the adaptive signal processor may be of interest in relation to the possibility of epileptiform activity in the cerebral (though not in the cerebellar) cortex. Detailed comparisons of internal and external connectivity might be of some interest.

C Placement of Scalp Electrodes

The placement of scalp electrodes according to the International Federation of Societies of Electroencephalography and Clinical Neurophysiology (IFSECN) is illustrated in figure C.1. The Rolandic and sylvian fissures are shown in outline. *Nasion* and *inion* refer respectively to the depression at the base of the

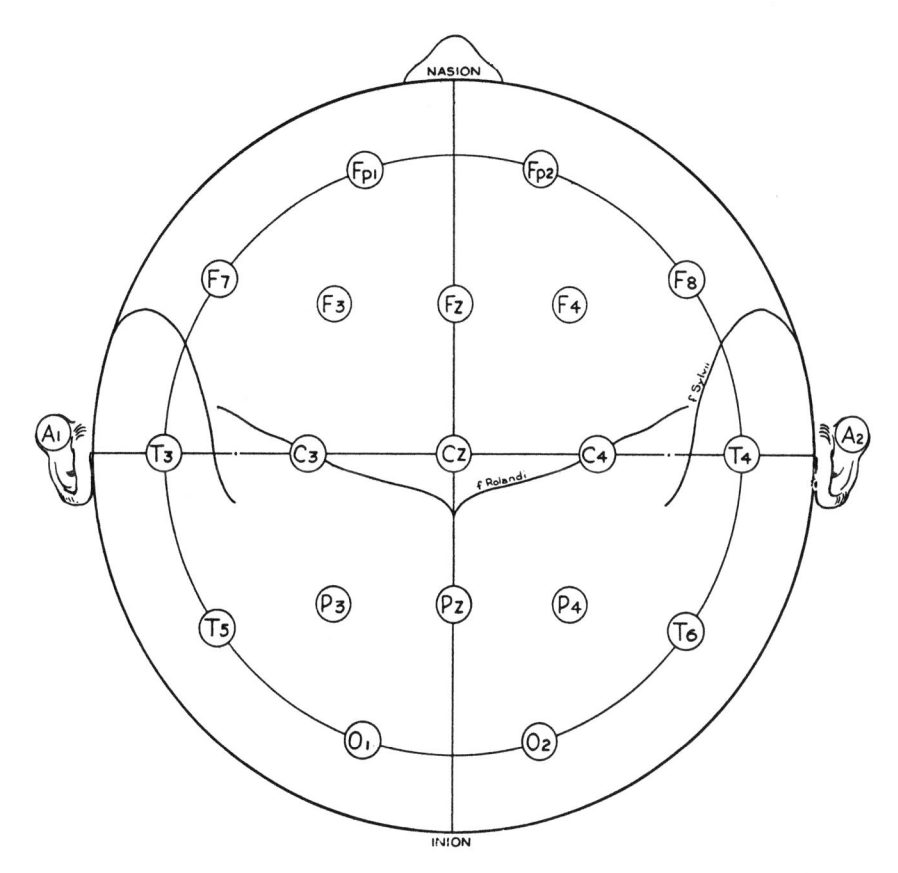

Figure C.1 Placement of scalp electrodes according to the Ten-Twenty System of the International Federation of Societies for Electroencephalography and Clinical Neurophysiology. Fp: frontopolar. F: frontal. C: central. T: temporal. P: parietal. O: occipital. A: earlobe. (From Jasper 1958; reprinted in Jasper 1983.)

nasal ridge and the slight elevation at the back of the skull; these landmarks, together with additional ones just in front of the external auditory canals, form the basis of the measurement system (termed the *Ten-Twenty System*, after the percentages) used to place the electrodes irrespective of the size or shape of the head (see Jasper 1958 or Jasper 1983 for details).

Glossary

(Definitions of additional EEG terms can be found in Chatrian et al. 1974; additional definitions of computer terms can be found in Walter et al. 1972b and in Walter 1976.)

$\bar{a}$ *See* Running mean amplitude.

Aliasing   Spurious representation (masquerading) as lower frequencies by frequencies higher than the sampling frequency; arises as a result of failure to eliminate such higher frequencies by anti-alias filtering before sampling of an input signal.

Alpha band   EEG activity with frequencies in the range 8–13 Hz.

Alpha-coma EEG pattern   An EEG pattern, associated with coma instead of the waking eyes-closed relaxed state, in which there is no reactivity of the rhythm to sensory stimulation, the pattern appearing predominantly anteriorly on the scalp instead of posteriorly as with normal alpha.

Amplitude   The vertical extent or dimension of a wave, measured in (e.g.) volts or millimeters and expressed as (e.g.) peak-to-peak value, mean (after reversing the sign of any negative values), or root-mean-square (the square root of the mean squared voltage). *See also* Extrema *and* Instantaneous amplitude.

Amplitude modulation   Scaling of a wave to make the entire wave larger or smaller in voltage (vertical dimension) by a modulating signal; does not change the frequency or duration of the wave.

Analytic signal   A vector, spiraling around the time axis, whose length (magnitude) corresponds to the instantaneous envelope of a signal (which see) and whose angular position corresponds to the phase of a signal, the rate of change of angular position being the instantaneous frequency. The magnitude (the instantaneous envelope) of a narrow-band signal is the square root of the sums of the squares of the instantaneous (momentary) value of the original signal and of its Hilbert transform (which see).

Architectonics   The structure or construction of the brain.

Band-limited noise   Electronic noise intermediate in its bandwidth between wide-band noise and narrow-band noise; e.g., 6–12 Hz.

Beta band   EEG activity with frequencies in the range 14–35 Hz.

Burst   A group of waves appearing and disappearing abruptly, distinguished from background activity by differences in frequency, form, and/or amplitude. (Does not imply abnormality; see Paroxysm, not a synonym.)

$\bar{c}$ *See* Running mean curvature.

CD   *See* Coefficient of Determination.

Coefficient of Determination (CD) A measure of the degree of similarity of two signals without regard to sign; the square of the Pearson Product-Moment Correlation Coefficient; ranges in value between 1.0 and 0.

Coefficient of Variation (CV) The quotient of the standard deviation and the mean; the "normalized" standard deviation.

Constant slope Short form for "relatively constant running mean absolute slope"; used in reference to waves for which the variability of the running mean slope is appreciably less than the variability of the running mean amplitude, as evidenced from a difference in the respective short-term Coefficients of Variability (or their quotient or the logarithm of the latter) and/or from a difference in their longer-term trends. Constant-slope waves occur with extrema modulation (which see).

Contralateral Opposite side to.

Convolution A running multiplication, with summation of the resultant cross-products, of a fixed waveform with a continuous signal as the former is moved stepwise in a window along the latter. *See* Hilbert transform.

Curvature A measure of the sharpness of a signal (e.g., a spike); mathematically, the second time derivative of a signal, or, the first time derivative of its slope; expressed in units of (e.g.) V/sec^2 or mm/sec^2.

CV *See* Coefficient of Variation.

Decibel (dB) A unit for expressing power on a logarithmic scale; a 10-fold increase in power corresponds to a 20-dB increase in voltage (amplitude).

Delta band EEG activity of frequencies in the range 1–4 Hz.

Extrema The positive and negative peak points of a series of waves, including intermediate or secondary peaks. *See also* Amplitude modulation *and* Extrema modulation.

Extrema modulation (modulation of extrema) Modulation of positive and negative reversal points (e.g., of a triangular wave); results in variation of both amplitude and frequency of waves, in an inverse manner. Contrast with amplitude modulation (which see), which results in variation of amplitude only.

$\bar{f}$ *See* Running mean frequency.

Fourteen-and-six positive bursts Bursts of arch-shaped waves at 13–7 Hz and/or 5–7 Hz, but most commonly as 14 and/or 6 Hz, seen generally over the posterior temporal and adjacent areas of one or both sides of the head during sleep. The sharp peaks of the component waves are positive with respect to other regions. Generally considered a normal variant pattern.

Frequency modulation Variation of the frequency of a wave train according to the imposed modulation; does not change the amplitude of the waves.

Gain Synonymous with amplification factor, often expressed as a ratio (e.g., 100,000:1); not to be confused with sensitivity (which see).

Gamma band EEG activity of 35 Hz and up.

Gaussian noise Electronic noise having a normal or Gaussian (bell-shaped) distribution of its instantaneous amplitudes, so that the smaller the amplitude, the more probable its occurrence, zero being the most probable amplitude; bandwidth is unspecified.

Hilbert transform A transform such that each and every frequency component of a signal is shifted by 90°; obtainable by convolution (which see) of a signal with a pair of back-to-back hyperbolas, or by a combination of direct and inverse Fourier transforms of the original. *See also* Analytic signal *and* Instantaneous envelope.

Instantaneous amplitude The instantaneous or moment-to-moment course of a signal or a voltage-time graph; can have positive or negative values.

Instantaneous envelope   The (smooth) curve passing through the extrema of a signal after full-wave rectification (reversal of negative phases); in the case of a narrow-band signal (e.g., an alpha rhythm), it is obtainable as a continuous curve as the square root of the sums of the squares of the signal and its Hilbert Transform. *See also* Analytic signal *and* Hilbert transform.

Insilateral   Same side as (compare Contralateral).

Lennox-Gastaut syndrome   A type of childhood epilepsy involving severe seizures, mental retardation, and a distinctive EEG pattern termed the slow (1–2.5 Hz) spike-wave pattern.

Logarithm of the quotient of the Coefficient of Variation of the running mean slope and the Coefficient of Variation of the running mean amplitude   A dimensionless quantity indicating the relative short-term variability of slope and amplitude of a signal (an EEG) on a normalized linear scale; a value of 0 indicates equal variability, a value of -0.5 indicates indicates half as much variability of slope as of amplitude, and a value of $+0.5$ indicates twice as much variability of slope as of amplitude.

Mu rhythm   An arcuate-shaped rhythm in the alpha frequency range seen in the EEG overlying the motor cortex; characteristically disappears upon finger movement on the opposite side (so named because of resemblance to the Greek letter μ).

Narrow-band noise   Electronic noise made up of a very limited range (e.g., 9.5–10 Hz) of frequencies; its appearance can be that of rhythmic activity.

Oscillator model   A special analog electronic oscillator, the extrema and the slopes of the output waves of which can be modulated independently; the physical or "hardware" embodiment of the extrema-slope hypothesis, designed and implemented for testing the present extrema-slopes hypothesis.

Paroxysm   An EEG phenomenon characterized by abrupt onset, rapid attainment of a maximum, and sudden termination; distinguished from background activity. (Commonly refers to epileptiform or seizure patterns; see also Burst, not a synonym.)

Pearson Product-Moment Correlation Coefficient (PPMCC)   The correlation coefficient for two variables (signals) after removal of any DC component (the latter is removed in the computation); a measure of the degree of relatedness between two variables, including sign; ranges in value from 1.0 (for two identical sets of data points) to -1.0 (for two sets of data points identical except for sign).

Psychomotor variant EEG pattern   *See* Rhythmic temporal theta bursts of drowsiness.

Random noise   Synonymous with Gaussian noise, unless otherwise characterized.

Random rectangular noise   Electronic noise having a rectangular distribution of its instantaneous amplitude; within the positive and negative limits, all amplitudes (including 0) are equally probable.

Rhythmic temporal theta bursts of drowsiness   Characteristic bursts of 4–7-Hz waves, frequently notched by faster waves, occurring over the temporal regions of the head during drowsiness.

Running mean   The mean of some feature of a signal computed within a rectangular averaging window of a specified width (e.g., 0.5 sec); synonymous with moving average computed with a rectangular averaging window.

Running mean (absolute) amplitude ($\bar{a}$)   The mean amplitude of a signal after all negative waves are made positive (i.e., after full-wave rectification), computed over a rectangular averaging window (e.g., 0.5 sec) that moves along the signal.

Running mean (absolute) curvature ($\bar{c}$)   Same as running mean (absolute) amplitude except computed for the second derivative of a signal.

Running mean (absolute) slope ($\bar{s}$) Same as running mean (absolute) amplitude, except computed for the first derivative of a signal.

Running mean frequency ($\bar{f}$) Quotient of the running mean (absolute) slope and the running mean (absolute) amplitude.

$\bar{s}$ *See* Running mean slope.

Scale factor The degree of vertical enlargement (or contraction) employed for a display; can be arbitrary.

Sharp wave *See* Spike.

Sensitivity A measure of the scale of a write-out or a display, e.g., mV/mm or V/cm; not to be confused with gain.

Signal envelope The outline of a signal, obtained to a crude approximation by joining positive peaks (extrema), or successive positive and negative peaks after the latter have been reversed in sign.

Six-Hz spike waves A spike-wave pattern at 4–7 Hz, but mostly at 6 Hz, occurring in brief bursts bilaterally synchronously, symmetrically or asymmetrically, and either confined to or of larger amplitude over the posterior or anterior regions of the head. Generally considered a normal variant pattern.

Slope The steepness or degree of incline of a signal; mathematically, its first time derivative; expressed in units of, e.g., V/sec or mm/sec.

Slow spike-wave pattern A 1.5–2.5-Hz spike-wave pattern in which the second part or trailing edge of the slow wave is often prolonged; associated with Lennox-Gastaut syndrome.

Slopes modulation Modulation of the slopes of waves; the modulation can take on either positive or negative values (unlike frequency modulation, which is ordinarily limited to positive values).

Slowing A general term to indicate a decrease of frequency (e.g., (normal) hyperventilation-induced, slowing with drowsiness, abnormal or pathological slowing).

Spectral Purity Index (SPI) A measure of EEG rhythmicity; a dimensionless number that provides an index of the degree of spread of frequencies about the mean frequency of a signal; has a maximum value of 1.0 for a sine wave, and progressively smaller values for progressively greater spread of frequencies about the mean; defined as the quotient of the square of the running mean slope to the product of the running mean amplitude and the running mean curvature (steepness).

SPI *See* Spectral Purity Index.

Spike A transient, usually negative (relative to surrounding areas of the scalp), 20–70 msec in duration, clearly distinguishable from background EEG activity, differing from a sharp wave only in duration (the latter being 70–200 msec).

SSW Abbreviation for spike and/or sharp wave.

Theta band EEG activity of frequencies in the range 4–7 Hz.

Type 1 waves Output of the oscillator model in Mode 1 operation (modulation of extrema only); synonymous with constant-slope waves. The waves vary inversely in amplitude and frequency.

Type 2 waves Output of the oscillator model in Mode 2 operation (modulation of slopes only); synonymous with constant-amplitude waves. The waves are equivalent to those in conventional frequency modulation.

Type 3 waves Output of the oscillator model in Mode 3 operation (congruent or identical modulation of extrema and slopes); irrespective of the modulating input, the resultant waves are of constant frequency but variable amplitude, therefore resembling the waves of conventional amplitude modulation.

Type 4 waves Output of the oscillator model in Mode 4 operation (independent modulation of extrema and slopes); the waves are random, varying in amplitude, slope, and frequency.

Vertex sharp transient Sharp potential (i.e., duration of less than 200 msec), maximum at the vertex and negative relative to other areas, occurring apparently spontaneously during sleep or in response to a sensory stimulus during sleep or wakefulness. May be single or repetitive.

Wide-band noise Electronic noise made up of a wide range of frequencies (e.g., 1–100,000 Hz) and giving the appearance of a completely random signal.

Bibliography

The literature search was greatly facilitated by the combined extensive holdings and services of the Treadwell Library at Massachusetts General Hospital; the Countway Library at Harvard Medical School; the Widener Library and the Cabot Science Library at Harvard University; and the Science, Barker Engineering, and Schering-Plough (Brain and Cognitive Sciences) Libraries at the Massachusetts Institute of Technology.

Abbott, L. E., Marder, E., and Hooper, S. L. (1991) Oscillating networks: control of burst duration by electrically coupled neurons. *Neural Comput.* 3: 487–497.

Abraham, K., and Ajmone-Marsan, C. (1958) Patterns of cortical discharges and their relation to routine scalp electroencephalography. *Electroenceph. Clin. Neurophysiol.* 10: 447–461.

Adey, W. R. (1969) Spectral analysis of EEG data from animals and man during alerting, orienting and discriminative responses. In: C. R. Evans and T. B. Mulholland, eds., *Attention in Neurophysiology*. Butterworth.

Adey, W. R. (1972) Organization of brain tissue: Is the brain a noisy processor? *Int. J. Neurosci.* 3: 271–284.

Adey, W. R. (1988) Do EEG-like processes influence brain function at a physiological level? In: E. Başar, ed., *Dynamics of Sensory and Cognitive Processsing by the Brain*. Springer.

Adey, W. R., and Walter, D. O. (1963) Application of phase detection and averaging techniques in computer analysis of EEG records in cats. *Exp. Neurol.* 7: 186–209.

Adrian, E. D., and Matthews, B. H. C. (1934) The interpretation of potential waves in the cortex. *J. Physiol.* 81: 440–471.

Alger, B. E., and Nicoll, R. A. (1982) Pharmacological evidence for two kinds of GABA receptor on rat hippocampal pyramidal cells studied *in vitro*. *J. Physiol.* 328: 125–141.

Allen, P. J., Fish, D. R., and Smith, S. J. M. (1992) Very high-frequency rhythmic activity during SEEG suppression in frontal lobe epilepsy. *Electroenceph. Clin. Neurophysiol.* 81: 155–159.

an der Heiden, U., and Mackey, M. C. (1987) Mixed feedback: A paradigm for regular and irregular oscillations. In: L. Rensing, U. an der Heiden, and M. C. Mackey, eds., *Temporal Disorder in Human Oscillatory Systems*. Springer.

Andersen, P., and Andersson, S. A. (1968) *Physiological Basis of the Alpha Rhythm*. Appleton-Century-Crofts.

Andersen, P., and Andersson, S. A. (1974). Thalamic origin of cortical rhythmic activity. In: *Handbook of Electroencephalography and Clinical Neurophysiology*, vol. 2C. Elsevier.

Anninos, P. A., and Zenone, S. (1980) A neural net model for the alpha-rhythm. *Biol. Cybern.* 36: 187–191.

Arle, J. E., and Simon, R. H. (1990) An application of fractal dimension to the detection of transients in the electroencephalogram. *Electroenceph. Clin. Neurophysiol.* 75: 296–305.

Avoli, M. (1984) Penicillin induced hyperexcitability in the in vitro hippocampal slice can be unrelated to impairment of somatic inhibition. *Brain Res.* 323: 154–158.

Avoli, M. (1987) Mechanisms of generalized epilepsy with spike and wave discharge. In: R. J. Ellingson, N. M. F. Murray, and A. M. Halliday, eds., *The London Symposia* (EEG Suppl. 39). Elsevier.

Avoli, M., and Gloor, P. (1982a) Interaction of cortex and thalamus in spike and wave discharges of feline generalized penicillin epilepsy. *Exp. Neurol.* 76: 196–217.

Avoli, M., and Gloor, P. (1982b) Role of the thalamus in generalized penicillin epilepsy: Observations on decorticate cats. *Exper. Neurol.* 77: 386–402.

Avoli, M., Gloor, P., and Kostopoulos, G. (1990) Focal and generalized epileptiform activity in the cortex: In search of differences in synaptic mechanisms, ionic movements, and long-lasting changes in neuronal excitability. In: M. Avoli, P. Gloor, G. Kostopoulos, and R. Naquet, eds., *Generalized Epilepsy*. Birkhäuser.

Babloyantz, A. (1989) Estimation of correlation dimension from single and multichannel recordings: A critical view. In: E. Başar and T. H. Bullock, eds., *Brain Dynamics*. Springer.

Babloyantz, A. (1991) Evidence for slow brain waves: A dynamical approach. *Electroenceph. Clin. Neurophysiol.* 78: 402–405.

Babloyantz, A., and Destexhe, A. (1986) Low-dimensional chaos in an instance of epilepsy. *Proc. Natl. Acad. Sci. USA* 83: 3513–3517.

Babloyantz, A., and Destexhe, A. (1987) The Creutzfeldt-Jakob disease in the hierarchy of chaotic attractors. In: M. Markus, S. C. Müller, and G. Nicolis, eds., *From Chemical to Biological Organization*. Springer.

Babloyantz, A., Salazar, J. M., and Nicolis, C. (1985) Evidence of chaotic dynamics of brain activity during the sleep cycle. *Phys. Lett.* 111A: 152–156.

Balestra, V., Balzani, P., Cabri, M., Padovan, C., and Sannita, W. G. (1981) Standardization vs. normalization in the power spectral analysis of the EEG signal. *Bol. Soc. Ital. Biol. Sperimentale* 57: 1823–1829.

Ball, G. J., Gloor, P., and Schaul, N. (1977) The cortical electromicrophysiology of pathological delta waves in the electroencephalogram of cats. *Electroenceph. Clin. Neurophysiol.* 43: 346–361.

Barinaga, M. (1990) The mind revealed? *Science* 249: 856–858

Barlow, J. S. (1960) Rhythmic activity induced by photic stimulation in relation to intrinsic alpha activity of the brain in man. *Electroenceph. Clin. Neurophysiol.* 12: 317–326.

Barlow, J. S. (1962a) The relationship among "photic driving" responses to single flashes and the resting EEG. In: Quarterly Progress Report 64, Research Laboratory of Electronics, Massachusetts Institute of Technology.

Barlow, J. S. (1962b) Simulation of normal and abnormal electroencephalograms. In: Quarterly Progress Report 65, Research Laboratory of Electronics, Massachusetts Institute of Technology.

Barlow, J. S. (1962c) A phase-comparator model for the diurnal rhythm of emergence of Drosophila. *Ann. N.Y. Acad. Sci.* 98, Art. 4: 788–805.

Barlow, J. S. (1967a) Automatic curve reading by phase-modulated analog sampling. *Proc. IEEE* 55: 1079–1080.

Barlow, J. S. (1967b) Multichannel time-domain filtering employing time-division multiplexing and a magnetic delay drum. In: *Quarterly Progress Report 84*, Research Laboratory of Electronics, Massachusetts Institute of Technology.

Barlow, J. S. (1968) Computer analyses of clinical electroencephalographic ink tracings with the aid of a high-speed automatic curve reader. *IEEE Trans. Biomed. Eng.* 15: 54–61.

Barlow, J. S. (1971) Brain information processing during reading: Electrophysiological correlates. *Dis. Nerv. System* 32: 668–672.

Barlow, J. S. (1979) Computerized clinical electroencephalography in perspective. *IEEE Trans. Biomed. Eng.* 26: 377–391.

Barlow, J. S. (1984) Analysis of EEG changes with carotid clamping by selective analog filtering, matched inverse digital filtering and automatic adaptive segmentation: A comparative study. *Electroenceph. Clin. Neurophysiol.* 58: 193–204.

Barlow, J. S. (1985a) The human alpha rhythm as a brain clock. Commentary on [55e], [56e], [57e]. In: P. Masani, ed., *Norbert Wiener: Collected Works*, vol. 4. MIT Press.

Barlow, J. S. (1985b) Microwave/far-infrared radiation and biological macromolecules. Commentary on [60g], [65b]. In: P. Masani, ed., *Norbert Wiener: Collected Works*, vol. 4. MIT Press.

Barlow, J. S. (1985c) Methods of analysis of nonstationary EEGs, with emphasis on segmentation techniques: A comparative review. *J. Clin. Neurophysiol.* 2: 267–304.

Barlow, J. S. (1985d) Computer characterization of tracé alternant and REM sleep patterns in the neonatal EEG by adaptive segmentation: An exploratory study. *Electroenceph. Clin. Neurophysiol.* 60: 163–173.

Barlow, J. S. (1986) Artifact processing (rejection and minimization) in EEG data processing. In: F. H. Lopes da Silva, W. Storm van Leeuwen, and A. Rémond, eds., *Clinical Applications of Computer Analysis of EEG and Other Neurophysiological Signals (Handbook of Electroencephalography and Clinical Neurophysiology*, revised series, vol. 2). Elsevier.

Barlow, J. S. (1989) A new oscillator model for normal and abnormal EEG patterns. *Electroenceph. Clin. Neurophysiol.* 73: 42P.

Barlow, J. S. 1993. Tests of a new model for normal and abnormal EEG phenomena. In: St. Zschocke and E.-J. Speckmann, eds., *Basic Mechanism of the EEG*. Birkhäuser.

Barlow, J. S., and DiPerna, R. A. (1967) Analog inked-trace reader for automatic continuous high-speed multi-channel operation. *Electroenceph. Clin. Neurophysiol.* 23: 371–375.

Barlow, J. S., and DiPerna, R. A. (1968) A continuous multichannel automatic curve reader. *IEEE Trans. Biomed. Eng.* 15: 46–53.

Barlow, J. S., and Dubinsky, J. (1976) Some computer approaches to continuous automatic clinical EEG monitoring. In: P. Kellaway and I. Petersén, eds., *Quantitative Analytic Studies in Epilepsy*. Raven.

Barlow, J. S., and Estrin, T. (1971) Comparative phase characteristics of induced and intrinsic alpha activity. *Electroenceph. Clin. Neurophysiol.* 30: 1–9.

Barlow, J. S., and Trabka, J. (1961) The relationship between "photic driving" in the EEG and responses to single flashes. *Excerpta Medica*, International Congress Series no. 37 (Fifth International Congress of Electroencephalography and Clinical Neurophysiology, Rome) abstract 182.

Barlow, J. S., Brazier, M. A. B., and Rosenblith, W. A. (1959) The application of autocorrelation analysis to electroencephalography. In: H. Quastler and H. J. Morowitz, eds., *Proceedings of the First National Biophysics Conference*. Yale University Press.

Barlow, J. S., Creutzfeldt, O. D., Michael, D., Houchin, J., and Epelbaum, H. (1981) Automatic adaptive segmentation of clinical EEGs. *Electroenceph. Clin. Neurophysiol.* 51: 512–525.

Başar, E. (1990) Chaotic dynamics and resonance phenomena in brain function: Progress, perspectives, and thoughts. In: E. Başar, ed., *Chaos in Brain Function*. Springer.

Başar, E., and Bullock, T. H., eds. (1992) *Induced Rhythms of the Brain*. Birkhäuser.

Başar, E., Başar-Eroglu, C., and Röschke, J. (1987) Do coherent patterns of the strange attractor EEG reflect deterministic sensory-cognitive states of the brain? In: M. Markus, S. C. Müller, and G. Nicolis, eds., *From Chemical to Biological Organization*. Springer.

Bendat, J. L., and Piersol, A. G. (1966) *Measurement and Analysis of Random Data*. Wiley.

Berger, H. (1929) Über das Elektrenkephalogramm des Menschen. *Arch. Psychiat. Nervenkr.* 87: 527–570.

Berglund, K., and Elmqvist, D. (1975) Estimation of sleep depth using normalized slope descriptor quantification of the EEG (Hjorth Descriptors). In: *Sleep 1974* (Second European Congress on Sleep Research, Rome, 1974). Karger.

Berlyne, D. E., and McDonald, P. (1965) Effects of stimulus complexity and incongruity on duration of EEG desynchronization. *Electroenceph. Clin. Neurophysiol.* 18: 156–161.

Bernstein, N. (1927) Analyse aperiodischer trigonometrischer Reihen. *Z. angew. Math. Mech.* 7: 476–485.

Bertrand, I., and Lacape, R.-S. (1943) Théorie de l'électro-encephalogramme: États élémentaires. Paris: Doin.

Beurle, R. L. (1956) Properties of a mass of cells capable of regenerating pulses. *Phil. Trans. Roy. Soc.* 240A: 55–94.

Bickford, R. G., and Klass, D. W. (1963) Electroencephalography in children having seizures. In: Keith, H. M., ed., *Convulsive Disorders in Children*. Little, Brown.

Bindman, L., and Lippold, O. (1981) *The Neurophysiology of the Cerebral Cortex*. University of Texas Press.

Bingham, C., Godfrey, M. D., and Tukey, J. W. (1967) Modern techniques of power spectrum estimation. *IEEE Trans. Audio Electroacoustics* 15: 56–66.

Binnie, C. D. (1986) Computer applications in monitoring. In: F. H. Lopes da Silva, W. Storm van Leeuwen, and A. Rémond, eds., *Clinical Applications of Computer Analysis of EEG and Other Neurophysiological Signals* (Handbook of Electroencephalography and Clinical Neurophysiology, revised series, vol. 2). Elsevier.

Blomfield, S. (1974) Arithmetical operations performed by nerve cells. *Brain Res.* 69: 115–124.

Blume, W. T., and Lemieux, J. F. (1988) Morphology of spikes in spike-and-wave complexes. *Electroenceph. Clin. Neurophysiol.* 69: 508–515.

Blume, W. T., and Sharbrough, F. W. (1987) EEG monitoring during carotid endarterectomy and open heart surgery. In: E. Niedermeyer and F. Lopes da Silva, eds., *Electroencephalography*, second edition. Urban & Schwarzenberg.

Blume, W. T., Young, G. B., and Lemieux, J. F. (1984) EEG morphology of partial epileptic seizures. *Electroenceph. Clin. Neurophysiol.* 57: 295–302.

Bodenstein, G., and Praetorius, H. M. (1977) Feature extraction from the EEG by adaptive segmentation. *Proc. IEEE* 65: 642–652.

Bodenstein, G., Schneider, W., and von der Malsburg, C. (1985) Computerized EEG pattern classification by adaptive segmentation and probability-density-function classification: Description of the method. *Comput. Biol. Med.* 15: 297–313.

Bohlin, T. (1971) Analysis of EEG Signals with Changing Spectra. Technical Paper 18.212, IBM Nordic Lab, Lindigö, Sweden.

Bohlin, T. (1973) Comparison of two methods of modeling stationary EEG signals. *IBM J. Res. Dev.* 17: 194–205.

Bohlin, T. (1977) Analysis of EEG signals with changing spectra using a short-word Kalman estimator. *Math. Biosci.* 35: 221–259.

Bouyer, J. J., Montaron, M. F., and Rougeul, A. (1981) Fast fronto-parietal rhythms during combined focused attentive behaviour and immobility in cat: Cortical and thalamic localizations. *Electroenceph. Clin. Neurophysiol.* 51: 244–252.

Bouyer, J. J., Montaron, M. F., Vahnée, J. M. Albert, M. P., and Rougeul, A. (1987) Anatomical localization of cortical beta rhythms in cat. *Neuroscience* 22: 863–869.

Bracewell, R. N. (1986) *The Fourier Transform and Its Applications*, second edition, revised. McGraw-Hill.

Bradley, P. B. (1953) The effect of some drugs on the electrical activity of the brain in the cat. *Electroenceph. Clin. Neurophysiol.* 5: 471.

Bradley, P. B., and Elkes, J. (1957) The effects of some drugs on the electrical activity of the brain. *Brain* 80: 77–116.

Braitenberg, W. (1977) *On the Texture of Brains*. Springer.

Braitenberg, W. (1978) Cortical architectonics: General and areal. In: M. A. B. Brazier and H. Petsche, eds., *Architectonics of the Cerebral Cortex*. Raven.

Brenner, R. P., and Schaul, N. (1990) Periodic EEG patterns: Classification, clinical correlation, and pathophysiology. *J. Clin. Neurophysiol.* 7: 249–267.

Brodal, A. (1981) *Neurological Anatomy*. Oxford University Press.

Broughton, R. J. (1987) Polysomnography: Principles and applications in sleep and arousal disorders. In: E. Niedermeyer and F. Lopes da Silva, eds., *Electroencephalography*, second edition. Urban & Schwarzenberg.

Bullock, T. H. (1988a) Compound potentials of the brain, ongoing and evoked: Perspectives from comparative neurology. In: E. Başar, ed., *Dynamics of Sensory and Cognitive Processing by the Brain*. Springer.

Bullock, T. H. (1988b) Signs of dynamic processing in organized neural tissue: Extracting order from chaotic data. In: E. Başar and T. H. Bullock, eds., *Brain Dynamics*. Springer.

Bullock, T. H. (1990) An agenda for research on chaotic dynamics. In: E. Başar, ed., *Chaos in Brain Function*. Springer.

Bullock, T. H., and Başar, E. (1988) Comparison of ongoing compound field potentials in the brains of invertebrates and vertebrates. *Brain Res. Rev.* 13: 57–75.

Bullock, T. H., Iragui, V. J., and Alksne, J. F. (1990) Electrocorticogram coherence and correlation of amplitude modulation between electrodes both decline in millimeters in human as well as in rabbit brains. *Soc. Neurosci. Abstr.* 16: 1241.

Bullock, T. H., and McClune, M. C. (1989) Lateral coherence of the electrocorticogram: A new measure of brain synchrony. *Electroenceph. Clin. Neurophysiol.* 73: 479–498.

Burns, B. D. (1951) Some properties of isolated cerebral cortex in the unanesthetized cat. *J. Physiol. (Lond.)* 112: 156–175.

Buzsaki, G., Bickford, R. G., Ponomareff, G., Thal, L. J., Mandel, R., and Gage, F. H. (1988) Nucleus basalis and thalamic control of neocortical activity in the freely moving rat. *J. Neurosci.* 8: 4007–4026.

Caille, E. J., and Bassano, J. L. (1975) Value and limits of sleep statistical analysis: Objective parameters and subjective evaluations. In: G. Dolce and H. Künkel, eds., *CEAN: Computerized EEG Analysis*. Fischer.

Campbell, D., and Rose, H. (1983) *Order in Chaos*. North-Holland.

Carskadon, M. A., and Rechtschaffen, A. (1989) Monitoring and staging human sleep. In: M. H. Kryger, T. Roth, and W. C. Dement, eds., *Principles and Practice of Sleep Medicine*. Saunders.

Caton, R. (1875) The electric currents of the brain. *Brit. Med. J.* 2: 278.

Caveness, W. F. (1962) *Atlas of Electroencephalography in the Developing Monkey*. Addison-Wesley.

Celesia, G. C., and Jasper, H. H. (1966) Acetylcholine released from cerebral cortex in relation to state of activation. *Neurology (Minneapolis)* 16: 1053–1070.

Chatrian, G. E., Lettich, E., Wilkus, R. J., and Vallarta, J. (1982) Polygraphic and clinical observations on tonic-autonomic seizures. In: R. J. Broughton, ed., *Henri Gastaut and the Marseilles School's Contributions to the Neurosciences* (EEG Suppl. 35). Elsevier.

Chatrian, G. E., Petersen, M. C., and Lazarte, J. A. (1959) The blocking of the rolandic wicket rhythm and some central changes related to movement. *Electroenceph. Clin. Neurophysiol.* 11: 497–510.

Chatrian, G. E., Somasundaram, M., and Tassinari, C. A. (1968) DC changes recorded transcranially during "typical" three per second spike and wave discharges in man. *Epilepsia* 9: 185–209.

Chatrian, G. E., Bergamini, L., Dondey, M., Klass, D. W., Lennox-Buchthal, M., and Petersén, I. (1974) A glossary of terms most commonly used by clinical electroencephalographers. *Electroenceph. Clin. Neurophysiol.* 37: 538–548.

Chavance, M. (1976) L'analyse temporelle de l'EEG et ses quantifications. *Rev. Electroencephal. Neurophysiol. Clin* 6: 282–218.

Childers, D. G. (1973) Complex demodulation of visual evoked responses. *Electroenceph. Clin. Neurophysiol.* 34: 446–447.

Childers, D. G., and Pao, M.-T. (1972) Complex demodulation for transient wavelet detection and extraction. *IEEE Trans. Audio Electroacoustics* 20: 295–308.

Coben, L. A., Danziger, W. L., and Berg, L. (1983) Frequency analysis of the resting awake EEG in mild senile dementia of Alzheimer type. *Electroenceph. Clin. Neurophysiol.* 55: 372–380.

Cohn, R. (1954) Spike-dome complex in the human electroencephalogram. *Arch. Neurol. Psych. (Chicago)* 71: 699–706.

Cohn, R. (1964) DC recordings of paroxysmal disorders in man. *Electroenceph. Clin. Neurophysiol.* 15: 17–24.

Connors, B. W., and Gutnick, M. J. (1984) Cellular mechanisms of neocortical epileptogenesis in an acute experimental model. In: P. A. Schwartzkroin and H. V. Wheal, eds., *Electrophysiology of Epilepsy*. Academic Press.

Connors, B. W., Gutnick, M. J., and Prince, D. A. (1982) Electrophysiological properties of neocortical neurons *in vitro*. *J. Neurophysiol.* 48: 1302–1320.

Cooper, R., Winter, A. L., Crow, H. J., and Walter, W. G. (1965) Comparison of subcortical, cortical and scalp activity using chronically indwelling electrodes in man. *Electroenceph. Clin. Neurophysiol.* 18: 217–228.

Cooper, R., Osselton, J. W., and Shaw, J. C. (1981) *EEG Technology*, third edition. Butterworths.

Creutzfeldt, O. D. (1969) Neuronal mechanisms underlying the EEG. In: H. H. Jasper, A. A. Ward, Jr., and A. Pope, eds., *Basic Mechanisms of the Epilepsies*. Little, Brown.

Creutzfeldt, O. D. (1977) Generality of the functional structure of the neocortex. *Naturwissenschaften* 64: 507–517.

Creutzfeldt, O. D. (1978) The neocortical link: Thoughts on the generality of structure and function of the neocortex. In: M. A. B. Brazier and H. Petsche, eds., *Architectonics of the Cerebral Cortex*. Raven.

Creutzfeldt, O. D. (1983) *Cortex Cerebri*. Springer.

Creutzfeldt, O. D., and Houchin, J. (1974) Neuronal basis of EEG waves. In: *Handbook of Electroencephalography and Clinical Neurophysiology*, vol. 2C.

Creutzfeldt, O. D., and Meisch, J. J. (1963) Changes in cortical neuronal activity and EEG during hypoglycemia. *Electroenceph. Clin. Neurophysiol.* Suppl. 24: 154–171.

Creutzfeldt, O. D., Bodenstein, G., and Barlow, J. S. (1985) Computerized EEG pattern classification by adaptive segmentation and probability-density-function classification: Clinical evaluation. *Electroenceph. Clin. Neurophysiol.* 670: 373–393.

Creutzfeldt, O. D., Grünewald, G., Simonova, O., and Schmitz, H. (1969) Changes of the basic rhythms of the EEG during the performance of mental and visuomotor tasks. In: C. R. Evans and T. B. Mulholland, eds., *Attention in Neurophysiology*. Butterworth.

Creutzfeldt, O. D., Watanabe, S., and Lux, H. D. (1966) Relations between EEG phenomena and potentials of single cortical cells. II. Spontaneous and convulsoid activity. *Electroenceph. Clin. Neurophysiol.* 20: 19–37.

Crunelli, V., and Leresche, N. (1991) A role for $GABA_B$ receptors in excitation and inhibition of thalamocortical cells. *Trends Neurosci.* 14: 16–21.

Cvitanović, P. (1984) *Universality in Chaos*. Bristol: Adam Hilger.

Daly, D. D. (1979) Use of the EEG for diagnosis and evaluation of epileptic seizures and nonepileptic episodic disorders. In: D. W. Klass and D. D. Daly, eds., *Current Practice of Clinical Electroencephalography*. Raven.

Daly, D. D. (1990) Epilepsy and syncope. In: D. D. Daly and T. A. Pedley, eds., *Current Practice of Clinical Electroencephalography*, second edition. Raven.

Daly, D. D., and Pedley, T. A., eds. (1990) *Current Practice of Clinical Electroencephalography*. Raven.

Da Rosa, A. C., Kemp, B., Paiva, T., Lopes da Silva, F. H., and Kamphuisen, H. A. C. (1991) A model-based detector of vertex waves and K complexes in sleep electroencephalogram. *Electroenceph. Clin. Neurophysiol.* 78: 71–79.

Darrow, C. W., Vieth, R. N., Maller, J., and Wilson, J. (1960). The psychophysiological importance of a continuous EEG frequency index. *Electroenceph. Clin. Neurophysiol.* 12: 238.

Daube, J. R., Harper, C. M., Litchy, W. J., and Sharbrough, F. W. (1990) Intraoperative monitoring. In: D. D. Daly and T. A. Pedley, eds., *Current Practice of Clinical Electroencephalography*, second edition. Raven.

Davis, R. L., and Robertson, D. M. (1991) *Textbook of Neuropathology*, second edition. Williams and Wilkins.

Davenport, J., Schwindt, P. C., and Crill, W. E. (1979) Epileptogenic doses of penicillin do not reduce a monosynaptic GABA-mediated postsynaptic inhibition in the intact anesthetized cat. *Exper. Neurol.* 65: 552–572.

Dean, A. F., Hess, R. F., and Tolhurst, D. J. (1980) Divisive inhibition involved in directional selectivity. *J. Physiol. (London)* 308: 34–85.

DeFrance, J., and Sheer, D. E. (1988) Focused arousal, 40-Hz EEG, and motor programming. In: D. Giannitrapani and L. Murri, eds., *The EEG of Mental Activities*. Karger.

DeLucchi, M. R., Garoutte, B., and Aird, R. B. (1962) The scalp as an electroencephalographic averager. *Electroenceph. Clin. Neurophysiol.* 14: 191–196.

Dement, W., and Kleitman, N. (1957) Cyclic variations in EEG during sleep and their relation to eye movements, body motility, and dreaming. *Electroenceph. Clin. Neurophysiol.* 9: 673–690.

Dempsey, E. W., and Morison, R. S. (1942) The production of rhythmically recurrent cortical potentials after localized thalamic stimulation. *Amer. J. Physiol.* 135: 293–300.

Denoth, F. (1975). Some general remarks on Hjorth's parameters used in EEG analysis. In: G. Dolce and H. Künkel (eds.), *CEAN: Computerized EEG Analysis*. Stuttgart: Gustav Fischer.

Deschênes, M., Madariaga-Domich, A., and Steriade, M. (1985) Dendodendritic synapses in the cat reticularis thalami nucleus: A structural basis for thalamic spindle synchronization. *Brain Res.* 334: 165–168.

Détári, L., and Vanderwolf, C. H. (1987) Activity of identified cortically projecting and other basal forebrain neurones during large slow waves and cortical activation in anaesthetized rats. *Brain Res.* 437: 1–8.

Dewan, E. M. (1964) Nonlinear oscillations and electroencephalography. *J. Theoret. Biol.* 7: 141–159.

Devyatkov, N. D., Grindel, O. M., Kharchenko, I. F., Boldyreva, G. N., Betskii, O. V., and Gnezditskii, V. V. (1973) Investigation of the instability of temporal characteristics of the human EEG by the method of phase-frequency analysis. *Vestnik Akademii Meditsinskikh Nauk SSSR* 5: 41–45. (In Russian.)

Dichter, M. A., and Ayala, G. F. (1987) Cellular mechanisms of epilepsy: A status report. *Science* 237: 157–164.

Dick, D. E., and Vaughn, A. O. (1970) Mathematical description and computer detection of alpha waves. *Math. Biosci.* 7: 81–95.

Dietsch, G. (1932) Fourier-Analyze von Electroencephalogrammen. *Pflügers Arch. ges. Physiol.* 230: 106–112.

Dodge, P. R., Richardson, E. P., Jr., and Victor, M. (1954) Recurrent convulsive seizures as a sequel to cerebral infarction: A clinical and pathological study. *Brain* 77: 610–638.

Dubinsky, J., and Barlow, J. S. (1980) A simple dot-density topogram for EEG. *Electroenceph. Clin. Neurophysiol.* 48: 473–477.

Duffy, F. H., ed. (1986) *Topographic Mapping of Brain Electrical Activity*. Butterworth.

Dumermuth, G. (1977) Fundamentals of spectral analysis in electroencephalography. In: A. Rémond, ed., *EEG Informatics*. Elsevier.

Dumermuth, G., and Molinari, L. (1987) Spectral analysis of EEG background activity. In: A. S. Gevins and A. Rémond, eds., *Methods of Analysis of Brain Electrical and Magnetic Signals* (Handbook of Electroencephalography and Clinical Neurophysiology, revised series, vol. 1). Elsevier.

Dumermuth, G., Lange, B., and Herdan, M. (1983) Analyse spectral de l'activité EEG rapide (béta). *Rev. EEG Neurophysiol.* 13: 122–128.

Dumermuth, G., Lange, B., Lehmann, D., Meier, C. A., Dinkelmann, R., and Molinari, L. (1983) Spectral analysis of all-night sleep EEG in healthy adults. *Europ. Neurol.* 22: 322–339.

Duquesnoy, A. (1976) Segmentation of EEGs by means of Kalman filtering. Progress Report 5, Institute of Medical Physics, Utrecht.

Dutertre, F. (1977) Origin and transformation of the electrical activities which result in the electroencephalogram. In: *Handbook of Electroencephalography and Clinical Neurophysiology*, vol. 11A. Elsevier, pp. 5–24.

Duyckaerts, C., Hauw, J.-J., Bastenaire, F., Piette, F., Poulain, C., Rainsard, V., Javoy-Agid, F., and Berthaux, P. (1986) Laminar distribution of neocortical senile plaques in senile dementia of the Alzheimer's type. *Acta Neuropathol.* (Berlin) 70: 249–256.

Dvořák, I., and Siska, J. (1986) On some problems encountered in the estimation of the correlation dimension of the EEG. *Phys. Lett.* A 118: 63–66.

Eccles, J. C. (1951) Interpretation of action potentials evoked in the cerebral cortex. *Electroenceph. Clin. Neurophysiol.* 3: 449–464.

Eccles, J. C. (1984) The cerebral neocortex: A theory of its operation. In: E. G. Jones and A. Peters, eds., *Cerebral Cortex*, vol. 2. Plenum.

Eckhorn, R., Bauer, R., Jordan, W., Brosch, M., Kruse, W., Munk, M., and Reitboeck, H. J. (1988) Coherent oscillations: A mechanism of feature linking in the visual cortex: Multiple electrode and correlation analyses in the cat. *Biol. Cybern.* 60: 121–130.

Ehret, C. F., and Barlow, J. S. (1960) Toward a realistic model of a biological period-measuring mechanism. *Cold Spring Harbor Symp. Quant. Biol.* 25: 217–220.

Elul, R. (1969). Gaussian behavior of the electroencephalogram: Changes during mental task. *Science* 164: 328–331.

Elul, R. (1972a) Randomness and synchrony in the generation of the electroencephalogram. In: H. Petsche and M. A. B. Brazier, eds., *Synchronization of EEG Activities in Epilepsies*. Springer.

Elul, R. 1972b. The genesis of the EEG. *Int. Rev. Neurobiol.* 15: 227–272.

Engel, A. K., König, P., Gray, C. M., and Singer, W. (1990) Stimulus-dependent neuronal oscillations in cat visual cortex: Inter-columnar interaction as determined by cross-correlation analysis. *Europ. J. Neurosci.* 2: 588–606.

Ermentrout, G. B., and Cowan, J. D. (1980) Secondary bifurcation in neuronal nets. *SIAM J. Appl. Math.* 39: 323–340.

Étévenon, P. (1977) Étude Methodologique de l'Encéphalographie. Quantitative Application à Quelques Exemples. Doctoral dissertation, Paris.

Étévenon, P. (1987) Du Rêve à l'Éveil. Paris: Albin Michel.

Étévenon, P., and Giannella, F. (1980) Waking and sleeping states in the rat from an EEG data analysis point of view. *Waking and Sleeping* 4: 33–45.

Étévenon, P., and Guillou, S. (1986) EEG cartography of a night of sleep and dreams. *Neuropsychobiol.* 16: 146–151.

Étévenon, P., Giannella, F., and Abarnou, F. (1980) Modèle d'É.E.G. par modulation radioélectrique d'amplitude et de phase. *Revue EEG Neurophysiol.* 10: 69–80.

Fairén, A., DeFelipe, J., and Regidor, J. (1984) Nonpyramidal neurons. In: A. Peters and E. G. Jones, eds., *Cerebral Cortex*, vol. 1. Plenum.

Fariello, R. G., Orrison, W., Blanco, G., and Reyes, P. F. (1982) Neuroradiological correlates of frontally predominant intermittent rhythmic delta activity (FIRDA). *Electroenceph. Clin. Neurophysiol.* 54: 194–202.

Farley, B. G. (1965) A neural network model and the "slow potentials" of electrophysiology. In: R. W. Stacy and B. D. Waxman, eds., *Computers in Biomedical Research*, vol 1. Academic Press.

Farley, B. G., and Clark, W. A. (1954) Simulation of self-organizing systems by digital computer. *Trans. IRE Profess. Group on Infor. Theory* 4: 76–84.

Feldman, M. L. (1984) Morphology of the neocortical pyramidal neuron. In: A. Peters and E. G. Jones, eds., *Cerebral Cortex*, vol. 1. Plenum.

Fenwick, P. B. C., Michie, P., Dollimore, J., and Fenton, G. W. (1971) Mathematical simulation of the electroencephalogram using an autoregressive series. *Biomed. Comput.* 2: 281–307.

Fitzhugh, R. (1961) Impulses and physiological states in theoretical models of nerve membrane. *Biophys. J.* 1: 445–464.

Flytzanis, N., Yiachnakis, E., and Micheloyannis, J. (1991) Analysis of EEG signals and their spatial correlation over the scalp surface. In: A. V. Holden, M. Markus, and H. G. Othmer, eds., *Nonlinear Wave Processses in Excitable Media*. Plenum.

Franaszczuk, P. J., and Blinowska, K. J. (1985) Linear model of brain electrical activity—EEG as a superposition of damped oscillatory modes. *Biol. Cybern.* 53: 19–25.

Freedman, N. L., Hafer, B. M., and Daniel, R. S. (1966) EEG arousal decrement during paired-associate learning. *J. Comp. Physiol. Psychol.* 61: 15–19.

Freeman, W. J. (1975) *Mass Action in the Nervous System: Examination of the Neurophysiological Basis of Adaptive Behavior through the EEG*. Academic Press.

Freeman, W. J. (1987) Simulation of chaotic EEG patterns with a dynamic model of the olfactory system. *Biol. Cybern.* 56: 139–150.

Freeman, W. J. (1989) Analysis of strange attractors in EEGs with kinesthetic experience and 4-D computer graphics. In: E. Başar and T. H. Bullock, eds., *Brain Dynamics*. Springer.

Freeman, W. J. (1990) Nonlinear neural dynamics in olfaction as a model for cognition. In: E. Başar, ed., *Dynamics of Sensory and Cognitive Processing by the Brain*. Springer.

Freeman, W. J., and Skarda, C. A. (1985) Spatial EEG patterns, nonlinear dynamics and perception: The neo-Sherringtonian view. *Brain Res. Rev.* 10: 147–175.

Freeman, W. J., and van Dijk, B. W. (1987) Spatial patterns of visual cortical fast EEG during conditioned reflex in a rhesus monkey. *Brain Res.* 422: 267–276.

Friedrich, R., Fuchs, A., and Haken, H. (1991) Synergetic analysis of spatio-temporal EEG patterns. In: A. V. Holden, M. Markus, and H. G. Othmer, eds., *Nonlinear Wave Processes in Excitable Media*. Plenum.

Froehling, H., Crutchfield, J. P., Farmer, D., Packard, N. H., and Shaw, R. (1981) On determining the dimension of chaotic flows. *Physica* 3D: 605–617.

Frolov, A. A., and Medvedev, A. V. (1986) Substantiation of the "point approximation" for describing the total electrical activity of the brain with use of a simulation model. *Biophysics* 31: 332–337. Original Russian publication: *Biofizika* 31 (1986): 304–308.

Frolov, A. A., Medvedev, A. V., Dolina, S. A., Kuznetsov, G. D., and Shulgina, G. I. (1984) Modeling different types of bioelectrical "convulsivity" by means of a "neuronal" network. *Zh. Vyssh. Nerv. Deiatel.* 34: 527–536. (In Russian.)

Frost, J. D., Jr. (1968) EEG–intracellular potential relationships in isolated cerebral cortex. *Electroenceph. Clin. Neurophysiol.* 24: 434–443.

Frost, J. D., Jr. (1976) Physiological bases of normal EEG rhythms. In: *Handbook of Electroencephalography and Clinical Neurophysiology*, vol. 6A. Elsevier.

Frost, J. D., Jr. (1979) Microprocessor-based EEG spike detection and quantification. *Int. J. BioMed. Comput.* 10: 357–373.

Frost, J. D., Jr. (1985) Automatic recognition and characterization of epileptiform discharges in the human EEG. *J. Clin. Neurophysiol.* 2: 231–249.

Frost, J. D., Jr. (1987) Mimetic techniques. In: A. S. Gevins and A. Rémond, eds. *Methods of Analysis of Brain Electrical and Magnetic Signals (Handbook of Electroencephalography and Clinical Neurophysiology,* revised series, vol. 1). Elsevier.

Frost, J. D., Jr., and Gol, A. (1966) Computer determination of relationships between EEG activity and single unit discharge in isolated cerebral cortex. *Exp. Neurol.* 14: 506–519.

Frost, J. D., Jr., Kellaway, P., and Gol, A. (1966) Single-unit discharges in isolated cerebral cortex. *Exp. Neurol.* 14: 305–316.

Frost, J. D., Jr., and Kellaway, P. (1981) Changes in epileptic spike configuration associated with achievement of clinical seizure control. *Electroenceph. Clin. Neurophysiol.* 51: 20p–21p.

Frost, J. D., Jr., Kellaway, P., Hrachovy, R. A., Glaze, D. G., and Mizrahi, E. M. (1986) Changes in epileptic spike configuration associated with attainment of seizure control. *Ann. Neurol.* 20: 723–726.

Gaenshirt, H., Krenkel, W., and Zylka, W. (1954) The electrocorticogram of the cat's brain at temperatures between 40°C and 20°C. *Electroenceph. Clin. Neurophysiol.* 6: 409–413.

Galambos, R., Makeig, S., and Talmachoff, P. J. (1981) A 40-Hz auditory potential recorded from the human scalp. *Proc. Natl. Acad. Sci. USA* 78: 2643–2647.

Garfinkel, A. (1983) A mathematics for physiology. *Amer. J. Physiol.,* 245 (*Regulatory Integrative Comp. Physiol.* 14): R455–R466.

Garoutte, W., and Aird, R. B. (1958) Synchrony and asynchrony of bilateral alpha activity. *Electroenceph. Clin. Neurophysiol.* 10: 259–268.

Garthwaite, J. (1991) Glutamate, nitric oxide and cell-cell signalling in the nervous sytem. *Trends Neurosci.* 14(2): 60–67.

Gasser, T. (1977) General characteristics of the EEG as a signal. In: A. Rémond, ed., *EEG Informatics.* Elsevier.

Gavrilova, N. A., and Aslanov, A. S. (1968) Application of electronic computing techniques to the analysis of clinical electroencephaloscopic data. In: M. N. Livanov and V. S. Rusinov, eds., *Mathematical Analysis of the Electrical Activity of the Brain.* Harvard University Press. Original Russian publication: *Matematicheskii Analiz Electricheskikh Iavlenii Golovnovo Mosga.* Izdatel'stvo "Nauka," 1965.

Geissler, C. D., and Gerstein, G. L. (1961) The surface EEG in relation to its sources. *Electroenceph. Clin. Neurophysiol.* 13: 927–934.

Gersch, W. (1970) Spectral analysis of EEGs by autoregressive decomposition of time series. *Math. Biosci.* 7: 205–222.

Gersch, W. (1987) Non-stationary multichannel time series analysis. In: A. S. Gevins and A. Rémond, eds., *Methods of Analysis of Brain Electrical and Magnetic Signals (Handbook of Electroencephalography and Clinical Neurophysiology,* revised series, vol. 1). Elsevier.

Gevins, A. S. (1987) Correlation analysis. In: A. S. Gevins and A. Rémond, eds., *Methods of Analysis of Brain Electrical and Magnetic Signals (Handbook of Electroencephalography and Clinical Neurophysiology,* revised series, vol. 1). Elsevier.

Gevins, A. S., and Illes, J. (1991) Neurocognitive networks of the human brain. *Ann. N.Y. Acad. Sci.* 620: 22–44.

Gevins, A. S., and Rémond, A., eds. (1987) *Analysis of Brain Electrical and Magnetic Signals* (*Handbook of Electroencephalography and Clinical Neurophysiology*, revised series, vol. 1). Elsevier.

Gidlöf, A., and Söderberg, U. (1964) The activity of the cat's neuronally isolated cerebral cortex between 25° and 40°C. *Electroenceph. Clin. Neurophysiol.* 17: 531–539.

Gilbert, C. D., Bourgeois, J.-P., Eckhorn, R., Goldman-Rakic, P. S., Jones, E. G., Krüger, J., Luhmann, H. J., Lund, J. S., Orban, G. A., Prince, D. A., Sillito, A. M., Somogyi, P., Toyama, K., and van Essen, D. C. (1988) Group report: Neuronal and synaptic organization in the cortex. In: P. Rakic and W. Singer, eds., *Neurobiology of Neocortex*. Wiley.

Glass, A. (1969) Changes in the amplitude probability function of the EEG under varying normal conditions. *Electroenceph. Clin. Neurophysiol.* 26: 534–540.

Glass, L., Shrier, A., and Bélair, J. J. (1986) Chaotic cardiac rhythms. In: A. V. Holden, ed., *Chaos*. Manchester University Press.

Glaze, D. G. (1990) Drug effects. In: D. D. Daly and T. A. Pedley, eds., *Current Practice of Clinical Electroencephalography*, second edition. Raven.

Gleick, J. (1987) *Chaos: Making a New Science*. Viking.

Glenn, L. L., and Steriade, M. (1982) Discharge rate and excitability of cortically projecting intralaminar thalamic neurons during waking and sleep states. *J. Neurosci* 2: 1387–1404.

Gloor, P. (1969) Hans Berger on the electroencephalogram: The fourteen original reports on the human electroencephalogram. *Electroenceph. Clin. Neurophysiol. Suppl.* 28.

Gloor, P. (1972) Generalized spike and wave discharges: A consideration of cortical and subcortical mechanisms of their genesis and synchronization. In: H. Petsche and M. A. B. Brazier, eds., *Synchronization of EEG Activities in Epilepsies*. Springer.

Gloor, P. (1975) Contributions of electroencephalography and electrocorticography to the neurosurgical treatment of the epilepsies. *Adv. Neurol.* 8: 59–105.

Gloor, P. (1977) The EEG and differential diagnosis of epilepsy. In: H. van Duijn, D. N. J. Donker, and A. C. van Huffelen, eds., *Current Concepts in Clinical Neurophysiology*. The Hague: Trio.

Gloor, P. (1984) Electrophysiology of generalized epilepsy. In: P. A. Schwartzkroin and H. V. Wheal, eds., *Electrophysiology of Epilepsy*. Academic Press.

Gloor, P. (1985) Neuronal generators and the problem of localization in electroencephalography: Application of volume conductor theory to electroencephalography. *J. Clin. Neurophysiol.* 2: 327–354.

Gloor, P. (1987) Volume conductor principles: Their application to the surface and depth electroencephalogram. In: H. G. Wieser and C. E. Elger, eds., *Presurgical Evaluation of Epileptics*. Springer.

Gloor, P. (1988) Neurophysiological mechanism of generalized spike-and-wave discharge and its implication for understanding absence seizures. In: M. S. Myslobodsky and A. F. Mirsky, eds., *Elements of Petit Mal Epilepsy*. Peter Lang.

Gloor, P. (1989) Epilepsy: Relationships between electrophysiology and intracellular mechanisms involving second messengers and gene expression. *Can. J. Neurol. Sci.* 16: 8–21.

Gloor, P., and Fariello, R. G. (1988) Generalized epilepsy: Some of its cellular mechanisms differ from those of focal epilepsy. *Trends Neurosci.* 11(2): 63–68.

Gloor, P., Avoli, M., and Kostopoulos, G. (1990) Thalamocortical relationships in generalized epilepsy with bilaterally synchronous spike-and-wave discharge. In: M. Avoli, P. Gloor, G. Kostopoulos, and R. Naquet, eds., *Generalized Epilepsy*. Birkhäuser.

Gloor, P., Ball, G., and Schaul, N. (1977) Brain lesions that produce delta waves in the EEG. *Neurology* 27: 326–333.

Gloor, P., Kalabay, O., and Giard, N. (1968) The electroencephalogram in diffuse encephalopathies: Electroencephalographic correlates of grey and white matter lesions. *Brain* 91: 779–802.

Glover, J. R., Jr., Raghavan, N., Ktonas, P. Y., and Frost, J. D., Jr. (1989) Context-based automated detection of epileptogenic sharp transients in the EEG: Elimination of false positives. *IEEE Trans. Biomed. Eng.* 36: 519–527.

Goldbeter, A., and Moran, F. (1988) Dynamics of a biochemical system with multiple oscillatory domains as a clue for multiple modes of neuronal oscillations. *Eur. Biophysics. J.* 15: 277–287.

Goldensohn, E. S. (1979a) Use of the EEG for evaluation of focal intracranial lesions. In: D. W. Klass and D. Daly, eds., *Current Practice of Clinical Electroencephalography*. Raven.

Goldensohn, E. S. (1979b) Neurophysiologic substrates of EEG activity. In: D. W. Klass and D. D. Daly, eds., *Current Practice of Clinical Electroencephalography*. Raven.

Goldensohn, E. S., and Purpura, D. P. (1963) Intracellular potentials of cortical neurons during focal epileptogenic discharges. *Science* 139: 840–842.

Goldman, P. S., and Nauta, W. J. H. (1977) Columnar distribution of cortico-cortical fibers in the frontal association, limbic, and motor cortex of the developing rhesus monkey. *Brain Res.* 122: 393–413.

Goldman-Rakic, P. S. (1988a) Topography of cognition: Parallel distributed networks in primate association cortex. *Ann. Rev. Neurosci.* 11: 137–156.

Goldman-Rakic, P. S. (1988b) Changing concepts of cortical connectivity: Parallel distributed cortical networks. In: P. Rakic and W. Singer, eds., *Neurobiology of Neocortex*. Wiley.

Goldman-Rakic, P. S., and Selemon, L. D. (1984) Topography of corticostriatal projections in nonhuman primates and implications for functional parcellation of the neostriatum. In: E. G. Jones and A. Peters, eds., *Cerebral Cortex*, vol. 5. Raven.

Goldstein, S. (1970) Phase coherence of the alpha rhythm during photic blocking. *Electroenceph. Clin. Neurophysiol.* 29: 127–136.

Goncharova, I. I., and Barlow, J. S. (1990) Changes in EEG mean frequency and spectral purity during spontaneous alpha blocking. *Electroenceph. Clin. Neurophysiol.* 76: 197–204.

Goodman, N. R. (1960) Measuring amplitude and phase. *J. Franklin Inst.* 270: 437–450.

Goodwin, G. C., and Sin, K. S. (1984) *Adaptive Filtering Prediction and Control*. Prentice-Hall.

Gotman, J. (1980) Quantitative measurements of epileptic spike morphology in the human EEG. *Electroenceph. Clin. Neurophysiol.* 48: 551–557.

Gotman, J. (1982) Automatic recognition of epileptic seizures in the EEG. *Electroenceph. Clin. Neurophysiol.* 54: 530–540.

Gotman, J. (1985) Practical use of computer-assisted EEG interpretation in epilepsy. *J. Clin. Neurophysiol.* 2: 251–265.

Gotman. J. (1986) Computer analysis of the EEG in epilepsy. In: F. H. Lopes da Silva, W. Storm van Leeuwen, and A. Rémond, eds., *Clinical Applications of Computer Analysis of EEG and Other Neurophysiological Signals (Handbook of Electroencephalography and Clinical Neurophysiology*, revised series, vol. 2). Elsevier.

Gotman, J. (1990a) Automatic seizure detection: Improvements and evaluation. *Electroenceph. Clin. Neurophysiol.* 76: 317–324.

Gotman, J. (1990b) The use of computers in analysis and display of EEG and evoked potentials. In: D. D. Daly and T. A. Pedley, eds., *Current Practice of Clinical Electroencephalography*. Raven.

Gotman, J., and Wang, L. Y. (1991) State-dependent spike detection: Concepts and preliminary results. *Electroenceph. Clin. Neurophysiol.* 79: 11–19.

Gotman, J., Ives, J. R., and Gloor, P., eds. (1985) *Long-Term Monitoring in Epilepsy. Electroenceph. Clin. Neurophysiol.* Suppl. 37.

Grass, A. M., and Gibbs, F. A. (1938) A Fourier transform of the electroencephalogram. *J. Neurophysiol.* 1: 521–526.

Grassberger, P. (1983) Generalized dimensions of strange attractors. *Phys. Lett.* 97A: 227–230.

Grassberger, P., and Procaccia, I. (1983) Characterization of strange attractors. *Phys. Rev. Lett.* 50: 346–349.

Gray, C. M., and Singer, W. (1989) Stimulus-specific neuronal oscillations in orientation columns of cat visual cortex. *Proc. Natl. Acad. Sci. USA* 86: 1698–1702.

Gray, C. M., König, P., Engel, A. K., and Singer, W. (1989) Oscillatory responses in cat visual cortex exhibit inter-columnar synchronization which reflects global stimulus properties. *Nature* 338: 334–337.

Gumnit, R. J. (1974) DC shifts accompanying seizure activity. In: *Handbook of Electroencephalography and Clinical Neurophysiology*, vol. 10A. Elsevier.

Gumnit, R. J., and Takahashi, T. (1965) Changes in direct current activity during experimental focal seizures. *Electroenceph. Clin. Neurophysiol.* 19: 63–74.

Gutnick, M. J., Connors, B. W., and Prince, D. A. (1982) Mechanisms of neocortical epileptogenesis *in vitro*. *J. Neurophysiol.* 48: 1321–1335.

Hao, Bai-lin. (1984) *Chaos*. Singapore: World Scientific.

Hartley, R. V. L. (1928) Modulation System. U.S. Patent 1,666,205.

Hendrix, C. E. (1965) Transmission of electric fields in cortical tissue: A model for the origin of the alpha rhythm. *Bull. Math. Biophysics* 267: 197–213.

Hendry, S. H. C., Schwark, H. D., Jones, E. G., and Yan, J. (1987) Numbers and proportions of GABA-immunoreactive neurons in different areas of monkey cerebral cortex. *J. Neurosci.* 7: 1503–1519.

Hileman, R. E., and Dick, D. E. (1971) Detection of phase characteristics of alpha waves in the electroencephalogram. *IEEE Trans. Biomed. Eng.* 18: 379–382.

Hjorth, B. (1970) EEG analysis based on time domain properties. *Electroenceph. Clin. Neurophysiol.* 29: 306–310

Hjorth, B. (1973) The physical significance of time domain descriptors in EEG analysis. *Electroenceph. Clin. Neurophysiol.* 34: 321–325.

Hjorth, B. (1975) Time domain descriptors and their relation to a particular model for generation of EEG activity. In: G. Dolce and H. Künkel, eds., *CEAN: Computerized EEG Analysis*. Stuttgart: Gustav Fischer.

Hoagland, H. (1936a) Temperature characteristics of the "Berger rhythm" in man. *Science* 83: 84–85.

Hoagland, H. (1936b) Pacemakers of human brain waves in normals and in general paretics. *Am. J. Physiol.* 116: 604–615.

Hoagland, H. (1936c) Some pacemaker aspects of rhythmic activity in the nervous system. *Cold Spring Harbor Symp. Quant. Biol.* 4: 267–276.

Hobson, J. A., and Steriade, M. (1986) Neuronal basis of behavioral state control. In: V. B. Mountcastle, ed., *Handbook of Physiology*, vol. 4. American Physiological Society.

Hof, P. R., Cox, K., and Morrison, J. H. (1990) Quantitative analysis of a vulnerable subset of pyramidal neurons in Alzheimer's disease. I. Superior frontal and inferior temporal cortex. *J. Comp. Neurol.* 301: 44–54.

Hoovey, Z. B., Heinemann, U., and Creutzfeldt, O. D. (1972) Inter-hemispheric "synchrony" of alpha waves. *Electroenceph. Clin. Neurophysiol.* 32: 337–347.

Houser, C. R., Vaughn, J. E., Hendry, S. H. C., Jones, E. G., and Peters, A. (1984) GABA neurons in the cerebral cortex. In: E. G. Jones and A. Peters, eds., *Cerebral Cortex*, vol. 2. Plenum.

Hrachovy, R. A., Mizrahi, E. M., and Kellaway, P. (1990) Electroencephalography of the newborn. In: D. D. Daly and T. A. Pedley, eds., *Current Practice of Clinical Electroencephalography*, second edition. Raven.

Hubel, D. H., and Wiesel, T. N. (1962) Receptive fields, binocular interaction and functional architecture in the cat's visual cortex. *J. Physiol.* 160: 106–154.

Hubel, D. H., and Wiesel, T. N. (1977) Functional architecture of macaque monkey cortex. *Proc. Roy. Soc. Lond.* B198: 1–59.

Huberman, B. A., and Zisook, A. B. (1981) Power spectra of strange attractors. *Phys. Rev. Lett.* 46: 626–628.

Iasemidis, L. D., Sakellares, J. C., Zaveri, H. P., and Williams, W. J. (1990) Phase space topography and the Lyapunov exponent of electrocorticograms in partial seizures. *Brain Topography* 2: 187–201.

Ingber, L. (1982) Statistical mechanics of neocortical interactions. I. Basic formulation. *Physica* 5D: 83–107.

Ingber, L. (1984) Statistical mechanics of neocortical interactions. Derivation of short-term-memory capacity. *Phys. Rev. A* 29: 3346–3358.

Ingber, L. (1985) Statistical mechanics of neocortical interactions: EEG dispersion relations. *IEEE Trans. Biomed. Eng.* 32: 91–94.

Ingber, L., and Nunez, P. L. (1990) Multiple scales of statistical physics of the neocortex: Application to electroencephalography. *Math. Comput. Modelling* 13: 83–95.

Ingvar, D. H., Sjölund, B., and Ardö, A. (1976) Correlation between dominant EEG frequency, cerebral oxygen uptake and blood flow. *Electroenceph. Clin. Neurophysiol.* 41: 268–276.

Innocenti, G. M. (1984) General organization of callosal connections in the cerebral cortex. In: E. G. Jones and A. Peters, eds., *Cerebral Cortex*, vol. 5. Plenum.

Isaksson, A., and Wennberg, A. (1976) Spectral properties of nonstationary EEG signals evaluated by means of Kalman filtering. Application examples from a vigilance test. In: P. Kellaway and L. Petersén, eds., *Quantitative Analytic Studies in Epilepsy*. Raven.

Jahnsen, H., and Llinás, R. (1984a) Electrophysiological properties of guinea-pig thalamic neurones: An *in vitro* study. *J. Physiol.* 349: 205–226.

Jahnsen, H., and Llinás, R. (1984b) Ionic basis for the electroresponsiveness and oscillatory properties of guinea-pig thalamic neurones *in vitro*. *J. Physiol.* 349: 227–247.

Jasper, H. H. (1936a) Cortical excitatory state and variability in human brain rhythms. *Science* 83: 259–260.

Jasper, H. H. (1936b) Cortical excitatory state and synchronism in the control of bioelectric autonomous rhythms. *Cold Spring Harbor Symp. Quant. Biol.* 4: 320–332.

Jasper, H. H. (1949) Diffuse projection systems: The integrative action of the thalamic reticular system. *Electroenceph. Clin. Neurophysiol.* 1: 405–420.

Jasper, H. H. (1958) The Ten-Twenty Electrode System of the International Federation. *Electroenceph. Clin. Neurophysiol.* 10: 371–375.

Jasper, H. H. (1969) Neurochemical mediators of specific and non-specific cortical activation. In: C. R. Evans and T. B. Mulholland, eds., *Attention in Neurophysiology*. Butterworth.

Jasper, H. H. (1981) Problems of relating cellular or modular specificity to cognitive function: Importance of state-dependent reactions. In: F. O. Schmitt, F. G. Worden, G. Adelman, and S. G. Dennis, eds., *The Organization of the Cerebral Cortex*. MIT Press.

Jasper, H. H. (1983) The Ten-Twenty Electrode System of the International Federation. In: *Recommendations for the Practice of Clinical Neurophysiology made by the International Federation of Societies for Electroencephalography and Clinical Neurophysiology*. Elsevier. (Reprint of Jasper 1958.)

Jasper, H. H. (1991) Current evaluation of the concepts of centrencephalic and cortico-reticular seizures (guest editorial). *Electroenceph. Clin. Neurophysiol.* 78: 2–11.

Jasper, H. H., and Droogleever-Fortuyn, J. (1947) Experimental studies on the functional anatomy of petit mal epilepsy. *Res. Publ. Ass. Nerv. Ment. Dis.* 26: 272–298.

Jasper, H. H., and Penfield, W. (1949) Zur Deuting des normalen Elektrencephalogramms und seiner Veränderungen. *Archiv. Psych. Z. Neurol.* 183: 163–174.

Jasper, H., and van Buren, J. (1953) Interrelationship between cortex and subcortical structures: Clinical electroencephalographic studies. *Electroenceph. Clin. Neurophysiol.* (Suppl). 4: 168–188.

Johnson, B. W., Weinberg, H., Ribary, U., Cheyne, D. O., and Ancill, R. (1988) Topographic distribution of the 40 Hz auditory evoked-related potential in normal and aged subjects. *Brain Topography* 1: 117–121.

Johnson, L. C. (1972) Computers in sleep research. In: M. H. Chase, ed., *The Sleeping Brain*. Brain Information Service/Brain Research Institute, UCLA.

Johnson, L. C. (1977) The EEG during sleep as viewed by a computer. In: A. Rémond, ed., *EEG Informatics: A Didactic Review of Methods and Applications of EEG Data Processing*. Elsevier.

Johnson, L., Lubin, A., Naitoh, P., Nute, C., and Austin, M. (1969) Spectral analysis of the EEG of dominant and non-dominant alpha subjects during waking and sleeping. *Electroenceph. Clin. Neurophysiol.* 26: 361–370.

Johnston, D., and Brown, T. H. (1984) Mechanisms of neuronal burst generation. In: P. A. Schwartzkroin and H. V. Wheal, eds., *Electrophysiology of Epilepsy*. Academic Press.

Jones, E. G. (1984). Laminar distribution of cortical efferent cells. In: E. G. Jones and A. Peters, eds., *Cerebral Cortex*, vol. 1. Plenum.

Jones, E. G. (1985) *The Thalamus*. Plenum

Jones, E. G. (1986) Neurotransmitters in the cerebral cortex. *J. Neurosurg.* 65: 135–153.

Jones, E. G. (1987) GABA-peptide neurons of the primate cerebral cortex. *J. Mind Behav.* 8: 519–536.

Jones, E. G. (1988) What are the local circuits? In: P. Rakic and W. Singer, eds., *Neurobiology of the Neocortex*. Wiley.

Jones, E. G., and Peters, A. (1984) *Cerebral Cortex*, vol. 2: *Functional Properities of Cortical Cells*. Plenum.

Jonkman, E. J., van Huffelen, A. C., and Pfurtscheller, G. (1986) Quantative EEG in cerebral ischemia. In: F. H. Lopes da Silva, W. Storm van Leeuwen, and A. Rémond, eds., *Clinical*

Applications of Computer Analysis of EEG and Other Neurophysiological Signals (Handbook of Electroencephalography and Clinical Neurophysiology, revised series, vol. 2). Elsevier.

Kanai, T., and Szerb, J. C. (1965) Mesencephalic reticular activating system and cortical acetylcholine output. *Nature* 205: 80–82.

Kandel, E. R., Schwartz, J. H., and Jessell, T. M., eds., (1991) *Principles of Neural Science,* third edition. Elsevier.

Kaplan, P. W., and Lesser, R. P. (1990) Long-term monitoring. In: D. D. Daly and T. A. Pedley, eds., *Current Practice of Clinical Electroencephalography,* second edition. Raven.

Katz, A., Marks, D. A., McCarthy, G., and Spencer, S. S. (1991) Does interictal spiking change prior to seizures? *Electroenceph. Clin. Neurophysiol.* 79: 153–156.

Katznelson, R. D. (1981) Normal modes of the brain: Neuroanatomical basis and a physiological theoretical model. In: P. L. Nunez, ed., *Electric Fields of the Brain: The Neurophysics of the EEG.* Oxford University Press.

Kawahara, T. (1980) Coupled Van der Pol oscillators: A model of excitatory and inhibitory neural interactions. *Biol. Cybern.* 39: 37–43.

Kawakami, M., and Gellhorn, E. (1963) The influence of temperature on the balance between the excitatory and inhibitory cerebral systems. A contribution to the caudate-hypothalamic antagonism. *Electroenceph. Clin. Neurophysiol.* 15: 230–237.

Kellaway, P. (1990) An orderly approach to visual analysis: Characteristics of the normal EEG of adults and children. In: D. D. Daly and T. A. Pedley, eds., *Current Practice of Clinical Electroencephalography.* Raven.

Kellaway, P., Frost, J. D., Jr., and Crawley, J. W. (1980) Time modulation of spike-and-wave activity in generalized epilepsy. *Ann. Neurol.* 8: 491–500.

Kellaway, P., Gol, A., and Proler, M. (1966) Electrical activity of the isolated cerebral hemisphere and isolated thalamus. *Exp. Neurol.* 14: 281–304.

Kellaway, P., Hrachovy, R. A., Frost, J. D., Jr., and Zion, T. (1979) Precise characterization and quantification of infantile spasms. *Ann. Neurol.* 6: 214–218.

Kemp, B., and Blom, H. A. P. (1981) Optimal detection of the alpha state in a model of the human electroencephalogram. *Electroenceph. Clin. Neurophysiol.* 52: 222–225.

Kemp, B., Gröneveld, E. W., Janssen, A. J. M. W., and Franzen, J. M. (1987) A model-based monitor of human sleep stages. *Biol. Cybern.* 57: 365–378.

Kemp, B., Jaspers, P., Franzen, J. M., and Janssen, A. J. M. W. (1985) An optimal monitor of the electroencephalographic sigma sleep state. *Biol. Cybern.* 51: 263–270.

Kepler, T. B., Marder, E., and Abbott, L. F. (1990) The effect of electrical coupling on the frequency of model neuronal oscillators. *Science* 248: 83–85.

Klass, D. W. (1975) Electroencephalographic manifestations of complex partial seizures. *Adv. Neurol.* 11: 113–140.

Knott, J. R. (1939) Some effects of "mental set" on the electrophysiological processes of the human cerebral cortex. *J. Exp. Psychol.* 24: 384–405.

Knott, J. R., and Travis, L. E. (1937) A note on the relationship betweeen duration and amplitude of cortical potentials. *J. Psychol.* 3: 169–172.

Kornmüller, A. E. (1933) Die Ableitung bioelektrischer Effekte architektonischer Rindenfelder vom uneröffneten Schädel. *J. f. Psychol. u. Neurol.* 45: 172–184.

Kornmüller, A. E. (1935) Die bioelektrischen Erscheinungen architektonischer Felder der Grosshirnrinde. *Biol. Rev.* 10: 383–426.

Kozelka, J. W., and Pedley, T. A. (1990) Beta and mu rhythms. *J. Clin. Neurophysiol.* 7: 191–207.

Kozhevnikov, V. A. (1958) Some methods of automatic measurement of the electroencephalogram. *Electroenceph. Clin. Neurophysiol.* 10: 269–278.

Kreifeldt, J. (1970) Ensemble entrainment of self-sustaining oscillators: A possible application to neural signals. *Math. Biosci.* 8: 425–436.

Krnjević, K. (1980) Neurobiology: General principles related to epilepsy. In: G. H. Glaser, J. K. Penry, and D. M. Woodbury, eds., *Antiepileptic Drugs: Mechanisms of Action.* Raven.

Krnjević, K. (1984) Neurotransmitters in cerebral cortex: A general account. In: E. G. Jones and A. Peters, eds., *Cerebral Cortex,* vol. 2. Plenum.

Krnjević, K., and Phillis, J. W. (1963a) Acetylcholine-sensitive cells in the cerebral cortex. *J. Physiol. (London)* 166: 296–327.

Krnjević, K., and Phillis, J. W. (1963b) Pharmacological properties of acetylcholine-sensitive cells in the cerebral cortex. *J. Physiol. (London)* 166: 328–350.

Ktonas, P. Y. (1987) Automated spike and sharp wave (SSW) detection. In: A. S. Gevins and A. Rémond, eds., *Methods of Analysis of Brain Electrical and Magnetic Signals (Handbook of Electroencephalography and Clinical Neurophysiology,* revised series, vol. 1). Elsevier.

Ktonas, P. Y., and Papp, N. (1980) Instantaneous envelope and phase extraction from real signals: Theory, implementation, and an application to EEG analysis. *Signal Processing* 2: 373–385.

Ktonas, P. Y., Luoh, W. M., Kejariwal, M. L., Reilly, E. L., and Seward, M. A. (1981) Computer-aided quantification of EEG spike and sharp wave characteristics. *Electroenceph. Clin. Neurophysiol.* 51: 237–243.

Kubie, L. S. (1930) A theoretical application to some neurological problems of the properties of excitation waves which move in closed circuits. *Brain* 53: 166–177.

Kuhlman, W. N. (1978) EEG feedback training: Enhancement of somatosensory cortical activity. *Electroenceph. Clin. Neurophysiol.* 45: 290–294.

Lagerlund, T. D., and Sharbrough, F. W. (1988) Computer simulation of neuronal circuit models of rhythmic behavior in the electroencephalogram. *Comput. Biol. Med.* 18: 267–304.

Lagerlund, T. D., and Sharbrough, F. W. (1989) Computer simulation of the generation of the electroencephalogram. *Electroenceph. Clin. Neurophysiol.* 72: 31–40.

Lansing, R. W., and Barlow, J. S. (1972) Rhythmic after-activity to flashes in relation to the background alpha which precedes and follows the photic stimuli. *Electroenceph. Clin. Neurophysiol.* 32: 149–160.

Lee, Y. W. (1960) *Statistical Theory of Communication.* Wiley.

Leissner, P., Lindholm, L.-E., and Petersén, I. (1970) Alpha amplitude dependence on skull thickness as measured by ultrasound technique. *Electroenceph. Clin. Neurophyslol.* 29: 392–399.

Lemieux, J. F., and Blume, W. T. (1983) Automated morphological analysis of spikes and sharp waves in human electrocorticograms. *Electroenceph. Clin. Neurophysiol.* 55: 45–50.

Levine, D. A., Elashoff, R., Callaway, E. III, Payne, D., and Jones, R. T. (1972) Evoked potential analysis by complex demodulation. *Electroenceph. Clin. Neurophysiol.* 32: 513–520.

Lévy, J.-C. (1970) Modèle explicatif des ondes électro-encephalographiques du type alpha et théta. *C. R. Acad. Sci. Paris* 270 D: 859–861.

Lévy, J.-C. (1971a) Un modèle théoretique simulant les fuseaux d'ondes alpha de l'électro-encéphalogramme. *C. R. Acad. Sci. Paris* 272 D: 1163–1165.

Lévy, J.-C. (1971b) Complément à un modèle simulant les ondes électroencéphalographiques. *C. R. Acad. Sci. Paris* 272 D: 2954–2956.

Lévy, J.-C. (1974) Une propriété théorique des fuseau d'ondes alpha de l'électroencephalogrammme. *C. R. Acad. Sci. Paris* 279 D: 947–950.

Lion, K. S., and Winter, D. F. (1953) A method for the discrimination between signal and random noise of electrobiological potentials. *Electroenceph. Clin. Neurophysiol.* 5: 109–111.

Llinás, R. (1988) The intrinsic electrophysiological properties of mammalian neurons: Insights into central nervous system function. *Science* 242: 1654–1664.

Llinás, R., Grace, A. A., and Yarom, Y. (1991) *In vitro* neurons in mammalian cortical layer 4 exhibit intrinsic oscillatory activity in the 10- to 50-Hz frequency range. *Proc. Natl. Acad. Sci. USA* 88: 891–901.

Llinás, R., and Jahnsen, H. (1982) Electrophysiology of mammalian thalamic neurones *in vitro*. *Nature* 297: 406–408.

Llinás, R., and Yarom, Y. (1986) Oscillatory properties of guinea-pig inferior olivary neurons and their pharmacological modulation: An *in vitro* study. *J. Physiol.* 376: 163–182.

Lloyd, D. S. L., and Binnie, C. D. (1972) Pattern recognition in EEG. *Adv. Behav. Biol.* 5: 153–166.

Lombroso, C. T. (1987) Neonatal electroencephalography. In: E. Niedermeyer and F. Lopes da Silva, eds., *Electroencephalography*. Urban & Schwarzenberg.

Lopes da Silva, F. H. (1981) Analysis of EEG ongoing activity: Rhythms and nonstationarities. In: N. Yamaguchi and K. Fujisawa, eds., *Recent Advances in EEG and EMG Data Processing*. Elsevier.

Lopes da Silva, F. (1987a) Dynamics of EEGs as signals of neuronal populations: Models and theoretical considerations. In: E. Niedermeyer and F. Lopes da Silva, eds., *Electroencephalography*, second edition. Urban & Schwarzenberg.

Lopes da Silva, F. (1987b) EEG analysis: Theory and practice. In: E. Niedermeyer and F. Lopes da Silva, eds., *Electroencephalography*, second edition. Urban & Schwarzenberg.

Lopes da Silva, F. (1987c) Computer-assisted EEG diagnosis: Pattern recognition techniques. In: E. Niedermeyer and F. Lopes da Silva, eds., *Electroencephalography*, second edition. Urban & Schwarzenberg.

Lopes da Silva, F. (1991) Neural mechanism underlying brain waves: From neural membranes to networks. *Electroenceph. Clin. Neurophysiology* 79: 81–93.

Lopes da Silva, F., and Mars, N. J. I. (1987) Parametric methods in EEG analysis. In: A. S. Gevins and A. Rémond, eds., *Methods of Analysis of Brain Electrical and Magnetic Signals (Handbook of Electroencephalography and Clinical Neurophysiology*, revised series, vol. 1). Elsevier.

Lopes da Silva, F. H., and Storm van Leeuwen, W. (1978) The cortical alpha rhythm in dog: The depth and surface profile of phase. In: M. A. B. Brazier and H. Petsche. eds., *Architectonics of the Cerebral Cortex*. Raven.

Lopes da Silva, F. H., van Lierop, T. H. M. T., Schrijer, C. F., and Storm van Leeuwen, W. (1973a) Organization of thalamic and cortical alpha rhythms: Spectra and coherences. *Electroenceph. Clin. Neurophysiol.* 35: 627–639.

Lopes da Silva, F. H., van Lierop, T. H. M. T., Schrijer, C. F., and Storm van Leeuwen W. (1973b) Essential differences between alpha rhythms and barbiturate spindles: Spectra and thalamo-cortical coherences. *Electroenceph. Clin. Neurophysiol.* 35: 641–645.

Lopes da Silva, F. H., Hoeks, A., Smits, H., and Zetterberg, L. H. (1974) Model of brain rhythmic activity: The alpha-rhythm of the thalamus. *Kybernetik* 15: 27–37.

Lopes da Silva, F. H., van Rotterdam, A., Barts, P., van Heusden, E., and Burr, W. (1976) Models of neuronal populations: The basic mechanisms of rhythmicity. *Progr. Brain Res.* 45: 281–308.

Lopes da Silva, F. H., Vos, J. E., Mooibroek, J., and van Rotterdam, A. (1980a) Relative contributions of intracortical and thalamo-cortical processes in the generation of alpha rhythms, revealed by partial coherence analysis. *Electroenceph. Clin. Neurophysiol.* 50: 449–456.

Lopes da Silva, F. H., Vos, J. E., Mooibroek, J., and van Rotterdam, A. (1980b) Partial coherence analysis of thalamic and cortical alpha rhythms in dog: A contribution towards a general model of the cortical organization of rhythmic activity. In: G. Pfurtscheller, P. Buser, and F. H. Lopez da Silva, eds., *Rhythmic EEG Activities and Cortical Functioning.* Elsevier.

Lopes da Silva, F. H., Storm van Leeuwen, W., and Rémond, A., eds. (1986) *Clinical Applications of Computer Analysis of EEG and Other Neurophysiological Signals (Handbook of Electroencephalography and Clinical Neurophysiology,* revised series, vol. 2). Elsevier.

Lopes da Silva, F., Pijn, J. P., and Boeijinga, P. (1989) Interdependence of EEG signals: Linear vs. nonlinear associations and the significance of time delays and phase shifts. *Brain Topography* 2: 9–18.

Lorente de Nó, R. (1933) Studies on the structure of the cerebral cortex. *J. f. Psychol. u. Neurol.* 45: 420–438.

Lowenberg, E. C. (1959) An experimental EEG function generator. *Electroenceph. Clin. Neurophysiol.* 11: 355–357.

Lund, J. S. (1984) Spiny stellate neuron. In: A. Peters and E. G. Jones, eds., *Cerebral Cortex,* vol. 1. Plenum.

Ma, K. M., Celesia, G. G., and Birkemeier, W. P. (1976) Cluster analysis and spike detection in EEG. In: D. Janz, ed., *Epileptology: Proceedings of the 7th International Symposium on Epilepsy, Berlin, June 1975.* Stuttgart: Thiem.

Macchi, G., and Bentivoglio, M. (1984) The thalamic intralaminar nuclei and the cerebral cortex. In: E. G. Jones and A. Peters, eds., *Cerebral Cortex,* vol. 5. Plenum.

Mäkelä, J. P., and Hari, R. (1987) Evidence for cortical origin of the 40 Hz auditory evoked response in man. *Electroenceph. Clin. Neurophysiol.* 66: 539–546.

Mandell, A. J. (1983) From intermittency to transitivity in neuropsychobiological flows. *Am. J. Physiol.* 245 *(Regulatory Integrative Comp. Physiol.* 14): R484–R494.

Marder, E. (1991) Plateaus in time. *Current Biol.* 1: 326–327.

Marder, E., and Meyrand, P. (1989) Chemical modulation of an oscillatory neural circuit. In: J. W. Jacklet, ed., *Neuronal and Cellular Oscillators.* Dekker.

Markand, O. N. (1990a) Organic brain syndromes and dementias. In: D. D. Daly and T. A. Pedley, eds., *Current Practice of Clinical Electroencephalography,* second edition. Raven.

Markand, O. N. (1990b) Alpha rhythms. *J. Clin. Neurophysiol.* 7: 163–189.

Martin, J. H. (1991) The collective electrical behavior of cortical neurons: The electroencephalogram and the mechanisms of epilepsy. In: E. R. Kandel, J. H. Schwartz, and T. M. Jessell, eds., *Principles of Neural Science,* third edition. Elsevier.

Martin, K. A. C. (1984) Neuronal circuits in cat striate cortex. In: E. G. Jones and A. Peters, eds., *Cerebral Cortex,* vol. 2. Plenum.

Martin, W. B., Johnson, L. C., Viglione, S. S., Naitoh, P., Joseph, R. D., and Moses, J. D. (1972) Pattern recognition of EEG-EOG as a technique for all-night sleep stage scoring. *Electroenceph. Clin. Neurophysiol.* 32: 417–427.

Matsumoto, H., and Ajmone-Marsan, C. (1964a) Cortical cellular phenomena in experimental epilepsy: Interictal manifestations. *Exper. Neurol.* 9: 286–304.

Matsumoto, H., and Ajmone-Marsan, C. (1964b) Cortical cellular phenomena in experimental expilepsy: Ictal manifestations. *Exper. Neurol.* 9: 305–326.

Matthis, P., Scheffner, D., and C. Benninger (1981) Spectral analysis of the EEG: Comparison of various spectral parameters. *Electroenceph. Clin. Neurophysiol.* 52: 218–221.

Mayer-Kress, G., and Holzfuss, J. (1987) Analysis of the human electroencephalogram with methods from nonlinear dynamics. In: L. Rensing, U. an der Heiden, and M. C. Mackey, eds., *Temporal Disorder in Human Oscillatory Systems*. Springer.

Mayer-Kress, G., and Layne, S. P. (1987) Dimensionality of the human electroencephalogram. *Ann. N.Y. Acad. Sci.* 504: 62–87.

McCormick, D. A. (1992a) Neurotransmitter actions in the thalamus and cerebral cortex. *J. Clin. Neurophysiol.* 9: 212–223

McCormick, D. A. (1992b) Neurotransmitter actions in the thalamus and cerebral cortex and their role in neuromodulation of thalamocortical activity. *Progr. Neurobiol.* 39: 337–388.

McCormick, D. A., and von Krosigk, M. (1992) Corticothalamic activation modulates thalamic firing through glutamate "metabotropic" receptors. *Proc. Natl. Acad. Sci. USA* 89: 2774–2778.

McCormick, D. A., and Williamson, A. (1989) Convergence and divergence of neurotransmitter action in human cerebral cortex. *Proc. Natl. Acad. Sci. USA* 86: 8098–8102.

McEwen, J. A., and Anderson, G. B. (1975) Modeling the stationarity and gaussianity of spontaneous electroencephalographic activity. *IEEE Trans. Biomed. Eng.* 22: 361–369.

McWhorter, A. L. (1957) $1/f$ noise and germanium surface properties. In: R. H. Kinston, ed., *Semiconductor Surface Physics*. University of Pennsylvania Press.

Mergenhagen, D., Creutzfeldt, O., and Neuweiler, G. (1968) Beziehungen zwischen Aktivität corticaler Neurone und EEG-Wellen im motorischen Cortex der Katze bei Hypoglykämie. *Archiv. f. Psychiat. u. Z. f. d. ges. Neurol.* 211: 43–62.

Mesulam, M.-M. (1986) Frontal cortex and behavior. *Ann. Neurol.* 19: 320–325.

Mesulam, M.-M. (1990) Large-scale neurocognitive networks and distributed processing for attention, language, and memory. *Ann. Neurol.* 28: 597–613.

Michael, D., and Houchin, J. (1979) Automatic EEG analysis: A segmentation procedure based on the autocorrelation function. *Electroenceph. Clin. Neurophysiol.* 46: 232–235.

Michenfelder, J. D., and Theye, R. A. (1968) Hypothermia: Effect on canine brain and whole-body metabolism. *Anesthesiology* 29: 1107–1112.

Middleton, D. (1960) *An Introduction to Statistical Communication Theory*. McGraw-Hill. Reprint: Peninsula, 1987.

Minorsky, N. (1962) *Nonlinear Oscillations*. Van Nostrand.

Morison, R., and Dempsey, E. W. (1942) A study of thalamocortical relations. *Am. J. Physiol.* 135: 281–292.

Morrone, M. C., Burr, D. C., and Maffei, L. (1982) Functional implications of cross-orientation inhibition of cortical visual cells. I. Neurophysiological evidence. *Proc. R. Soc. Lond.* B 216: 335–354.

Moruzzi, G. (1964) The historical development of the deafferentation hypothesis of sleep. *Proc. Am. Philosoph. Soc.* 108: 19–28.

Moruzzi, G., and Magoun, H. W. (1949) Brain stem reticular formation and activation of the EEG. *Electroenceph. Clin. Neurophysiol.* 1: 455–473.

Mountcastle, V. B. (1957) Modality and topographic properties of single neurons of cat's somatic sensory cortex. *J. Neurophysiol.* 20: 408–434.

Mountcastle, V. B. (1978) An organizing principle for cerebral function: The unit module and the distributed system. In: V. B. Mountcastle and G. M. Edelman, The Mindful Brain. MIT Press.

Mulle, C., Madariaga, A., and Deschênes, M. (1986) Morphology and electrophysiological properties of reticularis thalami neurons in cat: *In vivo* study of a thalamic pacemaker. *J. Neurosci.* 6: 2134–2145.

Naitoh, P., and Lewis, G. W. (1981) Statistical analysis of extracted features. In: N. Yamaguchi and K. Fujisawa, eds., *Recent Advances in EEG and EMG Data Processing*. Elsevier.

Nakagawa, T., and Ohashi, A. (1980) A spatio-temporal filter approach to synchronous brain activities. *Biol. Cybern.* 36: 33–39.

Narasimhan, S. V., and Dutt, D. N. (1985) Software simulation of the EEG. *J. Biomed. Eng.* 7: 275–281.

Niedermeyer, E. (1987a) The normal EEG of the waking adult. In: E. Niedermeyer and F. Lopes da Silva, eds., *Electroencephalography*, second edition. Urban & Schwarzenberg.

Niedermeyer, E. (1987b) Maturation of the EEG: Development of waking and sleep patterns. In: E. Niedermeyer and F. Lopes da Silva, eds., *Electroencephalography*, second edition. Urban & Schwarzenberg.

Niedermeyer, E. (1987c) Abnormal EEG patterns (epileptic and paroxysmal). In: E. Niedermeyer and F. Lopes da Silva, eds., *Electroencephalography*, second edition. Urban & Schwarzenberg.

Niedermeyer, E. (1987d) EEG and dementia. In: E. Niedermeyer and F. Lopes da Silva, eds., *Electroencephalography*, second edition. Urban & Schwarzenberg.

Niedermeyer, E. (1987e) Epileptic seizure disorders. In: E. Niedermeyer and F. Lopes da Silva, eds., *Electroencephalography*, second edition. Urban & Schwarzenberg.

Niedermeyer, E., and Lopes da Silva, F., eds. (1987) *Electroencephalography: Basic Principles, Clinical Applications and Related Fields*, second edition. Urban & Schwarzenberg.

Niedermeyer, E., and Lopes da Silva, F., eds. (1993) *Electroencephalography: Basic Principles, Clinical Applications and Related Fields*, third edition. Williams and Wilkins.

Nogawa, T., Katayama, K., Tabata, Y., Ohshio, T., and Kawahara, T. (1976) Changes in amplitude of the EEG induced by a photic stimulus. *Electroenceph Clin. Neurophysiol.* 40: 78–88.

Nogawa, T., Katayama, K., Tabata, Y., Kawahara, T., and Ohshio, T. (1977) Dynamics of neuronal population. *Electroenceph. Clin. Neurophysiol.* 43: 543.

Nunez, P. L. (1974) The brain wave equation: A model for the EEG. *Math. Biosci.* 21: 279–297.

Nunez, P. L. (1981) *Electric Fields of the Brain*. Oxford University Press.

Nunez, P. L. (1988) Global contributions to cortical dynamics: Theoretical and experimental evidence for standing wave phenomena. In: E. Başar, ed., *Dynamics of Sensory and Cognitive Processing by the Brain*. Springer.

Nunez, P. L. (1989) Generation of human EEG by a combination of long and short range neocortical interactions. *Brain Topography* 1: 199–215.

Nunez, P. L., and Pilgreen, K. L. (1991) The spline-Laplacian in clinical neurophysiology: A method to improve EEG spatial resolution. *J. Clin. Neurophysiol.* 8: 397–413.

Nunez, P. L., Reid, L., and Bickford, R. G. (1978) The relationship of head size to alpha frequency with implications to a brain wave model. *Electroenceph. Clin. Neurophysiol.* 44: 344–352.

Ohara, P. T. (1988) Synaptic organization of the thalamic reticular nucleus. *J. Electron Microscopy Technique* 10: 283–292.

Oken, B. S., Chiappa, K. H., and Salinsky, M. (1989) Computerized EEG frequency analysis: Sensitivity and specificity in patients with focal lesions. *Neurology* 39: 1281–1287.

O'Leary, J. L., and Goldring, S. (1964) D-C potentials of the brain. *Physiol. Rev.* 44: 91–125.

O'Leary, J. L., and Goldring, S. (1976) *Science and Epilepsy: Neuroscience Gains in Epilepsy Research.* Raven.

Olson, G. E., and Schadé, J. P. (1965) A tribute to Norbert Wiener. *Progr. Brain Res.* 17: 1–8.

Osovets, S. M., Ginsburg, D. A., Gurfinkel', V. S., Zenkov, L. R., Latash, L. P., Malkin, V. B., Mel'nichuk, P. V., and Pastemak, E. B. (1983) Electrical activity of the brain: Mechanisms and interpretation. *Sov. Phys. Usp.* 26: 801–828. Original Russian Publication: *Usp. Fiz. Nauk* 141 (1983): 103–150.

Osovets, S. M., Gurfinkel', V. S., Ginsburg, D. A., Latash, L. P., Malkin, V. B., Mel'nichuk, P. V., and Pastemak, E. B. (1977) Mechanism of onset of generalized paroxysmal EEG rhythms. *Human Physiol.* 3: 389–398. Original Russian publication: *Fiziol. Cheloveka* 3 (1977): 482–492.

Panet-Raymond, D., and Gotman, J. (1990) Can slow waves in the electrocorticogram (ECoG) help localize epileptic foci? *Electroenceph. Clin. Neurophysiol.* 75: 464–473.

Pantev, C., Makeig, S., Hoke, M., Galambos, R., Hampson, S., and Gallen, C. (1991) Human auditory evoked gamma-band magnetic fields. *Proc. Natl. Acad. Sci. USA* 88: 8996–9000.

Pasquali, E. (1969) Alpha envelope detection and distortion: A polyphase rectifier circuit. *Electroenceph. Clin. Neurophysiol.* 26: 106–109.

Pavlidis, T. (1965) A new model for simple neural nets and its application in the design of a neural oscillator. *Bull. Math. Biophys.* 27: 215–229.

Pedley, T. A. (1984) Epilepsy and the human electroencephalogram. In: P. A. Schwartzkroin and H. V. Wheal, eds., *Electrophysiology of Epilepsy.* Academic Press.

Pedley, T. A., and Traub, R. D. (1990) Physiological basis of the EEG. In: D. D. Daly and T. A. Pedley, eds., *Current Practice of Clinical Electroencephalography.* Raven.

Perkel, D. H. (1987) Chaos in brains: fad or insight. *Behav. Brain Sci.* 10: 180–181.

Peters, A. (1984) Chandelier cells. In: A. Peters and E. G. Jones, eds., *Cerebral Cortex*, vol. 1. Plenum.

Peters, A., and Jones, E. G. (1984) Classification of cortical neurons. In: A. Peters and E. G. Jones, eds., *Cerebral Cortex*, vol 1. Plenum.

Petsche, H. (1962) Pathophysiologie und Klinik des Petit Mal. *Wiener Z. Nervenheilkunde u. Grenzgebiete* 19: 345–442.

Petsche, H., and Rappelsberger, P. (1970) Influence of cortical incision on synchronization pattern and travelling waves. *Electroenceph. Clin. Neurophysiol.* 28: 592–600.

Petsche, H., Pockberger, H., and Rappelsberger, P. (1984) On the search for the sources of the electroencephalogram. *Neuroscience* 11: 1–27.

Pfurtscheller, G. (1981) Central beta rhythm during sensorimotor activities in man. *Electroenceph. Clin. Neurophysiol.* 51: 253–264.

Pfurtscheller, G., and Cooper, R. (1975) Frequency dependence of the transmission of the EEG from cortex to scalp. *Electroenceph. Clin. Neurophysiol.* 38: 93–96.

Pijn, J. P., and Lopes da Silva, F. H. (1991) Chaos analysis, nonlinear associations and delay estimates for the dynamical analysis of the spread of an epileptic seizure. In: I. Dvořák and V. Holden, eds., *Mathematical Approaches to Brain Functioning Diagnostics*. Manchester University Press.

Pijn, J. P., van Neerven, J., Noest, A., and Lopes da Silva, F. H. (1991) Chaos or noise in EEG signals; dependence on state and brain site. *Electroenceph. Clin. Neurophysiol.* 79: 371–381.

Pollen, D. A. (1964) Cellular studies of cortical neurons during thalamic induced wave and spike. *Electroenceph. Clin. Neurophysiol.* 17: 398–404.

Pollen, D. A. (1968) Experimental spike and wave responses and petit mal epilepsy. *Epilepsia* 9: 221–232.

Pollen, D. A. (1969) On the generation of neocortical potentials. In: H. H. Jasper, A. A. Ward, and A. Pope, eds., *Basic Mechanisms of the Epilepsies*. Little, Brown.

Powell, T. P. S. (1981) Certain aspects of the intrinsic organization of the cerebral cortex. In: O. Pompeiano and C. Ajmone-Marsan, eds., *Brain Mechanisms and Perceptual Awareness*. Raven.

Praetorius, H. M., Bodenstein, G., and Creutzfeldt, O. D. (1977) Adaptive segmentation of EEG records: A new approach to automatic EEG analysis. *Electroenceph. Clin. Neurophysiol.* 42: 84–94.

Prast, J. W. (1949) An interpretation of certain EEG patterns as transient responses of a transmission system. *Electroenceph. Clin. Neurophysiol.* 1: 370.

Pratt, H., Rogowski, Z., and Bental, E. (1982) Analog delay line artifact rejector for evoked potential studies. *Electroenceph. Clin. Neurophysiol.* 53: 565–567.

Prince, D. A., and Connors, B. W. (1984) Mechanisms of epileptogenesis in cortical structures. *Ann. Neurol.* 16 (suppl.): S59–S64.

Pritchard, W. S., and Duke, D. W. (1992) Measuring chaos in the brain: A tutorial review of nonlinear dynamical EEG analysis. *Intern. J. Neuroscience* 67: 31–80.

Pronk, R. A. F. (1986) Peri-operative monitoring. In: F. H. Lopes da Silva, W. Storm van Leeuwen, and A. Rémond, eds., *Clinical Applications of Computer Analysis of EEG and Other Neurophysiological Signals* (Handbook of Electroencephalography and Clinical Neurophysiology, revised series, vol. 2). Elsevier.

Pronk, R. A. F., and Simons, A. J. R. (1982) Automatic recognition of abnormal EEG activity during open heart surgery. In: P. A. Buser, W. A. Cobb and T. Okuma, eds., *Kyoto Symposia* (*Electroencephal. Clin. Neurophysiol.* Suppl. 36). Elsevier.

Pronk, R. A. F., and Simons, A. J. R. (1984) Processing of the electroencephalogram in cardiac surgery. *Comp. Progr. Biomed.* 18: 181–190.

Purpura, D. P. (1959) Nature of electrocortical potentials and synaptic organizations in cerebral and cerebellar cortex. In: C. C. Pfeiffer and J.R. Smythies, eds., *International Review of Neurobiology*, vol. 1. Academic Press.

Qian, J., Barlow, J. S., and Beddoes, M. P. (1988) A simplified arithmetic detector for EEG sharp transients—preliminary results. *IEEE Trans. Biomed. Eng.* 35: 11–18.

Radtke, R. A. (1990) Sleep disorders: Laboratory evaluation. In: D. D. Daly and T. A. Pedley, eds., *Current Practice of Clinical Electroencephalography*, second edition. Raven.

Raeva, S., Lukashev, A., and Lashin, A. (1991) Unit activity in human thalamic reticular nucleus. I. Spontaneous activity. *Electroenceph. Clin. Neurophysiol.* 79: 133–140.

Rashevsky, N. (1971) A note on nonperiodic undamped oscillations, with special reference to brain waves. *Bull. Math. Biophys.* 33: 281–293.

Rechtschaffen, A., and Kales, A., eds. (1968) *A Manual of Standardized Terminology, Techniques and Scoring System for Sleep States of Human Subjects.* UCLA Brain Information Service/Brain Research Institute/NINDB Neurological Information Network.

Rempel, B., and Gibbs, E. L. (1936) The Berger rhythm in cats. *Science* 84: 334–335.

Ribak, C. E., Haris, A. B., Vaughn, J. E., and Roberts, E. (1979) Inhibitory, GABAergic nerve terminals decrease at sites of focal epilepsy. Science 205: 211–214.

Ribak, C. E., Hunt, C. A., Bakay, R. A. E., and Oertel, W. H. (1986) A decrease in the number of GABAergic somata is associated with the preferential loss of GABAergic terminals at epileptic foci. *Brain Res.* 363: 78–90.

Richardson, E. P., Jr., and Dodge, P. R. (1954) Epilepsy in cerebral vascular disease. *Epilepsia* (series III) 3: 1–26.

Riehl, J.-L. (1963) Analog analysis of EEG activity. *Electroenceph. Clin. Neurophysiol.* 15: 1039–1042.

Riekkinen, P., Buzsaki, G., Riekkinen, P., Jr., Soininen, H., and Partanen, J. (1991) The cholinergic system and EEG slow waves. *Electroenceph. Clin. Neurophysiol.* 78: 89–96.

Rinaldi, P., Juhasz, G., and Verzeano, M. (1977) Circulation of cortical and thalamic neuronal activity in wakefulness and in sleep. *Electroenceph. Clin. Neurophysiol.* 43: 248–259.

Rinzel, J., and Ermentrout, G. B. (1989) Analysis of neural excitability and oscillations. In: C. Koch and I. Segev, eds., *Methods in Neuronal Modeling: From Synapses to Networks.* MIT Press.

Roberts, E. (1976) Disinhibition as an organizing principle in the nervous system—the role of the GABA system. Application to neurologic and psychiatric disorders. In: E. Roberts, T. N. Chase, and D. B. Tower, eds., *GABA in Nervous System Function.* Raven.

Roberts, E. (1980) Prospectus. Epilepsy and epileptic drugs: A speculative synthesis. *Adv. Neurol.* 27: 667–713.

Roberts, G. W., Crow, T. J., and Polak, J. M. (1985) Location of neuronal tangles in somatostatin neurones in Alzheimer's disease. *Nature* 314: 92–94.

Rockel, A. J., Hiorns, R. W., and Powell, T. P. S. (1980) The basic uniformity in structure of the neocortex. *Brain* 103: 221–244.

Rogers, J., and Morrison, J. H. (1985) Quantitative morphology and regional and laminar distributions of senile plaques in Alzheimer's disease. *J. Neurosci.* 2801–2808.

Rohracher, H. (1937) Über die Kurvenform cerebraler Potentialschwankungen. *Pflüger's Archiv Ges. Physiol.* 238: 535–545.

Rohracher, H. (1938) Weitere Untersuchungen über die Kurvenform cerebraler Potentialschwankungen. *Pflüger's Archiv Ges. Physiol.* 239: 191–196.

Rose, D. (1977) On the arithmetical operation performed by inhibitory synapses onto the neuronal soma. *Exp. Brain Res.* 28: 221–223.

Rose, R. M., and Hindmarsh, J. L. (1985) A model of a thalamic neuron. *Proc. R. Soc. Lond.* B 225: 161–193.

Rössler, O. E., and Hudson, J. L. (1989) Self-similarity in hyperchaotic data. In: E. Başar and T. H. Bullock, eds., *Brain Dynamics.* Springer.

Rougeul, A., Bouyer, J. J., Dedet, L., and Debray, O. (1979) Fast somatoparietal rhythms during combined focal attention and immobility in baboon and squirrel monkey. *Electroencephal. Clin. Neurophysiol.* 46: 310–319.

Rougeul-Buser, A., Bouyer, J. J., Montaron, M. F., and Buser, P. (1983) Patterns of activities in the ventrobasal thalamus in the awake cat: Focal rhythms. In: J. Massion, J. Paillard, W. Schultz, and M. Wiesendanger, eds., *Neural Coding of Motor Performance* (*Exp. Brain Res.* Suppl 7). Springer.

Roux, J.-C., Simoyi, R. H., and Swinney, H. L. (1983) Observation of a strange attractor. *Physica* 8D: 257–268.

Rutecki, P. A. (1992) Neuronal excitability: Voltage-dependent currents and synaptic transmission. *J. Clin. Neurophysiol.* 9: 195–211.

Saltzberg, B., and Burch, N. R. (1971) Period analytic estimates of movements of the power spectrum: A simplified EEG time domain procedure. *Electroenceph. Clin. Neurophysiol.* 30: 568–570.

Saltzberg, B., Burton, W. D., Jr., Barlow, J. S., and Burch, N. R. (1985) Moments of the power spectral density estimated from samples of the autocorrelation function (a robust procedure for monitoring changes in the statistical properties of lengthy non-stationary time series such as the EEG). *Electroenceph. Clin. Neurophysiol.* 61: 89–93.

Santamaria, J., and Chiappa, K. H. (1987) *The EEG of Drowsiness*. Demos.

Saunders, M. G. (1963) Amplitude probability density studies on alpha and alpha-like patterns. *Electroenceph. Clin. Neurophysiol.* 15: 761–767.

Schaul, N. (1990) Pathogenesis and significance of abnormal nonepileptiform rhythms in the EEG. *J. Clin. Neurophysiol.* 7: 229–248.

Schaul, N., Gloor, P., Ball, G., and Gotman, J. (1978) The electromicrophysiology of delta waves induced by systemic atropine. *Brain Res.* 143: 475–486.

Schaul, N., Lueders, H., and Sachdev, K. (1981) Generalized, bilaterally synchronous bursts of slow waves in the EEG. *Arch. Neurol.* 38: 690–692.

Schetzen, M. (1960) Statistical behavior of coupled oscillators. In: Quarterly Progress Report 58, Research Laboratory of Electronics, Massachusetts Institute of Technology.

Schetzen, M. (1961) Statistical model of coupled oscillators. In: Quarterly Progress Report 61, Research Laboratory of Electronics, Massachusetts Institute of Technology.

Schlag, J. (1958) A differentiation of spontaneous unit firing in subcortical structures of the cat's brain. *Science* 127: 1184–1185.

Schlag, J. (1974) Reticular influences on thalamo-cortical activity. In: *Handbook of Electroencephalography and Clinical Neurophysiology*, vol. 2C. Elsevier.

Schwartz, J. H. (1991) Chemical messengers: Small molecules and peptides. In: E. R. Kandel, J. H. Schwartz, and T. M. Jessell, eds., *Principles of Neural Science*, third edition. Elsevier.

Schwartzkroin, P. A. (1984) Epileptogenesis in the immature central nervous system. In: P. A. Schwartzkroin and H. V. Wheal, eds., *Electrophysiology of Epilepsy*. Academic Press.

Schwartzkroin, P. A. (1987) *In vivo* and *in vitro* microphysiology of focal epilepsy. In: R. J. Ellingson, N. M. F. Murray, and A. M. Halliday, eds., *The London Symposia* (*Electroenceph. Clin. Neurophysiol.* Suppl. 39). Elsevier.

Segen, J., and Sanderson, A. C. (1979) Piece-wise stationary models of biomedical signals. In: Proceedings of the Tenth Modeling Simulation Conference, Pittsburgh.

Sharbrough, F. W. (1987) Nonspecific abnormal EEG patterns. In: E. Niedermeyer and F. H. Lopes da Silva, eds., *Electroencephalography*, second edition. Urban & Schwarzenberg.

Sharpless, S., and Jasper, H. (1956) Habituation of the arousal reaction. Brain 79: 655–680.

Shaw, J. C. (1971) An EEG signal generator with variable time delayed output. *Med. Biol. Eng.* 9: 71–73.

Shepherd, G. M., Brayton, R. K., Miller, J. P., Segev, I., Rinzel, J., and Rall, W. (1985) Signal enhancement in distal cortical dendrites by means of interactions between active dendritic spines. *Proc. Natl. Acad. Sci. USA* 82: 2192–2195.

Sie, G., Jasper, H., and Wolfe, L. (1965) Rate of ACh release from cortical surface in *encephale* and *cerveau isolé* cat preparations in relation to arousal and epileptic activation of the ECoG. *Electroenceph. Clin. Neurophysiol.* 18: 206.

Siebert, W. M. (1986) *Circuits, Signals, and Systems.* MIT Press.

Siegel, A. (1981) Stochastic aspects of the generation of the electroencephalogram. *J. Theor. Biol.* 92: 317–339.

Siggins, G. R., and Gruol, D. L. (1986) Mechanisms of transmitter action in the vertebrate central nervous system. In: F. E. Bloom, ed., *Handbook of Physiology*, section 1, vol. IV. American Physiological Society.

Simon, O., Müllner, E., and Heinemann, U. (1976) Relationship between background activity and subclinical seizure pattern. *Electroenceph. Clin. Neurophysiol.* 40: 449–455.

Skarda, C. A., and Freeman, W. J. (1987) How brains make chaos in order to make sense of the world. *Behav. Brain Sci.* 10: 161–195.

Sloper, J. J., Johnson, P., and Powell, T. P. S. (1980) Selective degeneration of interneurons in the motor cortex of infant monkeys following controlled hypoxia: A possible cause of epilepsy. *Brain Res.* 198: 204–209.

Smith, J. R. (1972) Discussion of: Johnson, L. C., Computers in sleep research. In: M. H. Chase, ed., *The Sleeping Brain.* Brain Information Service/Brain Research Institute, UCLA.

Smith, J. R. (1986) Automated analysis of sleep EEG data. In: F. H. Lopes da Silva, W. Storm van Leeuwen, and A. Rémond, eds., *Clinical Applications of Computer Analysis of EEG and Other Neurophysiological Signals (Handbook of Electroencephalography and Clinical Neurophysiology,* revised series, vol. 2). Elsevier.

Soininen, H., Partanen, V. J., Helkala, E.-L., and Riekkinen, P. J. (1982) EEG findings in senile dementia and normal aging. *Acta Neurol. Scandinav.* 65: 59–70.

Sokal, R. R., and Rohlf, F. J. (1973) *Introduction to Biostatistics.* Freeman.

Speckmann, E.-J., and Elger, C. E. (1987) Introduction to the neurophysiological basis of the EEG and DC potentials. In: E. Niedermeyer and F. Lopes da Silva, eds., *Electroencephalography,* second edition. Urban & Schwarzenberg.

Speckmann, E.-J., Caspers, H., and Janzen, R. W. C. (1972) Relations between cortical DC shifts and membrane potential changes of cortical neurons associated with seizure activity. In: H. Petsche and M. A. B. Brazier, eds., *Synchronization of EEG Activity in Epilepsies.* Springer.

Spydell, J. D., Pattee, G., and Goldie, W. D. (1985) The 40 Hz auditory event-related potential: Normal values and effects of lesions. *Electroenceph. Clin. Neurophysiol.* 62: 193–202.

Starzl, T. E., and Magoun, H. W. (1951) Organization of the diffuse thalamic projection system. *J. Neurophysiol.* 14: 133–146.

Steriade, M., and Deschênes, M. (1984) The thalamus as a neuronal oscillator. *Brain Res. Rev.* 8: 1–63.

Steriade, M., and Llinás, R. R. (1988) The functional states of the thalamus and the associated neural interplay. *Physiol. Reviews* 68: 649–742.

Steriade, M., Curró Dossi, R., and Nuñez, A. (1991) Network modulation of a slow intrinsic oscillation of cat thalamocortical neurons implicated in sleep delta waves: Cortically induced synchronization and brainstem cholinergic suppression. *J. Neurosci.* 11: 3200–3217.

Steriade, M., Domich, L., and Oakson, G. (1986) Reticularis thalami revisited: Activity changes during shifts of states of vigilance. *J. Neurosci.* 6: 68–81.

Steriade, M., Domich, L., Oakson, G., and Deschênes, M. (1987) The deafferented reticular thalamic nucleus generates spindle rhythmicity. *J. Neurophysiol.* 57: 260–273.

Steriade, M., Jones, E. G., and Llinás, R. R. (1990a) *Thalamic Oscillations and Signaling*. Wiley.

Steriade, M., Oakson, G., and Ropert, N. (1982) Firing rates and patterns of midbrain reticular neurons during steady and transitional states of the sleep-waking cycle. *Exp. Brain Res.* 46: 37–51.

Steriade, M., Gloor, P., Llinás, R. R., Lopes da Silva, F. H., and Mesulam, M.-M. (1990b) Basic mechanisms of cerebral rhythmic activities (Report of IFCN Committee on Basic Mechanisms). *Electroenceph. Clin. Neurophysiol.* 76: 481–508.

Stewart, D. J., MacFabe, D. F., and Vanderwolf, C. H. (1984) Cholinergic activation of the electrocorticogram: Role of the substantia innominata and effects of atropine and quinuclidinyl benzilate. *Brain Res.* 322: 219–232.

Storm van Leeuwen, W. (1978) The alpha rhythm. In: W. A. Cobb and H. Van Duijn, eds., *Contemporary Clinical Neurophysiology* (*Electroenceph. Clin. Neurophysiol.* Suppl. 34). Elsevier.

Swinney, H. L. (1983) Observations on order and chaos in nonlinear systems. *Physica* 7D: 3–15.

Symonds, C. (1962) Discussion. *Proc. Roy. Soc. Med.* 55: 314–315.

Szentágothai, J. (1978a) The local neuronal apparatus of the cerebral cortex. In: P. Buser and A. Rougeul-Buser, eds., *Cerebral Correlates of Conscious Experience*. Elsevier.

Szentágothai, J. (1978b) The neuron network of the cerebral cortex: A functional interpretation (The Ferrier Lecture). *Proc. Roy. Soc. Lond.* B 201: 219–248.

Szentágothai, J. (1983) The modular architectonic principle of neural centers. *Rev. Physiol. Biochem. Pharmacol.* 98: 35–61.

Takahashi, T. (1987) Activation methods. In: E. Niedermeyer and F. Lopes da Silva, eds., *Electroencephalography*, second edition. Urban & Schwarzenberg.

Tatsuno, J. (1981) Analysis of basic rhythm from the viewpoint of the EEG envelope. In: N. Yamaguchi and K. Fujisawa, eds., *Recent Advances in EEG and EMG Data Processing*. Elsevier.

Tatsuno, J., Mori, J., Ashida, H., and Maru, E. (1980) Changes in alpha band activities during alpha blocking induced by flash stimulation. In: G. Pfurtscheller, P. Buser, and F. H. Lopes da Silva, eds., *Rhythmic EEG Activities and Cortical Functioning*. Elsevier.

Terry, R. D., Masliah, E., Salmon, D. P., Butters, N., DeTeresa, R., Hill, R., Hansen, L., A., and Katzman, R. (1991) Physical basis of cognitive alterations in Alzheimer's disease: Synapse loss is the major correlate of cognitive impairment. *Ann. Neurol.* 30: 572–580.

Testa, J., Perez, J., and Jeffries, C. (1982) Evidence for universal chaotic behavior of a driven nonlinear oscillator. *Phys. Rev. Lett.* 48: 517–521.

Thom, R. (1987) Chaos can be overplayed. *Behav. Brain Sci.* 10: 182–183.

Tolonen, U., and Sulg, I. A. (1981) Comparison of quantitative EEG parameters from four different analysis techniques in evaluation of relationships between EEG and CBF in brain infarction. *Electroenceph. Clin. Neurophysiol.* 51: 177–185.

Tourenne, C. J. (1985) A model of the electric field of the brain at EEG and microwave frequencies. *J. Theoret. Biol.* 116: 495–507.

Trabka, J. (1962) High frequency components in brain wave activity. *Electroenceph. Clin. Neurophysiol.* 14: 453–464.

Traub, R. D., Knowles, W. D., Miles, R., and Wong, R. K. S. (1984) Synchronized after-discharges in the hippocampus: Simulation studies of the cellular mechanism. *Neurosci.* 12: 1191–1200.

Tsutsumi, K., and Matsumoto, H. (1984) Ring neural network qua a generator of rhythmic oscillation with period control mechanism. *Biol. Cybern.* 51: 181–194.

Tyner, F. S., Knott, J. R., and Mayer, W. B., Jr. (1983) *Fundamentals of EEG Technology*, vol. 1: *Basic Concepts and Methods*. Raven.

Tyner, F. S., Knott, J. R., and Mayer, W. B., Jr. (1989) *Fundamentals of EEG Technology*, vol. 2: *Clinical Correlates*. Raven.

van der Pol, B. (1926) On "relaxation-oscillations." *Phil. Mag.* 2: 978–992.

van der Pol, B., and van der Mark, J. (1928) The heartbeat considered as a relaxation oscillation, and an electrical model of the heart. *Phil. Mag.* 6: 763–775.

van Gelder, N. M., Janjua, N. A., Metrakos, K., MacGibbon, B., and Metrakos, J. D. (1980) Plasma amino acids in 3/sec spike-wave epilepsy. *Neurochem. Res.* 5: 659–671.

van Rotterdam, A., Lopes da Silva, F. H., van den Ende, J., Viergever, M. A., and Hermans, A. J. (1982) A model of the spatial-temporal characteristics of the alpha rhythm. *Bull. Math. Biol.* 44: 283–305.

Vas, G. A., and Cracco, J. B. (1990) Diffuse encephalopathies. In: D. D. Daly and T. A. Pedley, eds., *Current Practice of Clinical Electroencephalography*, second edition. Raven.

Verzeano, M. (1972) Pacemakers, synchronization, and epilepsy. In: H. Petsche and M. A. B. Brazier, eds., *Synchronization of EEG Activity in Epilepsies*. Springer.

Verzeano, M., and Negishi, K. (1960) Neuronal activity in cortical and thalamic networks. *J. Gen. Physiol.* 43 (6), part 2: 177–195.

von der Malsburg, C., and Schneider, W. (1986) A neural cocktail-party processor. *Biol. Cybern.* 54: 29–40.

Walma, A. A. (1980) On the superposition of relaxation spectra as an explanation for $1/f$ noise. *Rev. Phys. Appl.* 15: 1435–1443.

Walmsley, M. (1984) On the normalized slope descriptor method of quantifying electroencephalograms. *IEEE Trans. Biomed. Eng.* 31: 720–723.

Walter, D. O. (1968) The method of complex demodulation. In: D. O. Walter and M. A. B. Brazier, eds., *Advances in EEG Analysis (Electroenceph. Clin. Neurophysiol.* suppl. 27).

Walter, D. O. (1972) Discussion of: Johnson, L. C., Computers in sleep research. In: M. H. Chase, ed., *The Sleeping Brain*. Brain Information Service/Brain Research Institute, UCLA.

Walter, D. O. (1976) Glossary of computer terminology. In: *Handbook of Electroencephalography and Clinical Neurophysiology*, vol. 4A. Elsevier.

Walter, D. O. (1987) Introduction to computer analysis in electroencephalography. In: E. Niedermeyer and F. Lopes da Silva, eds., *Electroencephalography*, second edition. Urban & Schwarzenberg.

Walter, D. O., Cooper, R., and Frost, J. D., Jr. (1972a) Specific means of data processing. In: *Handbook of Electroencephalography and Clinical Neurophysiology*, vol. 4B. Elsevier.

Walter, D. O., Cooper, R., and Frost, J. D., Jr. (1972b) Glossary. In: *Handbook of Electroencephalography and Clinical Neurophysiology*, vol. 4B. Elsevier.

Walter, D. O., Rhodes, J. M., Brown, D., and Adey, W. R. (1966) Comprehensive spectral analysis of human EEG generators in posterior cerebral regions. *Electroenceph. Clin. Neurophysiol.* 20: 224–227.

Walter, W. G. (1943a) An automatic low frequency analyser. *Electron. Eng.* 16: 3–13.

Walter, W. G. (1943b) An improved low frequency analyser. *Electron. Eng.* 16: 236–240.

Walter, W. G. (1959) Intrinsic rhythms of the brain. In: *Handbook of Physiology*, section 1: *Neurophysiology*, vol. 1. American Physiological Society.

Walter, W. G. (1962) Oscillatory activity in the nervous system. In: R. G. Grenell, ed., *Neural Physiopathology*. Hoeber/Harper.

Weir, B. (1965) The morphology of the spike-wave complex. *Electroenceph. Clin. Neurophysiol.* 19: 284–290.

Wennberg, A., and Zetterberg, L. H. (1971) Applications of a computer-based model for EEG analysis. *Electroenceph. Clin. Neurophysiol.* 31: 457–468.

Wescoe, W. C., Green, R. E., McNamara, B. P., and Krop, S. (1948) The influence of atropine and scopolamine on the central effects of DFP. *J. Pharm. Exp. Therapeutics* 92: 63–72.

Westmoreland, B. F. (1990) Benign EEG variants and patterns of uncertain clinical significance. In: D. D. Daly and T. A. Pedley, eds., *Current Practice of Clinical Electroencephalography*, second edition. Raven.

Westmoreland, B. F., and Klass, D. W. (1990) Unusual EEG patterns. *J. Clin. Neurophysiol.* 7: 209–228.

White, R. P., and Boyajy, L. D. (1960) Neuropharmacological comparison of atropine, scopolamine, benactyzine, diphenhydramine and hydroxyzine. *Arch. Int. Pharmacodyn.* 127: 260–273.

Widrow, B., and Stearns, S. D. (1985) *Adaptive Signal Processing*. Prentice-Hall.

Wiener, N. (1955) Time and Organization (Second Fawley Foundation Lecture, University of Southampton). Reprinted in: P. Masani, ed., *Norbert Wiener: Collected Works*, vol. IV. MIT Press, 1985.

Wiener, N. (1956) Brain waves and the interferometer. *J. Phys. Soc. Japan* 18: 499–507. Reprinted in: P. Masani, ed., *Norbert Wiener: Collected Works*, vol. IV. MIT Press, 1985.

Wiener, N. (1957) Rhythms in physiology with particular reference to electroencephalography. *Proc. Rudolf Virchow Med. Soc. (N.Y.)* 16: 109–124. Reprinted in: P. Masani, ed., *Norbert Wiener: Collected Works*, vol. IV. MIT Press, 1985.

Wiener, N. (1958) *Nonlinear Problems in Random Theory*. MIT Press.

Wiener, N. (1961) *Cybernetics: or Control and Communication in the Animal and the Machine*, second edition. MIT Press.

Wilson, H. R., and Cowan, J. D. (1972) Excitatory and inhibitory interactions in localized populations of model neurons. *Biophys. J.* 12: 1–24.

Wilson, H. R., and Cowan, J. D. (1973) A mathematical theory of the functional dynamics of cortical and thalamic nervous tissue. *Kybernetik* 13: 55–80.

Wilson, N. J., and Wilson, W. P. (1959) The duration of human electroencephalographic arousal responses elicited by photic stimulation. *Electroenceph. Clin. Neurophysiol.* 11: 85–91.

Witte, H., Eiselt, M., Patakova, I., Petranek, S., Griessbach, G., Krajca, V., and Rother, M. (1991) Use of discrete Hilbert transformation for automatic spike mapping: A methodological investigation. *Med. Biol. Eng. Comput.* 29: 242–248.

Witte, H., Stallknecht, K., Ansorg, J., Griessbach, G., Petranek, S., Rother, M. (1990) Using Discrete Hilbert Transformation to realize a general methodical basis for dynamic EEG mapping: A methodical investigation. *Automedica* 13: 1–13.

Woodbury, J. W. (1965) Potentials in a volume conductor. In: T. C. Ruch and H. D. Patton, eds., *Medical Physiology and Biophysics*, 19th edition. Saunders.

Wright, J. J., and Kydd, R. R. (1984) A linear theory for global electrocortical activity and its control by the lateral hypothalamus. *Biol. Cybern.* 50: 75–82.

Xu, N., and Xu, J.-H. (1988) The fractal dimension of EEG as a physical measure of conscious human brain activities. *Bull. Math. Biol.* 50: 559–565.

Yarom, Y. (1991) Rhythmogenesis in a hybrid system: Interconnecting an olivary neuron to an analog network of coupled oscillators. *Neuroscience* 44: 263–275.

Zeeman, E. C. (1976) Duffing's equation in brain modelling. *Bull. Inst. Math. Appl.* 12: 207–214. Reprinted in: Zeeman, E. C., *Catastrophe Theory*. Addison-Wesley, 1977.

Zetterberg, L. H. (1973) Experience with analysis and simulation of EEG signals with parametric description of spectra. In: P. Kellaway and I. Petersén, eds., *Automation of Clinical Electroencephalography*. Raven.

Zetterberg, L. H. (1977) Experiments with a model for a neuron population. *Electroenceph. Clin. Neurophysiol.* 43: 480.

Zetterberg, L. H., and Ahlin, K. (1975) Analog simulator of EEG signals based on spectral components. *Med. Biol. Eng.* March: 272–278.

Zetterberg, L. H., Kristiansson, L., and Mossberg, K. (1978) Performance of a model for a local neuron population. *Biol. Cybern.* 31: 15–26.

Zhadin, M. N. (1984) Rhythmic processes in the cerebral cortex. *J. Theor. Biol.* 108: 565–595.

Zhadin, M. N. (1991) Biophysical mechanisms of the EEG formation. In: Dvořák, I., and Holden, A.V., eds., *Mathematical Approaches to Brain Functioning Diagnostics*. Manchester University Press.

Zifkin, B. G., and Cracco, R. Q. (1990) An orderly approach to the abnormal EEG. In: D. D. Daly and T. A. Pedley, eds., *Current Practice of Clinical Electroencephalography*, second edition. Raven.

Index

Abnormal EEG patterns, 168
Abnormal random delta slowing, 85
Acetylcholine, 170, 232
  cortical arousal and, 170
  delta waves and, 176
  substantia innominata (nucleus basalis of Meynert) and, 154
Activating system, 153
Activation
  cortical excitatory state and, 150
  excitatory and inhibitory drives and, 151
  of EEG, 153
Adaptive segmentation, 6, 88, 196, 238, 247, 261, 281
  epileptiform activity and, 104
  probability-density-function classification and, 54
Adaptive signal processing, 400–407
Adaptive signal processor
  cortical columns and, 408
  epilepsy and, 408
  finite impulse response (FIR) type, 404
  infinite impulse response (IIR) type, 404
Afterhyperpolarization, 161, 179
  delta waves and, 173
Alpha activity, 3, 20, 283 (*see also* Alpha rhythm; Alpha waves)
  complex demodulation of, 361
  corticocortical and corticothalamic circuits and, 152
  idling cortex and, 168
  minimal drowsiness and, 168
  origins of, 152
  Type 3 waves and, 53
  waking relaxed state and, 71
  waxing and waning of, 7
Alpha blocking, 164, 251, 275
  reading and, 64
Alpha coma, 122

Alpha envelope, 355–356
Alpha frequency
  evaluation by phase-locked loop demodulation, 356
  head size and, 204
Alpha-generating mechanisms, temperature compensation of, 174
Alpha rhythm, 9, 223 (*see also* Alpha activity; Alpha waves)
  in dogs, 162, 199
  ensemble of generators of, 277
  neocortex and, 161
  origin of, 147
  stability of, 280
  standing waves and, 203
  temperature compensation of, 235
  waxing and waning of, 6
Alpha waves, 7 (*see also* Alpha activity; Alpha rhythm)
  frequency-amplitude interdependence of, 54, 57
Alzheimer's disease, 187, 222, 285
  infrequency of epileptiform activity in, 175
Amphetamine, 173
Amplitude modulation, 197, 218, 281
  vs. Type 3 waves, 55
Amplitude-frequency characteristic, in random delta slowing, 88, 91
Amplitude-frequency combined modulation, 219
  vs. constant-slope waves, 19
Analytic signal, 357
  magnitude of. *See* Instantaneous envelope
Arousal, 151, 251
Ascending reticular activating system, 153
  cholinergic nature of, 173
Aspartate, 170
Association fibers, 141
Atropine, delta waves and, 172, 176

Attractors
  point, 208
  simple, 206
  strange, 207–208
Attractor region, of an oscillator, 206
Autocorrelation, 50, 190, 238, 386–387
  polarity conservation and, 125
Autocorrelation function(s), 6, 88, 247, 281
  comparisons using, 117
Autoregressive analysis, 238
Autoregressive coefficients, 195–196
Autoregressive filter, 196
Autoregressive modeling, 50, 195, 400

Background activity, 6
Barbiturates, 169, 171
Basal forebrain nucleus (structures), 154
  acetylcholine and, 170
  cholinergic fibers (pathways) and, 154, 164
Basin of attraction, 207
Benign epileptiform transients, 275
Benign patterns with "epileptiform morphology," 43
Benign sporadic sleep spikes, 275
Benzodiazepines, 169, 171
Berger, Hans, 1
Bicuculline, 171, 180, 227
Bispectral analysis, 245
Bispectrum, alpha variants and, 214
"Black box," source of EEG as, 3, 127, 133, 189, 284
"Brain clock" hypothesis, 9, 277
Brain mechanisms of EEG, 9
Brain, oscillator systems of, 6
Brain stem, 143
Brain-stem nuclei, 145
Brain-stem reticular formation, 227
Burst-suppression patterns, simulation of, 38

Calcium spike, low-threshold, 203
Callosal fibers, 141
Carotid endarterectomy, 256
Carrier modulation, suppressed, 239
Catecholamines, 171
Caton, Richard, 1
Central Limit Theorem, 67, 68, 131, 192
Cerebellar cortex, 179
Cerebellum, 407
Cerebral cortex, 147
  EEG and, 2
  oscillatory systems of, 6
Cerebral oxygen uptake, 163
Chandelier cells, inhibitory activity of, 144

Chaos, deterministic, 204–211
Cholinergic mechanisms, cortical, 184
Cholinergic pathways, 160
Classical transmitters, 171
Clinical EEG, 1
Closed neural chains, 147
Clustering of like EEG segments, after adaptive segmentation, 6, 89
Coefficient of Determination, 25, 129
  comparisons using, 118
  derivation of, 331
  Type 4 waves evaluated by, 61, 67
Coefficient of Variation, 25, 128
  as normalized standard deviation, 25
  derivation of, 327
Coherence, 152, 190
  corticorcortical vs. corticothalamic, 162–163
  lateral, 163
Coherence function, 331
Coherent rejection of artifact, 394–400
Coherent stimulus-evoked resonances, 165
Colored noise, spectrum and, 214
Complex demodulation, 357, 360, 362
Compressed spectral arrays, 255, 385
Computer techniques, 1
Computerized axial tomography (CAT), 1
Constant-amplitude waves, 16
Constant-frequency waves, 19
Constant-slope waves, 281
  inverse relation of amplitude and frequency in, 16, 18, 20
  non-REM sleep and, 75
  Stage 1 sleep and, 71
  Stage 2 sleep and, 76
  Stage 3–4 sleep onset and, 78
Corpus callosum, 163
Correlation dimension, 205, 208–210
  cerebellar, 179
  cerebral, 2, 6, 147
  synchronization in, 153
Cortex, undercutting of, 162, 177
  visual, 154
Cortical column(s), 142, 145, 163, 165, 200, 204, 221, 285
Cortical excitatory state, 191
Corticocortical disconnection, 188
Corticocortical fibers, 142
  vs. thalamocortical fibers, relative preponderance of, 148
Corticostriatal projections, 145
Creutzfeldt, Otto, 29
Creutzfeldt-Jakob disease, 175, 187, 222
  nonlinear dynamics and, 208, 210

Cross-correlation, 163, 190, 238
    evaluation of, 386–387
Cumulative distribution function, 345

Database, EEG, 29
DC aspects
    of EEG, 153
    of human epileptogenic neocortex, 153
DC changes, in epilepsy, 185
Delta activity (waves)
    frontal intermittent rhythmic, 176
    hyperventilation-induced, and constant-slope (Type 1) waves, 85, 100
    hypoglycemia and, 176
    monomorphic (rhythmic), 175
    polymorphic (random), 175
    Stage 3–4 sleep and, 71
    thalamocortical neurons and, 161
    white-matter lesions and, 164
Dendrites
    active regions on, 202
    apical, of pyramidal cells, 137–139
    basal, of pyramidal cells, 139
Dendrodendritic synapses, 158, 161
Density spectral array, 261
Desynchronization, neurophysiology of, 151
Desynchronized EEG, 3, 283–284
    and integrative functions, 151
    during mental activity, 149
    randomly recurring postsynaptic potentials and, 147
    REM sleep and, 166
    Type 4 waves and, 57
Di-isopropyl flurophosphate, 173
Diffuse encephalopathies, 175
Discrete Fourier transform, 383
Divisive function of basket-cell synapses on pyramidal-cell bodies, 143–144
Divisive processes, 233
Dopamine, 171, 221
Dopamine-containing fibers, 154
Double-bouquet cells, minicolumns and, 144
Drowsinesss, 6, 13
Dual modulation, of extrema and slopes, 13, 224
Dual-modulation oscillator, 4

Electrocorticogram, 153, 273
Electrodecremental pattern, simulation of, 45
Electrogenesis, in cortical neurons, 153
Electromyographic monitoring, Stage REM sleep and, 71
Electro-oculographic monitoring, Stage REM sleep and, 71

Encephalopathies
    metabolic, 176
    toxic, 176
Entrainment, mutual, 3
Envelope, of EEG, 6
    inhibition and, 3, 224, 285
Envelope of first derivative of EEG, 6
    excitation and, 3, 224, 285
Ephaptic transmission, epileptic discharges and, 145
Epilepsy
    brain maturation and, 185
    EEG in, 1
    primary generalized, 103
    rhythmic slowing and, 97
Epileptiform discharge(s)
    basic mechanisms of, 186
    vs. interictal discharge, 178–179
    sleep and, 184, 230
Epileptiform patterns, 1, 3, 24, 168
    interictal, 264–268, 270
Epinephrine, 171
Event-related potentials, 275
    averaging of, 386
Excitation, 151
Excitatory cortical input, 221–222
Excitatory-inhibitory imbalance, focal epilepsy and, 180
Extracellular current flow, 149
Extrema (extremes), modulation of, 6, 281
    vs. amplitude modulation, 13
Extrema-slopes hypothesis (of EEG), 13, 213–214, 221, 282
    data-processing techniques for testing of, 24
    EEG patterns and, 24
    EEG sleep patterns and, 234
    methods based on, 237
    methods of testing, 23
    nonlinear dynamics and, 219
    origins of, 6
    predictions from, 21
    significant parameters in, 6
    as two-parameter model, 286
Extrema-slopes modulation, 218

Fast Fourier transform, 383
Feedback loops, 225
Feline generalized penicillin epilepsy, 180–181
Filters
    in-phase and in-quadrature, 357, 360
    low-pass RC, 308
    transversal (rectangular), 307–308

Fourier analysis, 189–190
  sensitivity of to amplitude variations, 118
Fourier inverse transformation, 133
Fourier sine and cosine components, 133
Fourier transformation, 133
Fractal dimension, 207
Fractals, 210
Frequency modulation, 6, 16, 19, 197, 218
  vs. slopes modulation, 13

GABA, 232
  -A, 144
  -B, 144
  divisive function and, 144
  as inhibitory transmitter, 145, 171
GABAergic neurons, 145
GAD, 145
Gamma-aminobutyric acid. *See* GABA
Gamma rhythms, 165
Gaussian amplitude distribution, 69, 192, 345
Gaussian noise, 67
General anesthesia, EEG in, 204
  nonlinear dynamics and, 210
Generalized bilaterally synchronous slow burst, 176
Generalized tonic-clonic convulsions (seizures), 178, 186, 274
Generating mechanisms, EEG, 31
Glutamate, 170
Glutamic acid decarboxylase (GAD), 145
Glutamic acid, feline generalized penicillin epilepsy and, 183
Glutamine, 232
Glycine, 171

Habituation, 406
Hanning window, 383
Herpes encephalitis, 187
Hidden variables, 225, 286
Hilbert transform, 357, 360, 362, 363
Hippocampal neurons, 202
Hippocampus, 178
Hjorth's normalized slope descriptors, 246, 250, 287
Hypothalamus, 195
Hypoxia, 180

Inferior olivary nucleus, 203
Inhibition
  divisive, 146
  subtractive, 146
Inhibitory loops, alpha activity and, 152
Instantaneous envelope(s), 222, 237, 249, 273, 285, 298
  by conventional Hilbert transform, 363–366
  derivation of, 356–377
  epileptiform activity and, 109
  interfacing with oscillator model, 377–379
  by paired integration and differentiation, 366–371
  reconstitution of EEGs and, 26–27
  of relatively wide-band signals, 373–377
  spike-and-slow-wave activity and, 111
  spike-wave activity and, 111
Instantaneous frequency, 123, 224, 360
  derivation of, 371
  EEG patterns and, 225
  excitation-inhibition and, 232, 285
  normal variant patterns and, 233
  variability of and information-processing rate, 286
Integrative functions, desynchronization and, 151
Intermittent patterns, simulation of, 38
Interneurons, 141, 145
Interpolation, by transversal filter, 310
Intracerebral recordings, 166
Intracortical inhibitory activity, 222
Intracortical neurons, 148
Intralaminar thalamic nuclei, 153, 154, 160
Inverse autoregressive filtering, spike detection and, 247
Ionotropic receptors, 170
Irregular activity, low-voltage, 36
Irregular waves, of oscillator model, 16

Joint probability density function, 345–346

Kalman filtering, 196, 400–407
K complexes, simulation of, 194
Kolmogorov entropy, 208

Lambda waves, reading and, 64
Learning curve, in adaptive signal processing, 406
Lennox-Gastaut Syndrome, 178, 187, 274
Limit cycle, 206
  spike-like waves and, 200
Limit-cycle activity, 198
Linear system, EEG as output of, 196
Lissajous pattern, 205
Locus ceruleus, 145, 154
Lyapunov exponent, 205, 208

Magnetic resonance imaging (MRI), 1
Maturation, of EEG, 264
Maturational changes in EEG, 2

Membrane potential fluctuations, subthreshold, 203
Memory, 407
Metabolic diseases, 177
Metabotropic receptors, 170
Metrazol, 153, 180
Microwave frequencies, 202
Midbrain
 dorsal nucleus of, 154
 ventral tegmental area of, 154
Mimetic analysis, 238
Model(s)
 distributed, 197
 filtered noise, 192, 205, 213
 lumped, 197
 modulation, 196–197
 nerve net, 197
Modulation. *See* Amplitude modulation; Extrema modulation; Frequency modulation; Slopes modulation
Mu rhythm, 164, 213, 245
 alpha rhythm and, 41
 feedback enhancement of, 165
 simulation of, 33, 41
Multi-channel EEG recordings, 264
Multiple sleep latency test, REM sleep and, 80, 82
Mutual entrainment, oscillator model and, 273

N-methyl-D-aspartate receptors, 186
Neocortex, basic architecture of, 137
 epileptogenic, 153
Neocortical cells, nonspiny, 137
Nerve net(s), 189, 201
 deterministic modeling of, 208
Neuroactive substances, 169
Neurogliaform cells, 144
Neuromodulators, 171, 221, 232
Neurons having quasi-bistable states, 221
 intrinsic (local-circuit), 141
 pedunculopontine tegmental, 159
Neuropeptides, 171
Neuropharmacological substances, 169
Neurotransmitters, 169, 221, 232
Nitric oxide, 170
Noise generators, 345–353
Noise, random, 207
Nonlinear dynamics, 210
Nonlinear mechanisms, 214
Nonlinear methods of EEG analysis, 238
Nonlinear oscillators, mutual entrainment of, 202
Non-REM sleep, 147, 282

Nonstationarity, 196
Nonstationary EEGs, methods for, 238
Noradrenaline, 221
 fibers containing, 154
Norepinephrine, 171
Normal distribution function, Type 4 waves and, 64
Normal variant patterns, 2, 168, 231–232
 simulation of, 33
Nucleus basalis of Meynert, 154, 159, 173
Nucleus centralis lateralis-paracentralis, 160
Nucleus ventralis posterolateralis, 198
Nyquist frequency, 394

Olfactory cortex, 209
Oscillators
 dual-modulation, 213
 Duffing, 202
 hybrid electronic neuronal, 203
 nonlinear, 133, 205–206
 relaxation, 17, 190–191, 161, 225
 simple harmonic, 191, 205–206
 van der Pol, 206
Oscillator model, 6, 293
 as analog counterpart of the extrema-slopes hypothesis, 15
 dual-modulation feature of, 7
 EEG pattern simulation and, 34
 evolution of, 281–282
 modes of oscillation of, 16, 27–28
 reconstitution of EEGs and, 15
 simulation of EEG patterns and, 50
 special features of output waves of, 18–19
 types of waves in, 27–28

Pacemaker, thalamic, 158, 161, 201, 278
Parabolic approximation, of sine waves, 17
Paroxysmal activity, 6
Paroxysmal depolarizing shift, 179
Paroxysmal negative shift, topography of, 185
Paroxysmal slow waves, detection of, 255
Pearson Product-Moment Correlation Coefficient, 25
 comparisons using, 118
 derivation of, 329
 ordinary correlation coefficient and, 27
Penicillin, 180, 186, 227
Penicillin focus, 153
Period-doubling, 209, 211
Periodogram analysis, 189
Perioperative monitoring, 250, 256
Phantom variables, 232
Phase-modulated analog sampling, 335

Phase modulation, 197, 218
Phase-plane plot, 27
Phase space, 205
Phase-space trajectory, 205
Phenytoin, 171
Photo-optical scanning, 335
Physostygmine, activated EEG and, 172
Picrotoxin, 171, 180, 227
Pink noise, spectrum and, 214
Poincaré, Henri, 205, 206
Poisson distribution, 199
Polarity ambiguity of reconstituted EEGs, 125, 379
Polyspike-and-slow-wave complexes, 49
  Type 4 waves and, 49
Positron emission tomography (PET), 1
Posterior rhythm, slowing of, 177
Posterior rhythmic (alpha) activity, 149
Postictal slowing, 186, 274
Postsynaptic potentials, 147, 161
Power (density) spectra
  via autoregressive modeling, 403
  correlation dimension and, 208
  random slowing and, 89
  of spikes, 247
Predictor coefficients, 401
Presynaptic dendrites, 158
Probability density function
  classification by, 247
  plots of, 218
  random slowing and, 89
  rectangular, 304–306
Psychomotor variant pattern, simulation of, 40
Pulvinar nucleus, 177
Purkinje cells, 179
Pyramidal cells
  hippocampal, 182
  neocortical, 137–139

Raleigh distribution, 192
Random signals, low-frequency, 23
Random-noise generators, 345–353
Raphe nuclei, 145
Reading, EEG during, 132
Reconstitution of EEGs, 7, 9, 219, 237, 273, 284
  instantaneous envelopes and, 26–27, 116, 127, 131
  intermittent patterns and, 38
  oscillator model and, 23
  polarity ambiguity of, 131
  running means and, 115

Rectangular amplitude distribution, 345
  vs. normal distribution function, 64
Rectifier, precision full-wave, 307
Regulation, degree of, 251
Relative variability, derivation of, 327–328
REM sleep, 282
  EEG in, 166
Repeller, of an oscillator, 206
Reticular formation, 153
Rhthmic theta activity of drowsiness, 53
Rhythmic activity
  in neocortex, 62
  as reverberating activity in corticocortical and corticothalamic circuits, 147, 151
  very-high-frequency, 166
Rhythmic fast activity, 53
Rhythmic temporal theta bursts, simulation of, 40
Rhythmicity, inherent, 147
Running mean amplitude of EEG, 6, 128, 282
  derivation of, 25
  sleep and, 71
Running mean amplitude of first derivative of EEG, 7
Running mean frequency, 7, 128, 249, 282
  derivation of, 25, 319
  limitations of, 246–247
  sleep and, 71
  3–Hz spike wave activity and, 112
Running mean slope, 17–18, 128, 282
  derivation of, 25
  sleep and, 71
Running means
  characteristics of for different patterns, 333
  derivation of, 317–318

Sawtooth waves, in REM sleep, 71, 81, 166
Scalp
  frequency-dependence of modifications by, 169
  modifications of the EEG by, 169
Scatter plot, 27
  amplitude vs. frequency, 89, 218
Seizure activity, nonlinear dynamics and, 210
Septohippocampal system, theta rhythm from, 154
Serotonin, 171, 221
Serotonin-containing fibers, 154
Siebert, W.M., 117
Simulation of EEG patterns, 23
Single neurons, intrinsic rhythm properties of, 159

Sinusoidality (regularity, rhythmicity) of a signal, 26
Sleep
 deafferentiation hypothesis of, 154
 disorders of, 1
 staging of, 194, 251–254
Sleep spindles, 234
 and complex demodulation of EEG, 361
 Stage 2 sleep and, 71
Slopes, modulation of, 6
Slow posterior rhythm, Type 3 waves and, 53
Slow spike-wave pattern, 178, 187, 274
 Lennox-Gastaut syndrome and, 43
 simulation of, 43
Slow waves, 164
Slow-wave sleep, Stage 3–4 sleep as, 71
Small sharp spikes, 275
Smoothing
 parabolic, 294
 parabolic plus quartic, 298
Spectra, autoregressive analysis and, 117
 Fourier analysis and, 117
 during reading, 61, 64, 66
 REM sleep and Stage 1 sleep and, 152
 sleep and, 83
Spectral analysis, 238, 383
 as linear method, 240
 basis of, 2
Spectral broadening, 240, 277–278
Spectral parameter analysis, 194, 214
Spectral Purity Index, 128, 240, 249, 282
 derivation of, 25, 320
 frequency spread and, 25
 limitations of, 246–247
 multiple simultaneous frequencies and, 104
Spike attenuation by the scalp, 169
Spike detection, 238
Spike parameters, clinical seizure control and, 269
Spike-and-slow-wave complex, 3, 178, 213, 228–230
 focal epilepsy and, 103
 as interictal pattern, 46
 simulation of, 45, 49
 Type 4 waves and, 46
Spikes, asymmetry of, 268
Spike-wave pattern, 3-Hz, 7, 43, 103, 105, 153, 178–183, 228–230, 274, 283
Spike wave, "phantom," 42
Spinal cord, 143
Spindle rhythmicity, barbiturate-induced, 158
Spindle-generating mechanisms, 160
Spiny stellate cells, 137, 144

State-setting substances, 171
States of consciousness, 71
Steady potential shift, 153
Strychnine, 171
Subacute sclerosing panencephalitis, 175
Subharmonic bifurcations, 211
Substantia innominata, 154, 173
Suppression-burst pattern, simulation of, 38
Synapses excitatory, 137
 inhibitory (GABAergic), 137
"Synaptic noise," 34
Synaptic strengths, 201
Synaptic vesicles, 158
Synchronized vs. desynchronized EEG, 149
Synergetic analysis, 209

Tapped delay line, 313
Temperature, effect of on EEG, 173
Temporal-lobe epilepsy, 178
Thalamectomy, 161
Thalamic neurons, burst-firing of, 160, 171
Thalamic nuclear groups, basic properties of, 137
Thalamic nuclei, midline, 154
Thalamic pacemaker, 152
Thalamic relay nuclei cells, 159
Thalamic reticular nucleus, 155–159, 173
 intrinsic rhythmic capabilities of, 160
 negative feedback and, 156
 spindle rhythmicity and, 154
 thalamocortical and corticothalamic fibers and, 155
Thalamocortical fibers, 141
Thalamocortical projection neurons, 143
Thalamocortical projection system/diffuse (nonspecific), 154
Thalamocorticothalamic loops, 161
Thalamus, 143
 medial dorsal nucleus of, 168
Theta activity
 in drowsiness, 53
 in Stage 1 sleep, 152
Time-scale converter ("time machine"), 341–343, 386, 387, 391
Topographic display, 264
Topography, 152
 of EEG, 167
Tracé alternant pattern, 238
Tracé discontinu pattern, 274
Trace-overlap compensation, 338
Trace-width compensation, 335
Transversal filter, time averaging and, 25
Traveling wave(s), 197, 199

Type 1 (constant-slope) waves, of oscillator model, 14, 293
  amplitude-frequency relationship in, 217
  general anesthesia and, 21
  hyperventilation-induced slowing and, 21
  non-REM sleep and, 21, 23, 129
  random (polymorphic delta) slowing and, 21, 33, 91, 129
  scatter diagram of, 28
  Stage 3–4 sleep and, 127, 129
Type 1–4 waves, spectra of, 302–306
Type 2 (constant-amplitude) waves, 14, 293
  epileptiform patterns and, 21, 33
  scatter diagram of, 28
  3-Hz spike wave and, 33, 120, 127, 129
Type 3 (constant-frequency) waves, 14, 294
  alpha activity and, 33, 130
  amplitude-frequency interdependence of, 36
  rhythmic activity and, 21, 128
  rhythmic slowing and, 99
  scatter diagram of, 28
  sleep spindles and, 33
Type 4 (irregular) waves, of oscillator model, 15, 294
  "desynchronized" EEG and, 21, 33, 128, 130
  evaluation by probability-density-function classification, 62, 64
  reading and, 66
  REM sleep and, 21, 33, 83, 130
  scatter diagram of, 28
  spike-and-slow-waves and, 128

van der Pol equations, 202
Vertex sharp waves, 234
  simulation of, 194
  Stage 2 sleep and, 71, 82
Voltage-controlled oscillator, 16, 19, 293

White matter
  lesions of, 222
  subcortical, 147
Wiener, Norbert, 9, 277, 287

Youth waves, as posterior slow waves, 64